Simple and Complex Fractures of the Humerus

Filippo Castoldi • Davide Blonna
Marco Assom
Editors

Simple and Complex Fractures of the Humerus

A Guide to Assessment and Treatment

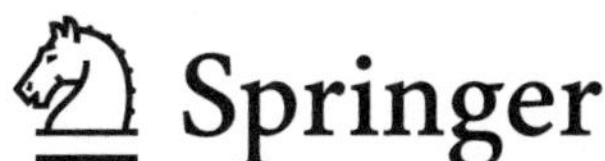

Editors
Filippo Castoldi
Department of Orthopaedics
and Traumatology
2nd University Clinic
CTO Hospital Turin
Turin
Italy

Marco Assom
Department of Orthopaedics
and Traumatology
Mauriziano-Umberto I Hospital
University of Turin Medical School
Turin
Italy

Davide Blonna
Department of Orthopaedics
and Traumatology
Mauriziano-Umberto I Hospital
University of Turin Medical School
Turin
Italy

ISBN 978-88-470-5838-5 ISBN 978-88-470-5307-6 (eBook)
DOI 10.1007/978-88-470-5307-6
Springer Milan Heidelberg New York Dordrecht London

Softcover reprint of the hardcover 1st edition 2015

Printed on acid-free paper

Springer is part of Springer Science+Business Media (www.springer.com)

To all my wonderful family, who always offer me such great support.

Filippo Castoldi

To my daughter, Eleanor, and my wife, Alessandra, for the time that I have stolen.

Davide Blonna

To my wife, Graziella, who is a constant source of support, my father, who raised me, and my mom and nan, who cannot be here.

Marco Assom

Foreword

The last 15–20 years have witnessed drastic changes in all surgical specialties, including orthopedics and, specifically, surgery of the upper extremity. The new horizons extend from endoscopic surgery of the rotator cuff to diverse options for prosthetic replacement of the shoulder and elbow and improved surgical management of both proximal humerus and distal radius fractures. These changes, and comparable advances in other surgical specialties, have initiated a clear trend toward superspecialization – a trend amplified, at least for complex pathologies, by data demonstrating a clear correlation between case load, (number of procedures performed by a single surgeon during a defined period), complications, and functional results. The interest of nonmedical professionals in these developments has been stimulated by publications showing the impact of complications on global health care costs and implying that hospitals might profit from more effective treatment of complications. Against this background it is imperative that efficacious learning instruments are made available, these being the basis of optimal surgical performance.

The evolution of information technology (IT) allows easy Internet access to almost all data. A few "mouse clicks" enable the user instantly to access the most recent papers from the most prestigious scientific journals. The same is true for video streams of surgical procedures performed by specialists from all over the world. It therefore seems legitimate to ask whether the era of conventional books has come to an end, particularly as these products are sometimes already obsolete by the time they are published and do not display the details expected by subspecialists.

The present monograph takes these facts fully into account. Traumatic and post-traumatic pathologies of a defined anatomic area are described in detail. Deep knowledge, experience, and balanced clinical judgment are the basis of this publication; they justify the publication of a book about fractures of a single skeletal segment in the era of IT. The description of validated solutions chosen by experts continues to have a clear didactic and educational value, including in comparison with Internet sources of information. Rightly or wrongly, today's generation of surgeons is asking for didactic material, which is immediately applicable in daily practice.

The monograph describes the entire spectrum of treatment options for fractures and post-traumatic conditions and illustrates them with images of high quality. It helps the reader to identify the problems, to consider different options, and to learn and understand the preferred solutions of experts.

Despite the eminent importance of the surgical procedure, it is mandatory to remember that prior to the surgical act – in all surgical specialties – there is the indication, an intellectual activity: “Decisions are more important than incisions.” Even for a passionate surgeon, the list of options has to include “the wisdom of surgical abstention”. Only by understanding the great importance of this process of reflection and the need for avoidance of excessively broad indications can the surgical community prevent further loss of decision-making power and reduction of its status to a level where it becomes simply the recipient of orders for a limited segment of the diagnostic and therapeutic supply chain.

I would like to thank Filippo Castoldi and his co-authors for having prepared a learning instrument that takes into account the above-mentioned lessons.

Pietro Regazzoni
Em. Chief of Trauma Surgery
University Hospital Basel
Basel, Switzerland

About the Editors

Filippo Castoldi, MD, is Associate Professor of Orthopedics and Traumatology at the University of Turin, Italy. His main interests are shoulder, elbow, and knee pathologies and their treatments – areas in which he undertook training during prolonged periods of study in Europe and the United States. Dr. Castoldi is the lead author of a number of scientific papers that have addressed the development of new techniques and clinical and basic science research. He is the winner of several international awards and has been a faculty member of national and international meetings and courses on surgery for the aforementioned pathologies. He is currently Chief of the 2nd Orthopedics and Traumatology University Clinic at the Orthopedics and Traumatology Center in Turin.

Davide Blonna, MD, has been a consultant in Orthopedics and Traumatology since 2008 and currently works as a shoulder and elbow surgeon at the Mauriziano Hospital, Turin, Italy. He has always been interested in shoulder and elbow surgery, conducting periods of study abroad, including in England and the United States. He is the lead author of various scientific articles focused primarily on minimally invasive treatment of fractures of the proximal humerus and elbow arthroscopy. Dr. Blonna has been the recipient of several international awards, including for best educational videos and best scientific papers. He is a member of the education committee of the European Shoulder and Elbow Society and the sport committee of SIGASCOT.

Marco Assom, MD, has been a consultant in Orthopedics and Traumatology since 1992. He has been interested especially in the shoulder since 1993, following periods of study in Lyon and Zurich, and he mainly performs open and arthroscopic surgeries for the treatment of shoulder and knee diseases. Dr. Assom is the lead author of publications on various new techniques and orthopedic implants that have become international landmarks in the treatment of proximal humeral fracture, tibial plateau fracture, and posterior shoulder dislocation. He currently works as a surgeon at the Mauriziano Hospital, Turin, Italy, where he is Chief of the Shoulder and Elbow unit.

Contents

Part I

Proximal Humerus

Surgical Main Anatomy of the Shoulder

1

Filippo Castoldi, Antonio Pastrone, and Antonio Marmotti

1.1 Surgical Main Anatomy of the Shoulder

The identification of skin landmarks is the first step in shoulder surgery. The most important landmarks are the anterior corner and the lateral margin of the acromion, the distal insertion of the deltoid, and the coracoid. The surgeon can draw these landmarks on the skin of the patient with a marker pen before surgery, in order to make easier the approach and to plan the procedure.

1.1.1 Superficial Layer

1.1.1.1 Deltoid Muscle

The deltoid is a large muscle that covers the shoulder anteriorly, laterally, and posteriorly. It is composed by three main raphes: the anterior, the middle, and the posterior. It is innervated by the axillary nerve.

The anterior deltoid takes its origin from the anterior corner of the acromion and from the inferior side of the clavicle; the middle one starts about 16 mm medially to the posterolateral corner of the acromion, while the posterior raphe originates from the posterolateral corner and from the scapular spine.

In the transdeltoid access and during the positioning of hardware for the external fixation of proximal humeral fracture, the surgeon must take care of the axillary nerve. This structure passes on average 60.8 mm below the anterior acromial margin and 48.7 mm below the posterior acromial corner [1]. The axillary nerve as it goes anteriorly reduces in size and gives rise to small and numerous branches that innervate the front portion of the deltoid. Therefore, when the surgeon proceeds to external fixation of the humeral fracture, it is suitable to introduce the wires anteriorly.

During shoulder motion the activation scheme of the deltoid is different between each raphe, and the direction of muscle fibers changes gradually with changing origins [2]. The fibers of the anterior and the posterior portions are parallel, while in the central one they are oblique and multi-pinnate. The medial fibers are oriented vertically, the anterior obliquely backward, and the posterior obliquely forward. The surgeon must consider these features during the incision of the muscle.

Each raphe forms an independent tendon, and they converge in a trapezoid shape insertion to the lateral aspect of the middle shaft of the humerus. The shape measures a height of 6 cm and a width of 2.1 cm proximally and 0.7 cm distally.

F. Castoldi
Department of Orthopaedics and Traumatology, 2nd University Clinic, CTO Hospital Turin, Largo Turati 62, Turin 10128, Italy
e-mail: filippo.castoldi@unito.it

A. Pastrone (✉) • A. Marmotti
Department of Orthopaedics and Traumatology, Mauriziano-Umberto I Hospital, Largo Turati 62, Turin 10128, Italy
e-mail: antonio.pastrone@gmail.com

F. Castoldi et al. (eds.), *Simple and Complex Fractures of the Humerus*,
DOI 10.1007/978-88-470-5307-6_1, © Springer-Verlag Italia 2015

The anterior band of the trapezoid shape insertion is separate from the posterior part. It accounts only for the anterior one fifth of the deltoid insertion (0.44 cm); therefore, the release of a small portion of the insertion can release all the anterior deltoid. It happens sometimes during internal fixation of proximal humerus fracture procedures.

The posterior part of the trapezoid insertion is composed by a wide and narrow band. The distance between the radial nerve and the posterior deltoid insertion averages on 2.4 cm proximally and 1.6 cm distally.

1.1.1.2 Pectoralis Major Muscle

The insertion of the pectoralis major muscle is located about 4.7 cm proximally to the deltoid insertion. The pectoralis major is a large triangular muscle, composed by a clavicular, a sternal, and a little abdominal portion. All these components converge laterally and insert on the humerus (Fig. 1.1). The distance between the upper border of the pectoralis major insertion and the top of the humeral head has been calculated and is on average 5.6 ± 0.5 cm. It is a landmark that could aid in accurate restoration of humeral anatomy when a reconstruction is difficult because of fragments comminution [3] (Fig. 1.2). Torrens and colleagues confirmed this relationship and added that also the rotation can be based on the insertion of the pectoralis major in case of arthroplasty or fixation. Furthermore, the authors found the distance from the upper margin of the insertion to be 17.55 % of the total humeral length [4].

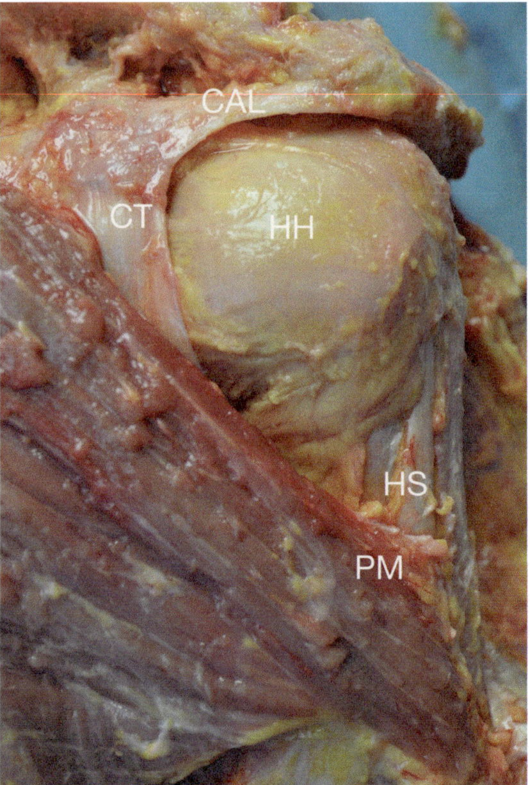

Fig. 1.1 The insertion of the pectoralis major (*PM*) on the humeral shaft (*HS*) (*HH* humeral head, *CAL* coracoacromial ligament, *CT* conjoint tendon). Specimen

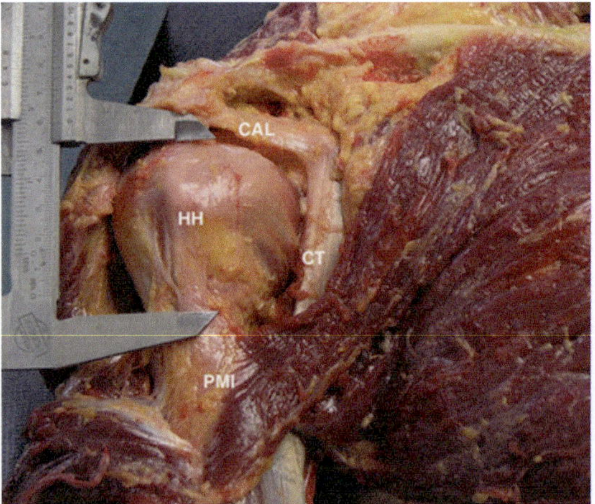

Fig. 1.2 The distance between the upper border of the pectoralis major insertion (*PMI*) and the top of the humeral head (*HH*) (*CT* conjoint tendon, *CAL* coracoacromial ligament). Specimen

1.1.1.3 Deltopectoral Interval

The space between the pectoralis and the deltoid is well known as the anterior shoulder approach. It is easier to identify this space proximally near the clavicle, where there is a natural triangular fat (Fig. 1.3).

The cephalic vein is the most important landmark for the deltopectoral interval and is absent in 4 % of cases. It has an intimate relationship with the deltoid artery that originates from the brachial artery and has two common variants. In type I (71 %) the deltoid artery crosses the interval without bumping into the cephalic vein. In type II (21 %) it crosses the interval, reaches the cephalic vein, and then runs down emitting several small arterial branches that return back to the pectoralis major across the interval [5]. Take care to these branches during the deltopectoral

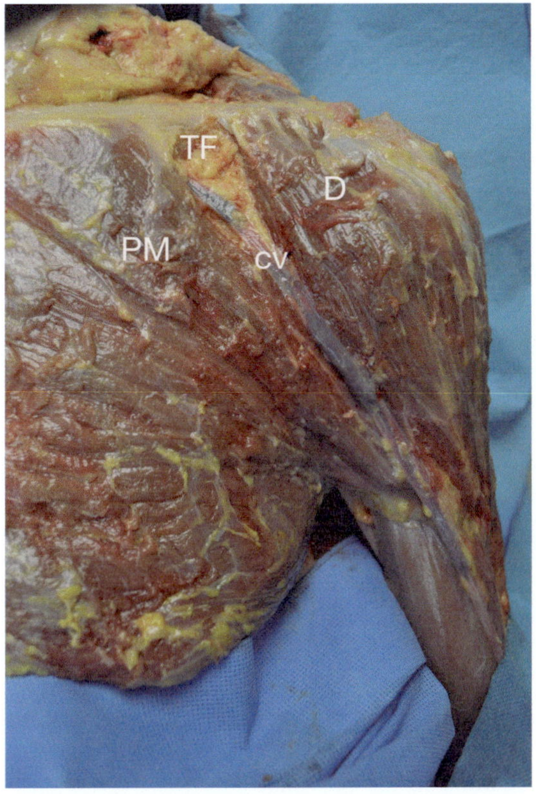

Fig. 1.3 The deltopectoral interval (*TF* triangular fat, *CV* cephalic vein, *D* deltoid, *PM* pectoralis major). Specimen

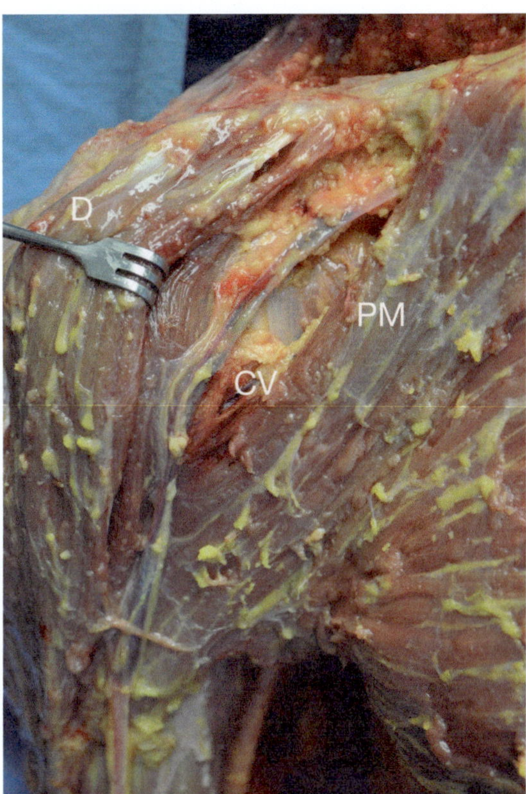

Fig. 1.4 The deltoid laterally retracted (*D* deltoid, *CV* cephalic vein, *PM* pectoralis major). Specimen

interval opening, in order to avoid bleeding. Consider that in the deltopectoral groove there are more lateral than medial feeder vessels to the cephalic vein, so splitting the pectoralis from the deltoid leaving the cephalic vein laterally can reduce hematoma after the surgical procedure [6] (Fig. 1.4).

To have a good view, the best way is to use Hohmann retractors on the coracoid and on the upper border of the pectoralis major. Two large retractors are useful to retract the deltoid and the pectoralis major. If we need more view the upper part of the pectoralis major can be released, as well as the resection of the coracoacromial ligament could be performed (Fig. 1.5).

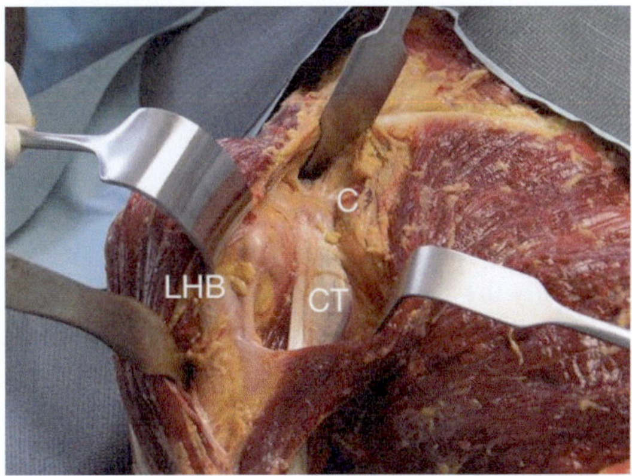

Fig. 1.5 Exposure of the deeper layer (*LHB* long head of biceps, *C* coracoid, *CT* conjoint tendon). Specimen

1.1.2 Deeper Layer

After muscle retraction it is possible to identify the coracoid process.

The coracoid can be considered as the center of a star composed by the coracoacromial ligament, the coracoclavicular ligaments, the pectoralis minor muscle, and the conjoint tendon. Deeper and medially to the conjoint tendon lies the musculocutaneous nerve. It enters into the coracobrachialis muscle in a very variable distance from 3.1 to 8.2 mm from the apex of the coracoid (Fig. 1.6).

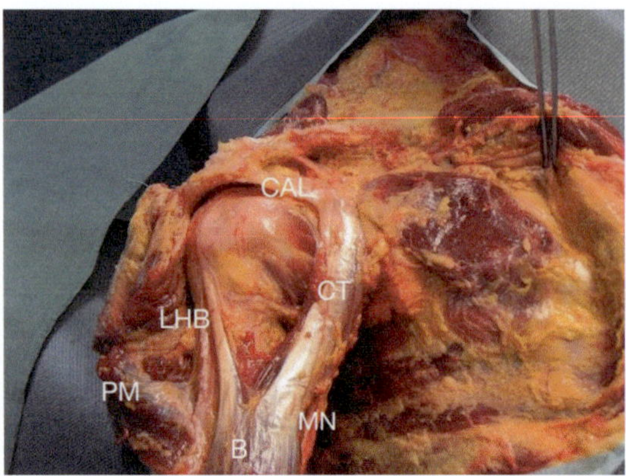

Fig. 1.6 The musculocutaneous nerve (*MN*) (*CAL* coracoacromial ligament, *LHB* long head of biceps, *B* biceps, *CT* conjoint tendon, *PM* pectoralis major). Specimen

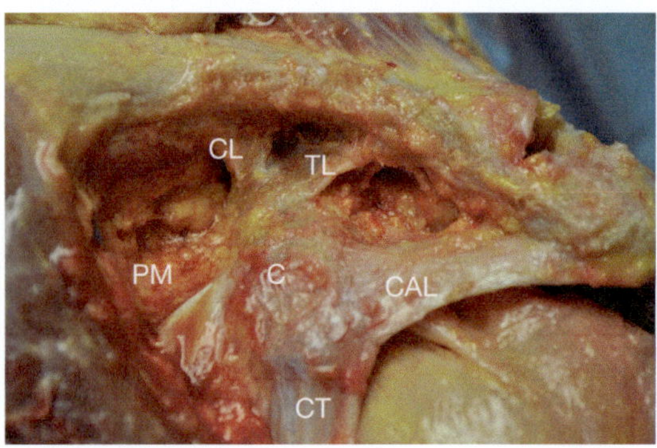

Fig. 1.7 The coracoid (*C*) and its ligaments (*CL* conoid ligament, *TL* trapezoid ligament, *CAL* coracoacromial ligament, *CT* conjoint tendon, *PM* pectoralis minor). Specimen

The coracoclavicular ligaments are deep on the basis of the coracoid. In the Latarjet procedure only the superficial part of the coracoid process is detached. The trapezoid ligaments begin about 2 cm from the central point of the distal coracoid process, while the conoid ligaments begin at the medial posterior margin [7] (Fig. 1.7).

The coracoacromial ligament can be identified more easily in its origin from the coracoid. It is important to recognize, and sometimes it is necessary to release, it to increase the visibility of the rotator cuff and the fracture.

Medially to the bicipital groove and distally to the subscapularis tendon, it is possible to recognize the anterior circumflex artery that originates from the axillary artery (Fig. 1.8).

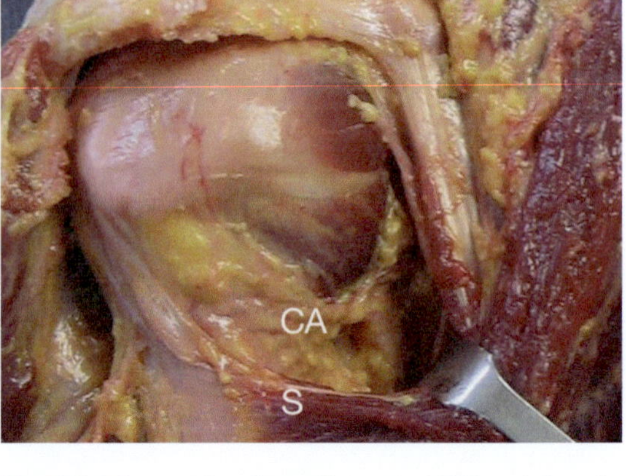

Fig. 1.8 The anterior circumflex artery (*CA*) and the subscapularis tendon (*S*). Specimen

The anterior circumflex artery emits an anterolateral ascending branch that crosses the subscapularis tendon anteriorly and runs superiorly along the lateral border of the intertubercular groove before terminating as the arcuate artery [8].

The anterior circumflex artery has been historically considered the most important blood contribution to the proximal humerus. Nevertheless lately some authors pointed out that the majority of the blood supply actually belongs to the posterior circumflex artery. The authors showed that 64 % of the humeral head blood supply arises from the posterior artery, while the anterior is responsible for 36 % of the humeral head perfusion [9].

The posterior circumflex artery passes with the axillary nerve through the quadrangular space, delimited by the humerus laterally, the subscapularis and teres minor superiorly, the teres major inferiorly, and the triceps medially. The posterior circumflex artery originates from the axillary artery and enters into the humeral head from 0 to 33 mm from the inferior border of the articular cartilage in conjunction with the posterior line of the capsular insertion (Fig. 1.9). It is important to know this landmark. It permits to understand what Hertel says about humeral head ischemia in case of fractures of the proximal humeral head: "take care of the integrity of the medial hinge" [10].

The common branch of the axillary nerve can be found more distally, under the anterior circumflex artery. The axillary nerve is the most frequently injured nerve in proximal humerus fractures. It

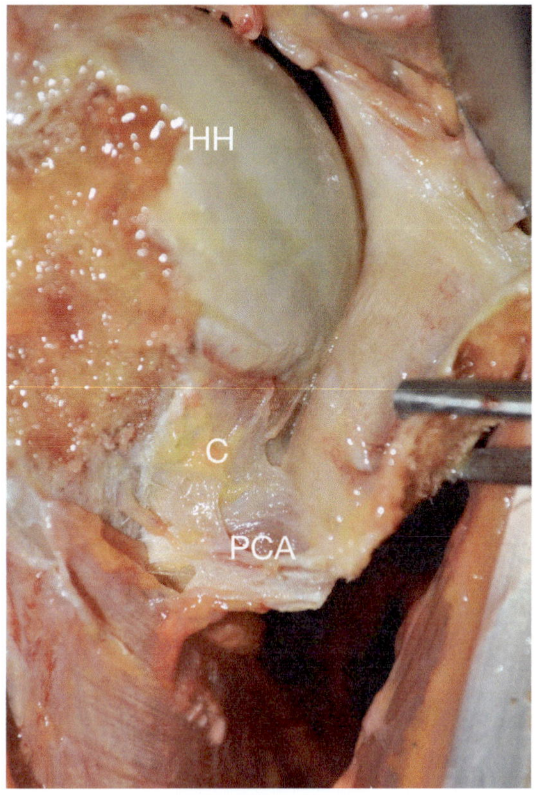

Fig. 1.9 The posterior circumflex artery (*PCA*) (*C* calcar, *HH* humeral head). Specimen

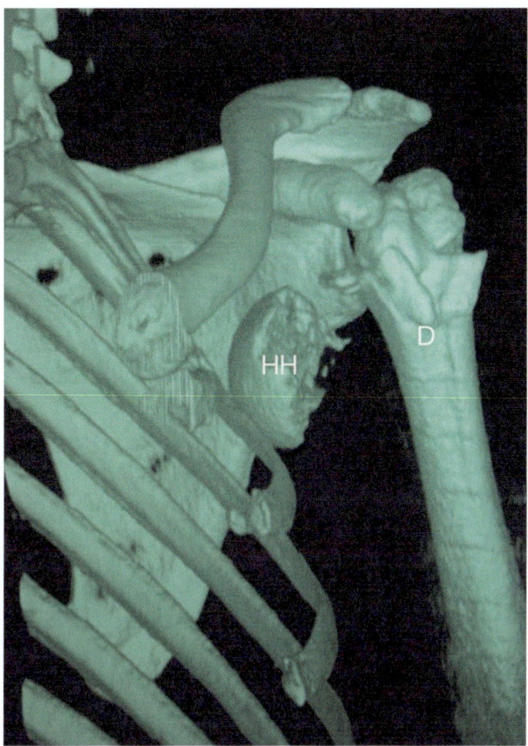

Fig. 1.10 Fracture and dislocation of the humeral head (*HH*) in the axillary fossa (*D* diaphysis). Specimen

enters the quadrangular space at an average distance of 1.7 cm from the surgical neck and divides into the anterior and posterior branches [11]. The lesion of the axillary nerve can cause paralysis of the teres minor muscle and deltoid muscle, resulting in loss of abduction of arm. It is very important to know the neurovascular structures of the axillary fossa, wherein the axillary artery, the anterior and the posterior circumflex arteries, and the nervous plexus lie. In case of dislocation of the humeral head anterior-inferiorly this structures may be damaged (Fig. 1.10). The plexus is very close to the coracoid process, in particular when the arm is abducted. In the Latarjet procedure the surgeon must pay attention during the coracoid osteotomy; the osteotome must be used from medial to lateral with the arm adducted (Fig. 1.11).

The axillary nerve passes beyond the lower edge of the subscapularis muscle, and the surgeon must be careful when operating in this zone in order to preserve it. Near the axillary nerve, medially to the conjoint tendon lies the musculocutaneous nerve as shown in the picture. It is the more medial nerve of the brachial plexus, and the risk of injury in open shoulder surgery is relatively high, especially in the Latarjet procedure. The conjoined tendon is the limit beyond which you should not proceed medially. Therefore, in the presence of a fracture-dislocation with humeral head in the anteroinferior fossa, it is important to observe its position relative to the coracoid.

Reflecting the pectoralis major, the tendons of the latissimus dorsi and the teres major appear. These are muscles coming from the back, very close to the neurovascular structures. With the shoulder flexed and internally rotated, the mean distance between the inferior tendon margin and the radial nerve, brachial artery, and profunda brachii artery is 18, 22, and 14 mm, respectively. Moving the arm to a neutral position reduces these distances [12].

Under the tendon of the pectoralis major runs the long head of the biceps. It passes between the two

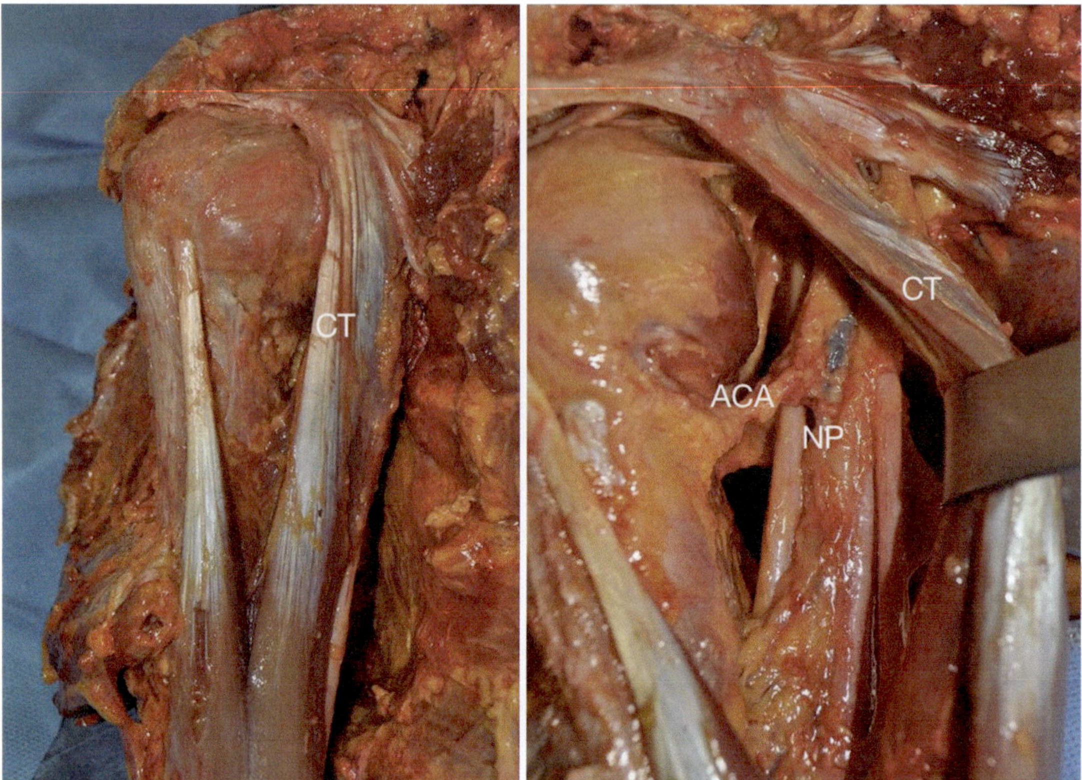

Fig. 1.11 The brachial plexus (*NP* brachial plexus, *ACA* anterior circumflex artery, *CT* conjoint tendon). Specimen

tuberosities in the bicipital groove, approximately 1 cm lateral to the midline of the humerus. It is defined as the polar star of the surgeon and can be a useful landmark during fracture reduction in case of severe comminution of the proximal humerus.

The retroversion of the proximal humeral articular surface ranges from 0° to 55° depending on the methodology used to measure and on the morphology. The head-shaft angle is also variable, ranging from 30° to 55° [13] (Fig. 1.12). The surgeon must remember that the bicipital groove rotates anteriorly about 9° from proximal to distal. It is important to remember when the anatomic retroversion of the humerus must be restored (Fig. 1.13).

Following the long head of biceps, it is easy to identify the space between the two tuberosities, the rotator interval, and then the boundary between the supraspinatus and subscapularis tendons.

In a deeper plan, after bursectomy, the rotator cuff can be exposed. It is composed by the teres minor and infraspinatus posteriorly, by the supraspinatus superiorly, and by the subscapularis anteriorly. The posterosuperior and the anterior part of the rotator cuff are separated by an interval between supraspinatus and subscapularis muscles. Its opening is useful for the humeral head exposure (Fig. 1.14).

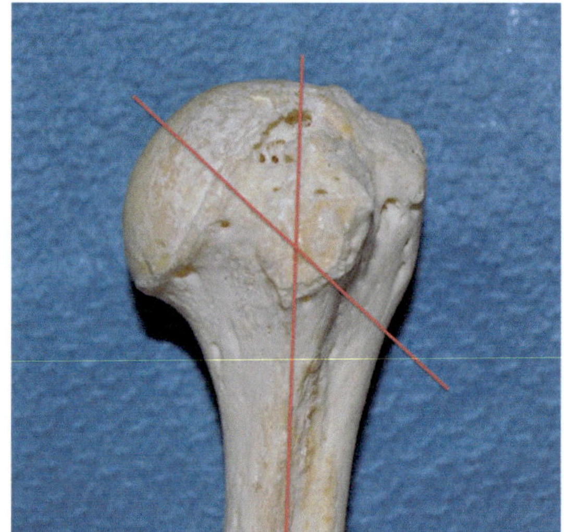

Fig. 1.12 The proximal humerus. The head-shaft angle ranges from 30° to 55°. Specimen

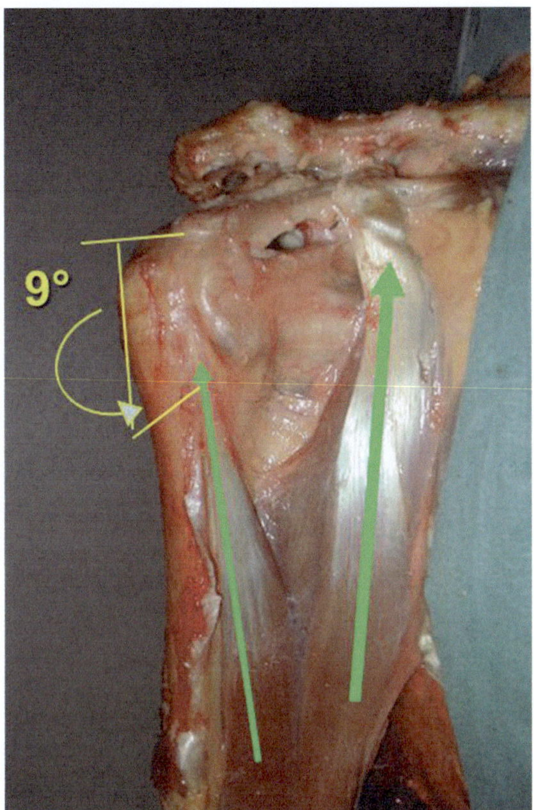

Fig. 1.13 The bicipital groove rotates anteriorly about 9° from proximal to distal (*yellow* lines). The long head of biceps and the conjoint tendons (*green* arrow). Specimen

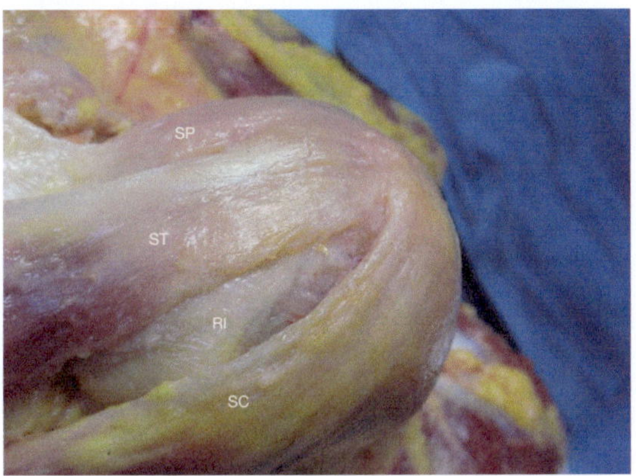

Fig. 1.14 The rotator cuff (*SP* infraspinatus, *ST* supraspinatus, *RI* rotator interval, *SC* subscapularis). Specimen

The supraspinatus and the infraspinatus muscles are both innervated by the suprascapular nerve. The insertion of the two tendons is posterior to the bicipital groove on the greater tuberosity,

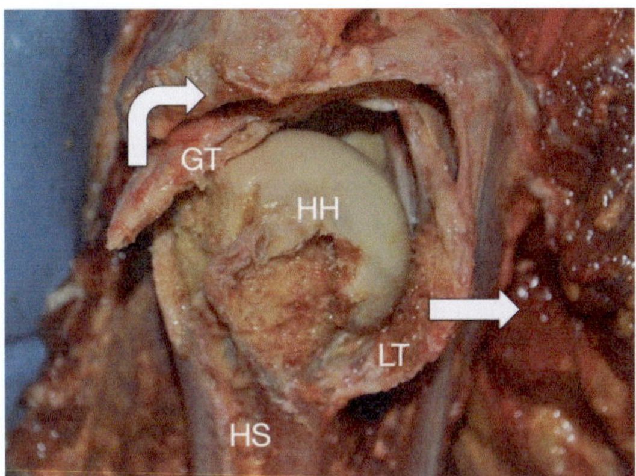

Fig. 1.15 Fragment dislocations after proximal humerus fracture. The grater tuberosity (*GT*) dislocates superiorly and posteriorly (curved *arrow*) and the lesser tuberosity (*LT*) anteriorly and inferiorly (*arrow*). (*HH* Humeral head, *HS* Humeral shaft). Specimen

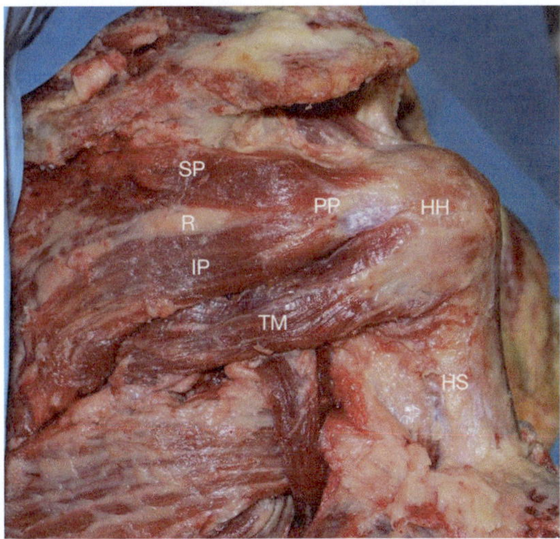

Fig. 1.16 The posterior portal (*PP*) lies between the superior (*SP*) and the inferior part (*IP*) of the infraspinatus (*R* raphe, *HH* humeral head, *HS* humeral shaft, *TM* Teres minor)

and it represents the entry point in case of intramedullary nailing.

It is important to know the anatomy of the insertion and the direction of the force vectors in order to reduce the fragments in case of fracture (Fig. 1.15).

The infraspinatus muscle is divided into a superior and inferior part by a raphe. During arthroscopic procedures the posterior portal passes through the infraspinatus between the raphes as shown in the picture (Fig. 1.16).

To reach posteriorly the medial third of the glenoid, it could be necessary to split the infraspinatus at the level of the raphe. No neurovascular structures are visible until 2 cm medial to the glenoid. At this level the suprascapular nerve lies between the suprascapular and the spinoglenoid notches. The nerve is particularly vulnerable to traction injury at two distinct locations: its branch point and at the suprascapular notch where it runs deep to the transverse scapular ligament [14]. An injury of the suprascapular nerve can cause palsy of the supraspinatus and infraspinatus muscles.

Anteriorly, the subscapularis, innervated by the upper and lower subscapular nerves, insert to the lesser tuberosity. The splitting of this muscle in a horizontal plane allows to reach the anterior part of the glenoid as it is required in the open Latarjet procedure.

The surgical access to the humeral head can vary, depending on the fracture features and on the displacement of the fragments. In case of multifragmental fracture of the humeral head, the line of fracture can be used as door to reach the deeper fragments. No neurovascular structure is at risk at this level.

References

1. Cetik O, Uslu M, Acar HI, Comert A, Tekdemir I, Cift H (2006) Is there a safe area for the axillary nerve in the deltoid muscle? A cadaveric study. J Bone Joint Surg Am 88:2395–2399
2. Sakoma Y, Sano H, Shinozaki N, Itoigawa Y, Yamamoto N, Ozaki T, Itoi E (2011) Anatomical and functional segments of the deltoid muscle. J Anat 218:185–190
3. Murachovsky J, Ikemoto RY, Nascimento LG, Fujiki EN, Milani C, Warner JJ (2006) Pectoralis major tendon reference (PMT): a new method for accurate restoration of humeral length with hemiarthroplasty for fracture. J Shoulder Elbow Surg 15(6):675–678
4. Torrens C, Corrales M, Melendo E, Solano A, Rodríguez-Baeza A, Cáceres E (2008) The pectoralis major tendon as a reference for restoring humeral length and retroversion with hemiarthroplasty for fracture. J Shoulder Elbow Surg 17(6):947–950
5. Bunker TD, Cosker TD, Dunkerley S, Kitson J, Smith CD (2013) Anatomical variations of the deltoid artery: relevance to the deltopectoral approach to the shoulder. Bone Joint J 95-B(5):657–659
6. Radkowski CA, Richards RS, Pietrobon R, Moorman CT 3rd (2006) An anatomic study of the cephalic vein in the deltopectoral shoulder approach. Clin Orthop Relat Res 442:139–142
7. Takase K (2010) The coracoclavicular ligaments: an anatomic study. Surg Radiol Anat 32(7):683–688
8. Terry GC, Chopp TM (2000) Functional anatomy of the shoulder. J Athl Train 35(3):248–255
9. Hettrich CM, Boraiah S, Dyke JP, Neviaser A, Helfet DL, Lorich DG (2010) Quantitative assessment of the vascularity of the proximal part of the humerus. J Bone Joint Surg Am 92(4):943–948
10. Hertel R, Hempfing A, Stiehler M, Leunig M (2004) Predictors of humeral head ischemia after intracapsular fracture of the proximal humerus. J Shoulder Elbow Surg 13(4):427–433
11. Gardner MJ, Griffith MH, Dines JS, Briggs SM, Weiland AJ, Lorich DG (2005) The extended anterolateral acromial approach allows minimally invasive access to the proximal humerus. Clin Orthop Relat Res 434:123–129
12. Henry PD, Dwyer T, McKee MD, Schemitsch EH (2013) Latissimus dorsi tendon transfer for irreparable tears of the rotator cuff: an anatomical study to assess the neurovascular hazards and ways of improving tendon excursion. Bone Joint J 95-B(4):517–522. doi:10.1302/0301-620X.95B4.30839
13. Boileau P, Walch G (1997) The three-dimensional geometry of the proximal humerus. Implications for surgical technique and prosthetic design. J Bone Joint Surg Br 79:857–865
14. Robinson CM, Seah M, Akhtar MA (2011) The epidemiology, risk of recurrence, and functional outcome after an acute traumatic posterior dislocation of the shoulder. J Bone Joint Surg 93:1605–1613

2 Proximal Humerus Fractures: Understanding and Managing the Fracture

Filippo Castoldi, Andrea Cimino, and Davide Bonasia

2.1 Introduction

The management of proximal humerus fractures has not yet been standardized. It is complex and there still remain a lot of disputes on which may be the best way to proceed depending on the fracture's patterns, type of patient, and bone quality.

Proximal humerus fractures comprise 4–5 % of all fractures and represent the most common humerus fracture (45 %). The proximal humerus is the second most frequently fractured upper limb bone. Their incidence has continued to increase, and some studies have predicted a threefold increase over the next three decades [1]. Their peak is after the fifth decade; the increased incidence in the older population is thought to be related to osteoporosis. Women are mostly affected; the 2:1 female-to-male ratio is likely related to issues of bone density [2].

Treatment should focus on maximizing the patient's functional outcome and minimizing pain. Intervention options range from nonoperative modalities to osteosynthesis and in selected cases arthroplasty. Understanding and handling the several factors that may influence the management of proximal humerus fractures is paramount to proceed in the right way.

The key point is the complex local anatomy: some fracture patterns can compromise the vascularity of the humeral head. The fracture patterns are often complex, complicated by poor bone quality, and may be difficult to reestablish the correct geometry of the proximal humerus.

2.2 Classification

A lot of classifications have been proposed along the years. The Neer classification of proximal humerus fracture is the most popular. It outlines the basic anatomic elements of proximal humerus fracture. These are identified in four segments: the humeral head, the greater tuberosity, the lesser tuberosity, and the humeral shaft. This classification is based on the degree of displacement of each of these segments, plus the presence of any associated dislocation, impaction, or splitting of the head.

The criteria to define displacement are distance >1 cm from the anatomic position and angulation >45°. The direction of displacement is mostly determined by muscle insertions. The humeral shaft is usually displaced anteromedially by the action of the pectoralis major. The greater tuberosity displaces posteriorly and superiorly pulled by the supraspinatus, infraspinatus, and teres minor. In three-part fractures involving the

F. Castoldi
Department of Orthopaedics and Traumatology, 2nd University Clinic, CTO Hospital Turin, Largo Turati 62, Turin 10128, Italy
e-mail: filippo.castoldi@unito.it

A. Cimino (✉) • D. Bonasia
Department of Orthopaedics and Traumatology, Mauriziano-Umberto I Hospital, Largo Turati 62, Turin 10128, Italy
e-mail: andreacimino87@gmail.com

F. Castoldi et al. (eds.), *Simple and Complex Fractures of the Humerus*, DOI 10.1007/978-88-470-5307-6_2, © Springer-Verlag Italia 2015

greater tuberosity, the humeral head may be anteriorly rotated by action of the subscapularis; the humeral head may be externally rotated by the supraspinatus whenever the lesser tuberosity is involved.

The understanding of proximal humerus fractures is complicated by variation in fracture patterns and by difficulties in interpreting two-dimensional radiographs in different positions of the arms. The common use of CT with three-dimensional reconstruction has powerfully increased the possibility of evaluation and treatment.

The classification developed by Neer in the 1970s continues to be the most popular; however, several studies have pointed out its low intraobserver and interobserver reliability. It is important to notice that the definition of displacement (>1 cm) and angulation (>45°) is in fact arbitrary. This classification is based on Codman's original drawings and was intended to help in understanding the pathological anatomy of different fracture patterns. However, the different fracture patterns depicted seem to be oversimplified, and some fracture plane combinations were not considered. This led to the search of developing alternative classifications [3–6] (Fig. 2.1).

The AO classification divided into type A (extra-articular—unifocal, lowest AVN risk), type B (extra-articular—bifocal, higher AVN risk), and type C (articular, highest AVN risk) also seems to have a rather low inter- and intraobserver agreement (Fig. 2.2). Recently, a system known as "binary classification" has been proposed by Hertel who associates the risk of ischemia to the pattern of fracture. As shown in Fig. 2.3, the Hertel classification is based on an analysis of fracture planes as opposed to fragment numbers as in Neer/Codman classification:

1. Between the greater tuberosity and the head
2. Between the greater tuberosity and the shaft
3. Between the lesser tuberosity and the head
4. Between the lesser tuberosity and the shaft
5. Between the lesser tuberosity and the greater tuberosity

2.3 Understanding the Fracture

The management of every kind of proximal humerus fracture makes mandatory the analysis of some essential features, depending on the patient, fracture's patterns, and bone quality:

1. Age and functional requirements of the patient
2. Integrity of calcar and medial hinge
3. Degree of displacement of tuberosities
4. Head impaction into valgus or varus
5. Displacement of humeral shaft
6. Head splitting or glenohumeral dislocation
7. Bone quality (comminution of tuberosities and surgical neck)

2.3.1 Age and Functional Requirements of the Patient

The age and functional requirements of the patient guide us to decide for the best treatment. The treatment could be simply a Desault bandage in the elderly patient with restricted or null functional requirements and poor bone quality.

The patient's functional requirements are an important element that must guide us in the choice of treatment. Nowadays we often find ourselves in front of an overweighing old man who still plays important daily activities such as driving, swimming, gardening, etc.

No less important is to consider the affected side: dominant or not.

2.3.2 Integrity of Calcar Medial Hinge

The evaluation of the fracture line extension length on the metaphyseal head is essential to assess the integrity of the calcar zone. Frequently, a head impaction into valgus or into varus has been observed. The head rotates into valgus when the greater tuberosity displaces posteriorly and superiorly and the below cancellous bone is compacted.

It is not uncommon that fractures with valgus head impaction have a low risk of osteonecrosis because the medial periosteal hinge is preserved.

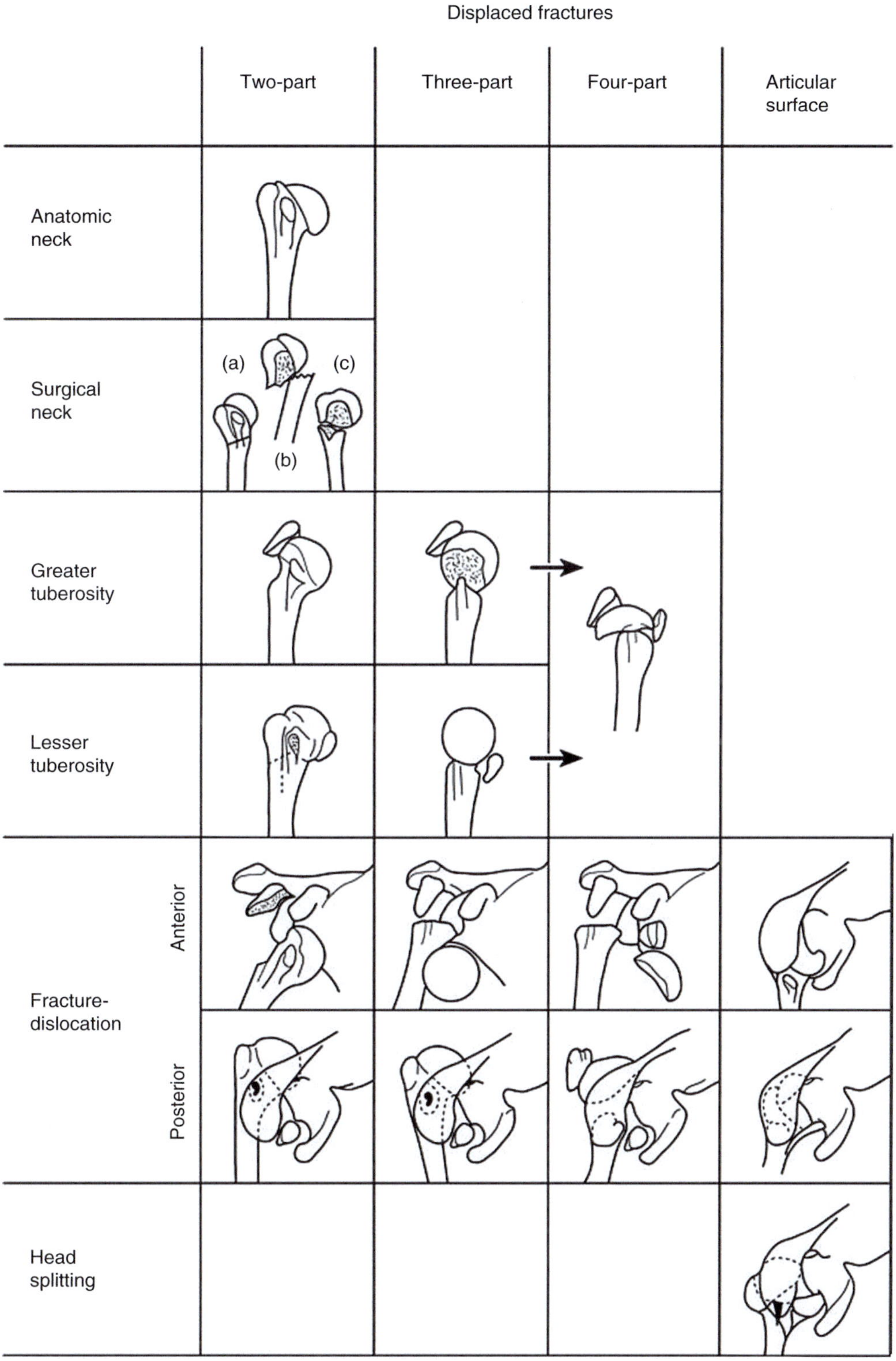

Fig. 2.1 Neer classification (Reproduced with permission from Neer [5])

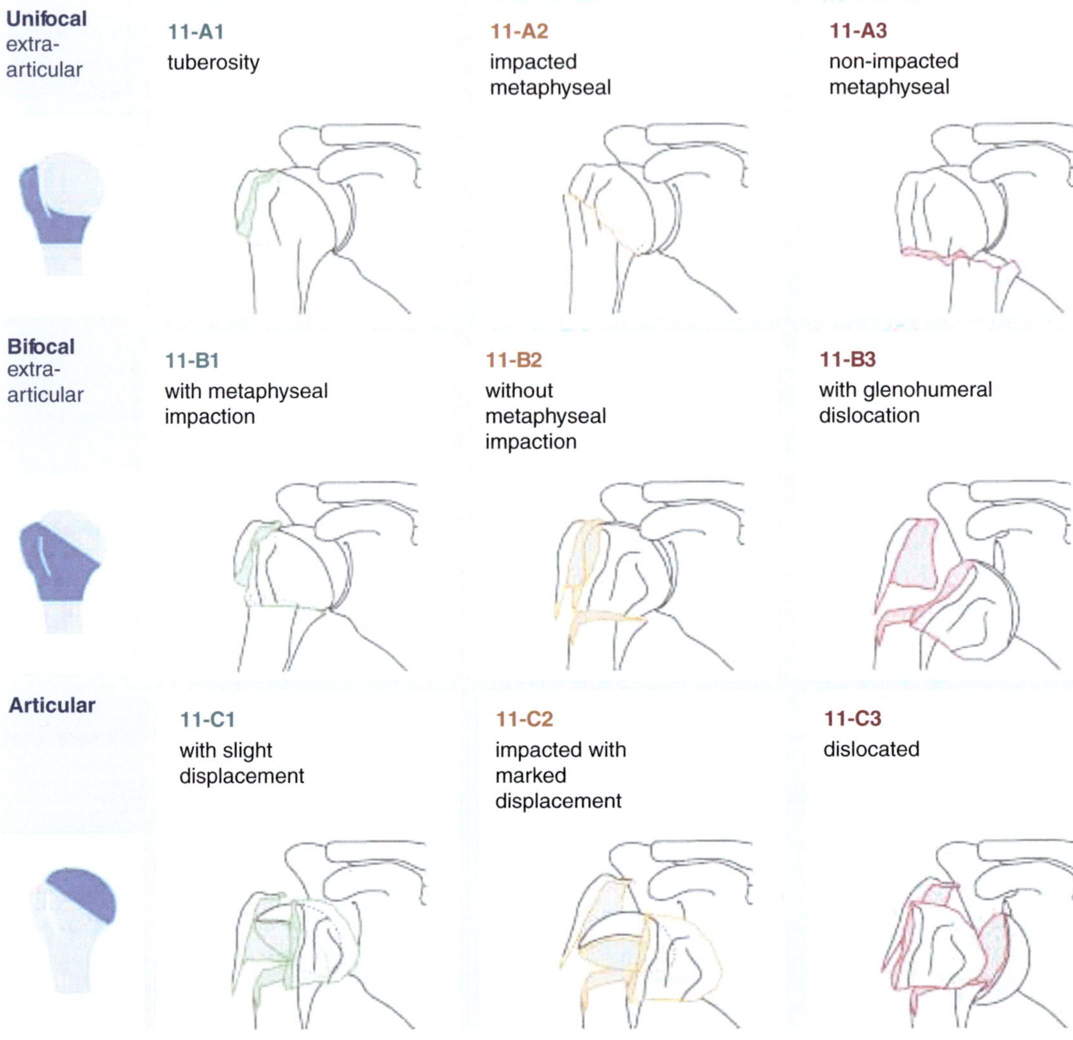

Fig. 2.2 AO classification

Most proximal humerus fractures occur in elderly patients with osteopenia; this can explain the high degree of comminution, the size of cancellous defects due to the impaction, and the potential risk for fixation failure and fracture redisplacement. The knowledge of differences of either bone quality or mineral density in different regions of proximal humerus guides us in reaching the best implant fixation and decreasing the potential failure [8] (Fig. 2.4).

2.3.2.1 Humeral Head Blood Supply

The major blood supply is from the anterior and posterior humeral circumflex arteries. The anterolateral branch of the anterior circumflex artery ascends parallel to the lateral aspect of the biceps tendon and through its terminal branch, the arcuate artery; it enters the head at the junction of the bicipital groove and the greater tuberosity and perfuses the head. Most contributions to the humeral head blood supply

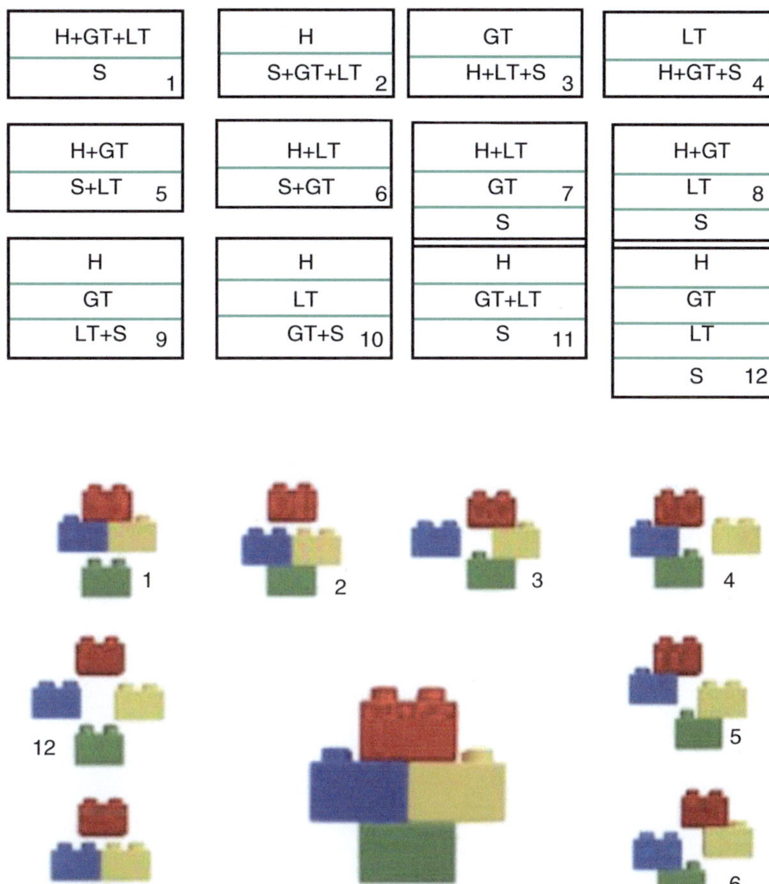

Fig. 2.3 Hertel classification *H* head humerus, *GT* greater tuberosity, *LT* lesser tuberosity, *S* shaft humerus (Reproduced with permission from Hertel et al. [7])

arise from the posterior humeral circumflex, reaching the humeral head via tendo-osseous anastomoses of the posterior and inferior capsule [9, 10].

This kind of knowledge is mandatory to understand and predict the probability of the most dangerous complication of proximal humerus fractures: osteonecrosis. It is a well-known condition which develops when fracture location and displacement compromise the humeral head vascularization. It may be associated with permanent disability. The risk of humeral head ischemia is related to fracture morphology [7] (Fig. 2.5).

Good ischemia predictors are (Fig. 2.6):

- Length of metaphyseal head extension (accuracy 0.84 for calcar segments <8 mm)
- Integrity of the medial hinge (accuracy 0.79 for disrupted hinge)
- Basic fracture pattern (accuracy 0.7 for fractures comprising the anatomic neck)

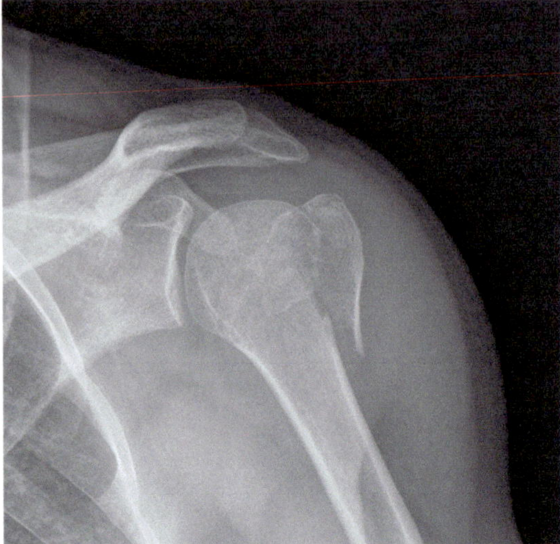

Fig. 2.4 Valgus head impaction fracture with a medial periosteal hinge preserved

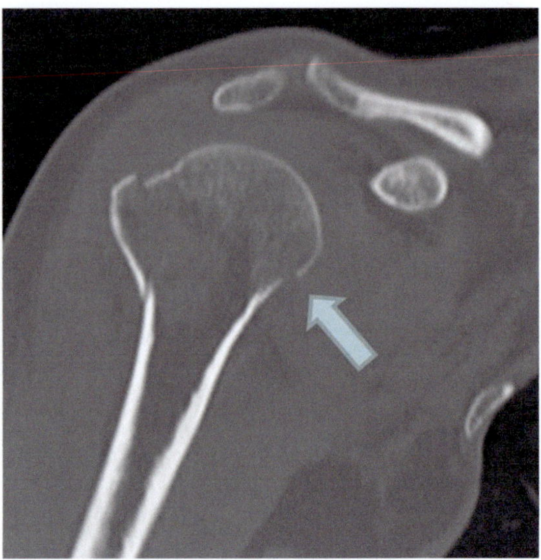

Fig. 2.6 Blue line intact and metaphyseal head extension <8 mm are good ischemia predictors

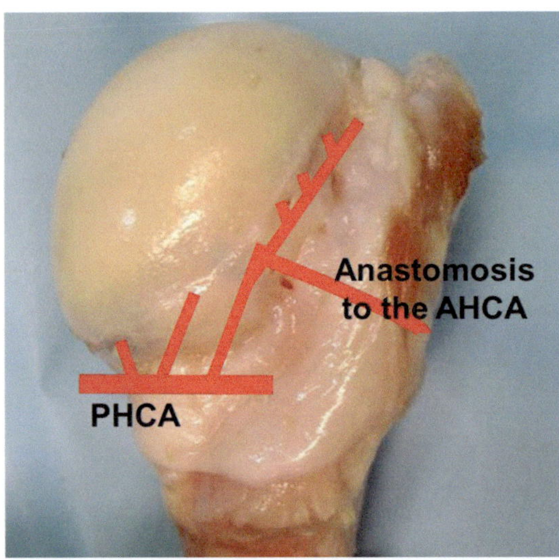

Fig. 2.5 Posterior humeral circumflex artery and posterior capsule

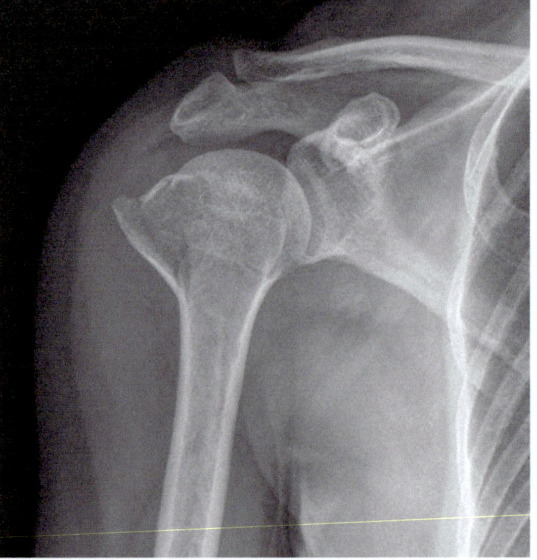

Fig. 2.7 In case of a valgus impacted head opposite to a preserved medial hinge, it will be easier to bring the head in anatomic position by exploiting the medial hinge effect

Poor ischemia predictors are:

- Angular displacement of the head (accuracy 0.62 for angulations over 45 deg)
- Extent of displacement of the tuberosities (displacement over 10 mm: accuracy 0.61)
- Glenohumeral dislocation (accuracy 0.49)
- Head-split components (accuracy 0.49)

The integrity of the medial hinge is also very important to plan reduction and synthesis. In fact, the hinge integrity makes definitely easier reestablishing the correct anatomy. In the case of a valgus impacted head opposite to a preserved medial hinge, in order to perform the reduction, it will be easier to bring the head in anatomic position by exploiting the medial hinge effect (Fig. 2.7). The management of the head can be

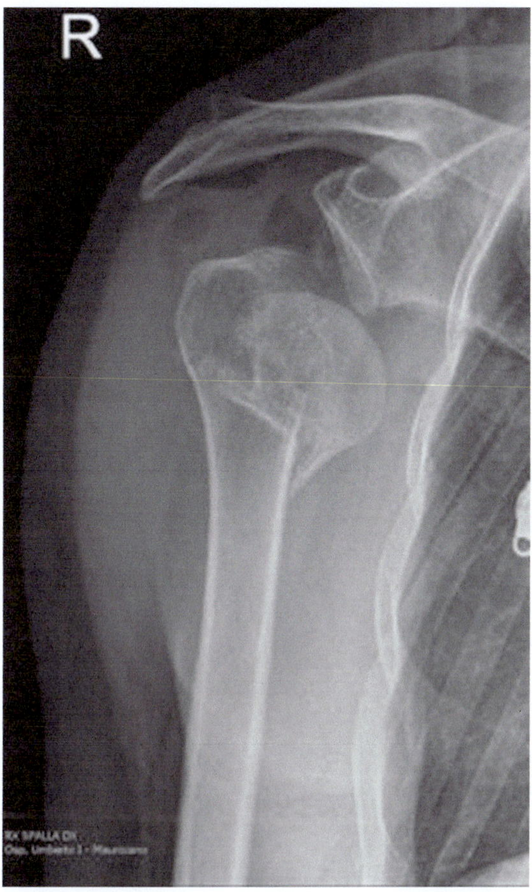

Fig. 2.8 In case of varus head, the medial hinge is frequently interrupted

extremely difficult and could fail, whenever the medial hinge is interrupted. In the event of a varus head, the medial hinge is more frequently interrupted.

A CT study in the frontal plane with 3D reconstructions can provide a complete view of the morphology of this region (Fig. 2.8).

The anatomic calcar reconstruction is the key point in this procedure; the calcar reduction must be carefully planned to obtain a stable synthesis (Fig. 2.9).

2.3.3 Degree of Tuberosities Displacement

In fractures involving the tuberosities, it is of fundamental importance to identify the number of fragments. For this reason, instrumental radiographic study of the fracture should always be on the two planes of space for getting the glenoid and axillary AP projection. The latter is sometimes difficult to perform due to poor patient cooperation especially in more complex cases. Therefore, the alternative is a projection in the scapular plane (*Y* view). However, it could be difficult to identify the fragment number of the epiphysis. This kind of imaging lets us clarify the shaft relationship and alignment with his head.

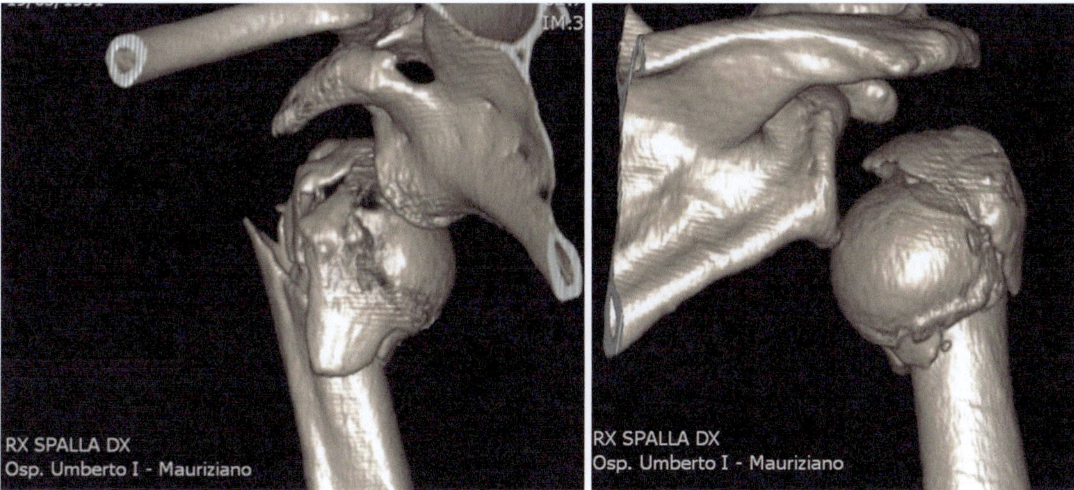

Fig. 2.9 A complete view of the calcar region

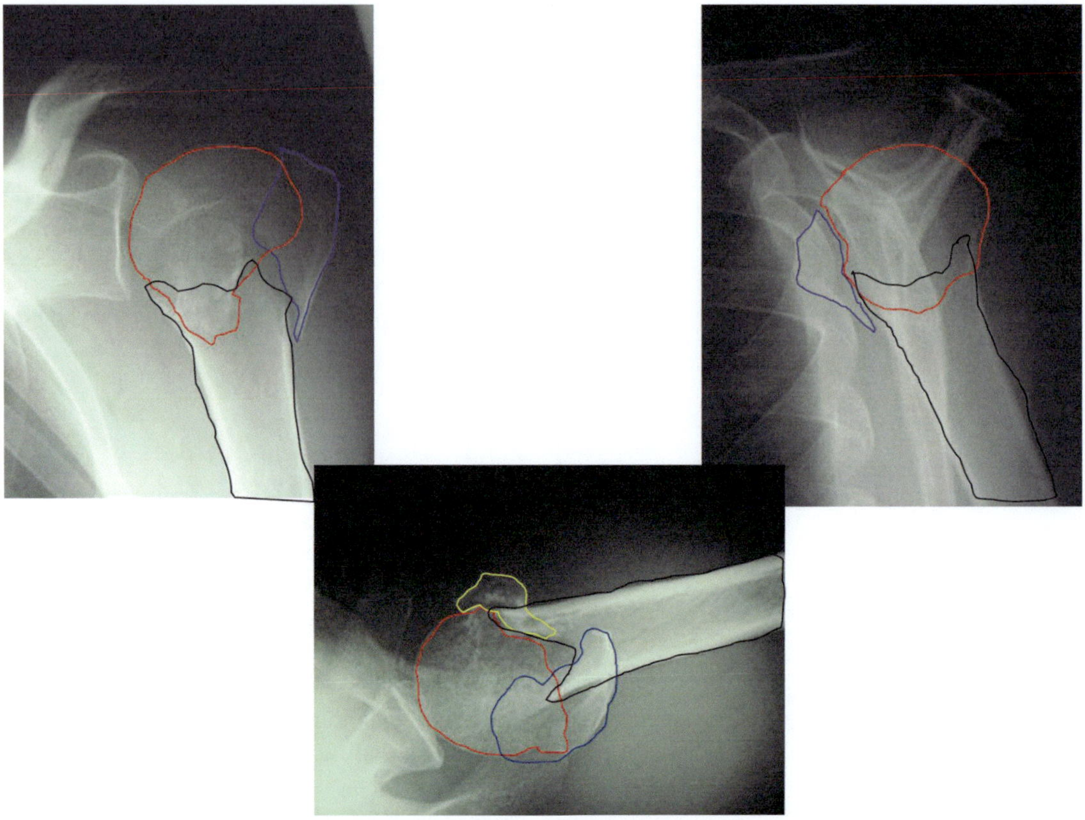

Fig. 2.10 A complete X-ray trauma series for the shoulder. Fragments of fracture. *red head*, blue *greater tuberosity*, yellow *lesser tuberosity*, black *diaphysis*

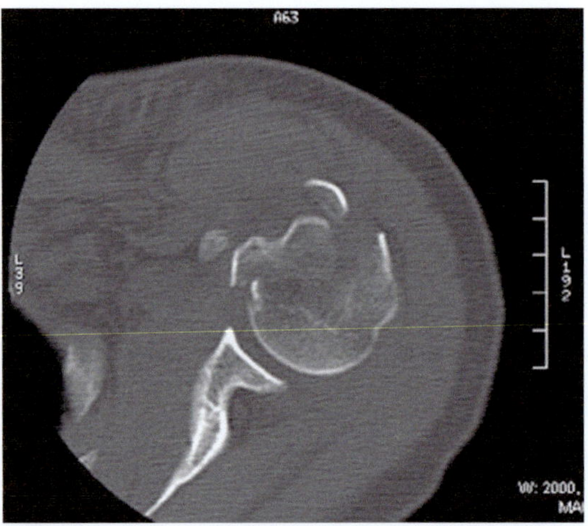

Fig. 2.11 A CT scan clarifying the true facture morphology and the number of fragments

If radiographic study highlights the proximal humerus involvement and shows the involvement of both tuberosity and head, further CT study is indicated to clarify the true fracture morphology (Fig. 2.10).

The tuberosity evaluation must identify its position. Normally, the greater tuberosity migrates posterosuperiorly when submitted to the traction of the posterosuperior cuff tendons. The surgeon should therefore plan the reduction maneuvers that neutralize the traction forces on the tuberosity to bring it back in the anatomic position, performing a proper reduction and synthesis (Fig. 2.11). At the same time, it is essential to observe the quality of the tuberosities in terms of bone quality and comminution (Fig. 2.12), in other words, to evaluate whether the reduction is possible and the healing is potentially reliable. At the same time each landmark that would allow to obtain an anatomic reconstruction should be identified, for example, points of contact between the lower edge of the tuberosity fragment and the diaphysis as in a puzzle (Fig. 2.13).

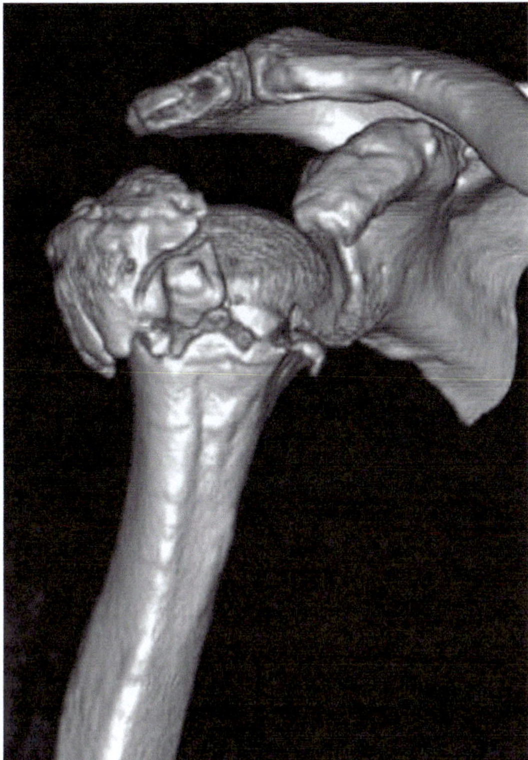

Fig. 2.12 Ct scan permits to plan the reduction maneuvers that neutralize the traction forces on the tuberosity and to bring it back in the anatomic position, performing a proper reduction and synthesis

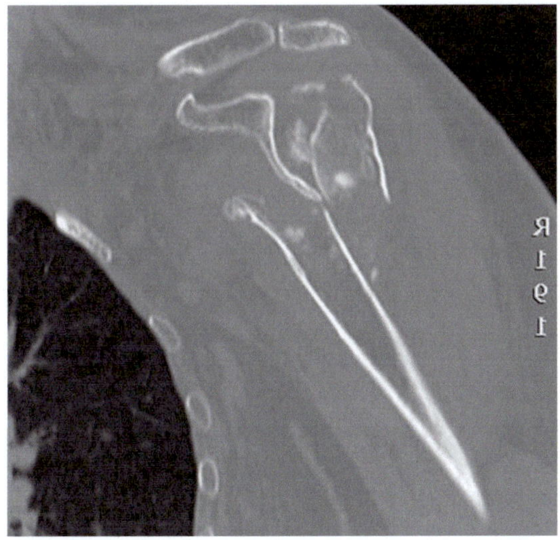

Fig. 2.13 The quality of the tuberosities in terms of bone quality and comminution in this case is low

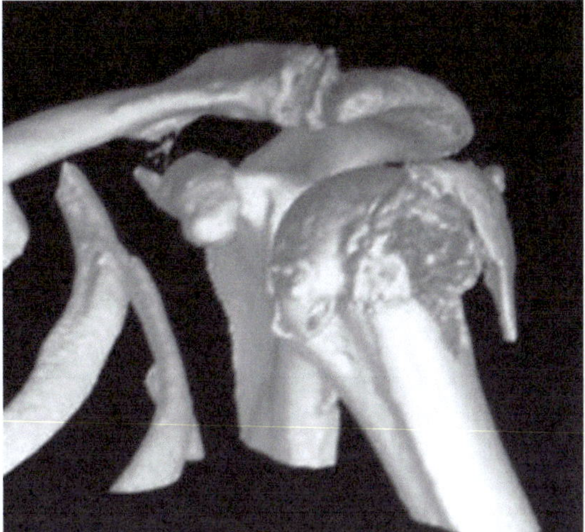

Fig. 2.14 Points of contact between the lower edge of the tuberosity fragment and the diaphysis should be identified to obtain an anatomic reconstruction

The lesser tuberosity should be inspected to see whether it remains adherent to the head or it is isolated from it. In the first case, the management of the lesser tuberosity and the subscapularis also allows the surgeon to maneuver the head if he needs to reduce it (Figs. 2.14 and 2.15).

It is also important to identify the plane that divides the two tuberosities. The fracture line that separates them can be in front of or behind the bicipital groove. When reduction of the head is needed, it might be necessary to use the fracture line to access the head (Fig. 2.16).

2.3.4 Head Impaction into Valgus or Varus

The alignment in the frontal plane of the epiphysis to the shaft is an important fact that must be well evaluated.

In fact, it is known that valgus is better tolerated even in case of nonoperative treatment. In this case it will be the position of the tuberosity that will guide us in the choice. In particular, if the greater tuberosity is high and posterior, it will alter the biomechanics of the cuff and of the subacromial space. In this case a surgical reduction will be the choice to restore anatomy and function (Fig. 2.17).

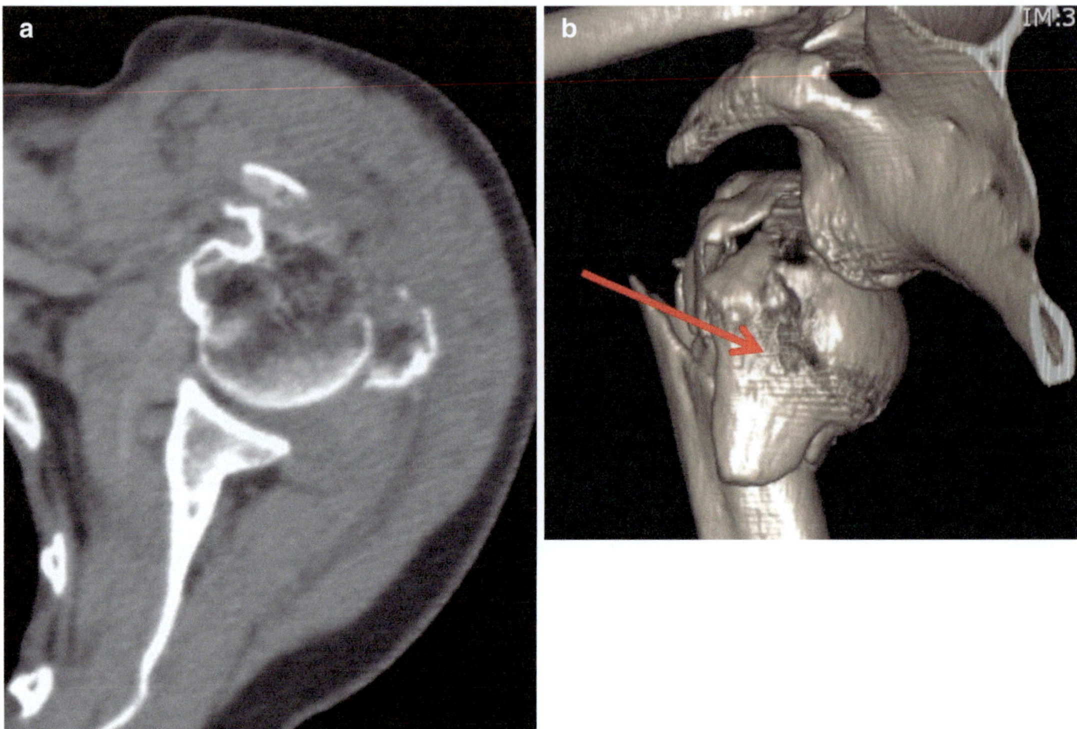

Fig. 2.15 The lesser tuberosity should be inspected to see whether it remains adherent to the head or it is isolated from it

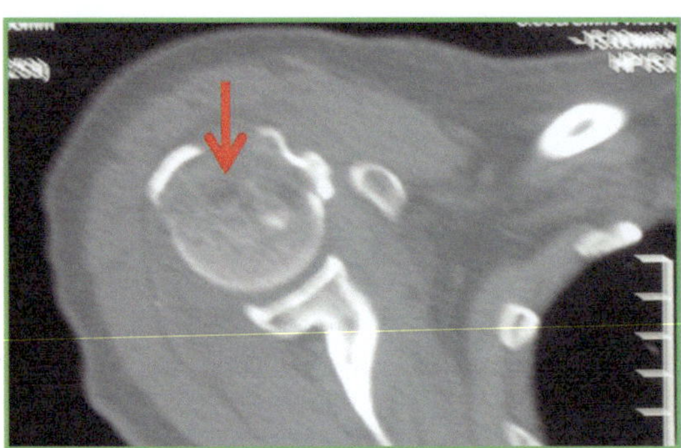

Fig. 2.16 The fracture line that separates the tuberosities can be in front of or behind the bicipital groove. When reduction of the head is needed, it might be necessary to use the fracture line to access the head

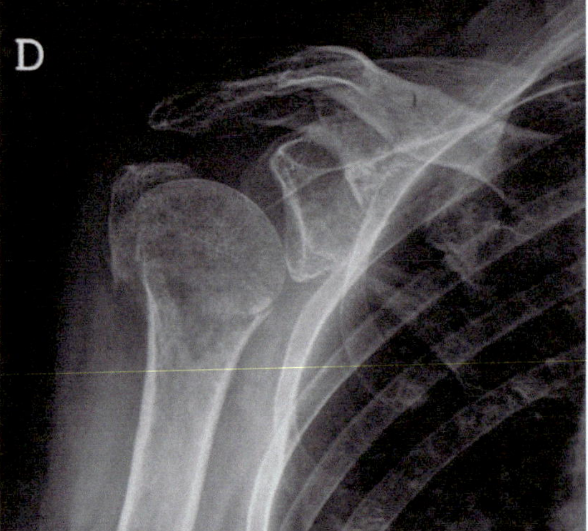

Fig. 2.17 In case of valgus impacted head the height of the greater tuberosity must be observed

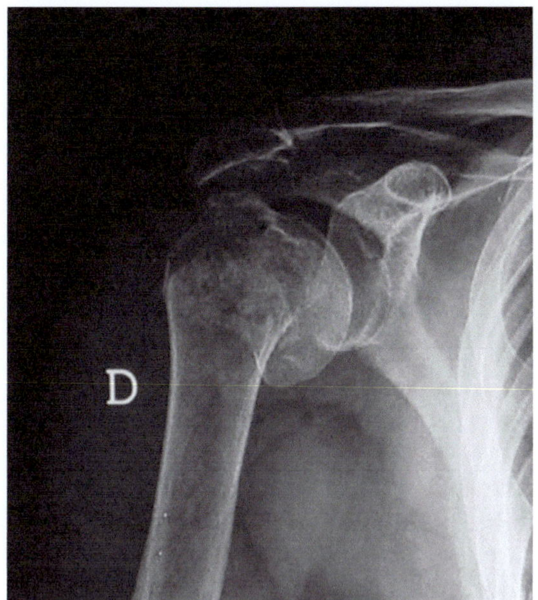

Fig. 2.18 Varus deformity poorly tolerated

The varus deformity is poorly tolerated, and therefore it is always worth the reduction (Fig. 2.18).

In case of a two-part fracture, you can schedule a closed reduction as will be described in the following chapters.

2.3.5 Displacement of Humeral Shaft

The humeral shaft is subjected to tensile forces by the pectoralis major traction in a medial and anterior direction, while the latissimus dorsi and the teres major act with a posterior direction, and the deltoid pulls the diaphyseal stump in a cranial direction.

The shaft is dislocated in the anterior and medial direction by the prevalent strength of the pectoralis major that is not neutralized by the other carriers acting on the shaft. This can be quite easily seen on the X-ray in the lateral plane (axillary or *Y* view) and CT scan.

This should be taken into account in planning the reduction maneuvers needed to realign the diaphysis. They must neutralize the force vectors of the pectoralis major (Fig. 2.19).

2.3.6 Head Splitting or Glenohumeral Dislocation

There are few absolute indications for the implantation of a prosthesis in the case of fracture of the proximal third of the humerus: one of these is the head splitting and/or fracture-dislocation (Fig. 2.20).

It is necessary to diagnose when an involvement of the articular surface of the humeral head is suspected. This suspicion can arise only if the radiographic study is carried out in two orthogonal planes. When this procedure is not applied, it is mandatory to add the CT study which obviously clears up any doubt.

CT will be required in case of fracture-dislocation to understand the morphology of the fracture, to plan when possible a closed reduction, and to better understand the relationship among the humeral head and the medial vascular and nervous structures (Fig. 2.21).

2.3.7 Bone Quality (Comminution of Tuberosities and Surgical Neck)

The quality of the bone is of extreme importance for the prognosis of the fracture. Considering that in the elderly there is a high frequency of these fractures, we have to deal with a poor quality bone.

There are no secure systems that allow us to quantify the quality that we have to face.

The X-rays, CT scans, and when possible the medical history of the patient can help us about this issue. The thin corticals, the severe comminution of both tuberosities and surgical neck, as well as an "empty" head should raise our suspicion.

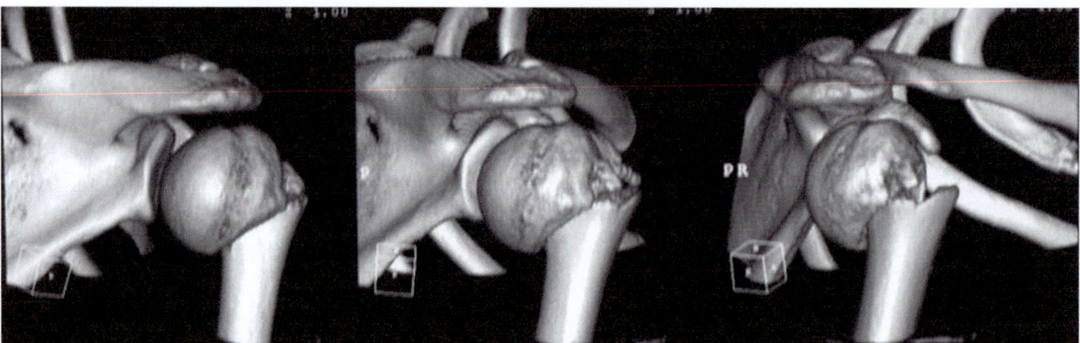

Fig. 2.19 3D CT scan helps us to plan the reduction maneuvers needed to realign the diaphysis. They must neutralize the force vectors of the pectoralis major

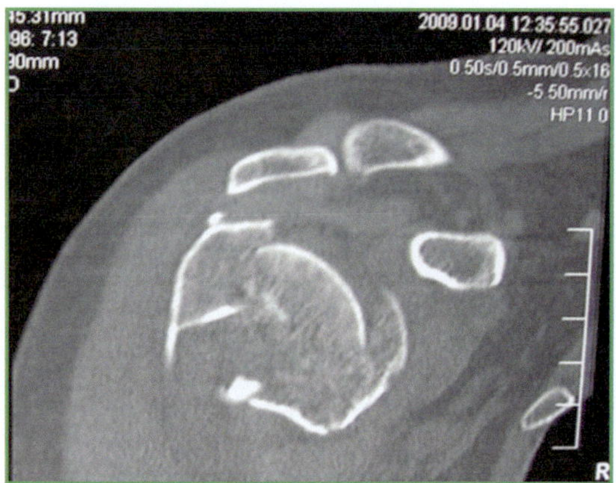

Fig. 2.20 The head splitting is one of the absolute indications for the implantation of a prosthesis

Understanding the fracture means planning the most suitable kind of treatment in relation to the quality of the bone.

2.4 Conclusive Remarks

Understanding the fracture is the key point of our treatment and our success.

Many factors are indispensable. Today there are no classifications that allow us to associate a type of fracture to a single type of treatment. The classification systems surely enable us to speak a common language and standardize our results.

To define the requested type of treatment, we have to involve in our algorithm several elements which include the type of the patient, his age, his expectations, the type of fracture, and bone quality.

Last but not least, the experience of the surgeon plays an important role.

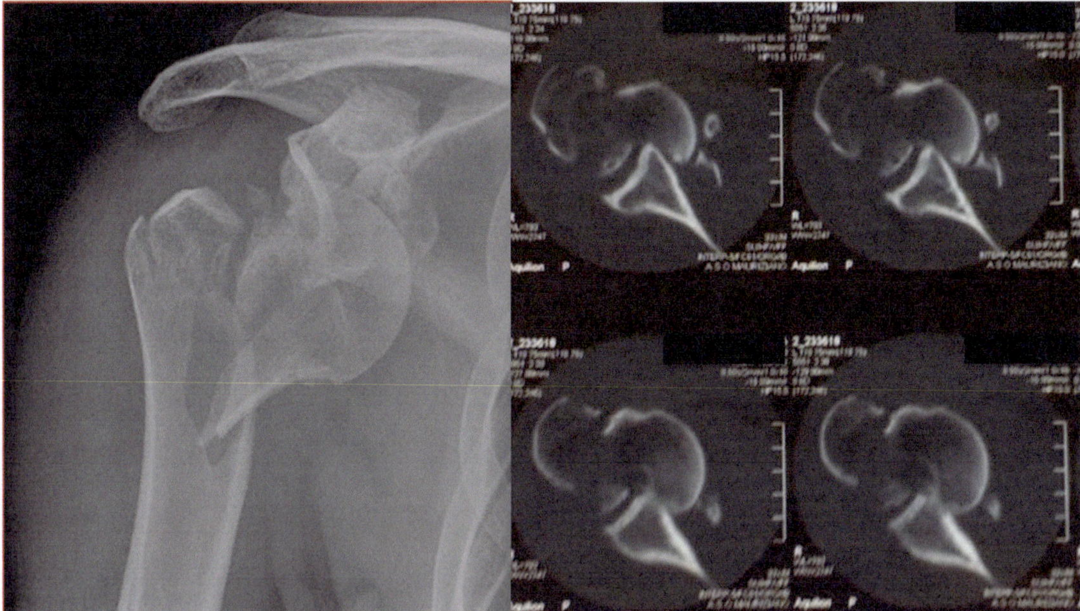

Fig. 2.21 CT in case of fracture-dislocation permits to better understand the relationship among the humeral head and the medial vascular and nervous structures

References

1. Kannus P, Palvanen M, Niemi S, Parkkari J, Jarvinen M, Vuori I (2000) Osteoporotic fractures of the proximal humerus in elderly Finnish persons: sharp increase in 1970–1998 and alarming projections for the new millennium. Acta Orthop Scand 71:465–470
2. Koval KJ, Zuckerman JD (2006) Handbook of fractures, 3rd edn. Lippincott Williams & Wilkins, Philadelphia
3. Sidor ML, Zuckerman JD, Lyon T, Koval K, Cuomo F, Schoenberg N (1993) The Neer classification system for proximal humeral fractures. An assessment of interobserver reliability and intraobserver reproducibility. J Bone Joint Surg Am 75:1745–1750
4. Siebenrock KA, Gerber C (1993) The reproducibility of classification of fractures of the proximal end of the humerus. J Bone Joint Surg Am 75:1751–1755
5. Neer CS II (1970) Displaced proximal humeral fractures. I. Classification and evaluation. J Bone Joint Surg Am 52:1077–1089
6. Neer CS II (2002) Four-segment classification of proximal humeral fractures: purpose and reliable use. J Shoulder Elbow Surg 11:389–400
7. Hertel R, Hempfing A, Stiehler M, Leunig M (2004) Predictors of humeral head ischemia after intracapsular fracture of the proximal humerus. J Shoulder Elbow Surg 13:427–433
8. Sanchez-Sotelo J (2006) Proximal humerus fractures. Clin Anat 19:588–598
9. Gerber C, Hersche O, Berberat C (1998) The clinical relevance of posttraumatic avascular necrosis of the humeral head. J Shoulder Elbow Surg 7:586–590
10. Gerber C, Schneeberger AG, Vinh TS (1990) The arterial vascularization of the humeral head. An anatomical study. J Bone Joint Surg Am 72:1486–1494

Operating Theater Setup

3

Enrico Bellato, Umberto Cottino, and Eleonora Marini

The surgical treatment of a proximal humeral fracture is not something that should be improvised: everything needs to be carefully planned to achieve an optimal result. Just like preparing a successful show requires effort and a meticulous preparation, the same goes for a well-executed surgical operation. This chapter will provide the information to standardize the treatment of the patient and his/her pathology. Let us consider the standardization of the surgical technique, even in its most banal aspects, as the only way to strive for excellence in the treatment and for the patient's complete satisfaction. In doing so, surgeons can concentrate their efforts solely on the surgical motions with the flexibility necessary to face potential complications.

E. Bellato (✉) • U. Cottino
Department of Orthopaedics and Traumatology, University of Turin, Medical School, CTO-Maria Adelaide Hospital, Via Zuretti 29, Turin 10126, Italy
e-mail: bellatoenrico@gmail.com; umberto.cottino@gmail.com

E. Marini
Oncologic Orthopaedic Center, University of Milan, Medical School, "Gaetano Pini Hospital", Piazza Ferrari 1, Milan, 20122, Italy
e-mail: eleonoramarini21@gmail.com

3.1 Preparing the Script

It is important not to be caught off guard or unprepared in any situation. When entering the operating room, surgeons, anesthesiologists, surgical technicians, and other nurses need to have clearly in mind the type of operation that will be performed. It is customary to discuss the operating list of the week in a meeting involving all the members of the surgical team: this briefing provides an opportunity for the surgeons to examine the cases and exchange ideas. The anesthetic consultation and preoperative examinations must take place just prior to the surgery in order to portray a general clinical picture that is both up to date and accurate for the surgical procedure: the patient could present an unstable clinical condition that needs to be carefully monitored. After completing this step, the anesthesiologist must communicate the findings to the surgeon, and the two of them should discuss the priorities.

Through a thorough knowledge of the patient's anamnesis, it will be possible to choose the appropriate antibiotic prophylaxis and whether to start thromboprophylaxis as well. We have recently completed a multicenter retrospective study [1] aimed at researching the risk factors associated with the outbreak of surgical site infections following reduction and fixation procedures for proximal humeral fractures. The study included 452 patients, of which 209 treated with percutaneous pinning, 197 with plate and

F. Castoldi et al. (eds.), *Simple and Complex Fractures of the Humerus*,
DOI 10.1007/978-88-470-5307-6_3, © Springer-Verlag Italia 2015

screws, and 46 with other devices (excluding prosthetic implants). Based on our results, we suggest using third-generation cephalosporin or vancomycin. There has been an increasing attention in the literature to the use of thromboprophylaxis in patients undergoing upper limb surgery. Often, however, these publications present only sporadic cases and cannot therefore serve as a model when deciding for the indiscriminate use of low-molecular-weight heparin (LMWH) [2–4]. This is not devoid of complications, so it would be best to select which patients this prophylaxis is administered to, especially for subjects at risk and in case of prosthetic implants.

In our experience, the study of proximal humeral fractures should be accompanied by CT scans in almost every case. Additionally, 3D reconstructions can also be very useful [5]. CT scans make it possible to evaluate specific elements like the integrity of the medial hinge [6], the number of fragments, and whether it affects the joint surface in order to select the correct procedure to perform before surgery. It is important, however, to have the option of changing strategy midcourse: we believe that every team that is about to engage in the surgical treatment of a proximal humeral fracture should have ready at its disposal the tools to perform to perform either an osteosinthesis or a hemiarthroplasty [7].

Being aware of the chance of changing treatment during surgery makes it possible to correctly inform the patient about the procedure. The informed consent process consists in establishing a treatment agreement with a patient so that the person concerned is also directly involved in the choice. The involvement of patients in the decision stream protects them and gives them the opportunity to express their preferences or refusals concerning surgery. Similarly, this direct exchange between a surgeon and a patient also helps the doctor evaluate the subject's general characteristics and his/her compliance to the subsequent rehabilitation treatment: attempting high levels of physiotherapy would be counterproductive for patients lacking motivation [8].

Based on the preoperative complete blood count and the surgery that will be performed, blood type and packed red blood cells will have to be prepared. This is recommended in case of internal fixations or prosthetic implants and especially in the case of a fracture-dislocation where the humeral head is displaced in the axilla.

In summary:

1. Admission to the emergency room
2. Diagnostic imaging techniques (including 3D CT scan)
3. Discussing case during the weekly meeting
4. Deciding best treatment options
5. Preanesthesia evaluation
6. Signing of the informed consent to the surgical procedure
7. Preparing the patient: antibiotic prophylaxis (ATB), possible thromboprophylaxis (ATE), washing the axilla

3.2 Set Design

The patient's position is crucial. It is extremely important to keep the upper arm free and mobile on all planes to allow for an adequate surgical exposition, as well as to obtain high-quality X-ray images. There are fundamentally two options:

- Beach-chair position. This position has two main advantages: it allows the shoulder a greater range of movement, and it is compatible with every type of operation. Some authors prefer the supine position to perform an osteosynthesis with plate and screws; nevertheless, we believe that the beach-chair position should be favored because it is more suitable in case the surgeon decides to resort to a prosthetic implant while the procedure is taking place. Being able to hyperextend the arm to gain access to the medullary canal is fundamental when performing an implant or an intramedullary nailing.

  It is important to set up the modular operating table correctly: the various components need to be placed following a specific order to prevent the patient from falling, slouching, or sliding to the end of the table (Fig. 3.1).

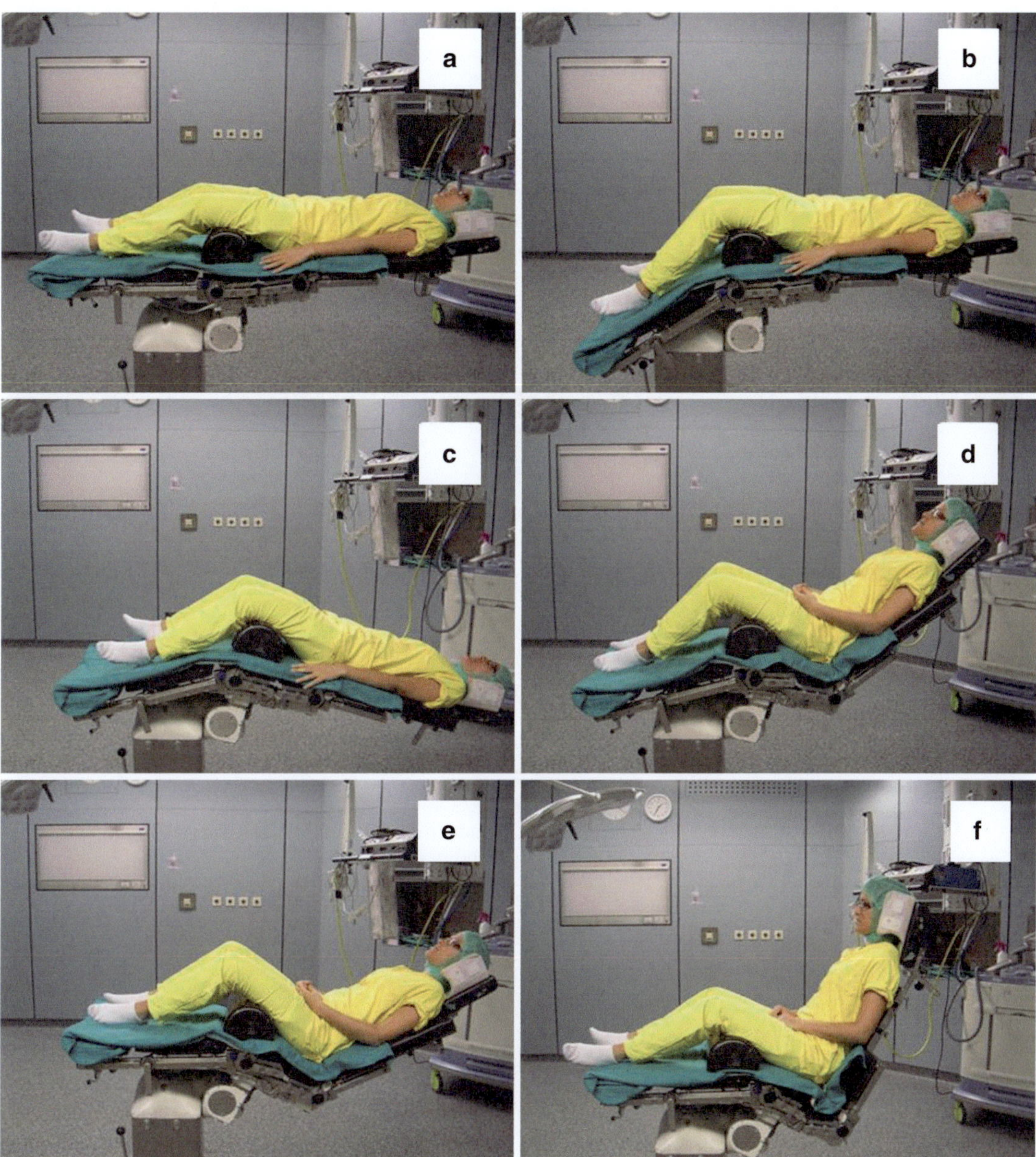

Fig. 3.1 Images (**a**–**f**) illustrate the sequence of steps to correctly position the patient on the modular operating table. It is important to note that, in (**f**), the support behind the operative shoulder has been removed to guarantee a greater inter-operatory mobility of the limb

Alternatively, the standard operating table can also be used by adding an appropriate trapezoidal wedge pillow (Fig. 3.2). The head should be secured with a proper head positioner (Fig. 3.3), which is instrumental in gaining sufficient operating space and to avoid lesions caused by brachial plexus injuries during the surgery. The headrest should keep the head in a neutral position: the head should be aligned with the neck and the neck slightly bent over the chest. The contralateral inclination of the head in relation to the affected limb

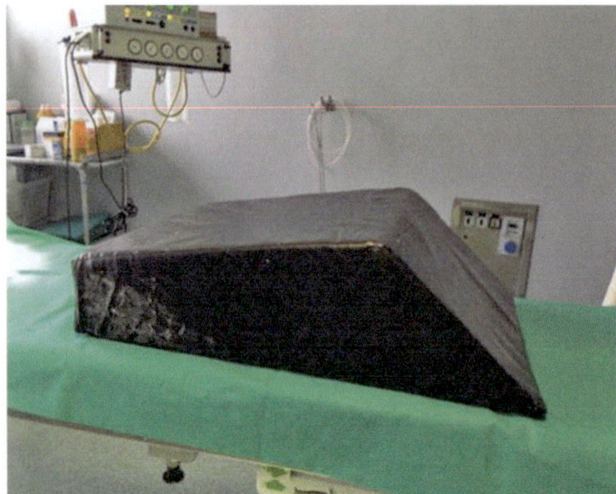

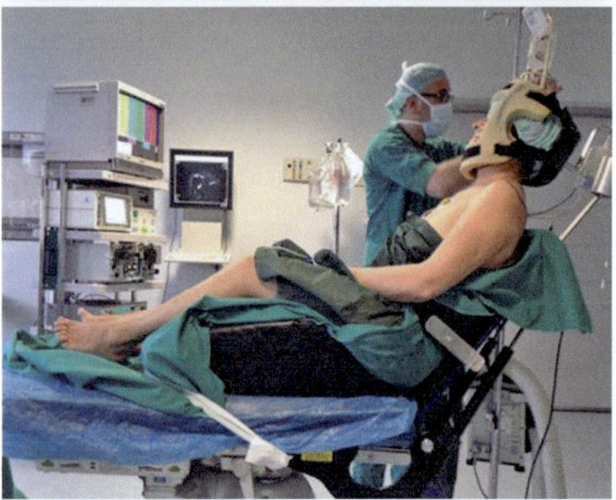

Fig. 3.2 A trapezoidal wedge pillow can serve in lieu of the modular operating table

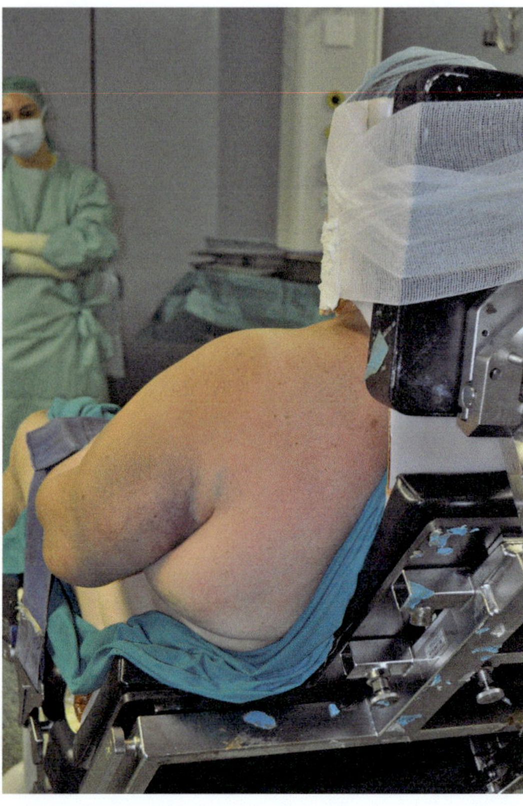

Fig. 3.4 The table segment that supports the operative shoulder can be removed to achieve a greater degree of mobility of the limb

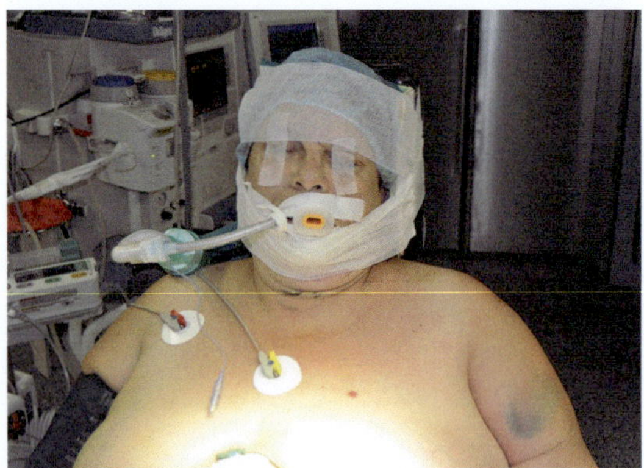

Fig. 3.3 It is of paramount importance to have a proper head positioner to keep the patient's head firmly in place during the operation. The endotracheal tube for respirator and anesthesia should be placed on the side opposite to the shoulder that will be operated

should be avoided; the head should also not lean forward or backward compared to the neck.

The mobility of the arm can be improved if the table segment that supports the operative shoulder is removed (Fig. 3.4). According to the surgeon's preference, an arm holder can also be useful to rest the forearm of the operative limb at the level of the elbow.

The greatest disadvantage of the beach-chair position is the difficulty in obtaining a full axillary projection with the C-arm. Furthermore, beach-chair positioning is recommended for arthroscopic fixations of fractures to the greater tuberosity of the humerus [9–12].

- Supine position. This has the advantage of keeping the limb in a position that permits a

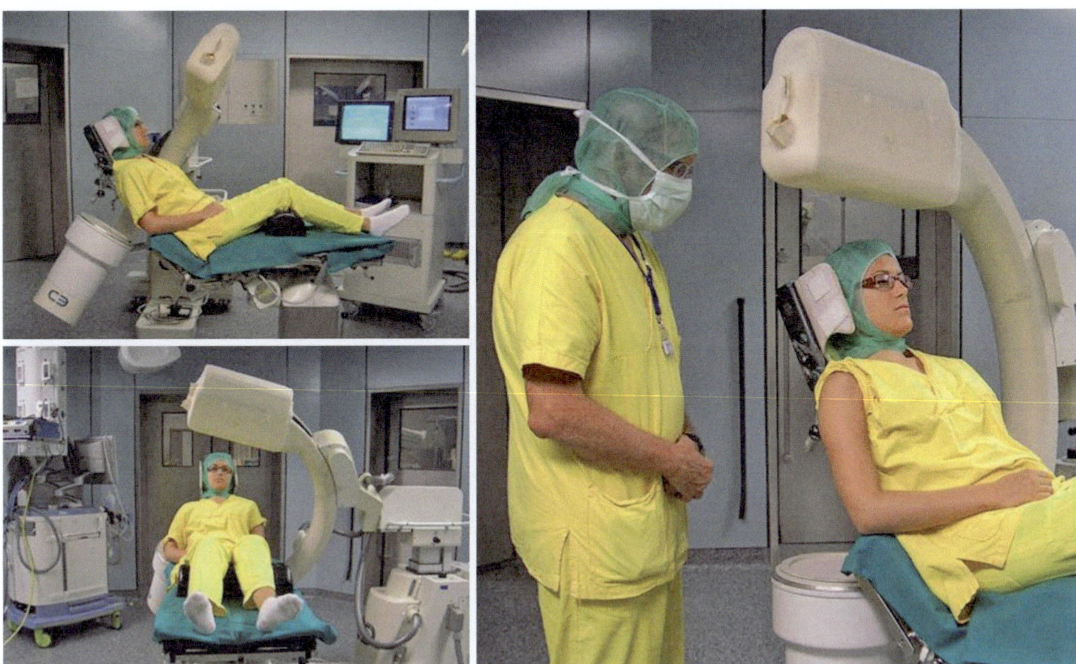

Fig. 3.5 The image intensifier should be positioned contralateral to the operative limb in order to get the best visualizations without getting in the way of the surgical team

true axial visualization without moving the arm (which is very useful for unstable fractures). However, the shoulder has a smaller range of movement compared to the beach-chair position. In our opinion, this surgical position is better suited for cases of percutaneous fixations after a closed reduction. It could be useful to shift the patient laterally so that the operative shoulder is toward the outside of the Table. A radiolucent table could then possibly be used to provide additional support.

The image intensifier needs to always be present in the operating room when performing an osteosynthesis, and it should be available also during a prosthetic replacement. The correct placement of the image intensifier is fundamental: even though it is usually placed behind the patient's head [13–17] or on the side being operated on [18], in our opinion the most functional position is contralateral to the fracture. This makes it possible to obtain a good visualization without the C-arm getting in the surgical team's way (Fig. 3.5). It is of paramount importance that the lower operating part of the table be cleared so that the C-arm can pass unobstructed. After placing the patient on the table, but before preparing the surgical site, a few tests should be carried out to ensure that the image intensifier can access every plane. Moreover, correctly defining the orientation of the C-arm is also useful in obtaining a true anteroposterior (AP) view.

The same preliminary tests should be performed if the C-arm is positioned behind the patient's head (parallel to the longitudinal axis of the patient), making sure the image intensifier does not get in the anesthesiologist's way. As a matter of fact, the anesthesiologist usually stands behind the patient's head: this place is both convenient and strategic in case a rapid intervention is required because it does not interfere with the surgeons, who can keep on working unobstructed and at their best. The endotracheal tube for the anesthesia should be positioned in the corner of the mouth opposite to the side that is being operated on (Fig. 3.3).

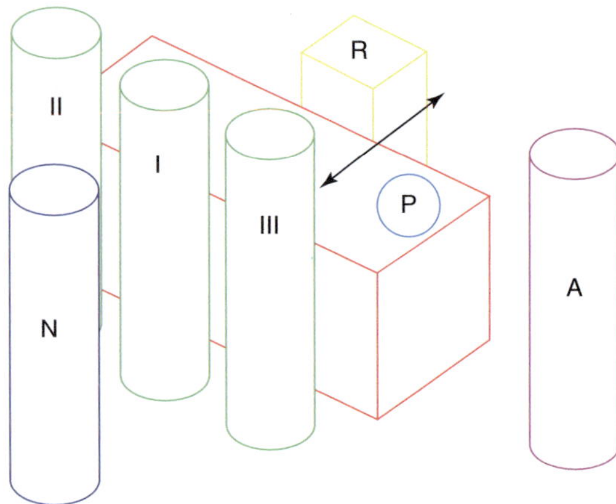

Fig. 3.6 *I* first surgeon, *II* second surgeon, *III* third surgeon, *A* anesthesiologist, *N* operating nurse, *P* patient, *R* image intensifier. The *black arrow* indicates that the position of the third surgeon can be on either side of the patient depending on the type of surgery

Most of the cases only require two surgeons; in case a third one is needed, this additional member of the surgical team usually stands on the other side of the table by the nonoperative limb. In this way, the anesthesiologist is placed between the surgeons; however, it could also be useful for the anesthesiologist to stand by the patient's healthy side, leaving the place behind the subject's head for the third surgeon (Fig. 3.6).

The type of anesthesia needs to be discussed with the patient. The options available are either general anesthesia or brachial plexus block that can be potentially accompanied by sedation [13, 16, 19, 20]. Because of the close proximity of the surgical site to the subject's head, we prefer the former option; furthermore, general anesthesia also ensures a greater degree of tranquility in case the operation lasts longer than expected or if a minor surgery turns into a prosthetic replacement or in an open reduction and internal fixation.

3.3 Costumes and Props

A dermographic marker can be helpful to draw the approach and the useful landmarks (Fig. 3.7). For a transdeltoid approach, the longitudinal lateral axis of the humerus and the lateral contour of the acromion should be drawn; from this point distally measure 5 cm and trace a line perpendicular to the humeral diaphysis: the axillary nerve is usually located in this area [21]. For the deltopectoral approach, the useful landmarks are the acromion and the coracoid process. For the anterolateral approach, instead, only the contour of the acromion, the acromioclavicular joint, and the longitudinal lateral axis of the humerus need to be traced. When performing a fixation with percutaneous pinning, it can be very useful to mark the intersection of the deltoid with the humeral diaphysis (the axillary nerve branches in front of the deltoid tuberosity and it will be harder to damage it with the pins) and the coracoid process (which tells us the correct direction to insert the pins). The lines traced with the dermographic marker can be useful for surgeons to help them orient themselves during the procedure; they are also helpful to those who have to prepare the operating field by giving them an idea of the area they need to circumscribe with sterile drapes.

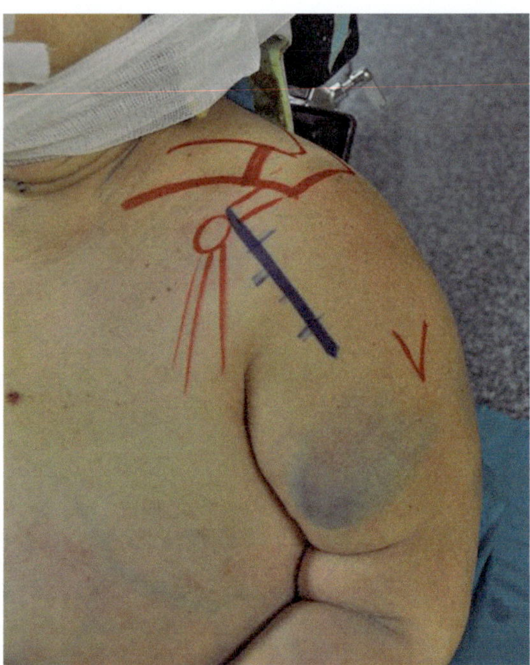

Fig. 3.7 With the appropriate dermographic marker, trace the landmarks useful to the specific surgical procedure: for the deltopectoral approach (*blue line*), highlight the site of the coracoid, of the conjoint tendon, of the coracoacromial ligament, of the deltoid insertion, of the acromion, and of the acromioclavicular joint (*red lines*)

Before preparing the surgical site, we recommend washing the axilla with chlorhexidine and a sponge. From our multicenter study mentioned in the beginning of this chapter, we can infer that the preoperative washing of the site can significantly reduce the risks of postsurgical infections (ODDS 0.13, $p=0.008$) [1].

The drapes to prepare the operating field should not be chosen at random. Surgical drapes with circular aperture should only be used if there is the certainty that the procedure that will be performed is a closed reduction and percutaneous fixation. With this type of drape, in fact, it is not possible to perform a deltopectoral approach, which could be necessary if, during the procedure, the surgeons decided not to perform a closed reduction and internal fixation, opting instead for an open reduction and internal fixation or a prosthetic replacement. When using a U-drape, a sufficient portion of the mammary surface should remain exposed (Fig. 3.8a).

The use of Steri-Drape (3M, Maplewood, Minnesota, St. Paul I-94 at McKnight Road) is debatable. It is better not to use it in cases involving percutaneous fixation because it could get in the way of the insertion point for the pins. Conversely, we recommend using it for open reductions and especially for prosthetic replacements. The complete coverage of the axilla can be achieved with the double layering technique used in hip surgery.

We suggest using a stockinette (Fig. 3.8); it should be unrolled no further than the distal extremity of the humerus, so as to isolate the hand and to allow for a safer procedure. It can be very helpful to wrap it with a cohesive bandage (e.g., Peha-haft, Paul Hartmann Ltd Heywood Distribution Park Pilsworth Road, Heywood, Lancashire) to prevent the stockinette from getting in the way or from unraveling; make sure the thumb is isolated, so the rotations during surgery can be controlled better.

As far as the instrumentation goes, we suggest preparing a range of equipment that would allow the surgical staff to deal with all surgical operations

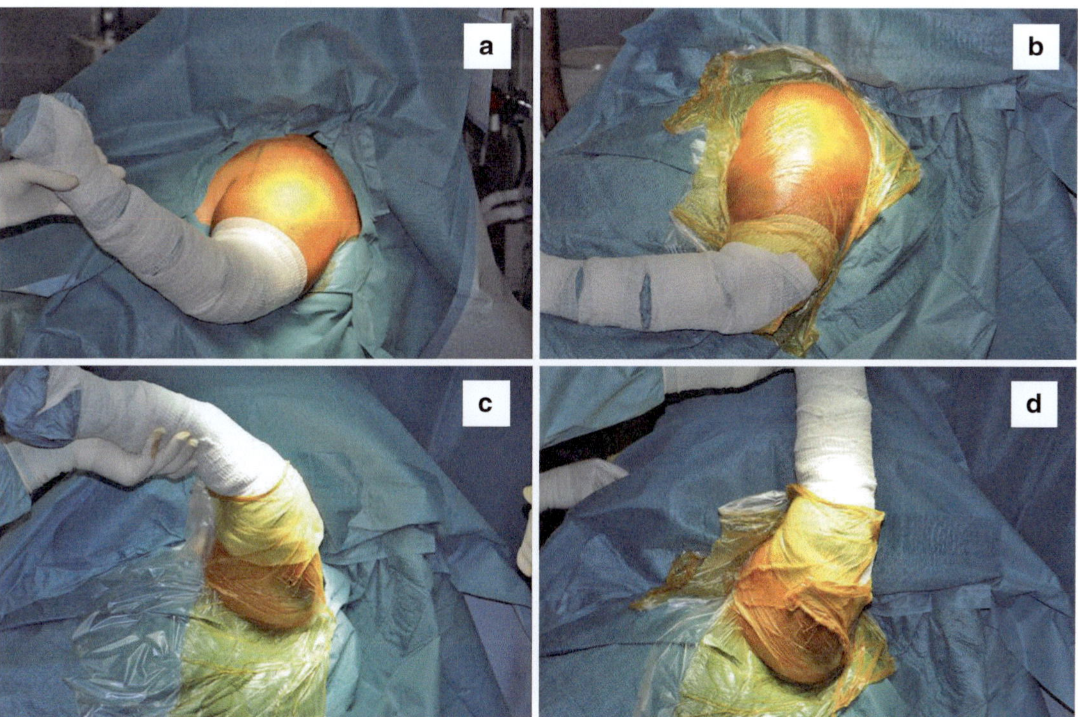

Fig. 3.8 (**a**) Preparing the surgical site can involve the use of a stockinette, which can be wrapped with a cohesive bandage; U-drapes need to be placed in such a way that a sufficient portion of the mammary surface remains exposed. (**b–d**) Steri-Drape can be useful to guarantee a safer procedure, but it must also ensure the shoulder's complete mobility

but which should be supplemented with specific items depending on the particular kind of surgery planned. The general tool kit should always include:

1. Self-retaining retractors (if there are not enough members in the surgical team)
2. Hohmann retractors of various sizes and one with a rounded end (to use on the humeral metaphysis)
3. Double hook retractors (to expose the glenoid cavity)
4. Fukuda retractors: two small and one large (to retract the humeral head without damaging it)
5. Electric drill and thread separator
6. Drills tips (a 2 mm and a 3.2 mm)
7. Richardson retractors (to retract muscle tissue and, in particular, the conjoint tendon toward the brachial plexus and deltoid)
8. Steinmann pins (to use as a joystick in case of a difficult reduction of multiple fragments)
9. Museaux clamps to clasp the humeral head in case it needs to be removed (especially if the dislocated head is in the axillary cavity)

Specific instruments will be then added to this list based on the surgeon's chosen procedure, which must obviously be known in detail. Before the operation, the first surgeon should also make sure that the implants are also present.

The surgeon should also have nonabsorbable braided surgical threads for osteosutures (e.g., Flexidene dec 5, B. Braun Milano Via Vincenzo da Seregno, 14-20161 Milano - Italia), which can be useful in the fixation of plate and screws to reinsert the tendons in the rotator cuff, or for prosthetic replacements to fixate the tuberosities.

Even if the surgery planned does not involve pinning, we still suggest keeping in the operating room some Steinmann pins: they can be useful to perform a temporary fracture fixation or to mobilize the fragments like with a joystick.

There should also be a sterile cover for the image intensifier to carry out monitoring procedures in complete safety.

3.4 Reviewing the Script

It is of paramount importance that the surgery be preceded by a series of procedures aimed at reducing to a minimum the risk of errors. It is a known fact that about half of all surgical complications are avoidable [22, 23]. It is estimated that, in the United States, surgery is performed on the wrong patient or on the wrong surgical site in one every 50,000–100,000 cases, amounting to 1,500–2,500 cases a year [24, 25]. Wrong-site surgery mistakes are typical errors for orthopedic surgeons: in a study published in 1998, Cowell underlines how 68 % of compensation claims made by patients after an orthopedic procedure are related to this type of mistake [26]. Wrong-site surgery has been classified as a "never event" by the NHS's National Patient Safety Agency [27]. The American Academy of Orthopedic Surgeons has launched the "Sign Your Site" campaign [28], and the WHO has issued the guidelines "Ten essential objectives for safe surgery" [29]: the first of these objectives states that "the team will operate on the correct patient at the correct site." The suggested protocol envisages three steps:

- *Verification*: this step involves verifying that the patient, the surgical site, and type of procedure are all correct, as well as checking whether the patient has any allergies to drugs or metals. It is important that this step be carried out when the patient's procedure is scheduled, at the time of admission or entry to the operating theater, every time the responsibility for the care of the patient is transferred from one team to another, and from the preoperative area to the surgical room.
- *Marking*: the site or sites to be operated must be marked; it is important not to mark nonoperative sites and to avoid using ambiguous markings: the National Patient Safety Agency and the Royal College of Surgeons of England recommend against using crosses (which could be used to denote a site that should not be operated on), opting instead for drawing arrows [30]. The markings need to be made by one of the surgeons, preferably when the patient is awake.
- *Time out*: a brief pause just before the beginning of the actual surgery to confirm the name of the patient, the type of procedure, and the surgical site. This moment is also useful to verify that the antibiotic prophylaxis has been administered, that the doors of the operating theater are closed, and that the X-ray images

have been displayed correctly in the surgery room and to provide an accurate surgery start time.

To achieve those ten objectives correctly, the WHO formulated a checklist divided in three phases: before the induction of anesthesia, before the skin incision, and before the patient leaves the operating room. The checklist used by the authors is based on this model, and it is illustrated in Table 3.1.

In 2009, *The New England Journal of Medicine* published a multicenter prospective

Table 3.1 Authors' preferred surgical safety checklist

Patient: **Born on:** **In:**	**Surgical procedure**	**Date --/--/20--**
	SURGICAL SAFETY CHECKLIST	
Sign in Before induction of anesthesia	**Time out** Before skin incision	**Sign out** Before the patient leaves the operating room
1. Has the patient confirmed: □ Wristband identification □ His/her identity □ Surgical site □ Surgical procedure □ Informed consents (anesthesia, surgery, etc.)	1. Have the surgeon, the anesthesiologist, and the nurses confirmed: □ Identity □ Surgical site □ Surgical procedure	1. Confirm that the instrument, sponge, and needle counts have been completed and is correct: □ Yes □ No
2. Is the surgical site marked? □ Yes □ No	2. Has the patient's surgical position been checked? □ Yes □ No	2. Confirm that surgical specimens have been identified and containers are labeled correctly (patient name and specimen description): □ Yes □ n/a
3. Difficult airway or aspiration risk? □ Yes □ No □ Anesthesia and equipment safety check completed	3. Bovie settings check? □ Yes □ n/a	3. Were there problems related to the use of any medical equipment? □ Yes □ No Which?
4. Patient's risk identification: □ Allergy risk checked?	4. Antibiotic prophylaxis administered within 60 min before incision? □ Yes □ n/a	4. Were there any intraoperative critical events? □ Yes □ No Have they been communicated to the ward? □ Yes □ No
5. Patient monitoring □ Yes □ No	5. Has the diagnostic imaging been displayed and viewed? □ Yes □ n/a	5. Is postoperative thromboembolism prophylaxis required? □ Yes □ No
6. Risk of blood loss >500 ml (700 ml/kg in children)? □ Yes □ No		6. Is postoperative analgesia required? □ Yes □ No
7. TS opening procedure? □ Yes □ No Blood □ Available □ Not requested		
8. Is the necessary equipment present? Has it been checked? □ Yes □ No		

study based on the 2008 WHO guidelines, which took in consideration all types of surgical procedures with the exception of heart surgeries. It assessed the impact of introducing a preoperative checklist by comparing two groups of patients (3,733 vs 3,955): after implementing this protocol, the mortality rate decreased from 1.5 to 0.8 % ($p=0.003$) and the complications from 11 to 7 % ($p<0.001$) [31]. It is therefore fundamental for every surgical team to have its checklist to ensure that they all follow the same steps [32].

References

1. Blonna D, Barbasetti N, Banche G, Cuffini AM, Bellato E, Massè A, Marenco S, Battiston B, Castoldi F (2014) Incidence and risk factors for acute infection after proximal humeral fractures: a multicenter study. J Shoulder Elbow Surg 23(4):528–35
2. Yamamoto T, Tamai K, Akutsu M, Tomizawa K, Sukegawa T, Nohara Y (2013) Pulmonary embolism after arthroscopic rotator cuff repair: a case report. Case Rep Orthop 2013:801752
3. Edgar R, Nagda S, Huffman R, Namdari S (2012) Pulmonary embolism after shoulder arthroscopy. Orthopedics 35:e1673–e1676
4. Garofalo R, Notarnicola A, Moretti L, Moretti B, Marini S, Castagna A (2010) Deep vein thromboembolism after arthroscopy of the shoulder: two case reports and a review of the literature. BMC Musculoskelet Disord 11:65
5. Edelson G, Kelly I, Vigder F, Reis ND (2004) A three-dimensional classification for fractures of the proximal humerus. J Bone Joint Surg Br 86:413–425
6. Hertel R (2005) Fractures of the proximal humerus in osteoporotic bone. Osteoporos Int 16(Suppl 2): S65–S72
7. Magovern B, Ramsey ML (2008) Percutaneous fixation of proximal humerus fractures. Orthop Clin North Am 39:405–416, v
8. Porcellini G, Campi F, Paladini P, Rossi P, Lollino N (2008) Informed consent in shoulder surgery. Chir Organi Mov 91:103–107
9. Lee SU, Jeong C, Park IJ (2012) Arthroscopic fixation of displaced greater tuberosity fracture of the proximal humerus. Knee Surg Sports Traumatol Arthrosc 20:378–380
10. Ji JH, Moon CY, Kim YY, Shafi M (2009) Arthroscopic fixation for a malunited greater tuberosity fracture using the suture-bridge technique: technical report and literature review. Knee Surg Sports Traumatol Arthrosc 17:1473–1476
11. Wang YP, Zhao JZ, Huangfu XQ et al (2012) Arthroscopic reduction and fixation for isolated greater tuberosity fractures. Chin Med J (Engl) 125:1272–1275
12. Gartsman GM, Taverna E, Hammerman SM (1999) Arthroscopic treatment of acute traumatic anterior glenohumeral dislocation and greater tuberosity fracture. Arthroscopy 15:648–650
13. Soete PJ, Clayson PE, Costenoble VH (1999) Transitory percutaneous pinning in fractures of the proximal humerus. J Shoulder Elbow Surg 8: 569–573
14. Fenichel I, Oran A, Burstein G, Perry Pritsch M (2006) Percutaneous pinning using threaded pins as a treatment option for unstable two- and three-part fractures of the proximal humerus: a retrospective study. Int Orthop 30:153–157
15. Seyhan M, Kocaoglu B, Nalbantoglu U, Aydin N, Guven O (2012) Technique of Kirschner wire reduction and fixation of displaced two-part valgus angulated proximal humerus fractures at the surgical neck. J Orthop Trauma 26:e46–e50
16. Resch H, Hübner C, Schwaiger R (2001) Minimally invasive reduction and osteosynthesis of articular fractures of the humeral head. Injury 32(Suppl 1):SA25–SA32
17. Yu Z, Zheng L, Wang Y, Zhang Y, Zhang X, Ma B (2010) Functional and radiological evaluations of unstable displaced proximal humeral fractures treated with closed reduction and percutaneous pinning fixation. Eur Surg Res 45:138–145
18. Williams GR, Wong KL (2000) Two-part and three-part fractures: open reduction and internal fixation versus closed reduction and percutaneous pinning. Orthop Clin North Am 31:1–21
19. Resch H, Povacz P, Fröhlich R, Wambacher M (1997) Percutaneous fixation of three- and four-part fractures of the proximal humerus. J Bone Joint Surg Br 79:295–300
20. Carbone S, Tangari M, Gumina S, Postacchini R, Campi A, Postacchini F (2012) Percutaneous pinning of three- or four-part fractures of the proximal humerus in elderly patients in poor general condition: MIROS® versus traditional pinning. Int Orthop 36:1267–1273
21. Kamineni S, Ankem H, Sanghavi S (2004) Anatomical considerations for percutaneous proximal humeral fracture fixation. Injury 35:1133–1136
22. Gawande AA, Thomas EJ, Zinner MJ, Brennan TA (1999) The incidence and nature of surgical adverse events in Colorado and Utah in 1992. Surgery 126: 66–75
23. Kable AK, Gibberd RW, Spigelman AD (2002) Adverse events in surgical patients in Australia. Int J Qual Health Care 14:269–276
24. Kwaan MR, Studdert DM, Zinner MJ, Gawande AA (2006) Incidence, patterns, and prevention of wrong-site surgery. Arch Surg 141:353–357; discussion 357–358
25. Seiden SC, Barach P (2006) Wrong-side/wrong-site, wrong-procedure, and wrong-patient adverse events: are they preventable? Arch Surg 141:931–939

26. Cowell HR (1998) Wrong-site surgery. J Bone Joint Surg Am 80:463
27. NHS National Patient Safety Agency (2011) Never events: wrong site surgery. http://www.nrls.npsa.nhs.uk/resources/collections/never-events/. Accessed 8 Jan 2013
28. American College of Surgeons (2002) Statement on ensuring correct patient, correct site, and correct procedure surgery. Bull Am Coll Surg 87:12
29. World Health Organization (2009) WHO guidelines for safe surgery. Safe surgery saves lives. World Health Organization, Geneva
30. National Patient Safety Agency and Royal College of Surgeons of England (2005) Patient briefing-correct site surgery. http://www.rcseng.ac.uk/publications/docs/patient_briefing.html/?searchterm=patient%20safety. Accessed 25 Jan 2008
31. Haynes AB, Weiser TG, Berry WR et al (2009) A surgical safety checklist to reduce morbidity and mortality in a global population. N Engl J Med 360: 491–499
32. Michaels RK, Makary MA, Dahab Y et al (2007) Achieving the National Quality Forum's "Never Events": prevention of wrong site, wrong procedure, and wrong patient operations. Ann Surg 245: 526–532

4 Closed Reduction Principles

Marco Assom and Enrico Bellato

Closed reduction of proximal humeral fractures is characterized by obvious advantages. Basically, it prevents damage to the soft tissues, and, as a consequence, the blood supply of the humeral head is usually preserved [1–5].

4.1 Anatomic Considerations

The proximal humerus can be divided into four main anatomic and functional segments, as described by Codman [6] and Neer [7]: the head, the greater tuberosity, the lesser tuberosity, and the diaphysis. Following a trauma, the various bone fragments variably displace according to the different traction forces and to the type of fracture. A deep knowledge of fracture pathology and of bone fragment behavior is mandatory when performing a correct closed reduction maneuver.

We can take a four-part fracture as an example: the diaphysis is typically medialized and internally rotated by the pectoralis major tendon; the greater tuberosity is posteriorly and superiorly displaced by the supraspinatus, infraspinatus, and teres minor tendons; the lesser tuberosity is medially dislocated by the subscapularis tendon. Then the humeral head is free and variably dislocates according to the leftover connections with other fragments or with the articular capsule. On the other hand, in the case of a three-part fracture involving the greater tuberosity, the head is medially rotated by the subscapularis tendon, while a three-part fracture involving the lesser tuberosity is characterized by a medial dislocation of the lesser tuberosity and an external rotation of the head [8, 9]. Figure 4.1 shows what happens in case of a two-part fracture.

However, it has been demonstrated that this description does not fully correspond to the real fracture morphology. The greater tuberosity is typically posteriorly and laterally dislocated, not superiorly. This can be explained by the work carried out by Mochizuki, who included 113 shoulders in his cadaver study; he demonstrated that the supraspinatus always inserted into the anteriormost area of the highest impression on the greater tuberosity, while the infraspinatus extended to the anterolateral area of the highest impression of the greater tuberosity [10].

Before performing surgery it is mandatory to study and thoroughly understand the pattern of fracture, but sometimes this cannot be achieved even with the use of imaging. Traditional X-ray imaging is almost always insufficient, even when particular tricks are employed [11, 12]. The CT scan is very helpful [13], and also 3D imaging

M. Assom
Department of Orthopaedics and Traumatology, University of Turin Medical School, Mauriziano-Umberto I Hospital, Largo Turati 62, Turin 10128, Italy
e-mail: dassom@libero.it

E. Bellato (✉)
Department of Orthopaedics and Traumatology, University of Turin Medical School, CTO-Maria Adelaide Hospital, Via Zuretti 29, Turin 10126, Italy
e-mail: bellatoenrico@gmail.com

F. Castoldi et al. (eds.), *Simple and Complex Fractures of the Humerus*, DOI 10.1007/978-88-470-5307-6_4, © Springer-Verlag Italia 2015

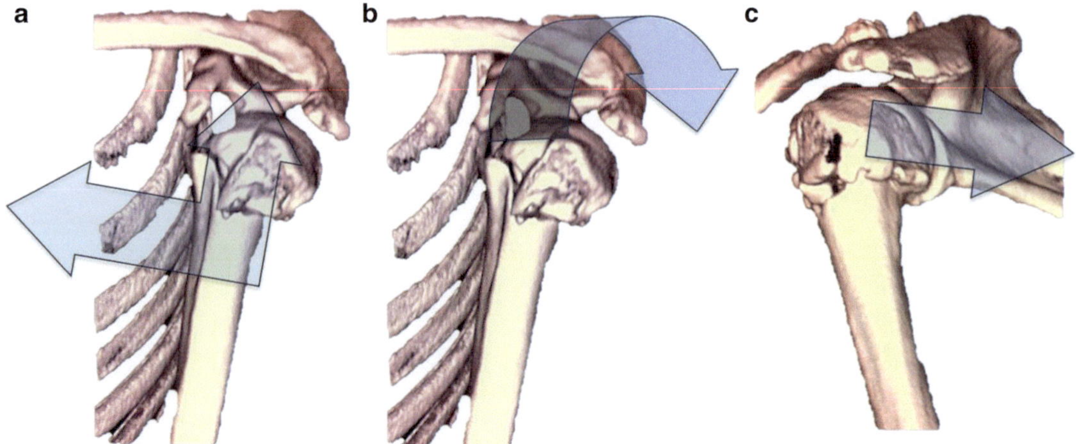

Fig. 4.1 A two-part fracture pattern. The fragments are dislocated by the pectoralis major and deltoid muscle (**a**, anterolateral view), by the supraspinatus and subscapularis tendon (**b**, anterolateral view), and by the infraspinatus tendon (**c**, posterior view)

reconstruction can greatly improve the quality of preoperative planning [14]. However, the correct analysis of the fracture is not easy, and even expert surgeons can remain at variance at the end of the preoperative phase. Nevertheless, we believe it is crucial to always evaluate the fracture with a standard X-ray view, a transthoracic lateral view, an axillary view and, where possible, a CT scan.

4.2 Which Type of Fracture?

Closed reduction procedure is mainly indicated in the case of two-segment fractures with dislocation or distal translation of the diaphysis and with varus impacted humeral fractures [15–18]. Good results can be achieved even in the event of associated greater tuberosity fracture.

4.3 Closed Reduction Technique

Proper positioning of the patient is vital. Several authors describe the lateral [19], the beach-chair [20–24], and the supine [15, 17, 25, 26] positions. The image intensifier positioning is also very important because it must provide good X-ray views without hindering the surgeons' work: it can be placed behind the patient's head [22, 23, 27, 28], on the side being operated on [29], or contralateral to the fracture. The surgical site must be prepared with attention to common landmarks such as the acromion, the coracoid, and the acromioclavicular joint which need to be easily palpable. The patient must be perfectly stable on the operating table, and the head should be secured with a proper head positioner.

Various authors describe the closed reduction maneuver in different ways. Several surgeons usually refer to the techniques previously described by Jaberg [15], who suggests carrying out the procedure with the shoulder abducted to 70–80°; then progressive longitudinal traction is performed to position the diaphysis slightly lateral to the humeral head; downward pressure against the anterior aspect of the arm completes the maneuver.

Some authors use devices to make the reduction easier. Calvo et al. [17], in medially translated fractures, used a post connected to the surgical table as a fulcrum in the medial side of the fracture while the arm was in adduction to help the reduction of the displaced humeral shaft. Williams and Wong [29] suggests the association of flexion, adduction, and slight internal rotation to relax the pectoralis major tendon; then a longitudinal traction of the arm is applied along with a posteriorly directed force. Seyhan et al. [24] believes that traction of the adducted arm is enough. Herscovici et al. [30] recommends that the forearm be kept supinated and the elbow extended while performing the longitudinal traction; a 45° abduction completes the maneuver. Other authors describe different maneuvers for each type of fracture. Magovern and Ramsey [16] differentiates between five possible situations:

- Two-part surgical neck fractures: the humeral head lies in a neutral position or is slightly varus dislocated because cuff tendons are intact; the shaft is medially and anteriorly dislocated and internally rotated because of the action of the pectoralis major tendon, while the humeral head is more retroverted than it is normally. Flexion together with adduction allows the surgeon to deal with the force of the pectoralis major tendon; traction and a posteriorly directed force applied to the arm complete the reduction maneuver.
- Two-part greater and lesser tuberosity fractures: a tuberosity percutaneous pin inserted just before starting the maneuver is needed (the greater tuberosity is typically more involved than the lesser, which is difficult and dangerous to fix with a pin); the following arm rotation helps to fully reduce the fracture.
- Three-part greater tuberosity fractures: the diaphysis is dislocated as mentioned above, so the maneuver implies flexion, adduction, and internal rotation followed by traction and a posteriorly directed force applied to the arm; once the surgical neck fracture has been fixated, the arm is externally rotated to achieve greater tuberosity reduction.
- Three-part lesser tuberosity fractures: the humeral head is abducted and externally rotated; the surgical neck fracture is reduced thanks to flexion and external rotation; external rotation and abduction follow traction and the posteriorly directed force applied to the arm.
- Four-part valgus impacted fractures: they need pins or blunt elevators inserted through mini-incisions.

Other authors suggest that mini-incisions be performed (also called "reduction portals") so that instruments which can help the surgeon may be inserted, in particular in cases of complex fractures [31].

No complications are reported in the literature after a closed reduction maneuver.

4.3.1 Authors' Preferred Technique

Whenever we have planned a closed reduction, we prefer the supine position. The image intensifier is contralateral to the fracture. As a consequence we can obtain both a good AP view and a good axial view without rotating the arm; moreover the C-arm does not get in the surgical team's way and the surgeons have enough room to perform the reduction maneuver and the following fixation. A proper shoulder operating table is very useful in obtaining good intraoperative X-rays (Fig. 4.2).

A two-part varus impacted fracture (Fig. 4.3) has been taken as an example. The closed reduction procedure is clearly illustrated step-by-step in the following sequence of photographs (Fig. 4.4):

A: The "resting" start position consists in the 30° abducted arm with 10–15° of external rotation.

B: When the arm is at 90° of abduction, the humeral head progressively becomes externally rotated, but the fracture displacement does not change.

C: By increasing arm abduction to more than 90°, the surgeon blocks the humeral head under the acromion, which acts as a fulcrum: so the shaft can be abducted even more than 120° and become separated from the humeral head.

D: The posteriorly directed force applied to the arm reduces the diaphysis under the humeral head.

E: Once back at the starting position, we can check the fracture reduction achieved.

Sometimes the closed reduction maneuver needs some small adjustments or improvements which can usually be obtained by repeating the procedure or by insisting on the posteriorly directed force applied to the arm.

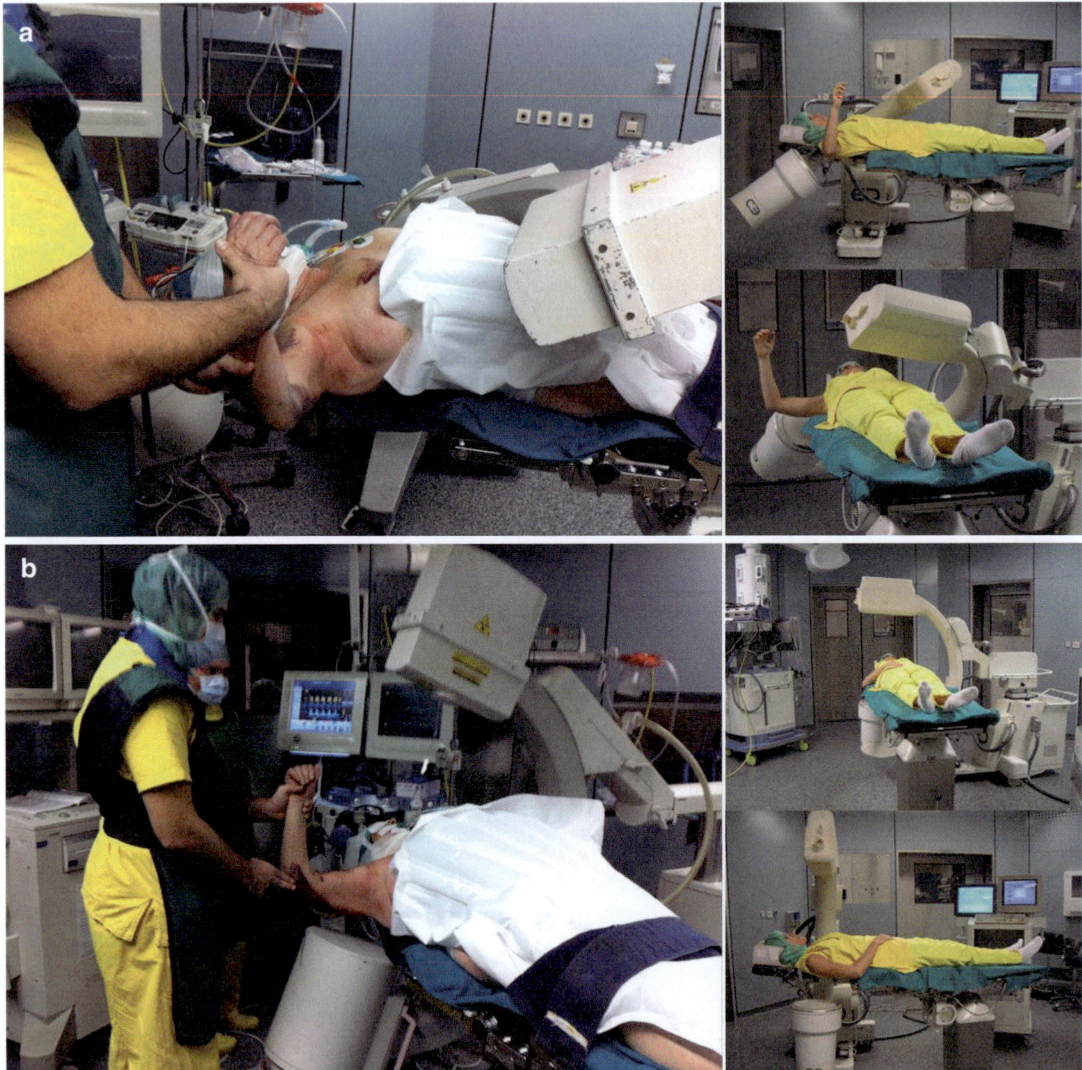

Fig. 4.2 (**a**) The C-arm position to achieve the AP view. (**b**) The C-arm position to achieve the axial view

Longitudinal traction of the arm is not necessary: the deltoid muscle does not interfere during the reduction, and, moreover, its action is reduced by abduction. Fragment reduction is usually associated with quite a loud sound, and the force needed for the maneuver is considerable.

Once the reduction has been obtained, the arm must be kept firmly abducted at 20–30° and slightly internally rotated, while the arm must be parallel to the floor: slight position modifications may improve or worsen alignment of the fracture fragments. The bicipital groove can be seen during fluoroscopic checks and can give important information about the correct humeral rotation: if it is too lateral, the arm needs to be slightly externally rotated, while a medial position can suggest that the surgeon internally rotate the arm. The diaphysis can be rarely displaced posteriorly to the humeral head. So the surgeon must carefully examine the CT scan: in this case the humeral diaphysis must be pushed anteriorly to obtain fracture reduction.

Once the reduction is deemed to be satisfactory, the surgeon can complete surgery with mini-invasive percutaneous fixation. Whenever the reduction cannot be achieved, we prefer to move the patient to a beach-chair position and perform an open reduction.

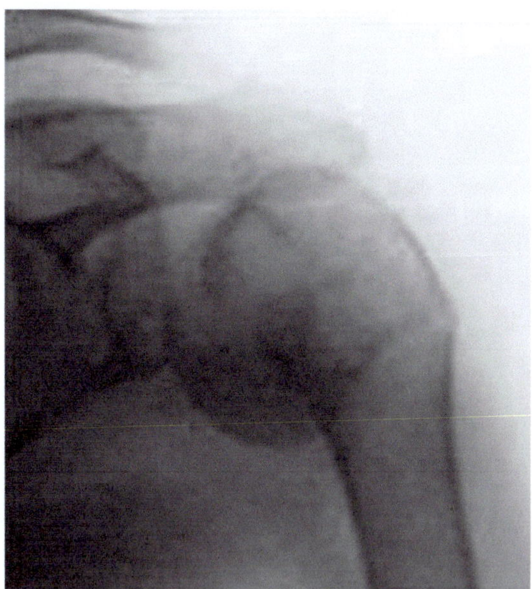

Fig. 4.3 A two-part varus impacted fracture

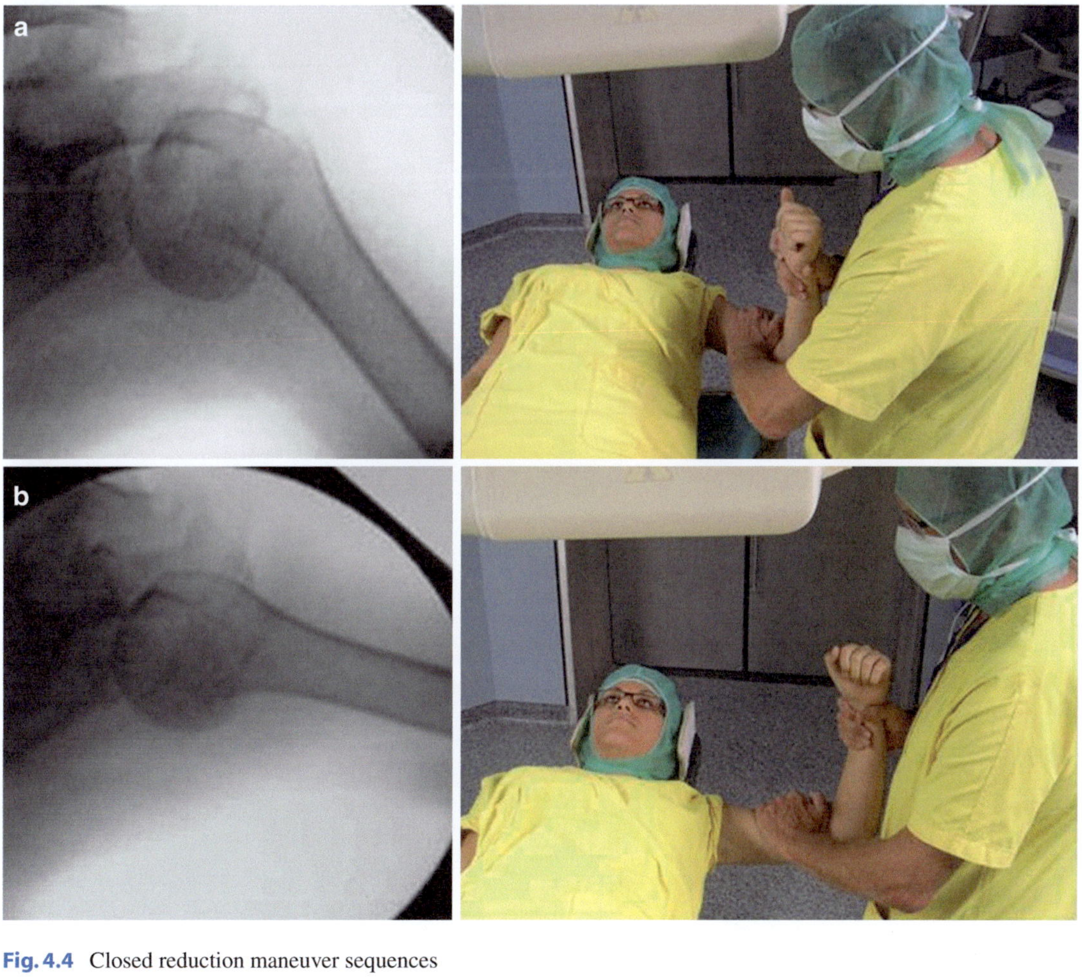

a

b

Fig. 4.4 Closed reduction maneuver sequences

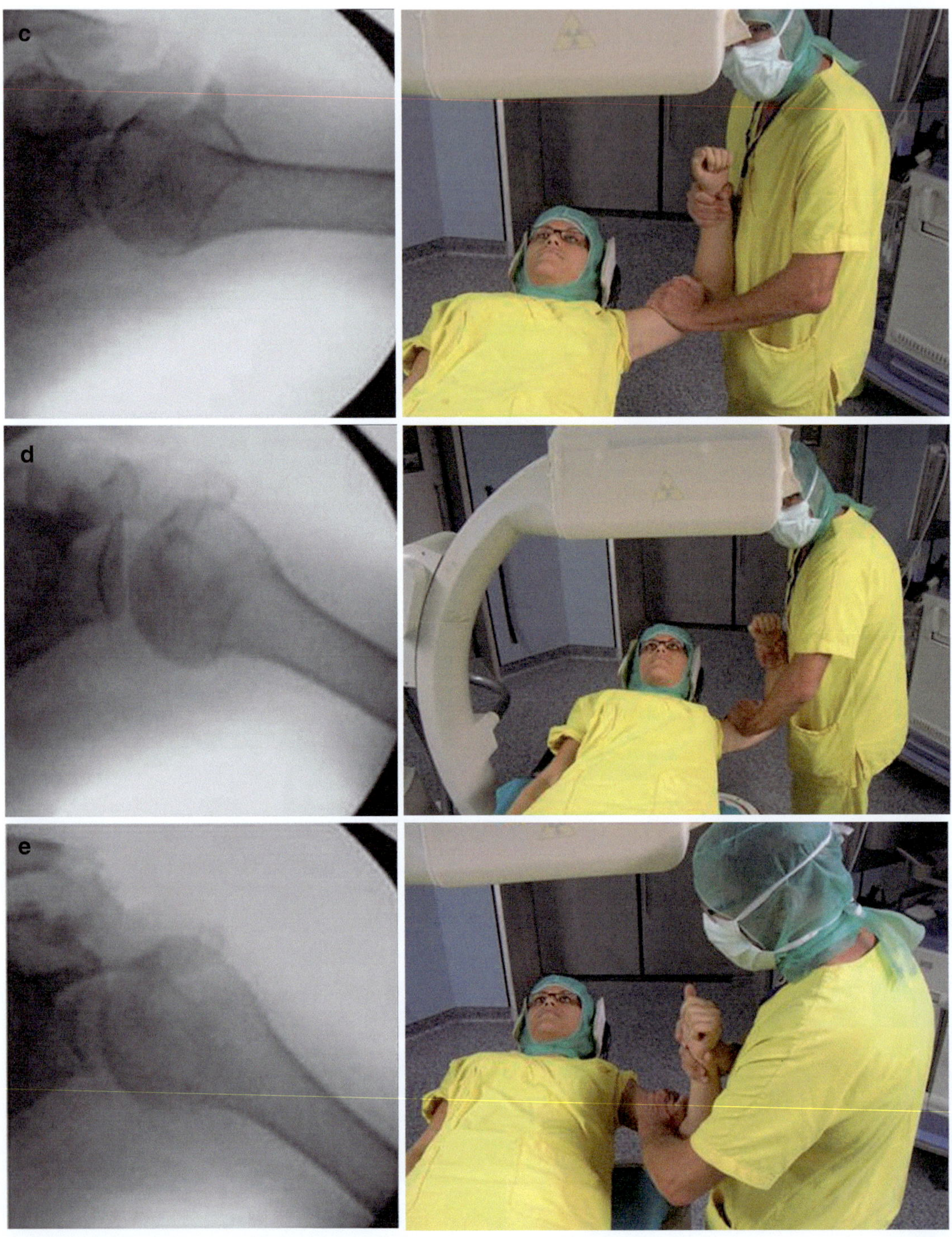

Fig. 4.4 (continued)

References

1. Hagg O, Lundberg B (1984) Aspects of prognostic factors in comminuted and dislocated proximal humerus fractures. In: Bateman JE, Welsh PR (eds) Surgery of the shoulder. BC Decker, Philadelphia
2. Hawkins RJ, Kiefer GN (1987) Internal fixation techniques for proximal humeral fractures. Clin Orthop Relat Res 223:77–85
3. Neer CS II (1984) Fractures about the shoulder. In: Rockwood CA Jr, Green DP (eds) Fractures in adults, vol I, 2nd edn. JB Lippincott, Philadelphia
4. Rose SH, Melton LJ, Morrey BF, Ilstrup DM, Riggs BL (1982) Epidemiologic features of humeral fractures. Clin Orthop Relat Res 168:24–30
5. Bohler J (1962) Percutane osteosynthese mit dem rontgenbildverstarker. Wien Klin Wochenschr 74:485–487
6. Codman EA (1934) Rupture of the supraspinatus tendon and other lesions in or about the subacromial bursa. In: The shoulder. Thomas Todd, Boston
7. Neer CS (1970) Displaced proximal humeral fractures. I. Classification and evaluation. J Bone Joint Surg Am 52:1077–1089
8. Neer CS (2002) Four-segment classification of proximal humeral fractures: purpose and reliable use. J Shoulder Elbow Surg 11:389–400
9. Sanchez-Sotelo J (2006) Proximal humerus fractures. Clin Anat 19:588–598
10. Mochizuki T, Sugaya H, Uomizu M et al (2008) Humeral insertion of the supraspinatus and infraspinatus. New anatomical findings regarding the footprint of the rotator cuff. J Bone Joint Surg Am 90:962–969
11. Bloom MH, Obata WG (1967) Diagnosis of posterior dislocation of the shoulder with use of Velpeau axillary and angle-up roentgenographic views. J Bone Joint Surg Am 49:943–949
12. Warner JJP (1998) Instability of the shoulder. Clinical diagnosis and imaging. Syllabus Course 425. American Academy of Orthopaedic Surgeons and American Shoulder and Elbow Surgeons, Rosemont, p 187–192
13. Kilcoyne RF, Shuman WP, Matsen FA, Morris M, Rockwood CA (1990) The Neer classification of displaced proximal humeral fractures: spectrum of findings on plain radiographs and CT scans. AJR Am J Roentgenol 154:1029–1033
14. Edelson G, Kelly I, Vigder F, Reis ND (2004) A three-dimensional classification for fractures of the proximal humerus. J Bone Joint Surg Br 86:413–425
15. Jaberg H, Warner JJ, Jakob RP (1992) Percutaneous stabilization of unstable fractures of the humerus. J Bone Joint Surg Am 74:508–515
16. Magovern B, Ramsey ML (2008) Percutaneous fixation of proximal humerus fractures. Orthop Clin North Am 39:405–416
17. Calvo E, de Miguel I, de la Cruz JJ, López-Martín N (2007) Percutaneous fixation of displaced proximal humeral fractures: indications based on the correlation between clinical and radiographic results. J Shoulder Elbow Surg 16:774–781
18. Clifford PC (1980) Fractures of the neck of the humerus: a review of the late results. Injury 12: 91–95
19. Kocialkowski A, Wallace WA (1990) Closed percutaneous K-wire stabilization for displaced fractures of the surgical neck of the humerus. Injury 21: 209–212
20. Harrison AK, Gruson KI, Zmistowski B et al (2012) Intermediate outcomes following percutaneous fixation of proximal humeral fractures. J Bone Joint Surg Am 94:1223–1228
21. Zhang J, Ebraheim N, Lause GE (2012) Surgical treatment of proximal humeral fracture with external fixator. J Shoulder Elbow Surg 21:882–886
22. Soete PJ, Clayson PE, Costenoble VH (1999) Transitory percutaneous pinning in fractures of the proximal humerus. J Shoulder Elbow Surg 8:569–573
23. Fenichel I, Oran A, Burstein G, Perry Pritsch M (2006) Percutaneous pinning using threaded pins as a treatment option for unstable two- and three-part fractures of the proximal humerus: a retrospective study. Int Orthop 30:153–157
24. Seyhan M, Kocaoglu B, Nalbantoglu U, Aydin N, Guven O (2012) Technique of Kirschner wire reduction and fixation of displaced two-part valgus angulated proximal humerus fractures at the surgical neck. J Orthop Trauma 26:46–50
25. Resch H, Povacz P, Fröhlich R, Wambacher M (1997) Percutaneous fixation of three- and four-part fractures of the proximal humerus. J Bone Joint Surg Br 79:295–300
26. Ebraheim NA, Patil V, Husain A (2007) Mini-external fixation of two- and three-part proximal humerus fractures. Acta Orthop Belg 73:437–442
27. Resch H, Hübner C, Schwaiger R (2001) Minimally invasive reduction and osteosynthesis of articular fractures of the humeral head. Injury 32(Suppl 1):SA25–SA32
28. Yu Z, Zheng L, Wang Y, Zhang Y, Zhang X, Ma B (2010) Functional and radiological evaluations of unstable displaced proximal humeral fractures treated with closed reduction and percutaneous pinning fixation. Eur Surg Res 45:138–145
29. Williams GR, Wong KL (2000) Two-part and three-part fractures: open reduction and internal fixation versus closed reduction and percutaneous pinning. Orthop Clin North Am 31:1–21
30. Herscovici D, Saunders DT, Johnson MP, Sanders R, DiPasquale T (2000) Percutaneous fixation of proximal humeral fractures. Clin Orthop Relat Res 375:97–104
31. Keener JD, Parsons BO, Flatow EL, Rogers K, Williams GR, Galatz LM (2007) Outcomes after percutaneous reduction and fixation of proximal humeral fractures. J Shoulder Elbow Surg 16:330–338

5 Proximal Humerus: Surgical Approaches

Giandomenico Logroscino, Ernesto Pagano, Vincenzo Campana, and Giuseppe Milano

5.1 Introduction

In 1961, De Palma defined the main surgical approaches to the shoulder. He described the scapulohumeral joint in detail and developed the current guidelines [1, 2].

The deltopectoral approach is the most popular route for large shoulder exposure. However, some alternative approaches have been introduced over time by several authors with the aim to minimize the dissection of soft tissues, to reduce the risk of neurovascular lesions, and also to adequately expose fractures and to provide a stable fixation.

Levy et al. [3] described a combined approach to the shoulder with an easy access to the anterior, the lateral, and the posterior shoulder. This approach is a combination of the deltopectoral and transdeltoid route, but with a single skin incision, thus avoiding muscle detachment and possible injuries to the deltoid muscle and to the axillary nerve.

Several modifications to the traditional approach by Judet [4] have been proposed to access the posterior scapula; these approaches are less invasive because the scapular muscles are only partially detached, but the quality of the exposure remains very high. Clinical experience has shown that these modified approaches can be used for most fractures of the body and of the neck of the scapula and of the glenoid [5].

Anatomic studies show that the blood supply to the humeral head is provided by the humeral anterior circumflex artery [6]; however, on the basis of the results of a new volumetric analysis performed by contrast MRI, the posterior circumflex artery of the humerus significantly contributes to the blood supply of the proximal humerus [7]. In this connection, the proximal part of the humerus can be accessed by means of lateral approaches through the raphe between the anterior and medial heads of the deltoid.

Whatever the approach to the humerus, it is fundamental to identify and protect the axillary nerve that runs on the deep surface of the deltoid in front of the humeral diaphysis at a certain distance from the lateral margin of the acromion [8]. In addition, a recent cadaver study [9] has indicated that the position of the nerve changes according to the abduction degree of the shoulder.

The literature describes several surgical approaches to the proximal humerus, as well as their variations. In order to simplify their description, they will be classified into four different types: anterior, lateral, posterior, and axillary approaches.

G. Logroscino • E. Pagano
V. Campana • G. Milano (✉)
Department of Orthopaedics, Catholic University, Largo A. Gemelli 8, Rome, RM 00168, Italy
e-mail: g.logroscino@fastwebnet.it; ern.pagano@libero.it; Dr.vincenzocampana@gmail.com; giuseppe.milano@rm.unicatt.it

F. Castoldi et al. (eds.), *Simple and Complex Fractures of the Humerus*,
DOI 10.1007/978-88-470-5307-6_5, © Springer-Verlag Italia 2015

5.2 Anterior Approaches

5.2.1 Deltopectoral Approach

5.2.1.1 Indications

This approach is used for any anterior procedure to the shoulder and the proximal humerus to address glenohumeral instability, to fix proximal humerus and anterior glenoid fractures, and to implant shoulder prostheses.

5.2.1.2 Technique

The patient is placed in a beach-chair position, with the head rotated in the opposite position with respect to the shoulder to be operated or in a neutral position. The upper limb is left free. The skin is incised 1 cm. below the middle third of the clavicle, passing above the coracoid up to the deltoid tuberosity. The deltopectoral sulcus is identified together with the cephalic vein. Once isolated, the latter can be retracted medially or laterally with the deltoid muscle. The clavipectoral fascia covering the biceps and the coracobrachialis muscles is identified and is then incised between the two heads of the biceps, by moving the short head medially and the long head laterally. It is necessary to isolate and protect the musculocutaneous nerve that penetrates the coracobrachialis muscle 6 cm distally from its origin. There are numerous anatomic variations to take into consideration, and the nerve can be divided into several branches. Traction of the coracobrachialis muscle has to be performed very carefully to avoid damage to the nerve. By externally rotating the arm, the subscapularis muscle is exposed. The anterior and posterior circumflex arteries of the humerus can be identified on the lower margin, where they are adjacent to the axillary nerve. The posterior circumflex artery runs with the axillary nerve in the quadrilateral space (the space bound by the teres minor and the teres major muscles, the long head of the triceps, and the humeral diaphysis) near the inferior margin of the glenohumeral capsule and firmly in contact with the humeral neck. The anterior circumflex artery crosses the humeral metaphysis and runs below the long head of the biceps. In general, it is accompanied by two veins, and the vascular complex is referred to as "three sisters." This is the origin of the arterial blood supply to the proximal humerus (arcuate arteries). If an intra-articular approach is required, after the maximum external rotation of the arm, the tendon of the subscapularis muscle is incised, 2 cm medially with respect to its insertion, so as to keep inside a sufficient amount of tissue for the suture; the tendon is cleaved from the anterior capsule only in its proximal three quarters in order to protect the axillary nerve (Fig. 5.1). Finally, a capsulotomy is performed longitudinally in order to expose the humeral head and the glenoid. In case of surgical procedures limited to the shoulder joint, the approach is still lateral and superior to the coracoid; in case of procedures on the brachial plexus or on the axillary artery, it is necessary to isolate and detach the pectoralis minor from the coracoid.

5.2.1.3 Limitations

In case of an intra-articular inspection, this approach requires the detachment of the subscapularis tendon. There are different detachment techniques (transosseous-lesser tuberosity, complete, L-shaped), but all of them carry the risk of inducing iatrogenic complications to the subscapularis muscle, such as re-rupture and fat degeneration, with the loss of strength in internal rotation and possible anterior instability [10].

5.2.1.4 Risks

Several neurovascular structures must be isolated and protected with this approach: the brachial plexus; the axillary artery, vein, and nerve; and the musculocutaneous nerve, as well as the anterior circumflex artery (in case of reduction and fixation of fractures).

Numerous anatomic studies on cadavers have tried to correctly define the safety margins of the deltopectoral structures [11]. Loomer and Graham [12] described the path of the axillary nerve, at about 3.5 mm inferiorly and laterally with respect to the myotendinous margin of the subscapular muscle and in contact with the inferior margin of the glenoid. Other studies have described the path of the axillary nerve, 3–8 mm from the inferior margin of the joint capsule [11, 13]. In a cadaver study, McFarland et al. [14] examined the relationships between the retractors

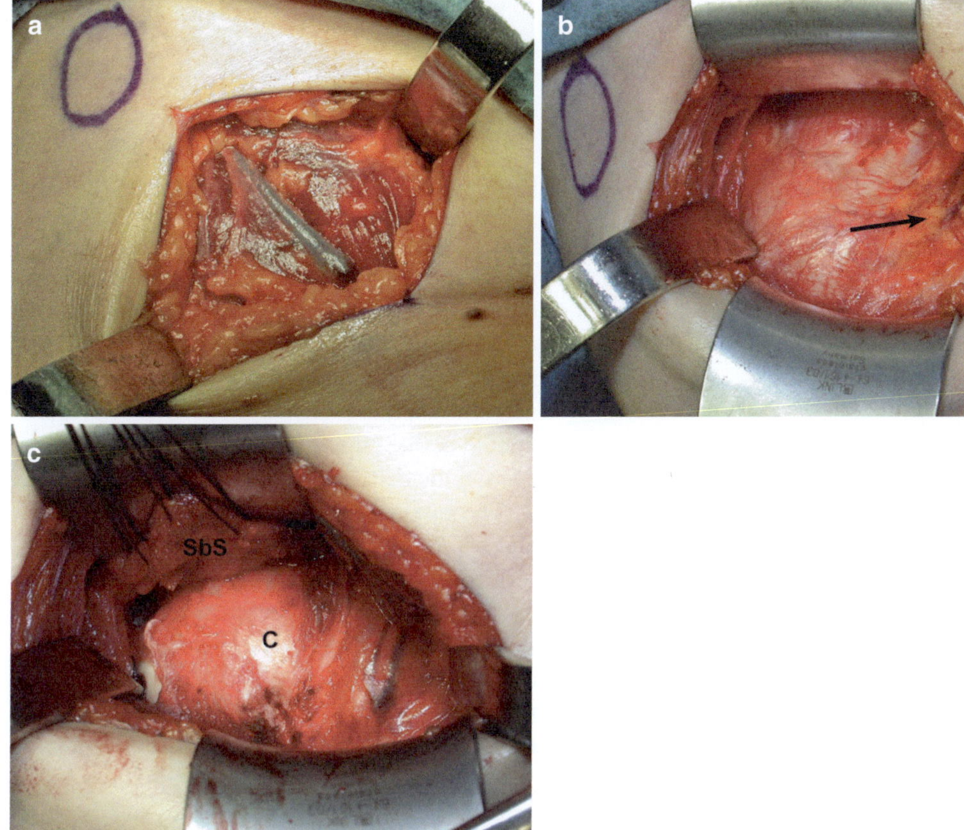

Fig. 5.1 Deltopectoral approach. (**a**) The deltopectoral sulcus is identified together with the cephalic vein. (**b**) The anterior circumflex artery crosses the humeral metaphysis and is accompanied by two veins. This vascular complex is referred to as "three sisters" (*arrow*). (**c**) Deltopectoral approach. The subscapularis muscle (*SbS*) is incised 2 cm medially with respect to its insertion, and the tendon is cleaved from the anterior capsule (*C*) only in its proximal three quarters in order to protect the axillary nerve

positioned during an anterior capsuloplasty and the adjacent nerve structures. In particular, this study showed that the brachial plexus is at about 2 cm distance from the glenohumeral joint and, in some cases, the variability amounted to 0.5 cm. The musculocutaneous nerve was found at about 1.5 cm from the articular rim. The posterior and medial cords were at about 1–2 cm from the articular rim. The minimum distance measured was about 5 mm for the axillary nerve, 7 mm for the posterior cord, and 9 mm from the medial one.

The deltopectoral approach requires the displacement or the ligation of the cephalic vein. Even though the ligation does not entail any major complications, it is better to preserve it. Generally, for practical purposes, it is better to retract it laterally together with the deltoid muscle since there are a higher number of collaterals laterally rather than medially [15]. However, the author's personal experience shows that medial retraction requires a longer preparation, but it does not overstretch the vein and so it is less traumatic.

Very often, this approach leaves an ugly scar because it does not follow the skin cleavage.

5.2.2 Anterior Extended Deltopectoral Approach

The deltopectoral approach can be extended distally along the arm down to the elbow. On the contrary, the proximal extension is infrequently used because it does not allow for an easy access to the subacromial space and to the rotator cuff

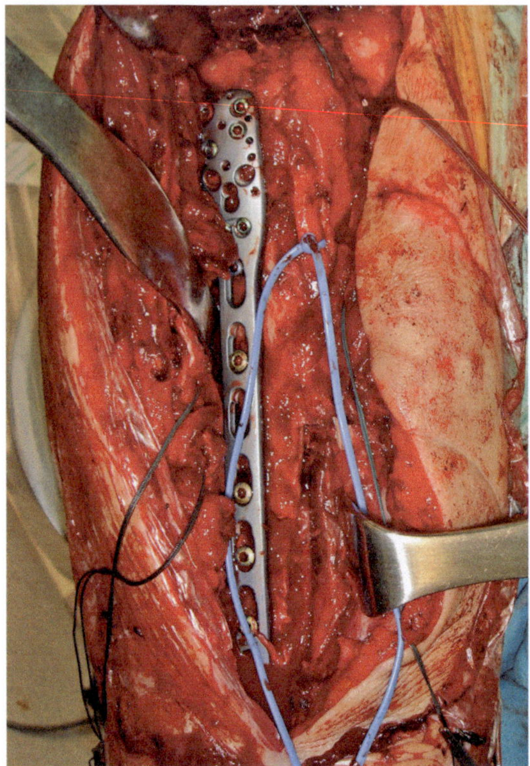

Fig. 5.2 The distal extension of the deltopectoral approach is used to treat complex fractures of the proximal humerus extending to the diaphysis. The route goes through the space between the deltoid and the biceps muscles proximally and through a split in the brachialis muscle distally

that are more easily reached with a transdeltoid or posterior approach.

The distal extension of the deltopectoral approach is performed through an anterolateral access to the humerus. The route goes through the space between the deltoid and the biceps muscles proximally and through a split in the brachialis muscle distally [16] (Fig. 5.2).

5.3 Variations to the Anterior Approach

5.3.1 Combined Anterior Approach

Several variations of the anterior approach have been described. Each of them provides a limited exposure of the shoulder joint. A combined anterior and posterior or anterior and lateral approach is required to treat complex injuries.

Sometimes, the deltopectoral approach does not allow for a complete exposure of the lateral and posterior parts of the proximal humerus and requires a partial detachment of the deltoid [17, 18]. This procedure can lead to a significant deterioration of the deltoid function, with a long and difficult postoperative rehabilitation.

The combined approach to the shoulder makes it possible to easily reach the anterior, lateral, and posterior regions of the shoulder, thus avoiding detachment of the deltoid muscle. This route results from the combination of an anterior deltopectoral approach and of a subcutaneous transdeltoid access. It uses a single skin incision thus sparing the deltoid [3].

The patient is placed in a beach-chair position, and a traditional deltopectoral approach is performed. If a lateral or posterior approach is necessary, the subcutaneous tissue is dissected laterally. Once the deltoid is exposed, it is incised along the acromion up to a maximum of 5 cm distally. If required, the deltoid can be dissected more anteriorly or posteriorly. Thanks to the rich vascularization of the skin on the shoulder and to its elasticity, both the intermuscular and the intramuscular approaches can be performed with a single skin incision.

During the procedure, it is possible to move from one approach to the other according to the need, without damaging the muscle insertions or neurovascular structures. This approach allows for the open reduction and the internal fixation of comminuted fractures of the humeral head with a good exposure of its lateral and posterior portion.

5.3.2 Anteromedial Approach

A skin incision is performed 1 cm laterally to the coracoid, and then it is extended to the clavicle and laterally along the anterior fibers of the deltoid [19] (Fig. 5.3). By carefully separating the subcutaneous layer, it is possible to identify the anterior acromion, the insertion of the deltoid on the lateral aspect of the clavicle, the anterior deltoid, and the deltopectoral interval. Gradually the deltoid is detached first from the lateral aspect of the clavicle, from the acromioclavicular (AC)

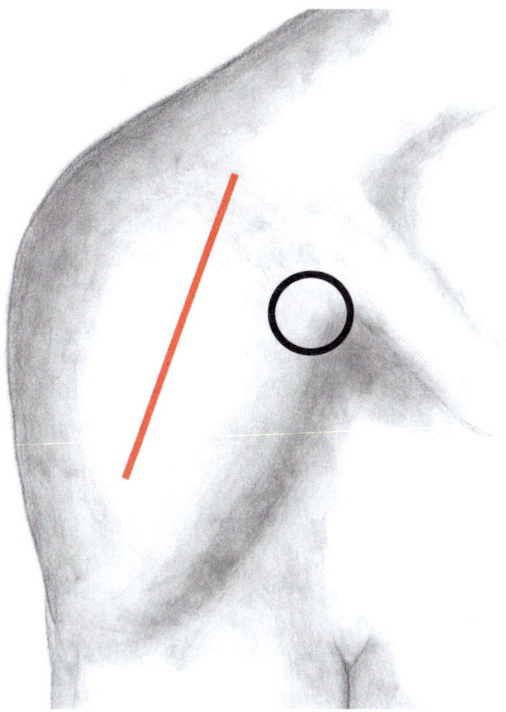

Fig. 5.3 Anteromedial approach. A skin incision (*red line*) is performed 1 cm laterally to the coracoid (*black circle*), and then it is extended to the clavicle and laterally along the anterior fibers of the deltoid

joint, trying to preserve the joint capsule and finally, from the anterior acromion, by incising the fascia and by lifting the muscle from the bone, thus preserving the coracoacromial ligament. The deltoid muscle is retracted laterally to expose the subacromial region. Once the procedure is over, the deltoid is reinserted with transosseous sutures to the acromion and to the clavicle and with simple sutures to the AC joint and to the fascia of the trapezius muscle.

This technique is safe and without complications [20] and is particularly indicated in the three following situations:

1. To implant a shoulder prosthesis and to repair a posterior rotator cuff tear with a single procedure
2. To protect the very fragile anterior deltoid that is not able to tolerate tractions or in a patient with severe osteopenia (e.g., in rheumatoid arthritis) so as to avoid iatrogenic fractures
3. In case of a shoulder arthroplasty revision surgery when the soft tissues are stiff and fragile

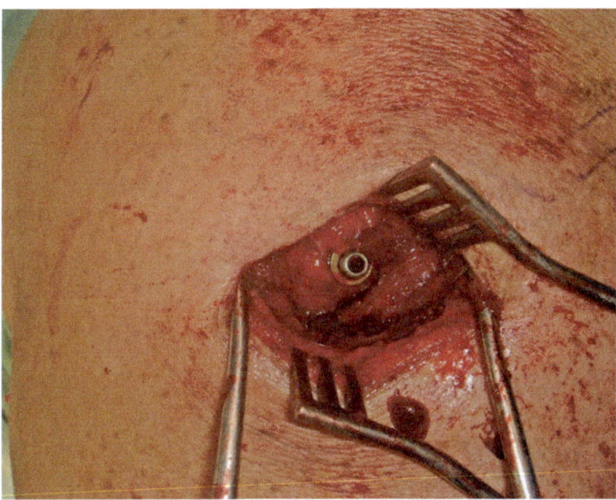

Fig. 5.4 The transdeltoid approach is used to treat the fractures of the greater tuberosity. A 5 cm longitudinal incision is made, starting 1 cm proximally to the lateral edge of the acromion. The subcutaneous tissue is incised together with the fascia above the deltoid, and its muscle fibers are split

5.4 Lateral Approaches

5.4.1 Transdeltoid or Lateral Approach

5.4.1.1 Indications

This approach is indicated to treat the fractures of the greater tuberosity and of the proximal humerus in general (Fig. 5.4). Moreover, it allows for the repair of the rotator cuff.

5.4.1.2 Technique

The patient is placed in a beach-chair position, with the arm on the edge of the Table. A 5 cm longitudinal incision is made, starting 1 cm proximally to the lateral edge of the acromion and with a distal extension.

The subcutaneous tissue is incised together with the fascia above the deltoid, and its muscle fibers are split. In order to protect the axillary nerve, an anchoring suture is applied on the inferior apex of the splitting so as to prevent the approach from extending distally. Once the subacromial bursa is removed, the rotator cuff is identified. By means of the subperiosteal detachment of the deltoid, both anteriorly and posteriorly, it is possible to obtain a large exposure. The repair of the deltoid is crucial for a good functional recovery. If necessary, it is possible to enlarge this approach with a proximal extension. The incision is prolonged superiorly and medially by passing over the acromion, then it is extended along the anterosuperior margin of the spine of the scapula for its two thirds laterally. The trapezius muscle along the spine of the scapula is detached and lifted. The supraspinatus muscle is exposed. The osteotomy of the acromion is performed in line with the skin incision. By retracting the stumps obtained, the supraspinatus muscle is completely exposed from its origin in the supraspinatus fossa up to its insertion on the greater tuberosity of the humerus [21]. If, on the one hand, this extended approach allows for a greater exposure with respect to the traditional transdeltoid route, on the other, it is more invasive, with a poor cosmetic result and an impact on the functional recovery and the risk of residual pain or poor strength.

5.4.1.3 Limitations

This approach allows for a good access to the greater tuberosity and to the supraspinatus tendon, while the exposure of the proximal humerus is limited.

5.4.1.4 Risks

The greatest risk of this approach is the excessive distal extension that can damage the axillary nerve if the incision is extended beyond 5 cm distally with respect to the acromion [22].

5.5 Variations to the Lateral Approach

5.5.1 Anterosuperior Approach

In1993, MacKenzie [23] described an anterosuperior approach that provides for a large and easy exposure of the glenoid and of the proximal humerus.

This approach is used to implant primary or inverse prostheses [24] and to address humeral head fractures.

The patient is placed in the same position as for the deltopectoral approach, but the elbow must be left without any support so as to allow the assistant to apply the force in the proximal direction. This is required to subluxate the humeral head. The surgeon moves laterally with respect to the shoulder, helped by two assistants on the two sides of the patient. The incision starts 1 cm medially to the anterior margin of the AC joint and continues along the anterior edge of the clavicle. The surgeon proceeds with the incision 5 mm. posteriorly to the anterior margin of the acromion and finally 4–5 cm distally with respect to the lateral margin of the acromion. The deltoid muscle is detached from the anterior margin of the acromion, and the splitting is prolonged distally for 5 cm. Then, the coracoacromial ligament is dissected.

Many authors use the anterosuperior approach to treat complex fractures of the proximal humerus in elderly patients [25–27]. In addition to the better exposure of the proximal humerus and of the glenoid, this approach makes it possible to detach and fix the greater tuberosity more easily with respect to the deltopectoral approach. Moreover, it is simple and preserves the subscapularis tendon with a low risk of postoperative anterior instability. However, the anterior deltoid may be weakened because of a mechanical injury or a lesion of the distal branches of the axillary nerve; moreover, the glenoid component of a prosthesis may be positioned incorrectly (too high or too low or too tilted superiorly).

5.5.2 Extended Anterolateral Approach

In 2004, Gardner et al. [28] described a lateral approach designed to treat complex fractures of the proximal humerus extending to the diaphysis. As shown by cadaver studies, the axillary nerve does not have any branches in the anterior portion of the deltoid muscle, before going through the fibrous raphe that separates the anterior head from the middle head of the muscle.

The technique envisages a conservative skin incision at the level of the anterolateral angle of

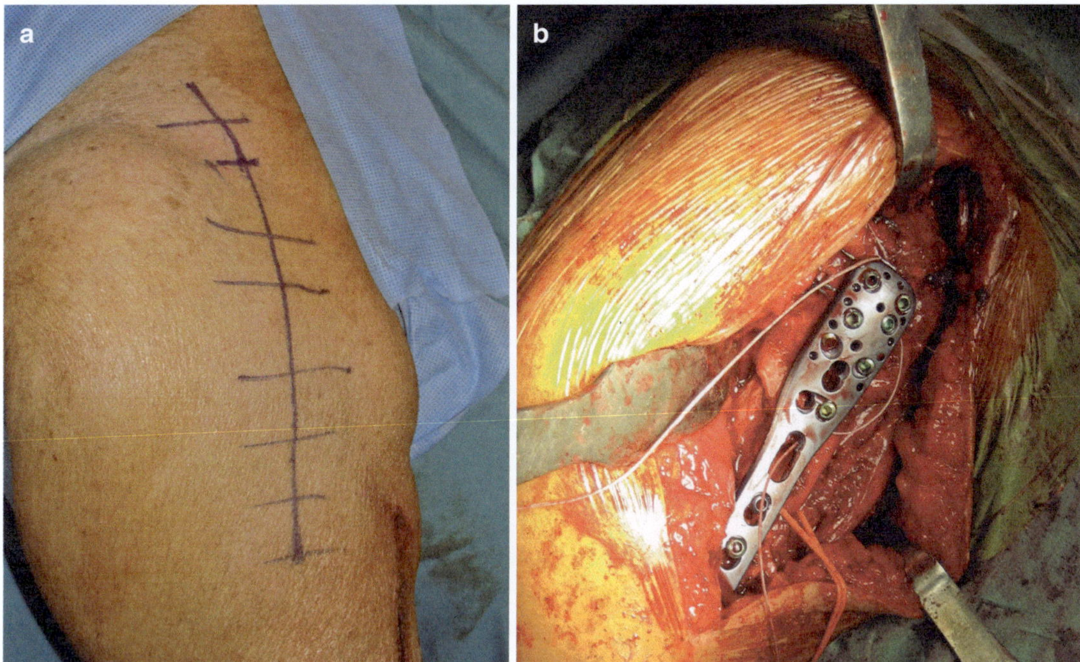

Fig. 5.5 Extended anterolateral approach. (**a**) Skin incision is performed at the level of the anterolateral angle of the acromion and is extended distally for about 5 cm. (**b**) The dissection can be extended distally up to the deltoid tuberosity in order to reduce and fix metaphyseal fractures of the humerus

the acromion, which is extended distally for about 5 cm. The fibrous raphe separating the anterior deltoid head from the medial one is identified and then incised for about 2 cm distally starting from the acromion. By palpating the deep surface of the deltoid, it is possible to identify the axillary nerve that feels like a "chord-like" structure. Then, the raphe is further dissected for about 6.5 cm from the acromion or for 3.5 cm from the greater tuberosity. The axillary nerve and the posterior circumflex vessels are isolated and protected. From here, the dissection can be extended distally up to the deltoid tuberosity without any risk in order to reduce and fix metaphyseal fractures of the humerus [28–30] (Fig. 5.5).

A very similar approach, with a different skin incision called "extended deltoid-splitting approach," has been recently proposed by Robinson [31, 32]. A suspender-like incision is performed, its apex centered over the tip of the acromion. This incision follows the tension lines of the relaxed skin around the shoulder [33] so as to obtain a good cosmetic result, as in the case of the traditional direct lateral approach; moreover, the surgical scar resulting from this route in women is easily hidden by the bra strap. The skin is incised and is detached en bloc with the subcutaneous tissue, and an elliptical flap is created and lifted in order to expose the superior part of the deltoid. A longitudinal split of this muscle is performed for about 3 cm at the origin of the anterior raphe. With the extension of the incision, the superior split of the deltoid muscle allows for a superior approach and so for the visualization of the whole anterolateral and posterolateral portion of the proximal humerus. By palpating the axillary nerve, it is possible to isolate and protect it with a portion of the deltoid muscle and to enlarge the split distally so as to expose the distal humerus.

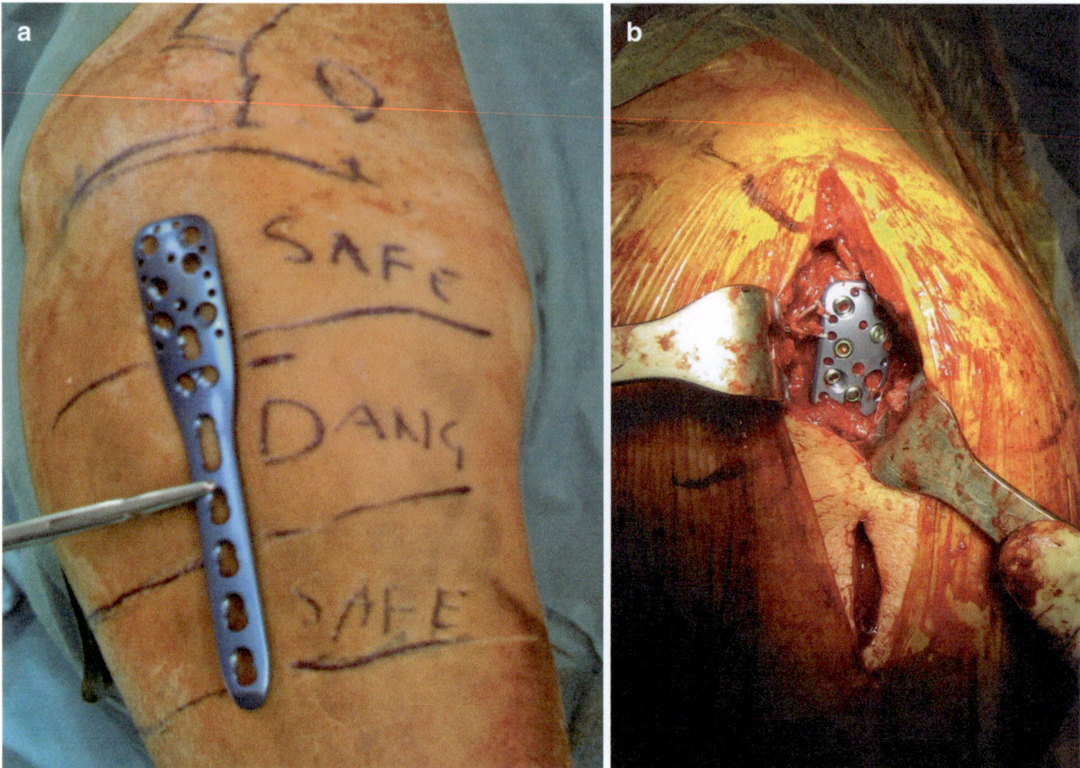

Fig. 5.6 The lateral mini approach is used to fix the fractures of the proximal third of the humerus through a minimally invasive plate osteosynthesis (MIPO) technique. (**a**) The approach avoids the dangerous zone where the axillary nerve is protected by the deltoid muscle. (**b**) A longitudinal proximal incision is performed for about 3–4 cm along the proximal and lateral portion of the arm. The second incision of about 5 cm is performed distally with respect to the proximal incision

5.5.3 Lateral Mini Approach

The lateral mini approach to the proximal humerus is designed to expose the head, the neck, and the proximal third of the humerus. It uses two routes, proximal and distal, located laterally along the proximal humerus. In its interval it is possible to find the axillary nerve that runs transversal to the arm deep to the deltoid muscle. The lateral mini approach is used to fix the fractures of the proximal third of the humerus through a minimally invasive plate osteosynthesis (MIPO) technique.

The patient is placed on the operating table in the same position as for the standard procedure. The lateral portion of the acromion is palpated, and a longitudinal incision is performed for about 3–4 cm along the proximal and lateral portion of the arm. Then, a second incision of about 5 cm is performed distally with respect to the proximal incision (Fig. 5.6). The position of this second incision depends on the site of the fracture and on the length of the implant to be used. From the proximal route, it is possible to expose the deltoid which is divided along its fibers up to a maximum of 5 cm from the lateral margin of the acromion. Once the axillary nerve is identified and isolated, an epi-periosteal plane is created on the lateral surface of the humerus. In the distal route, the subcutaneous tissue is incised, and the lateral fibers of the deltoid are identified and divided. With the finger, it is possible to identify the position of the axillary nerve. Then, an epi-periosteal plane is created and is carefully connected to the proximal one. The link between the epi-periosteal planes of the proximal and distal routes makes it possible not only to minimize the cosmetic damage but to avoid damaging the axillary nerve that will be adequately protected from the deltoid muscle.

5.6 Posterior Approach

The posterior approach to the shoulder is indicated in patients with a posterior glenohumeral instability and in glenoid fractures possibly associated to proximal humerus fractures. This approach is also utilized to treat malignant or suspicious tumors in order to avoid infiltrating the anterior neurovascular fascia.

5.6.1 Technique

The patient is placed in the lateral position or in the prone position with the shoulder and/or the superior part of the shoulder free. A vertical incision is performed from the posterolateral margin of the acromion by extending it for 6–10 cm slightly above the posterior axillary fold. The fibers of the deltoid are divided anteriorly, and the spine of the scapula is identified. The approach makes it possible to pass between the infraspinatus and the teres minor. If a larger exposure is needed, the infraspinatus and the teres minor tendons can be isolated and dissected [34].

When a larger exposure is required (fractures of the scapula and of the humerus), it is better to perform an S-shaped incision as described by Judet [4]. The incision starts at the level of the inferomedial angle of the scapular blade, and it continues with an arch-shaped line toward the medial part of the spine of the scapula. Then it follows the scapular spine laterally up to the margin of the acromion. This approach can be further extended superiorly above the clavicle, and it can continue anteriorly with the deltopectoral approach. Subperiosteal dissection of the trapezius and the posterior portion of the deltoid is performed so as to preserve the skin blood supply. The external rotators and the lateral and long head of the triceps are clearly identified. If an intra-articular approach is necessary, the interval between the teres minor and the infraspinatus muscle is identified. So it is possible to avoid damaging the suprascapular nerve which innervates the infraspinatus and the axillary nerve that innervates the teres minor. After separating the muscles from the joint capsule, the surgeon can access all the posterior parts of the glenohumeral joint. If it is necessary to reach the posterior part of the glenoid or the neck of the scapula, it is crucial to achieve a subperiosteal exposure so as to avoid damaging the intramuscular branches of the axillary nerves (teres minor) or of the suprascapular nerve (infraspinatus muscle). Otherwise, in order to obtain a better exposure, it is possible to perform a tenotomy at about 1 cm from the insertion of the infraspinatus and the teres minor trying to preserve the lower third as to avoid risks of injury to the axillary nerve (Fig. 5.7).

5.6.2 Limitations

The posterior vertical incision limits the surgical access to the neck of the scapula and to the posterior part of the glenohumeral joint. The deep dissection of the trapezius and deltoid muscles is designed to create a large flap to provide a blood supply to the skin.

5.6.3 Risks

With this approach, there are major risks for the suprascapular neurovascular bundle, for the posterior circumflex artery, for the axillary nerve, and for the radial nerve.

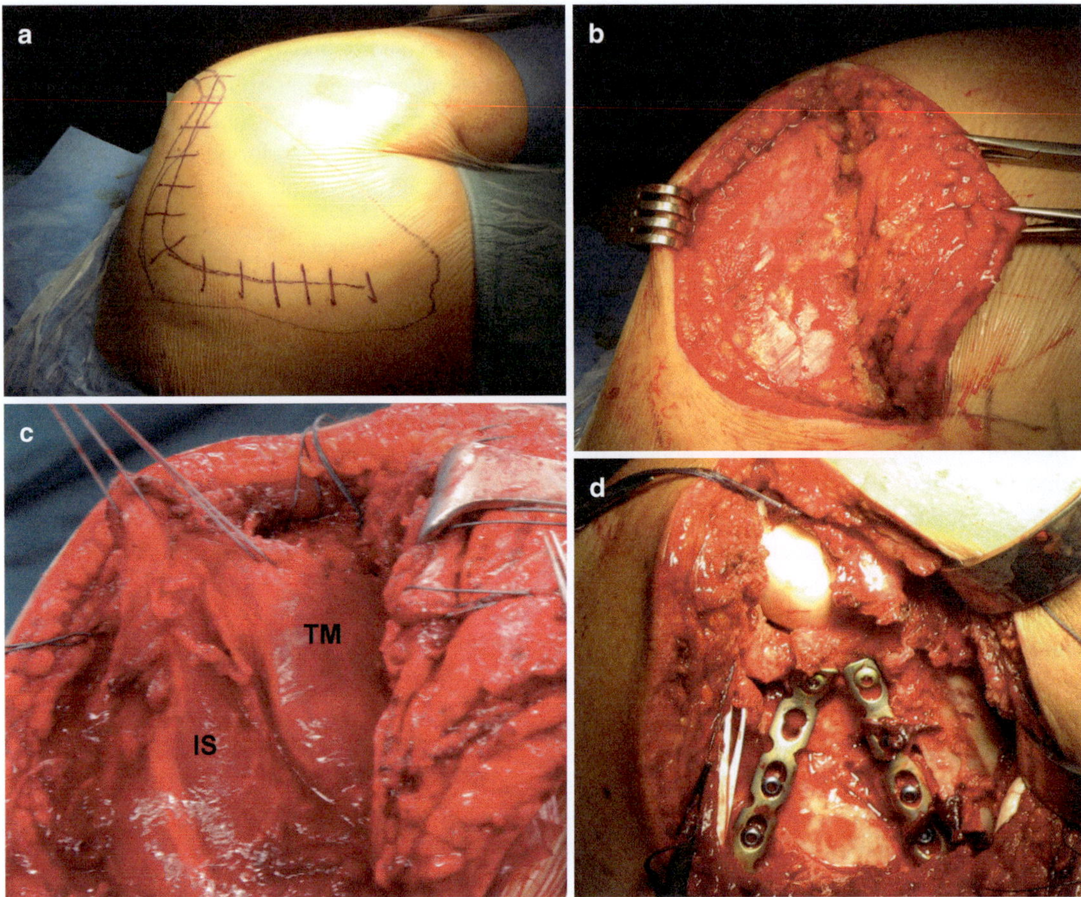

Fig. 5.7 Posterior approach. (**a**) The patient is placed in the lateral position. An S-shaped incision is performed, which starts at the level of the inferomedial angle of the scapular blade and continues with an arch-shaped line toward the medial part of the spine of the scapula and follows the scapular spine laterally up to the margin of the acromion. (**b**) Subperiosteal dissection of the trapezius and the posterior portion of the deltoid is performed so as to preserve the skin blood supply. (**c**) The interval between the teres minor (*TM*) and the infraspinatus (*IS*) muscle is identified. (**d**) Subperiosteal exposure and internal fixation of fractures of the scapular blade and glenoid neck. The infraspinatus and the teres minor tendons can be detached from their insertion in order to obtain a better exposure

5.7 Variations to the Posterior Approach

5.7.1 Extended Posterior Proximal Humeral Approach

This approach described by Berger and Buckwalter [35] allows for a posterior access into the proximal portion of the humerus, and it is an alternative with respect to the extended anterior deltopectoral approach. The route goes through the deltoid muscle supplied by the axillary nerve and the lateral head of the triceps supplied by the radial nerve.

The patient is placed in the lateral position, and the lateral incision starts three fingers distally with respect to the posterior margin of the acromion, in the palpable space between the deltoid and the triceps up to the deltoid tuberosity. The lateral head of the triceps is slightly retracted medially up to its proximal insertion. It is crucial to avoid damaging the radial nerve that is in contact with the humerus at about two fingers proximally with respect to the deltoid tuberosity. The deltoid is retracted laterally. Proximally, the approach is limited by the axillary nerve and by the posterior circumflex vessels, at about the intersection between the deltoid muscle and the lateral head of the triceps.

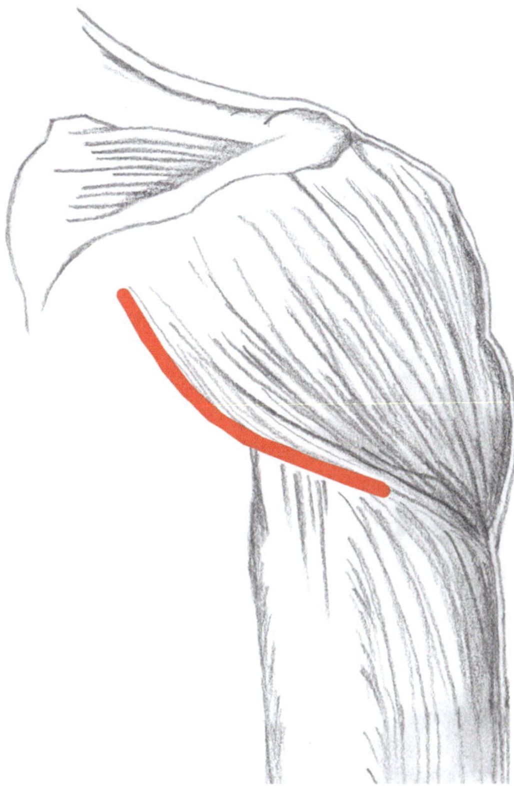

Fig. 5.8 Posterior subdeltoid approach. The skin is incised along the inferior margin of the spinal part of the deltoid muscle. The muscle is retracted superiorly and laterally

5.7.2 Posterior Subdeltoid Approach

The skin is incised along the inferior margin of the spinal part of the deltoid muscle. The muscle is retracted superiorly and laterally [36] (Fig. 5.8). This can be facilitated by slightly lifting the arm at a maximum of 60° to avoid dislocating and damaging the axillary nerve. Starting from its posteromedial margin, the deltoid muscle is carefully detached and lifted from its deep fascia. In this way, the axillary nerve is protected. So the external rotators are exposed and then retracted or dissected as already explained.

The posterior subdeltoid approach allows for an optimal exposure of the whole glenohumeral joint, of the posterior aspect of the scapular neck, of the posterior portion of the humeral head, and of the greater tuberosity. It is indicated for glenohumeral stabilizations, to remove benign soft tissue or bone tumors and to reduce and fix fractures of the humerus and the posterior glenoid. The main limitation of this approach is its high degree of invasiveness and its poor cosmetic outcome.

5.7.3 Posterolateral Approach

The patient is placed in the lateral position, with the arm free to move in all directions [37]. The surgeon is behind the patient, the first assistant to his side, and the second assistant in front. The skin incision is slightly curved; it follows the spine of the scapula and the tubercle of the trapezius muscle along the posterior margin of the acromion up to the deltoid for about 5 cm. The deltoid is detached from the spine of the scapula up the posterior margin of the acromion. Starting from the lateral margin of the acromion, the deltoid muscle is divided along its fibers into an anterior and posterior portion. If the incision of the muscle follows the convexity of the humeral head, there is no risk of damaging the axillary nerve. The subdeltoid bursa is largely detached to expose the external rotators. If it is necessary to access the joint, there are two possibilities: a less invasive one that uses the plane between the two external rotator muscles, by cleaving them from the capsule, or a more invasive one that envisages the detachment of the external rotators. Inferiorly, in order to avoid damaging the axillary nerve, the insertion of the teres minor is identified and partly dissected, by preserving the lower third. Then, the external rotators are detached through a 3 mm osteotomy from the posterior part of the greater tuberosity. The two muscles are cautiously retracted medially. The capsule is detached at the time of the osteotomy, and a capsulotomy can be performed so as to expose the humeral head. At the end of the procedure, the tendons of the external rotators are reinserted with transosseous sutures to the greater tuberosity. The deltoid is reinserted to the spine of the scapula and to the acromion with transosseous sutures.

This approach provides an intra-articular access that preserves the subscapularis muscle, thus reducing the risks of anterior instability.

5.7.4 Posterosuperior Approach

This approach makes it possible to obtain a large exposure of the posterior part of the glenoid and of the rotator cuff. In some selected cases, it is a valid alternative to an extended deltopectoral approach [38]. The patient is placed in the lateral position with the shoulder facing up. A Z-shaped incision is performed starting from the anterolateral corner and is continued posteriorly along the lateral border of the acromion, with a curved path over the scapula, and then it is extended downward on the posterior part of the shoulder. The acromion and the deltoid muscle are exposed. A special acromial plate is placed on the lateral margin of the acromion. The plate is anatomically adjusted to the profile of the acromion, and it is temporarily fixed with two Kirschner wires (K-wires) passed through the pin holes. A splitting of the deltoid fibers is performed for about 2 cm medially with respect to the posterior angle of the acromion, for about 5 cm. The anteromedial fibers of the deltoid are dissected from the anterolateral angle of the acromion, for about 2 cm. After establishing the osteotomy line, the K-wires are removed from the plate, and then an osteotomy of the acromion is conducted. A triangular bone segment, including the posterior three quarters of the lateral margin of the acromion and its posterior angle, is caudally dislocated, and the rotator cuff is exposed. In performing the osteotomy, the anterior part is treated with the utmost care to spare the anterior part of the acromion so as to avoid weakening the coracoacromial arch. Medially, near the suprascapular notch and the base of the acromion, it is easy to identify by palpation the interval between the muscular portions of the infraspinatus and of the supraspinatus as well as the anterior capsule. If the incision is extended too much medially beyond the glenoid margin, the suprascapular nerve can be damaged. The infraspinatus and part of the teres minor are detached from the greater tuberosity. Most often, it is preferable to detach the tendons with a bone chip to facilitate healing. Particular attention must be paid to the axillary nerve in the quadrilateral space and to the suprascapular nerve in the suprascapular notch [39]. At the end of the procedure, the infraspinatus and the teres minor tendons are reinserted into the greater tuberosity, and the acromion is fixed with an acromial plate with two 2.7 mm cannulated screws. Finally, the plate is further fixed to the spine of the scapula with two or three 2.7 mm screws.

This type of approach is not used on a routine basis in shoulder surgery. However, it provides an excellent exposure of the glenoid, which makes it ideal to reduce and fix intra-articular fractures.

5.8 Axillary Approach

5.8.1 Indications

This approach is rarely utilized because it requires the preparation of the neurovascular structures. However, it is not too aggressive and the scar is hardly visible. It gives the shoulder a good exposure for anterior stabilization and for capsular release.

5.8.2 Technique

The patient is placed in a beach-chair position with the arm in maximum abduction. The incision is performed on the tip of the axilla at the beginning of the anterior pillar and ends at the level of the posterior pillar. The skin is largely detached and retracted anteriorly and superiorly. The latissimus dorsi is identified inferiorly and the deltoid and the pectoralis major muscles superiorly. The axillary fat is removed with a blunt excision, thus exposing the neurovascular structures: the chords of the brachial plexus, the axillary artery, the circumflex nerve, and the anterior circumflex artery of the humerus. By retracting the neurovascular structures, the subscapularis muscle is exposed. Once the subscapularis tendon is dissected at 2.5 cm from its insertion and retracted medially, the glenohumeral joint capsule is exposed. It is possible to reach the glenohumeral joint with an incision that follows the posterior margin of the anterior axillary fold.

5.8.3 Limitations

This route allows for the anterior and inferior exposure of the shoulder joint, but it should be avoided in case of tumor biopsies, because of the adjacent neurovascular structures. The incision can be extended beyond the axillary fold but to the detriment of the cosmetic result.

References

1. De Palma AF (1961) Surgical approaches to the region of the shoulder joint. Clin Orthop Relat Res 20:163–184
2. Gruson KI (2011) 50 years Ago in CORR: surgical approaches to the region of the shoulder joint Anthony F. DePalma MD CORR 1961;20:163–184. Clin Orthop Relat Res 469:3515–3517
3. Levy O, Pritsch M, Oran A et al (1999) A wide and versatile combined surgical approach to the shoulder. J Shoulder Elbow Surg 8:658–659
4. Judet R (1964) Surgical treatment of scapular fractures. Acta Orthop Belg 30:673–678
5. Jones CB, Cornelius JP, Sietsema DL et al (2009) Modified Judet approach and minifragment fixation of scapular body and glenoid neck fractures. J Orthop Trauma 23:558–564
6. Gerber C, Schneeberger AG, Vinh TS (1990) The arterial vascularization of the humeral head: an anatomical study. J Bone Joint Surg Am 72:1486–1494
7. Hettrich CM, Borraiah S, Dyke JP et al (2010) Quantitative assessment of the vascularity of the proximal part of the humerus. J Bone Joint Surg Am 92:943–948
8. Burkhead WZ, Scheinberg RR, Box G (1992) Surgical anatomy of the axillary nerve. J Shoulder Elbow Surg 1:31–36
9. Cheung S, Fitzpatrick M, Lee TQ (2009) Effects of shoulder position on axillary nerve positions during the split lateral deltoid approach. J Shoulder Elbow Surg 18:748–755
10. Scheibel M, Habermeyer P (2008) Subscapularis dysfunction following anterior surgical approaches to the shoulder. J Shoulder Elbow Surg 17:671–683
11. Bryan WJ, Schauder K, Tullos HS (1986) The axillary nerve and its relationship to common sports medicine shoulder procedures. Am J Sports Med 14: 113–116
12. Loomer R, Graham B (1989) Anatomy of the axillary nerve and its relationship to inferior capsular shift. Clin Orthop Relat Res 243:100–105
13. McFarland EG, Caicedo JC, Kim TK et al (2002) Prevention of axillary nerve injury in anterior shoulder reconstructions use of a subscapularis muscle-splitting technique and a review of the literature. Am J Sports Med 30:601–606
14. McFarland EG, Caicedo JC, Guitterez MI et al (2001) The anatomic relationship of the brachial plexus and axillary artery to the glenoid implications for anterior shoulder surgery. Am J Sports Med 29:729–733
15. Radkowski CA, Richards RS, Pietrobon R et al (2006) An anatomic study of the cephalic vein in the deltopectoral shoulder approach. Clin Orthop Relat Res 442:139–142
16. Zlotolow DA, Catalano LW 3rd, Barron OA et al (2006) Surgical exposures of the humerus. J Am Acad Orthop Surg 14:754–765
17. Crenshaw AH (1992) Surgical techniques. In: Crenshaw AH (ed) Campbell's operative orthopaedics, vol 1, 8th edn. Mosby, St Louis, pp 88–95
18. Hoppenfeld S, de Boer P (1984) The shoulder. In: Hoppenfeld S, de Boer P (eds) Surgical exposures in orthopaedics. The anatomic approach. Lippincott Williams & Wilkins, Philadelphia, pp 1–45
19. Gill DR, Cofield RH, Rowland C (2004) The anteromedial approach for shoulder arthroplasty: the importance of the anterior deltoid. J Shoulder Elbow Surg 13:532–537
20. Foruria AM, Oh LS, Sperling JW et al (2010) Anteromedial approach for shoulder arthroplasty: current indications, complications, and results. J Shoulder Elbow Surg 19:734–738
21. Hoppenfield S, deBoer P, Buckley R (2009) Surgical exposures in orthopaedics: the anatomical approach, 4th edn. Lippincott Williams & Wilkins, Philadelphia, pp 34–35
22. Gardner MJ, Boraiah S, Helfet DL et al (2008) The anterolateral acromial approach for fractures of the proximal humerus. J Orthop Trauma 22:132–137
23. Mackenzie DB (1993) The antero-superior exposure for total shoulder replacement. Orthop Traumatol 2:71–77
24. Valenti P, Sauzieres P, Cogswell L et al (2008) The reverse shoulder prosthesis surgical technique. Tech Hand Up Extrem Surg 12:46–55
25. Bufquin T, Hersan A, Hubert L et al (2007) Reverse shoulder arthroplasty for the treatment of three- and four-part fractures of the proximal humerus in the elderly: a prospective review of 43 cases with a short-term follow-up. J Bone Joint Surg Br 89:516–520
26. Cazeneuve JF, Cristofari DJ (2009) Delta III reverse shoulder arthroplasty: radiological outcome for acute complex fractures of the proximal humerus in elderly patients. Orthop Traumatol Surg Res 95:325–329
27. Gallinet D, Clappaz P, Garbuio P et al (2009) Three or four parts complex proximal humerus fractures: hemiarthroplasty versus reverse prosthesis: a comparative study of 40 cases. Orthop Traumatol Surg Res 95:48–55
28. Gardner MJ, Griffith MH, Dines JS et al (2004) A minimally invasive approach for plate fixation of the proximal humerus. Bull Hosp Jt Dis 62:18–23
29. Gardner MJ, Griffith MH, Dines JS et al (2005) The extended anterolateral acromial approach allows minimally invasive access to the proximal humerus. Clin Orthop Relat Res 434:123–129

30. Hettrich CM, Paul O, Neviaser AS et al (2011) The anterolateral approach to the proximal humerus for nonunions and delayed unions. Int J Shoulder Surg 5:21–25
31. Robinson CM, Khan L, Akhtar A et al (2007) The extended deltoid-splitting approach to the proximal humerus. J Orthop Trauma 21:657–662
32. Robinson CM, Murray IR (2011) The extended deltoid-splitting approach to the proximal humerus: variations and extensions. J Bone Joint Surg Br 93:387–392
33. Borges AF (1989) Relaxed skin tension lines. Dermatol Clin 7:169–177
34. Brodsky JW, Tullos HS, Gartsman GM (1987) Simplified posterior approach to the shoulder joint. A technical note. J Bone Joint Surg Am 69:773–774
35. Berger RA, Buckwalter JA (1989) A posterior surgical approach to the proximal part of the humerus. J Bone Joint Surg Am 71:407–410
36. Jerosch J, Greig M, Peuker ET et al (2001) The posterior subdeltoid approach: a modified access to the posterior glenohumeral joint. J Shoulder Elbow Surg 10:265–268
37. Gagey O, Spraul JM, Vinh TS (2001) Posterolateral approach of the shoulder: assessment of 50 cases. J Shoulder Elbow Surg 10:47–51
38. Rozing PM (2008) A posterosuperior approach to the shoulder. J Shoulder Elbow Surg 17:431–435
39. Shaffer BS, Conway J, Jobe FW et al (1987) Infraspinatus muscle-splitting incision in posterior shoulder surgery. Am J Sports Med 22:113–120

6 Percutaneous Fixation: When and How

Marco Assom and Enrico Bellato

Closed reduction and percutaneous fixation in cases of proximal humeral fractures was first described by Bohler in 1962 in children [1]. Since then the literature has mainly focused on adults with a wide range of results. In fact this offers obvious advantages: the limited disruption of soft tissues and periosteum reduces the risk of avascular necrosis [2–8]; the articular surfaces and the rotator cuff are preserved, so the risk of fibrosis and stiffness is low [9]; the cosmesis is improved and this treatment is cheaper than others, so it can be a good choice in developing countries [10]. The disadvantages of this technique include the potential complications such as pin migration, loss of reduction, and pin-site infection; the learning curve is long, and an anatomic reduction is often not achieved; nevertheless, we have to state that good results are reported all the same [11–15]; moreover the revision rate is around 10 %, and some authors show a rate of 30 % [16–21].

The percutaneous treatment has been overlooked because of these negative aspects, and surgeons have been increasingly interested in other options such as the locking compression plate (LCP). However, this hardware has been recently criticized because of poor functional results, a high revision rate, and complications [22–25].

M. Assom
Department of Orthopaedics and Traumatology, University of Turin Medical School, Mauriziano-Umberto I Hospital, Largo Turati 62, Turin 10128, Italy
e-mail: dassom@libero.it

E. Bellato (✉)
Department of Orthopaedics and Traumatology, University of Turin Medical School, CTO-Maria Adelaide Hospital, Via Zuretti 29, Turin 10126, Italy
e-mail: bellatoenrico@gmail.com

6.1 Anatomic Considerations

Surgeons considering the closed reduction and internal fixation with pins need to have in-depth knowledge of both the musculoskeletal structures around the shoulder and their behavior in the event of fractures and the structures to be avoided so that damage is not caused and complications do not arise.

6.1.1 Relationship Between Humeral Diaphysis and Epiphysis, Anatomic Segments, and Their Displacement Direction

Before starting surgery the tridimensional geometry of the proximal humerus must be clear. Various authors have described the normal neck-shaft angle, which corresponds to pin direction in the frontal plane. We usually refer to Iannotti: the angle between the plane of the humeral articular margin and the longitudinal axis of the humeral diaphysis measures $45 \pm 5°$ [26].

Because of the retroversion angle, the humeral head lies posterior to the diaphysis in the frontal plane; the angle is determined in relation to the transepicondylar axis and is around 18° [27, 28].

F. Castoldi et al. (eds.), *Simple and Complex Fractures of the Humerus*, DOI 10.1007/978-88-470-5307-6_6, © Springer-Verlag Italia 2015

Regarding the anatomic segments and their displacement direction, we refer to the Chap. 4.

6.1.2 Vessels and Nerves

The axillary nerve and the circumflex arteries are the most important structures. Various authors have described superficial landmarks which can be useful to avoid vascular and nervous injuries during surgery. The lateral pins can cause injury in particular to the anterior branch of the axillary nerve and the posterior circumflex artery. Rowles states that the starting point of these pins should be at or distal to a point along the lateral aspect of the shaft equal to twice the distance from the top of the humeral head to the inferiormost margin of the articular cartilage of the humeral head [29]. Other authors showed that the distance between the lateral edge of the acromion and the anterior branch of the axillary nerve is around 5, 3.1 cm in some cases [30]; this is confirmed also by Kamineni, who identified the nerve 5.7 cm along the lateral aspect of the arm and 5.1 cm along the anterior aspect [31], while Burkhart demonstrated the nerve to be an average of 7.9 cm in males, and 6.9 cm in females, distal to the acromion in the anterior clavicular line [32].

The main trunk of the axillary nerve and the posterior humeral circumflex artery are particularly at risk from the greater tuberosity pins placed proximal to distal and lateral to medial. The surgeon should aim for a point >20 mm distal from the inferior extent of the humeral head and should place these pins with the shoulder in external rotation: so that the axillary nerve and the posterior humeral circumflex artery are relaxed and tend to move farther away from the pins [29].

The deltoid tuberosity is an important landmark and corresponds to the lateral edge of the acromion. Anterior to this landmark the axillary nerve is already split into distinct smaller branches. So the pins placed in this area can cause injury to just a few of these small branches [33]. Moreover a pin insertion point proximal to the deltoid tuberosity means that the radial nerve is avoided [12, 31]. In the case of anterior pin placement, the surgeon must keep in mind that there is no truly safe zone anteriorly: the long head of the biceps is between the cephalic vein (lateral) and the musculocutaneous nerve (medial) [29]. However, the effectiveness of anterior pins here is debatable.

6.2 Biomechanical Considerations

Percutaneous fixation with pins has been criticized because of lack of stability and, as a consequence, a high risk of loss of fixation and pin migration. Calvo reports a migration rate of 36 % [34], while the rates reported by Kocialkowski and Wallace [35] and Yu et al. [36] are 41 % and 24 out of 64 cases, respectively. In contrast other systems seem to be more stable and reliable. There are different biomechanical studies dealing with this matter. Koval in a cadaver study compares the T-plate with the Schantz pins: the pins provide less resistance, regardless of their configuration [37]. Wheeler compares the intramedullary nail with the percutaneous pinning in the case of three-fragment fractures created on cadavers and shows that the first implant provides higher stability and stiffness; however, the author also stated that if extensive comminution is present, the purchase provided by the interlocking screws of the intramedullary device may be inadequate, and percutaneous pinning may be more effective [38].

However, conflicting results and complications associated with rigid systems such as LCP have reduced the initial enthusiasm. The risk of hardware cutout significantly increases, overall in high osteopenic patients [37, 39]. Semirigid implants have been taken into consideration again [40].

Various tips and pearls are described to reduce the risk of pin migration:

- The surgeon must avoid using smooth pins, even though some authors state that they can be used successfully in young patients with high-quality bone [41]: the high migration rate reported by Kocialkowski is mainly caused by smooth pins [35].
- Terminally threaded pins are more reliable because both the cortical and the subchondral bones are engaged.

- Various authors recommend cutting the pins and bending them beneath the skin [19, 42, 43].
- Some authors describe the use of pins and screws together [15].
- Some other implants have been created such as the Humerusblock [16, 44, 45], the ButtonFix [46], and the Humerusblock NG [47].

Various authors have carried out biomechanical tests to find the best pin configuration. Jiang compares the box configuration with the fan-shaped configuration in cases of two-fragment fractures: the first one provides better torsional stability, in particular when 1 cm is used for the pin-to-pin distance [48]. Koval instead shows that three pins placed in a triangular configuration inserted from distal to proximal into the subchondral bone of the humeral head and one pin inserted from the greater tuberosity into the medial shaft provide the most stable configuration [37]. In the study by Naidu, the configuration with two retrograde lateral pins, one retrograde anterior pin, and two bicortical tuberosity pins is the best; moreover multiplanar pins increase torsional stiffness, while the bending rigidity mostly relies on the number of cortices engaged. However, the author stresses the importance of using threaded pins engaging both the lateral cortex and the subchondral bone: this is more important than pin configuration [49].

The plate is usually biomechanically superior to the percutaneous pinning [50]; however, some authors state that this is more stable than T-plate/screw fixation in cases of osteopenia [37].

6.2.1 Authors' Opinion

We planned a biomechanical study whose aim was to improve pin stability [51]. We compared different pin configurations, we evaluated the stabilization provided by an external fixator, and we compared the percutaneous pinning (with and without external fixation) with the LCP. Our results allow us to state that:

- The box configuration is the stiffest and strongest.
- Osteosynthesis is much more stable if we use fully threaded pins with wider diameter; the longer thread engages the lateral cortex: as a result the migration of the pins is difficult even without engaging the subchondral bone; as a consequence iatrogenic articular lesions decrease.
- Augmentation with external fixation (Fig. 6.1) makes the osteosynthesis more stable: the LCP is still more resilient than the percutaneous technique, but the stiffness and strength of the construct did not differ significantly from that of the LCP.

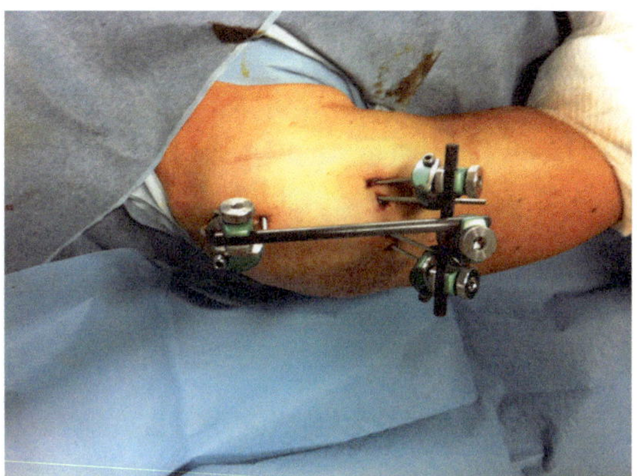

Fig. 6.1 An example of the "hybrid technique": pins, with a longer thread, are easily joined together by clamps and carbon rods

Going by the results described, we have modified the percutaneous technique: we have started using pins with a longer thread (7 cm), and we have stabilized the pins with an external fixator. These two changes increase the resistance to pullout by a factor of 8; moreover the external fixator reduces the importance of pin configuration in implant stability.

6.3 What Kind of Fractures?

The conditions required for a correct percutaneous technique are a stable closed reduction, a good bone stock, a minimal comminution (particularly involving the tuberosities), an intact medial calcar, and good patient compliance [52].

The two-fragment fractures involving the humeral surgical neck are the most suitable for treatment with this technique [12, 34, 52, 53]: it is reported by various authors that the worst results associated with percutaneous pinning are achieved in fractures involving the tuberosities [34, 54]. Even though different authors report bad results in displaced three to four-fragment fractures [55, 56], recently these fractures have been supposed to be increasingly suitable for the percutaneous technique [15, 42], especially in cases of valgus impacted fractures [57–60].

The patient's age is an important aspect. Some authors recommend this surgical treatment when the patient is young because of high bone quality [41]. But Calvo, referring to three-fragment fractures, states that young patients are better suited to open reduction and internal fixation because better reduction can be achieved, while for older patients closed reduction and external fixation may be sufficient [34]. Also Carbone, dealing with a particular implant called MIROS, states that percutaneous pinning is a good choice for older patients [61].

6.3.1 Authors' Opinion

We believe the majority of fractures can be treated with pins, either with a closed technique or with an open one: in fact, even in cases of complex fractures, the surgeon can perform an open reduction followed by percutaneous osteosynthesis. Hertel has focused our attention on the medial hinge [62], but its continuity does not strictly correlate with the humeral head blood supply [63], especially in young patients (up to the age of 60). In fact the possible avascular necrosis can be completely asymptomatic; in cases of disability it can be treated with a prosthesis. Moreover joint replacement is easier without any hardware to be removed.

This technique is contraindicated in cases of:

- Fractures without a good lateral cortex where the pins are introduced and engage.
- Splitting of the humeral head: it is a relative contraindication because the risk of avascular necrosis is high; however, Resch believes that young patients with an AOC3-type fracture deserve an attempt at osteosynthesis [33].
- Tuberosity highly comminuted: the fragments must keep their anatomic integrity.
- Fractures with diaphysis involvement: it is a relative contraindication because a different pin configuration described below can get round this problem.

6.4 Surgical Technique and Postoperative Care

The main steps of this procedure are two, as described by different authors: the closed reduction using the C-arm (we referred to the Chap. 4) and the percutaneous fixation.

The operation is usually performed under general anesthesia, but the interscalenic block is also a good option [15, 33, 42, 61].

Correct patient position is mandatory. Even though some surgeons prefer the lateral position [35], usually we have to choose between the supine position and the "beach-chair" position to perform the deltopectoral approach. Some authors use pins as joysticks during the reduction maneuvers [64–66].

Nowadays we know that pins must be terminally threaded. Different diameters are used: 2.5 mm pins are the most used [12, 31, 36, 41, 42, 52, 67], but also the 0.3 mm [43], 2 mm [31], 2.8 mm [9], and 3 mm [64] ones are suitable. Surgeons usually refer to Jaberg's technique regarding the number of pins to be placed: he states that the percutaneous osteosynthesis needs at least three pins (five pins in cases of three-fragment fractures involving the greater tuberosity), two laterally and one anteriorly [12]; the anterior pin is challenging, mainly because of the anterior structures it can injure [29]. Percutaneous pin placement options include retrograde lateral, retrograde anterior, retrograde anterolateral, antegrade through the humeral head, antegrade posterolateral through the greater tuberosity, and antegrade superomedial through the lesser tuberosity, depending on the fragments displaced [34]. Other authors use only antegrade pins [67].

Herscovici et al. [19] stresses three important technical points:

- The starting point of the pins should be at least 2 cm distal to the fracture.
- A wide pin spread should be performed.
- The pins should reach, but not go through, the subchondral bone.

The surgeon placing the pins must remember the humeral head retroversion (about 20°). They should be angled approximately 45° to the shaft in the coronal plane and 30° to the shaft in the sagittal plane [41]. Some authors suggest cutting and bending the pins beneath the skin to reduce the risk of infection and mobilization [19, 42, 43].

6.4.1 Augmentation of Pins by External Fixation

Pins can be used as external fixator fiches [68, 69], and this is a good option in cases of complex fractures [65]. Over the years we have stopped using bulky implants such as the Hoffman external fixator [49, 65, 68–70], and now we prefer more compact ones [64, 66]. The basic principle is still the classic external fixation as a bridge between the fracture stumps stabilizing after performing the reduction.

6.4.2 Authors' Opinion

Basing ourselves on the biomechanical study illustrated above [51], we have modified the percutaneous technique by introducing the so-called hybrid technique: it is based on the basic pinning principle (pins, with a longer thread, must go through the fracture) associated with an external fixator. Pins are easily joined together by clamps and carbon rods. Then we compared this surgical technique with the classic one in cases of two-/three-/four-fragment fractures: the results we achieved after 12 months of follow-up were statistically better in the group treated with the new technique, mainly with regard to complications (6 vs 16), revision rate (4 % vs 19 %), pin migration rate (1 vs 8), and modified Constant score (89±9 vs 77±14) [71].

6.4.2.1 Postoperative Care

The protocols described in the literature generally state that immediately after surgery, the arm is immobilized in adduction in a simple sling (an abduction sling does not seem necessary [15]) generally worn for 3–4 weeks [9, 12, 35, 36, 42]. Some authors postpone passive exercises until the patient stops wearing the sling, while other authors recommend passive exercises and pendulum exercises from the day after surgery [15, 41, 64, 67]. Instead there is considerable variability as regards the active exercises: from the first to third weeks [64], from the fourth [15], from the sixth [57], and from the seventh [34]; Ebraheim uses the mini-external fixator and lets the patient move their arm actively even from the first day after surgery [66].

Pins are usually removed in the outpatients' department, under local anesthesia if necessary [15], but some prefer to remove them in the operating room under sedation [9]. Removal is usually performed at 3–6 weeks postoperatively [9, 15, 33–35, 42]. Some authors describe removal on two different days, for example, Jaberg removes the tuberosity pins at 3 weeks postoperatively, while other pins at 6 weeks postoperatively [12]; Magovern removes tuberosity pins at 3–4 weeks postoperatively, while other pins are removed at 4–6 weeks postoperatively [52]; Seyhan places only four antegrade pins and removes two of them at 4 weeks postoperatively and the other 2 at 6 weeks after surgery [67]. Other authors describe pin removal at 6–8 weeks postoperatively [64] or even at 9–12 weeks [66]. However, there is no scientific rationale regarding either the best way to wear the sling or the best time to start passive/active mobilization, and no one knows whether late pin removal induces better healing of the fracture. The wide range of pin removal times may depend on the individual surgeon's familiarity with the fixation system.

6.4.2.2 Authors' Preferred Surgical Technique

An optimal patient resting position is mandatory and depends on the type of surgery to be performed: closed reduction (supine position) or open reduction (beach-chair position). The surgical field must be prepared so that the surgeon can fully move the shoulder and can see and palpate the acromioclavicular joint and the coracoid: these are very important landmarks for the osteosynthesis (Fig. 6.2).

An inaccurate surgical field usually leads to mistakes in the pin insertion point. Osteosynthesis starts after the reduction maneuvers which we have described in the previous chapter (Chap. 4). We prefer using self-drilling and self-tapping pins 300 mm long, 2.5 mm in diameter, and with a thread 7 cm long, even though the long thread has been blamed for causing soft tissue injuries [52]. Two lines on the pins (12 and 14 cm) are useful landmarks during the percutaneous insertion. The system is sold as the “Galaxy Shoulder” (Orthofix Srl, Via delle Nazioni 9, 37012 Bussolengo, Verona, Italy). The assistant must keep the arm parallel to the floor (which is our reference) while keeping the fracture reduced: so the humeral head is posterior to the diaphysis thanks to its own physiological offset. An adequate check with the C-arm is mandatory, mainly when the surgeon is placing the first retrograde pin and the antegrade pins. The first pin starting position is 9–10 cm distal to the lateral edge of the acromion, 4–5 cm proximal to the deltoid tuberosity and anterior to the lateral line parallel to the diaphysis and going through the lateral edge of the acromion (Fig. 6.2).

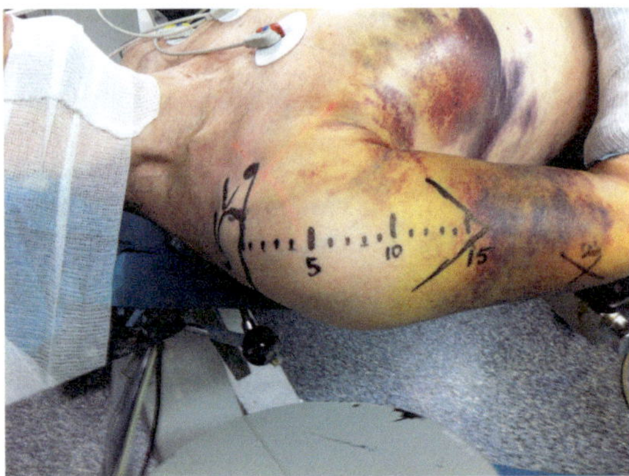

Fig. 6.2 With a dermographic marker the sites of the coracoid, of the coracoacromial ligament, of the deltoid insertion, of the acromion, and of the acromioclavicular joint are highlighted. The lateral longitudinal line is a very useful landmark for the axillary nerve (about 5 cm distal to the lateral edge acromion) and for the first pin starting position (9–10 cm distal to the lateral edge of the acromion, 4–5 cm proximal to the deltoid tuberosity and anterior to the line)

The pin is inserted 20–25° retroverted and pointing to the tip of the coracoid. The number and starting points of pins depend on fracture type. In the case of a two-fragment fracture, we use four retrograde pins (Fig. 6.3). In three- and four-fragment fractures (without or with low tuberosity dislocation), an attempt at closed reduction may be made; then we need two more antegrade pins to fix the humeral head and the greater tuberosity (Fig. 6.4). The starting point is just lateral to the lateral edge of the acromion and corresponds to the humeral footprint. One pin-points to the humeral head apex, the other one just beneath the medial hinge.

Our quite lengthy experience of percutaneous pinning has led us to consider it an alternative

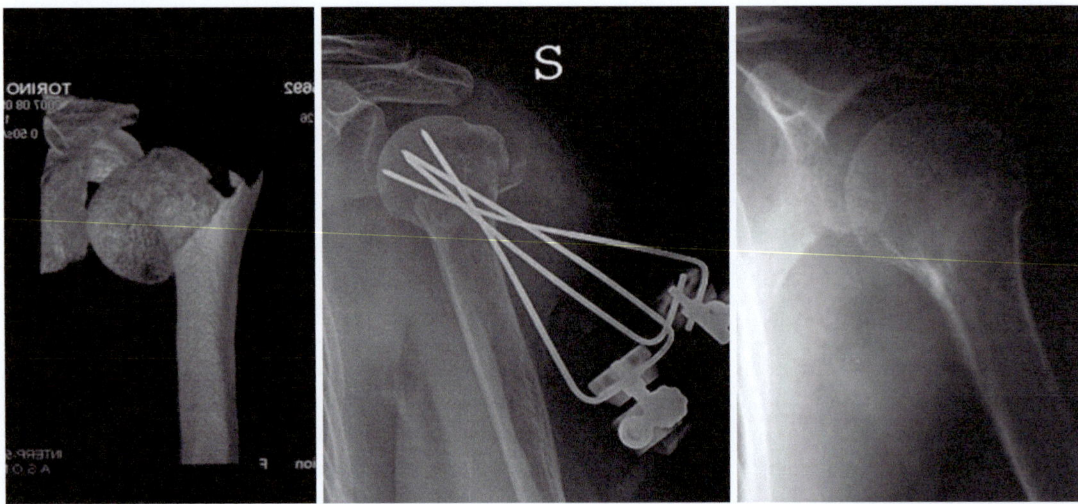

Fig. 6.3 An example of a two-fragment fracture before surgery (**a**), immediately after surgery (**b**), and after 1-year follow-up (**c**)

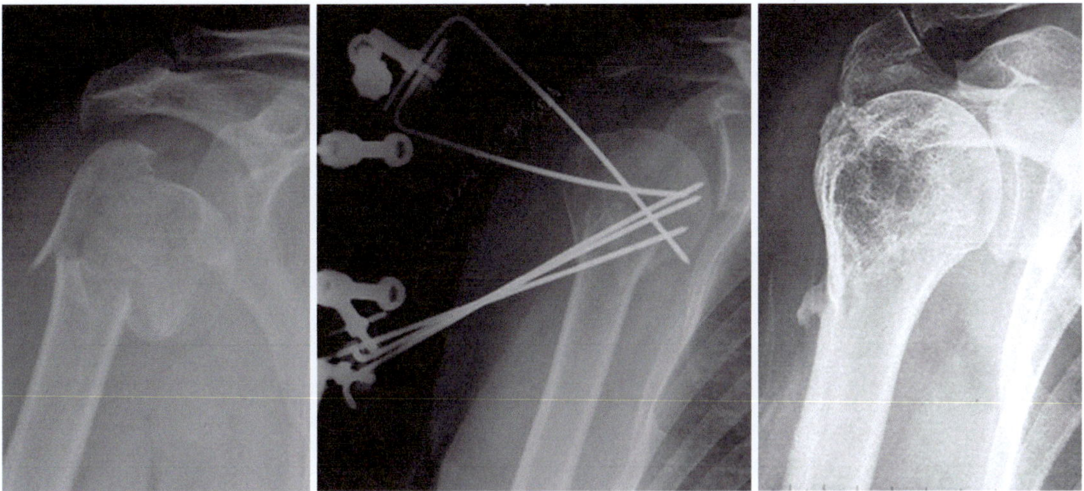

Fig. 6.4 An example of three-fragment fracture before surgery (**a**), immediately after surgery (**b**), and after 1-year follow-up (**c**)

treatment to internal fixation even in cases of complex fractures. Some fracture patterns, such as valgus impacted three-fragment fractures, fracture-dislocations, and four-fragment fractures, are best treated with the open approach. The integrity of each anatomic structure is mandatory: osteosynthesis can be performed only if tuberosities are not highly comminuted.

We start with the deltopectoral approach. The first step is to recognize the anatomic structures (long head of the biceps, lesser and greater tuberosity), and an accurate bursectomy can be helpful. The preoperative CT is very useful and helps us to plan surgery and to operate between bone fragments without further damage to the blood supply. In particular we have to look for the greater tuberosity posteriorly and superiorly to the long head of the biceps, while the lesser tuberosity is usually medial to it, often beneath the conjoint tendon. Tuberosities must be held by bioresorbable sutures through tendon insertion. This prevents further comminution of fracture fragments during reduction maneuvers. The correct anatomic reduction can be helped by landmarks such as the greater tuberosity height or the distance between the upper border of the pectoralis major tendon insertion on the humerus and the top of the humeral head (usually around 55 mm [72]). The humeral head is usually rotated showing the surgeon its articular surface and has to be properly replaced. The subsequent surgical steps are quite similar to those of any open reduction technique, but, after positioning the fragments correctly, the first two pins used to fix the head and the diaphysis together must be placed through the skin because they will take part in the definitive osteosynthesis. The C-arm lets the surgeon evaluate the initial correction achieved.

In the case of three- or four-fragment fractures, we augment the fixation with osteosutures of the tuberosities to oppose the traction forces caused by the supraspinatus and subscapularis tendons. We use three nonbioresorbable sutures dec 5: one for the supraspinatus tendon, one for the subscapularis tendon, and one to fix both tendons to the diaphysis (the hole in the diaphysis is made next to the tubercular groove, where bone quality is higher). Then percutaneous osteosynthesis is completed with four more pins: two from the diaphysis to the head with a distal to proximal direction and two from the greater tuberosity toward the medial hinge with a proximal to distal direction. The final fluoroscopic check and the wound suture complete the surgery. The pins are then joined together by the external fixator. Sometimes, depending on fracture type, two more pins can be used as a true external fixator fixing the system to the diaphysis (Fig. 6.5).

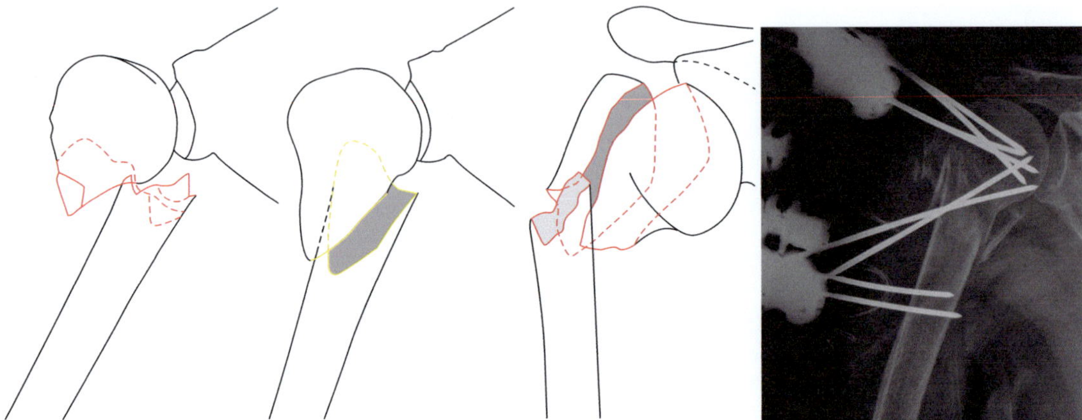

Fig. 6.5 In cases of fractures with diaphysis involvement or highly unstable fractures (shown in the pictures), the traditional pinning technique is contraindicated because pins cannot engage both the lateral cortex and the subchondral bone; pins can then be used as a true external fixator

Patients are usually discharged from the hospital within 2 or 3 days of surgery. They wear a shoulder sling which keeps the arm adducted until the pins are removed; this takes place in our outpatients' department without anesthesia. Active elbow and wrist mobilization is encouraged from the first day after surgery; patients can start pendulum exercises as soon as they can bear the pain. Even though there is insufficient evidence to say when to start mobilization (there is only some evidence to support earlier arm movement for less serious fractures [73]), we believe that, if the pain is controlled, patients should start rehabilitation as soon as possible. Patients undergo a weekly follow-up in our outpatients' department to have their surgical wounds dressed. Passive mobilization associated with external and internal rotations usually starts 3 weeks postoperatively, while patients are allowed to actively move their shoulder 6 weeks after surgery. X-rays are performed before discharge, 1 week, 6 weeks, and 3 months after surgery.

6.5 Complications

6.5.1 Pin Migration

First reported by Mazet [74], pin migration is probably what surgeons fear most. It rates between 0 and 41 % [9, 34–36, 67, 75]. However, Calvo et al. [34] emphasizes that pin migration resulted in loss of reduction of the fracture in 10 % of patients, and revision surgery was considered only in two patients, even though the migration rate is high in his study (36 %). We do not know why shoulder pins are so prone to mobilization: factors such as muscular activity, respiratory excursion, capillary action, electrolysis, regional resorption of bone, gravitational forces, and the great freedom of motion of the upper extremity are thought to be involved [74, 76, 77]. Cases of thoracic cavity migration have been reported [78], but it must be stressed that there are no reports of migrated Kirschner wires from the proximal humerus to the thoracic cavity causing cardiac tamponade and sudden death [79]. In studies involving an external fixator, the pin migration rate falls between 0 and 6 % [10, 61, 64, 66, 71].

6.5.2 Avascular Necrosis

The risk of avascular necrosis (AVN) is between 0 and 26 % [9, 12, 15, 19, 34, 42, 58, 61, 64], and symptoms or radiographic signs may also occur within 2 years after surgery; so patients should be followed for this length of time [9, 52]. We must keep in mind that:

- The development of AVN is determined largely by the injury itself and not necessarily by the course of treatment [80].

- The AVN can be absolutely asymptomatic or just partially symptomatic [81].
- Only in a few cases of AVN are the functional results so bad that further surgery is needed; Gerber reports that the clinical results for patients with AVN without malunion were as good as those for patients treated with hemiarthroplasty [82].

6.5.3 Infection

Infection rates are between 0 and 10 % for superficial infections and between 0 and 7 % for deep infections [10, 12, 34–36, 42, 43, 64–67, 70, 75, 83]. Usually sequelae do not result from superficial infections, and the problem is easily resolved by pin removal and by using antibiotics if necessary. Only a small number of deep infections usually have to be surgically treated [12, 66]: Shabtai focused his study on infections associated with the use of an external fixator in cases of proximal humeral fractures [83] and shows that all the infections (17 superficial and one deep among 46 patients) healed without surgery. Some authors state that pins should be placed under the skin [52].

Our preferred surgical technique has been criticized because of the risk of infection. So we planned a retrospective multicenter study examining the risk factors potentially associated with infection after various types of proximal humeral fracture fixation. Among the 209 patients who underwent pinning fixation, nine (4.3 %) showed a deep infection and one of these needed further surgery. The factors that correlated with infection were the length of surgery, the preoperative lavage with chlorhexidine gluconate, and the prophylactic antibiotic (it seems better to avoid the use of first-generation cephalosporin in favor of more effective prophylactic therapy). The type of fixation and the type of reduction (open vs closed) did not seem to affect the rate of infection. However, when patients who underwent a plate fixation were compared with those treated with percutaneous fixation, the rate of further surgery needed to treat the infection was lower in cases of percutaneous fixation. Of the five cases that needed further surgery, four had had a plate fixation and one a percutaneous fixation ($p=0.047$) [84].

6.5.4 Loss of Fixation

Loss of fixation is the main criticism of the pinning technique and relates to pin mobilization: in fact it usually arises in cases of osteopenic patients and comminuted fractures. Many authors show a rate of 0 % [67, 70], but in Jaberg's study the rate is 19 % (nine patients), and four cases needed a second closed fixation [12]. Soete et al. [42] and Fenichel et al. [43] report a 13 and 14 % rate, respectively, while Calvo et al. [34] shows five losses of fixation on 74 patients, with two patients who underwent further surgery (one closed fixation and one joint replacement with hemiarthroplasty). The rate of loss of fixation decreases if the surgeon uses the external fixator (0–9 %) [61, 64–66]. In our comparison study of the hybrid technique and the traditional pinning technique, the rate was 2 and 17 %, respectively [71].

6.5.5 Malunion

Malunion has been defined in various ways so it is difficult to compare patients across different studies. For example, Calvo reports a rate of 28 % [34], while Jaberg 19 % [12] and Keener 17 % [57]. The most common residual deformities include varus angulation of the head and posterosuperior displacement of the greater tuberosity [52]. Calvo et al. [34] and Yu et al. [36] performed a radiographic evaluation using a numeric scale: an angulation between 20° and 45° was scored as 1 point, and >45° was scored as 2 points; a displacement between 0.5 and 1 cm was scored as 1 point, and >1 cm was scored as 2 points; if the angulation and displacement were lower than 20° and 0.5 cm, respectively, the quality of reduction was considered excellent and scored as 0 points; the score in each case ranged from a minimum of 0 (in perfectly reduced fractures) to 12 points because the final score for each case was the sum of the scores allocated to each fragment. Calvo reported a mean score for residual deformity of 2.16 ± 1.8 and stated that the score was significantly higher in cases of reduction defects involving tuberosities [34]. Yu reported a mean value of 1.8 ± 1.3 and showed that there was no statistical difference between the immediate postoperative imaging and the final follow-up imaging [36]. It is important to remember that radiographic features may not correlate with clinical results: patients may well tolerate even quite significant failure of bone healing [12, 34, 36, 52].

6.5.6 Nonunion

The rates of pseudarthrosis are between 0 and 4.5 % [12, 34, 35, 42, 43, 66, 67, 70, 75], but this latter rate refers to the study performed by Kocialkowski and Wallace [35] who used smooth pins. Jaberg's patients developed nonunion in two cases out of 48, both surgical neck fractures. He supposed that there was unrecognized metaphyseal comminution leading to inadequate fixation of the fragment [12]. Apparently whether using an external fixator or not does not change the risk. Some authors believe that early removal of the fixator can contribute to the nonunion rate [10].

6.5.7 Peripheral Neurological Injury

These injuries are rare and can be avoided if the recommendations above are acted upon. Authors almost never report neurovascular lesions. They are very rare. Two patients included by Kristiansen in his study showed temporary paraesthesia of the brachial plexus postoperatively [65]. Kocialkowski reports one radial nerve palsy completely resolved [35].

6.6 Results

Several large series have reported the results after percutaneous pinning of proximal humeral fractures. Jaberg's results are the most cited, but date back to 1992 [12].

Seyhan et al. [67] has recently published his results of two-fragment valgus impacted fractures treated with four antegrade pins. According to the Constant scoring system, 21 patients (58 %) had excellent, nine patients (25 %) had good, and six patients (17 %) had fair results. He reports no cases of deep infection, nonunion, avascular necrosis, or implant failure.

Harrison et al. [9] describes his results after a 3-year follow-up. Some patients had already been included in a previous study [57]. The ASES score increased from 78.5 to 80.8, but the author focuses mainly on AVN and posttraumatic osteoarthritis. The AVN rate grew from 4.2 to 26 %, and ASES results were worse in cases of AVN (77 vs 84), but not significantly. Sixty percent of patients affected by four-part fractures, 33 % of patients affected by three-part fractures, and 0 % of patients who had two-part fractures showed posttraumatic osteoarthritis: the average ASES score for those patients without posttraumatic osteoarthritis was significantly better as compared with an average ASES score of 74 for those with posttraumatic osteoarthritis (87 vs 74).

Zhang et al. [64] has recently evaluated the outcomes of 32 patients (mean age of 56 years, range 23–81) treated with closed reduction and external fixation. The mean Neer score for injured shoulders improved from 53.2 ± 16.3 points at 8 weeks' follow-up to 83.2 ± 12.5 points at 1-year follow-up ($p < 0.001$). The rate of excellent and good results was 81 % (26 of 32) among all the cases. The incidence of excellent and good results in the subgroups with two-part, three-part, and four-part fractures was 91.7 % (11 out of 12), 80 % (12 out of 15), and 60 % (3 out of 5), respectively ($p = 0.0525$). Two patients had loosening of the pins, and one patient had a collapsed humeral head: all three patients eventually underwent hemiarthroplasty. There was no infection and impingement.

There are few studies comparing percutaneous pinning and other forms of treatment. Kralinger et al. [85] compared 12 patients treated with plate and screw with 71 patients treated with percutaneous pinning for two-/three-/four-part fractures and fracture-dislocations. Patients suffered significantly more AVN after open treatment: five patients (50 %) versus eight patients (12.7 %) in the percutaneous group.

We compared the results of two groups of 20 patients, one treated with percutaneous pinning and the other with hemiarthroplasty in complex three-/four-fragment fractures. Functional results were significantly better in the first group (Constant score 72.35 ± 13.26 vs 48.1 ± 16.26; modified Constant score 83 % ± 11 % vs 64 % ± 22 %) without the involvement of factors such as age, type of fracture, delay in surgery, and complications. As regards complications, in the first group we reported two cases of AVN (without symptoms) and one case of reflex sympathetic dystrophy, thrombophlebitis, nonunion, and one pin mobilization; in the second group we reported three cases of reflex sympathetic dystrophy, one thrombophlebitis, and one subscapularis deficit [86].

Conclusions

Even if proximal humeral fractures are among the most common fractures in the world, we are far from being able to define one particular treatment as the gold standard.

Recently the real necessity for surgical treatment has been discussed [87]. Surgeons' experience and confidence with a particular surgical technique are still very important aspects and often determine what type of surgery is performed. In fact it is difficult to evaluate the functional results. For example, Olerud, dealing with four-part fractures, compared functional results after nonsurgical treatment with those obtained after hemiarthroplasty at the final 2-year follow-up; the quality of life was significantly better in the second group compared to the first one, but there were no significant differences regarding the Constant score or range of motion [88].

Furthermore it is often hard to compare results between different studies. A proper evaluation is probably more accurate if we consider the complications associated with each type of surgery.

After the initial enthusiasm for LCP because of its high stability [89–91], many studies have been published stressing high complication rates [22–25, 92] and important rates of additional surgery, reaching even 30 % [93]. The articular screw perforation is the complication the surgeons fear most because of the possible disruption of the glenoid surface [92].

Moreover, there are some studies that are rediscovering the conservative treatment. A randomized controlled trial comparing tension-band wiring with nonoperative treatment found no significant difference in outcome at 1, 3, and 5 years of follow-up [94]. Fjalestad et al. [95] found no evidence of a difference in functional outcomes at 1-year follow-up between surgical treatment with LCP and conservative treatment of displaced proximal humeral fractures in elderly patients. Sanders reports that results of ASES and patient satisfaction scores were also tending toward nonsurgical treatment, and moreover surgical treatment had a higher complication rate, requiring more additional treatment [96].

Among the different treatment options, percutaneous pinning seems to be potentially associated with better functional results than conservative treatment but is also associated with lower complication risks than LCP. To be specific, it is known that varus impacted fractures usually have a poor prognosis if nonsurgically treated [75] and are prone to complications if treated with LCP [97–99]. Twenty-five degrees of varus displacement seems to be a reasonable indication for surgery [75].

We believe that what makes percutaneous pinning advantageous over other surgical treatments is the complete absence of hardware around the shoulder after the treatment has been completed: around 50 % of secondary surgery after LCP osteosynthesis is represented only by hardware removal and release [93]. Even if we cannot state that percutaneous pinning reduces AVN risk, it certainly does not lead to its increase, and patients better tolerate AVN without hardware such as plates and screws [9]. Even Humerusblock and Humerusblock NG are associated with these advantages, but they need surgery to remove the device screwed to the humeral shaft.

In order not to leave hardware in place permanently even in cases of complex fractures, open reduction followed by percutaneous pinning can be performed [100]. Even though several studies have shown that clinical results can be satisfactory even in the presence of a nonanatomic reduction of the fracture [11, 12, 15, 101], we believe that this is mandatory if good surgery is to be performed [52]: if the surgeon cannot achieve a good closed reduction, an open one must be performed.

The use of pins with a longer thread augmented by an external fixator has allowed us to feel increasingly confident about a surgical technique that is not widely used. We do believe it has advantages compared to internal fixation in cases of two- and three-part fractures, where there is a high risk of AVN and in patients below the age of 65.

References

1. Bohler J (1962) Percutane osteosynthese mit dem rontgenbildverstarker. Wien Klin Wochenschr 74: 485–487
2. Hawkins RJ, Kiefer GN (1987) Internal fixation techniques for proximal humeral fractures. Clin Orthop Relat Res 223:77–85
3. Angehrn F, Schultheiss HR (1986) Percutaneous drill wire osteosynthesis of fractures of the proximal humerus. Z Unfallchir Versicherungsmed Berufskr 79:155–160
4. Hagg O, Lundberg B (1984) Aspects of prognostic factors in comminuted and dislocated proximal humerus fractures. In: Bateman JE, Welsh PR (eds) Surgery of the shoulder. BC Decker, Philadelphia
5. Kristiansen B, Kofoed H (1988) Transcutaneous reduction and external fixation of displaced fractures of the proximal humerus. A controlled clinical trial. J Bone Joint Surg Br 70:821–824
6. Kristiansen B, Barfod G, Bredesen J et al (1987) Epidemiology of proximal humeral fractures. Acta Orthop Scand 58:75–77
7. Neer CS II (1984) Fractures about the shoulder. In: Rockwood CA Jr, Green DP (eds) Fractures in adults, vol I, 2nd edn, Neer CS II. JB Lippincott, Philadelphia
8. Court-Brown CM, Garg A, McQueen MM (2001) The epidemiology of proximal humeral fractures. Acta Orthop Scand 72:365–371
9. Harrison AK, Gruson KI, Zmistowski B et al (2012) Intermediate outcomes following percutaneous fixation of proximal humeral fractures. J Bone Joint Surg Am 94:1223–1228
10. Monga P, Verma R, Sharma VK (2009) Closed reduction and external fixation for displaced proximal humeral fractures. J Orthop Surg (Hong Kong) 17:142–145
11. Chen CY, Chao EK, Tu YK, Ueng SW, Shih CH (1998) Closed management and percutaneous fixation of unstable proximal humerus fractures. J Trauma 45:1039–1045
12. Jaberg H, Warner JJ, Jakob RP (1992) Percutaneous stabilization of unstable fractures of the humerus. J Bone Joint Surg Am 74:508–515
13. Misra A, Kapur R, Maffulli N (2001) Complex proximal humeral fractures in adults – a systematic review of management. Injury 32:363–372
14. Neer CS (1970) Displaced proximal humeral fractures. I. Classification and evaluation. J Bone Joint Surg Am 52:1077–1089
15. Resch H, Povacz P, Fröhlich R, Wambacher M (1997) Percutaneous fixation of three- and four-part fractures of the proximal humerus. J Bone Joint Surg Br 79:295–300
16. Bogner R, Hübner C, Matis N, Auffarth A, Lederer S, Resch H (2008) Minimally-invasive treatment of three- and four-part fractures of the proximal humerus in elderly patients. J Bone Joint Surg Br 90:1602–1607
17. Cuny C, Scarlat MM, Irrazi M et al (2008) The Telegraph nail for proximal humeral fractures: a prospective four-year study. J Shoulder Elbow Surg 17:539–545
18. Frangen TM, Müller EJ, Dudda M, Arens S, Muhr G, Kälicke T (2007) Proximal humeral fractures in geriatric patients. Is the angle-stable plate osteosynthesis really a breakthrough? Acta Orthop Belg 73:571–579
19. Herscovici D, Saunders DT, Johnson MP, Sanders R, DiPasquale T (2000) Percutaneous fixation of proximal humeral fractures. Clin Orthop Relat Res 375:97–104
20. Qidwai SA (2001) Treatment of proximal humeral fractures by intramedullary Kirschner wires. J Trauma 50:1090–1095
21. Smith AM, Mardones RM, Sperling JW, Cofield RH (2007) Early complications of operatively treated proximal humeral fractures. J Shoulder Elbow Surg 16:14–24
22. Greiner S, Kääb MJ, Haas NP, Bail HJ (2009) Humeral head necrosis rate at mid-term follow-up after open reduction and angular stable plate fixation for proximal humeral fractures. Injury 40: 186–191
23. Thanasas C, Kontakis G, Angoules A, Limb D, Giannoudis P (2009) Treatment of proximal humerus fractures with locking plates: a systematic review. J Shoulder Elbow Surg 18:837–844
24. Clavert P, Adam P, Bevort A, Bonnomet F, Kempf JF (2010) Pitfalls and complications with locking plate for proximal humerus fracture. J Shoulder Elbow Surg 19:489–494
25. Südkamp N, Bayer J, Hepp P et al (2009) Open reduction and internal fixation of proximal humeral fractures with use of the locking proximal humerus plate. Results of a prospective, multicenter, observational study. J Bone Joint Surg Am 91:1320–1328
26. Iannotti JP, Gabriel JP, Schneck SL, Evans BG, Misra S (1992) The normal glenohumeral relationships. An anatomical study of one hundred and forty shoulders. J Bone Joint Surg Am 74:491–500
27. Boileau P, Walch G (1997) The three-dimensional geometry of the proximal humerus. Implications for

surgical technique and prosthetic design. J Bone Joint Surg Br 79:857–865

28. Harrold F, Wigderowitz C (2012) A three-dimensional analysis of humeral head retroversion. J Shoulder Elbow Surg 21:612–617
29. Rowles DJ, McGrory JE (2001) Percutaneous pinning of the proximal part of the humerus. An anatomic study. J Bone Joint Surg Am 83-A: 1695–1699
30. Burkhead WZ, Scheinberg RR, Box G (1992) Surgical anatomy of the axillary nerve. J Shoulder Elbow Surg 1:31–36
31. Kamineni S, Ankem H, Sanghavi S (2004) Anatomical considerations for percutaneous proximal humeral fracture fixation. Injury 35: 1133–1136
32. Burkhart SS, Nassar J, Schenck RC, Wirth MA (1996) Clinical and anatomic considerations in the use of a new anterior inferior subaxillary nerve arthroscopy portal. Arthroscopy 12:634–637
33. Resch H, Hübner C, Schwaiger R (2001) Minimally invasive reduction and osteosynthesis of articular fractures of the humeral head. Injury 32(Suppl 1):SA25–SA32
34. Calvo E, de Miguel I, de la Cruz JJ, López-Martín N (2007) Percutaneous fixation of displaced proximal humeral fractures: indications based on the correlation between clinical and radiographic results. J Shoulder Elbow Surg 16:774–781
35. Kocialkowski A, Wallace WA (1990) Closed percutaneous K-wire stabilization for displaced fractures of the surgical neck of the humerus. Injury 21: 209–212
36. Yu Z, Zheng L, Wang Y, Zhang Y, Zhang X, Ma B (2010) Functional and radiological evaluations of unstable displaced proximal humeral fractures treated with closed reduction and percutaneous pinning fixation. Eur Surg Res 45:138–145
37. Koval KJ, Blair B, Takei R, Kummer FJ, Zuckerman JD (1996) Surgical neck fractures of the proximal humerus: a laboratory evaluation of ten fixation techniques. J Trauma 40:778–783
38. Wheeler DL, Colville MR (1997) Biomechanical comparison of intramedullary and percutaneous pin fixation for proximal humeral fracture fixation. J Orthop Trauma 11:363–367
39. Swiontkowski MF, Harrington RM, Keller TS, Van Patten PK (1987) Torsion and bending analysis of internal fixation techniques for femoral neck fractures: the role of implant design and bone density. J Orthop Res 5:433–444
40. Lill H, Hepp P, Korner J et al (2003) Proximal humeral fractures: how stiff should an implant be? A comparative mechanical study with new implants in human specimens. Arch Orthop Trauma Surg 123:74–81
41. Williams GR, Wong KL (2000) Two-part and three-part fractures: open reduction and internal fixation versus closed reduction and percutaneous pinning. Orthop Clin North Am 31:1–21
42. Soete PJ, Clayson PE, Costenoble VH (1999) Transitory percutaneous pinning in fractures of the proximal humerus. J Shoulder Elbow Surg 8:569–573
43. Fenichel I, Oran A, Burstein G, Perry Pritsch M (2006) Percutaneous pinning using threaded pins as a treatment option for unstable two- and three-part fractures of the proximal humerus: a retrospective study. Int Orthop 30:153–157
44. Aschauer E, Resch H, Hübner C (2007) Percutaneous osteosynthesis of humeral head fractures. Oper Orthop Traumatol 19:276–293
45. Brunner A, Weller K, Thormann S, Jöckel JA, Babst R (2010) Closed reduction and minimally invasive percutaneous fixation of proximal humerus fractures using the Humerusblock. J Orthop Trauma 24: 407–413
46. Jöckel JA, Brunner A, Thormann S, Babst R (2010) Elastic stabilisation of proximal humeral fractures with a new percutaneous angular stable fixation device (ButtonFix(®)): a preliminary report. Arch Orthop Trauma Surg 130:1397–1403
47. Brunner A, Resch H, Babst R et al (2012) The Humerusblock NG: a new concept for stabilization of proximal humeral fractures and its biomechanical evaluation. Arch Orthop Trauma Surg 132:985–992
48. Jiang C, Zhu Y, Wang M, Rong G (2007) Biomechanical comparison of different pin configurations during percutaneous pinning for the treatment of proximal humeral fractures. J Shoulder Elbow Surg 16:235–239
49. Naidu SH, Bixler B, Capo JT, Moulton MJ, Radin A (1997) Percutaneous pinning of proximal humerus fractures: a biomechanical study. Orthopedics 20:1073–1076
50. Kralinger F, Gschwentner M, Wambacher M, Smekal V, Haid C (2008) Proximal humeral fractures: what is semi-rigid? Biomechanical properties of semi-rigid implants, a biomechanical cadaver based evaluation. Arch Orthop Trauma Surg 128: 205–210
51. Castoldi F, Bonasia DE, Blonna D et al (2010) The stability of percutaneous fixation of proximal humeral fractures. J Bone Joint Surg Am 92(Suppl 2): 90–97
52. Magovern B, Ramsey ML (2008) Percutaneous fixation of proximal humerus fractures. Orthop Clin North Am 39:405–416
53. Clifford PC (1980) Fractures of the neck of the humerus: a review of the late results. Injury 12: 91–95
54. Roberts VI, Komarasamy B, Pandey R (2012) Modification of the Resch procedure: a new technique and its results in managing three- and four-part proximal humeral fractures. J Bone Joint Surg Br 94:1409–1413
55. Stableforth PG (1984) Four-part fractures of the neck of the humerus. J Bone Joint Surg Br 66:104–108
56. Svend-Hansen H (1974) Displaced proximal humeral fractures. A review of 49 patients. Acta Orthop Scand 45:359–364

57. Keener JD, Parsons BO, Flatow EL, Rogers K, Williams GR, Galatz LM (2007) Outcomes after percutaneous reduction and fixation of proximal humeral fractures. J Shoulder Elbow Surg 16: 330–338
58. Jakob RP, Miniaci A, Anson PS, Jaberg H, Osterwalder A, Ganz R (1991) Four-part valgus impacted fractures of the proximal humerus. J Bone Joint Surg Br 73:295–298
59. Resch H, Beck E, Bayley I (1995) Reconstruction of the valgus-impacted humeral head fracture. J Shoulder Elbow Surg 4:73–80
60. Robinson CM, Page RS (2003) Severely impacted valgus proximal humeral fractures. Results of operative treatment. J Bone Joint Surg Am 85-A:1647–1655
61. Carbone S, Tangari M, Gumina S, Postacchini R, Campi A, Postacchini F (2012) Percutaneous pinning of three- or four-part fractures of the proximal humerus in elderly patients in poor general condition: MIROS® versus traditional pinning. Int Orthop 36:1267–1273
62. Hertel R (2005) Fractures of the proximal humerus in osteoporotic bone. Osteoporos Int 16(Suppl 2): S65–S72
63. Bastian JD, Hertel R (2008) Initial post-fracture humeral head ischemia does not predict development of necrosis. J Shoulder Elbow Surg 17:2–8
64. Zhang J, Ebraheim N, Lause GE (2012) Surgical treatment of proximal humeral fracture with external fixator. J Shoulder Elbow Surg 21:882–886
65. Kristiansen B (1989) Treatment of displaced fractures of the proximal humerus: transcutaneous reduction and Hoffmann's external fixation. Injury 20:195–199
66. Ebraheim NA, Patil V, Husain A (2007) Mini-external fixation of two- and three-part proximal humerus fractures. Acta Orthop Belg 73:437–442
67. Seyhan M, Kocaoglu B, Nalbantoglu U, Aydin N, Guven O (2012) Technique of Kirschner wire reduction and fixation of displaced two-part valgus angulated proximal humerus fractures at the surgical neck. J Orthop Trauma 26:e46–e50
68. Kristiansen B, Kofoed H (1987) External fixation of displaced fractures of the proximal humerus. Technique and preliminary results. J Bone Joint Surg Br 69:643–646
69. Kristiansen B (1987) External fixation of proximal humerus fracture. Clinical and cadaver study of pinning technique. Acta Orthop Scand 58:645–648
70. Martin C, Guillen M, Lopez G (2006) Treatment of 2- and 3-part fractures of the proximal humerus using external fixation: a retrospective evaluation of 62 patients. Acta Orthop 77:275–278
71. Blonna D, Castoldi F, Scelsi M, Rossi R, Falcone G, Assom M (2010) The hybrid technique: potential reduction in complications related to pins mobilization in the treatment of proximal humeral fractures. J Shoulder Elbow Surg 19:1218–1229
72. Murachovsky J, Ikemoto RY, Nascimento LG, Fujiki EN, Milani C, Warner JJ (2006) Pectoralis major tendon reference (PMT): a new method for accurate restoration of humeral length with hemiarthroplasty for fracture. J Shoulder Elbow Surg 15:675–678
73. Handoll HH, Ollivere BJ, Rollins KE (2012) Interventions for treating proximal humeral fractures in adults. Cochrane Database Syst Rev (12): CD000434
74. Mazet R Jr (1943) Migration of a Kirschner wire from the shoulder region into the lung – report of two cases. J Boint Joint Surg Am 25:477–483
75. Blonna D, Rossi R, Fantino G, Maiello A, Assom M, Castoldi F (2009) The impacted varus (A2.2) proximal humeral fracture in elderly patients: is minimal fixation justified? A case control study. J Shoulder Elbow Surg 18:545–552
76. Glauser F, Kremens V (1956) Unusual sequela following pinning of medial clavicular fracture. Am J Roentgenol Radium Ther Nucl Med 76:1066–1069
77. Tristan TA, Daughtridge TG (1964) Migration of a metallic pin from the humerus into the lung. N Engl J Med 270:987–989
78. Lyons FA, Rockwood CA (1990) Migration of pins used in operations on the shoulder. J Bone Joint Surg Am 72:1262–1267
79. Freund E, Nachman R, Gips H, Hiss J (2007) Migration of a Kirschner wire used in the fixation of a subcapital humeral fracture, causing cardiac tamponade: case report and review of literature. Am J Forensic Med Pathol 28:155–156
80. Hertel R, Hempfing A, Stiehler M, Leunig M (2004) Predictors of humeral head ischemia after intracapsular fracture of the proximal humerus. J Shoulder Elbow Surg 13:427–433
81. Wijgman AJ, Roolker W, Patt TW, Raaymakers EL, Marti RK (2002) Open reduction and internal fixation of three and four-part fractures of the proximal part of the humerus. J Bone Joint Surg Am 84-A:1919–1925
82. Gerber C, Hersche O, Berberat C (1998) The clinical relevance of posttraumatic avascular necrosis of the humeral head. J Shoulder Elbow Surg 7:586–590
83. Shabtai L, Dolkart O, Chechik O et al (2013) Incidence and severity of infections after closed reduction and external fixation of proximal humeral fractures. J Orthop Trauma 27:e81–e86
84. Blonna D, Barbasetti N, Banche G, Cuffini AM, Bellato E, Massè A, Marenco S, Battiston B, Castoldi F (2014) Incidence and risk factors for acute infection after proximal humeral fractures: a multicenter study. J Shoulder Elbow Surg 23(4):528–35
85. Kralinger F, Irenberger A, Lechner C, Wambacher M, Golser K, Sperner G (2006) Comparison of open versus percutaneous treatment for humeral head fracture. Unfallchirurg 109:406–410
86. Bellato E, Scelsi M, Marini E, Mortera S, Marenco S, Blonna D, Assom M, Castoldi F (2011) Protesi versus sintesi nelle fratture complesse del terzo prossimale d'omero. Minerva Ortop Traumatol 62:19–27
87. Murray IR, Amin AK, White TO, Robinson CM (2011) Proximal humeral fractures: current concepts in classification, treatment and outcomes. J Bone Joint Surg Br 93:1–11

88. Olerud P, Ahrengart L, Ponzer S, Saving J, Tidermark J (2011) Hemiarthroplasty versus nonoperative treatment of displaced 4-part proximal humeral fractures in elderly patients: a randomized controlled trial. J Shoulder Elbow Surg 20:1025–1033
89. Moonot P, Ashwood N, Hamlet M (2007) Early results for treatment of three- and four-part fractures of the proximal humerus using the PHILOS plate system. J Bone Joint Surg Br 89:1206–1209
90. Fankhauser F, Boldin C, Schippinger G, Haunschmid C, Szyszkowitz R (2005) A new locking plate for unstable fractures of the proximal humerus. Clin Orthop Relat Res 430:176–181
91. Ricchetti ET, Warrender WJ, Abboud JA (2010) Use of locking plates in the treatment of proximal humerus fractures. J Shoulder Elbow Surg 19: 66–75
92. Jost B, Spross C, Grehn H, Gerber C (2013) Locking plate fixation of fractures of the proximal humerus: analysis of complications, revision strategies and outcome. J Shoulder Elbow Surg 22:542–549
93. Olerud P, Ahrengart L, Ponzer S, Saving J, Tidermark J (2011) Internal fixation versus nonoperative treatment of displaced 3-part proximal humeral fractures in elderly patients: a randomized controlled trial. J Shoulder Elbow Surg 20:747–755
94. Zyto K, Ahrengart L, Sperber A, Törnkvist H (1997) Treatment of displaced proximal humeral fractures in elderly patients. J Bone Joint Surg Br 79: 412–417
95. Fjalestad T, Hole M, Hovden IA, Blücher J, Strømsøe K (2012) Surgical treatment with an angular stable plate for complex displaced proximal humeral fractures in elderly patients: a randomized controlled trial. J Orthop Trauma 26:98–106
96. Sanders RJ, Thissen LG, Teepen JC, van Kampen A, Jaarsma RL (2011) Locking plate versus nonsurgical treatment for proximal humeral fractures: better midterm outcome with nonsurgical treatment. J Shoulder Elbow Surg 20:1118–1124
97. Solberg BD, Moon CN, Franco DP, Paiement GD (2009) Locked plating of 3- and 4-part proximal humerus fractures in older patients: the effect of initial fracture pattern on outcome. J Orthop Trauma 23:113–119
98. Hardeman F, Bollars P, Donnelly M, Bellemans J, Nijs S (2012) Predictive factors for functional outcome and failure in angular stable osteosynthesis of the proximal humerus. Injury 43:153–158
99. Krappinger D, Bizzotto N, Riedmann S, Kammerlander C, Hengg C, Kralinger FS (2011) Predicting failure after surgical fixation of proximal humerus fractures. Injury 42:1283–1288
100. Darder A, Sanchis V, Gastaldi E, Gomar F (1993) Four-part displaced proximal humeral fractures: operative treatment using Kirschner wires and a tension band. J Orthop Trauma 7:497–505
101. Neer CS (1970) Displaced proximal humeral fractures. II. Treatment of three-part and four-part displacement. J Bone Joint Surg Am 52:1090–1103

ORIF in Three-/Four-Part Fractures

7

Enrico Guerra, Daniele Fabbri, Graziano Bettelli, Alessandro Marinelli, Michele Cavaciocchi, and Roberto Rotini

7.1 Introduction

Proximal humerus fractures represent about 5 % of all fractures [1], and recent studies show that their incidence in the population over 75 years rises exponentially, with a probable increase of 250 % in the next 30 years [2–5]. Three-part and four-part fractures represent a share of 13–16 % of the total amount of proximal humerus fractures [4]. It is troublesome to indicate a universally accepted method of treatment, mainly because retrospective studies and meta-analyses have not yet clarified if one protocol of treatment is superior to others.

At the present time a number of treatments for displaced three- and four-part proximal humeral fractures are available, everyone with limits and advantages. The most employed are:

- *Conservative treatment*: This approach is reserved to patients in whom a surgical treatment would be hazardous. Kraulis and Hunter in 1977 and then Stableforth [6] have shown that in three- and four-part fractures healing can be hampered by the interposition of soft tissues, and the persistence of pain and functional limitation causes a delay in recovering a joint motion that can allow to perform the activities of daily living [6–10]. Moreover, worse clinical index results and lower ROM values have been recorded compared to the operated patients [11].
- *Reduction and fixation*: Several techniques can be employed, like open, or mini-open, or percutaneous pinning. Some authors advocate external fixation (in two-part or three-part fractures); others advise endomedullary nailing or plate fixation possibly together with bone sutures. Many cadaver studies have shown a superior stability and stress resistance of LCP compared to other fixation devices [7, 8, 12].
- *Shoulder prosthesis*: This option was indicated by Neer as the gold standard in four-part fractures, whereas nowadays it is usually considered as the last choice in case of severe comminution preventing a correct reconstruction of the joint surface or of too high risk of head necrosis. Hemiarthroplasty with a solid tuberosity reconstruction has been the traditional construct, while in the recent years an alternative option has been represented by reverse prosthesis, which allows more reproducible functional results and has to be reserved to elderly (over 70 years) patients [9, 13].

Having these premises in mind, it is essential to be able to correctly diagnose the type of fracture, to examine the vascular support and the level of head necrosis risk, to predict the advantages that the patient can take of the different

E. Guerra (✉) • D. Fabbri • G. Bettelli • A. Marinelli
M. Cavaciocchi • R. Rotini
Shoulder and Elbow Surgical Unit,
Rizzoli Orthopaedic Institute,
Via G.C. Pupilli, nr 1, Bologna 40136, Italy
e-mail: enrico.guerra@ior.it; graziano.bettelli@ior.it; alessandro.marinelli@ior.it; michele.cavaciocchi@ior.it; roberto.rotini@ior.it

F. Castoldi et al. (eds.), *Simple and Complex Fractures of the Humerus*,
DOI 10.1007/978-88-470-5307-6_7, © Springer-Verlag Italia 2015

treatments, and finally to indicate the best one. In this chapter, open reduction and internal fixation of three- and four-part fractures by plate and screws will be described.

7.2 Classifications

Codman was the first who described proximal humerus fractures according to the principle of division into four parts: humeral head, greater tuberosity, lesser tuberosity, and humeral shaft [14]. Neer in 1970, adopting this concept, developed a classification system describing as part of a fracture a fragment with dislocation of at least 1 cm and/or a rotation of at least 45° compared to the normal anatomic position. This classification, apparently easy and immediate, is based on the number of fragments, their position, the presence of glenohumeral dislocation, and the presence of lesions of the articular surface. In the conclusions of his work, Neer opened the questions about the treatment of the most difficult and displaced fractures, with the proposal of comparative studies among the different techniques of reduction and fixation for three-part fractures, while he advocated hemiarthroplasty for four-part fractures, which would otherwise benefit from "new techniques to be developed in the future" [3]. Neer's wise foresight is also evident in his final consideration: "comminuted fractures will grow in time, mainly because they will involve more and more elderly people, but apart from the technique to be chosen, a correct identification of the fracture remains unescapable" [3].

Neer's classification has long been criticized and revisited [15], but it is still now widely employed and appreciated in the clinical practice. After his work, several authors have developed more detailed and maybe complex classifications. A step forward is represented by the work by Hertel [5] who widened Codman classification (Lego description system) and described seven criteria to analyze the prognosis of proximal humerus fracture, obtaining a positive predictive power of 97 % [16]:

1. Length of metaphyseal calcar (limit 8 mm)
2. Integrity of the "medial hinge"
3. Amount of tuberosities displacement
4. Amount of varus or valgus angular displacement of the humeral head
5. Glenohumeral dislocation
6. Impacted fracture or head-splitting lesion involving over 20 % of the articular surface
7. Bone mechanical quality

The Association for the Study of Internal Fixation (AO-ASIF) [17] has developed an alphanumeric classification system which divides these fractures into articular and extra-articular. It is more complex than the systems by Neer and by Hertel, and its aim is to describe an international nomenclature of proximal humerus fractures. This classification takes into special account the vascular supply of the humeral head, separating fractures into three main groups (A, B, and C) based on an increasing risk of head necrosis. Each of these groups is divided into subgroups. Although this classification system allows a detailed description of each fracture pattern with a universal language, it is too complex to be used in the clinical practice; moreover, it is not correlated with the treatment indications [15]. Many studies have shown the low reliability and reproducibility of these systems [14–20].

It is also important to bear in mind that the classifications in use at present are mainly based on radiographic evaluation, whereas the important step forward in the study of complex proximal humerus fractures has been the use of CT scan with bi- and tridimensional rendering which allows to precisely know the number, size, and position of the fracture fragments.

The orthopedic surgeon who takes in charge these patients should consider all the abovementioned classifications applying them to a radiographic and CT study.

7.3 Plate Fixation

The rationale of the choice of plate and screw fixation is to seek a better alignment of the fracture fragments compared to what can be obtained with a closed technique and a more stable fixation compared to other systems like K-wires and endomedullary nails.

The first plates used in the past were not dedicated for the proximal humeral anatomy (e.g., AO T-plates); they were flat with oval 4.5 mm holes. During the operation it was necessary to bend them to adapt their shape to the humeral profile. Cancellous screws were used to obtain a better hold in the humeral head; however, the loss of stability frequently evolved in implant mobilization and varus deviation of the humeral epiphysis even without head necrosis.

Similar results were obtained with blade plates and with the first endomedullary nails. In the 1990s, several studies tried to demonstrate the superiority of blade plates or nails over plates or hemiarthroplasty (the only alternative to fixation and also the last resort in the treatment of these fractures) [20–22]. The principle emerging from these experiences was the need of a good reduction of the fragments, mainly the tuberosities, in order to obtain a satisfactory fracture healing [23].

In the early 2000s, the concept of internal fixator began to be applied to the proximal humerus with the appearance of the first dedicated locking plates having the following features:

- Precontoured, so that the surgeon has no longer to bend the plate to adapt it to the humeral anatomy; rather, the plate can act like a template for fracture reduction and anatomy reconstruction supporting the greater tuberosity at the same time.
- Locking screws: the screw head is threaded so that there is a stable connection between the screw and plate, avoiding any risk of screw loosening.
- Head screws are polyaxial in order to be fixed in different parts of the head, affording a superior stability.
- Holes for bone sutures are available, to fix smaller fragments and neutralize the rotator cuff tendon tensile strength; formerly used alone or in connection with endomedullary pins, bone sutures can be firmly connected to a stable construct like a locking plate.

The philosophy of locking plates is based on the point that stability does not rely on a strong hold of the screws in bone. The screws are locked on the plate so that they become part of an internal fixator. There is a definitely lower pullout of screws compared to previous fixation devices, with a relatively lower risk of loss of reduction, head displacement in varus, and nonunion. Specific screws reach the calcar region to support the head on its medial side without damaging the neurovascular structures lying at the inferior border of the subscapularis muscle. The results have been superior compared to non-locking plates: higher strength, less tissue dissection or cuff damage, shorter immobilization time, and lower risk of damage in case of implant removal [8, 23–30].

On these bases, several types of plates have been developed with different screw-plate locking systems or different shapes of the proximal part.

A final field of research in the development of fixation devices has been the study of biomaterials. The plates have been traditionally manufactured in metal alloys like cobalt-chrome, steel, or titanium. Cobalt-chrome assures a high mechanical resistance, but its elastic module is quite different from the bone, and there is a risk of immunologic reactions and release of metal ions [31] possibly leading to metallosis, osteolysis, and pseudotumors. A step forward has been obtained with stainless steel, which joins the qualities of cobalt-chrome with reduced risk of immune reactions or wear. With the advent of titanium however there has been a true step-up in biocompatibility. Titanium has an elastic modulus closer to the bone and a minor tendency to the "starburst artifact" (CT or MRI images distortion) and induces a lower production of granulation tissue. To these qualities unfortunately correspond a high cost, an excessive ductility that can cause complications when removing the locking screws, and a limited malleability in case of the need of intraoperative multiple bending (risk of hardware weakening and breakage).

Nowadays the polyether ether ketone (PEEK) is a new material used for plate manufacturing that the orthopedic surgeons already know (cages for vertebral fusion, bony anchors, etc.). This material can be produced with a variable rate of carbon fibers, modifying its structural properties. PEEK is light when added to 30 % of carbon and has a torsion strength similar to steel and an elastic modulus really close to the cortical bone.

In our department we have developed together with Lima Trauma Inc. a PEEK plate, launched on the market a few years ago, which has the following advantages:

- The holes for the screws are smooth, and there is no predetermined direction for the screw, as its self-threading head cuts a thread in the hole, so creating the locking configuration.
- PEEK is radiolucent, allowing a superior precision of intraoperative image intensifier checking and consolidation evaluation at follow-up.
- Hardware removal remains easy even years after implantation.

Unfortunately a PEEK plate cannot be contoured; therefore, it cannot be modified during surgery, and this makes it unfit for long constructs.

7.4 Surgical Technique

The patient is placed in the beach-chair position. It is unnecessary to have the trunk almost vertical, as for other surgical procedures like shoulder arthroscopy. The head support should be formfitting, best if helmet-shaped, in order to be safe even during traction maneuvers on the distal humerus to obtain fracture reduction. A counterforce support is placed on the iliac wing distal enough not to interfere with arm adduction. The surgical table should allow the removal of the posterior shoulder support so that intraoperative radiographic checking is simpler.

Before preparing the surgical field, it is a good practice to check the position of the patient on the table and of the anesthesiological equipment, to avoid interference with the X-ray machine C-arm and its movements.

When only few assistants are available, it is very useful to have a pneumatic arm holder, which allows to control the arm position during the fracture reduction and fixation.

7.4.1 Surgical Approaches

The surgical approaches described for ORIF of proximal humerus fractures are two: deltopectoral and transdeltoid approach.

7.4.1.1 Deltopectoral Approach

Anterior incision from the tip of the coracoid down to the humeral shaft, following the groove between deltoid and pectoralis major muscles and then the lateral border of the biceps muscle. The distal extension of the incision depends on the extension of the fracture below the surgical neck of the humerus; it is advisable to perform at first the proximal 10 cm of the incision, to dissect the deep layers, and then, once the fracture is exposed, to extend the incision distally as needed.

The cephalic vein once isolated can be displaced both medially (with the pectoralis major) and better laterally (with the deltoid) considering the lower number of collateral branches and the distal course of the vein, crossing the surgical field in case of distal extension of the approach.

The cephalic vein allows the identification of the plane between deltoid and pectoralis major. In young patients with well-developed muscles, it is sometimes more difficult to locate it, as it is deeper and the line of fat tissue surrounding it can be scarce. In case of intraoperative lesions the vein has to be ligated.

The clavipectoral fascia is then incised, and the conjoined tendon (formed by the short head of the biceps and the coracobrachialis) is located and displaced medially. The coracoid osteotomy has to be avoided, as it is worthless in order to enlarge the surgical space and bears a risk of traction and lesion on the musculocutaneous nerve. A smooth tip retractor is placed laterally to the conoid and trapezoid ligaments in the subacromial space to retract the deltoid avoiding its detachment from the clavicle. A partial resection of the coracoacromial ligament is useful to obtain a better view of the epiphyseal area corresponding to the rotator interval.

The lateral side of the humerus is exposed distally, and a partial subperiosteal detachment of the deltoid insertion is performed in order to create the space for the plate.

The tendon of the distal head of the biceps has to be identified just proximal to the pectoralis major insertion on the humerus and followed upward until the fracture fragments.

The subacromiondeltoid and *subscapularis* bursae, where the fracture hematoma is collected, have to be partially removed in order to expose the greater and the lesser tuberosities.

Anterolateral Deltoid Split

An anterolateral skin incision starts just inferior the anterior corner of the acromion and runs distally for about 10 cm. The raphe between the anterior and the lateral deltoid bellies has to be identified and opened. The axillary nerve has to be carefully identified 6–8 cm distal to the acromial edge. A further dissection of the deltoid fibers allows to reach its distal insertion on the humerus, then the tendon has to be subperiosteally detached to free the space for the plate.

Removing the hemorrhagic subacromion-deltoid bursa, a direct access to the proximal humerus is achieved.

7.4.1.2 Transdeltoid Approach

The transdeltoid approach allows an easier manipulation of the greater tuberosity and possibly a better respect of the vascular supply to the lesser tuberosity and the humeral head, as the anterior circumflex artery lies close to the lower edge of the subscapularis muscle as well as its ascendant anterolateral branch which runs proximally along the long head of the biceps groove. The downside/disadvantage of this approach however is a higher aggressiveness on the deltoid muscle, an increased risk of iatrogenic lesions of the axillary nerve, and the limited ability to control the calcar area, which is a key point of the fracture reduction.

None of the approaches has been demonstrated to be superior in terms of incidence of necrosis of the humeral head or of vascular or neurological complications; however, the deltopectoral approach allows a better conservation of the deltoid force as this muscle is less damaged [26, 32].

In our experience the deltopectoral approach has to be preferred as it is the most versatile approach to deal with all the different fracture patterns with a limited surgical aggressiveness. Also the possible future plate removal has to be considered, when the surgical scar makes identification and isolation of the axillary nerve more difficult and dangerous.

A new *double-incision mini-invasive approach* has been recently introduced. A smaller proximal, usually transdeltoid, incision allows to expose the fracture and to slide the plate in a subcutaneous and submuscular plane. The distal fixation of the plate takes place through a shorter direct incision on the humerus or through multiple stab wounds for percutaneous screw insertion. This less invasive technique needs a dedicated instrumentation, and many manufacturers nowadays have developed one. The main indication is a two-part fracture, which is not the subject of the present chapter. It should however be pointed out the lower invasiveness has to be intended not related to the length of the skin incisions, but to the anatomic damage that the surgeon can cause. The percutaneous technique is therefore in our opinion contraindicated in three- and four-part fractures, where the aim to obtain an anatomic reduction in the respect of the periosteal/tendon connections of the bony fragments often requires a series of adjustments of the surgical steps case by case.

7.4.2 Indications for Open Fracture Reduction and Internal Fixation with Plate and Screws (ORIF)

The indications for open reduction and internal fixation with plate and screws (ORIF) are in our opinion all the proximal humerus fractures in which the dislocation of the fragments does not allow to adopt a conservative treatment, considering the age of the patient and his or her functional needs.

The classification of proximal humeral fractures is a debated and complicated topic. The ideal classification system should allow to include whatever fracture in homogeneous groups according to prognosis and treatment and should be simple and reproducible. However, the wide variety of fractures together with the different classes of patients and the difficulties in interpreting the radiographic images make this task quite challenging.

In our unit we follow the Neer and the Codman Lego classifications for the decision-making and the AO Muller classification for scientific purposes of data collection. We examine the predictive factors of head necrosis as described by

Hertel (calcar length, integrity of the medial hinge, amount of tuberosities dislocation, valgus/varus deformity, dislocation of the humeral head, head splitting, bone quality).

Whenever the standard radiograms, even of adequate quality, do not allow a correct and safe evaluation, we elect to obtain a CT scan. Only the multiplanar renderings of CT allow in our opinion to identify the anatomic deformities and in the younger patients also to analyze fractures that had been judged as well aligned. A CT scan is also essential for surgical planning, and having in mind the aspects of a fracture enables the surgeon to foresee which maneuvers will be necessary for fragment reduction, which and how many fragments he will find, and where it will be necessary to place an osteosuture and to decide if bone grafts or a prosthesis equipment could be necessary.

A shoulder prosthesis should indeed always be available in the surgical theater, as also in relatively young patients with seemingly simple fractures, it may happen that intraoperative difficulties and low bone quality make this choice unavoidable.

7.4.3 Surgical Patterns

Three- or four-part fractures of the proximal humerus can grossly be separated in three different patterns:

1. Three- or four-part fracture without varus or valgus deviation
2. Three- or four-part fracture with valgus deviation
3. Three- or four-part fracture with varus deviation

7.4.3.1 Three- or Four-Part Fracture Without Varus or Valgus Deviation (Fig. 7.1)

The tendons of the rotator cuff dislocate the bone fragments. The deltoid and the pectoralis major muscles stabilize the position of the humeral shaft if there are no distal lines of fracture.

The shape and the position of the fragments have to be analyzed on CT scan before surgery.

In three-part fractures the humeral epiphysis is continuous with the greater or the lesser tuberosity, and this determines respectively an external or internal rotation, while the fractured tuberosities are dislocated along the line of traction of the supraspinatus-infraspinatus (greater tuberosity) or of the subscapularis (lesser tuberosity) (Fig. 7.1a).

After excision of the hemorrhagic bursal tissue, the fracture is opened. The hematoma should be gently removed, taking care not to discard minor bony fragments. If present, minor fragments are not always amenable to conservation and fixation, but it is important to consider them when performing the reduction to avoid the research of an impossible bone congruence. It should be borne in mind that the bone fragments are always brittle, and it is easy to further complicate the fracture pattern producing new lines of fracture during the reduction maneuvers, even in young patients.

Before attempting a reduction it is necessary to obtain the control of the greater and lesser tuberosities, placing sutures which can aid in tractioning the tuberosities to the shaft. For this purpose reinforced sutures size 2 (*FiberWire*, *HiFi*, *ORTHOCORD*, *ULTRABRAID*, etc.) can be used or in alternative nonresorbable sutures of higher caliber (size 5) which have the same resistance but lower cost and less tendency to cut the bony fragments when tractioned, due to the higher diameter.

When the tuberosities are consistent enough, the sutures are better placed through thin holes made in the bone by a 1.6 mm K-wire that allow an easier and less traumatic passage through. The fragments should be carefully debrided only along the fracture line, not to interfere with the healing process with a too aggressive debridement. Never tear out any rotator cuff tendon from the fragments in order to achieve a better reduction.

The next step is attempting the fracture reduction; for this purpose it is useful to place a Lambotte bone-holding forceps around the proximal humerus shaft. To do this it is useful to open

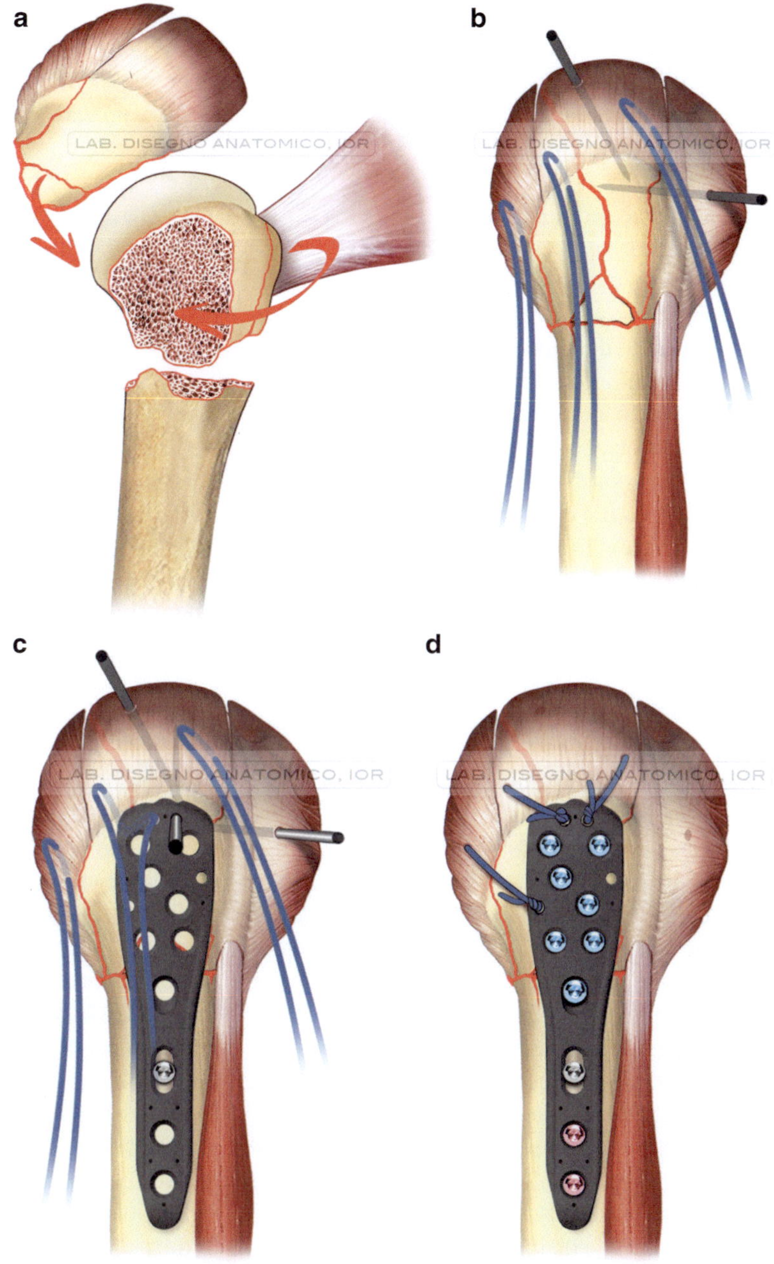

Fig. 7.1 Graphical representation of three- or four-part fracture without varus or valgus deviation. The DiPhos PEEK Lima Corporate plate is represented (Anatomical School of Anatomical Imaging, University of Bologna, Italy). (**a**) shows the reduction of the greater tuberosity and of the humeral head. Once an acceptable reduction is achived a temporary fixation is performed using wires. (**b**) The plate is then secured to the humerous using screws and non reabsorbable sutures

a narrow space in the area of insertion of the latissimus dorsi tendon, at the level of the released deltoid tendon, and to insert a 2.5 mm K-wire through the humeral head as a joystick to move it in a less traumatic way.

With a combined progressive action on the bone holder that tractions and rotates the shaft, on the sutures and on the joystick wire, the fracture fragments are reduced.

Once a satisfactory alignment is achieved, temporary K-wires can be employed to fix it (Fig. 7.1b) while the plate is applied. The K-wires can be drilled in several ways, but it is important to keep the space for the plate free. Percutaneous placement of the K-wires is discouraged, as this increases the risk of infection. By internal rotation of the limb, it is possible to place the plate on the lateral humeral surface, just lateral to the bicipital groove below the bone holder. Temporarily fix it by K-wires inserted through the plate dedicated holes.

The rotator cuff tendons hide the boundaries of the greater tuberosity, and this can induce the surgeon to place the plate too proximally. It is useful to probe the superior edge of the tuberosity by a needle through the supraspinatus tendon and put the plate at least 5 mm lower.

When the type of fracture does not allow to obtain a temporarily stable reduction by K-wires, it is possible to use the plate as a tool for the reduction (Fig. 7.1c). The bone sutures can be passed through the proximal holes of the plate if they are placed in the correct position. The plate should lie in the central part of the shaft; a screw is inserted in the oval hole and gradually tightened while the joystick wire controls the position of the humeral head; at the same time a traction on the bone sutures progressively pulls the tuberosities under the plate to the shaft. When the alignment of the fragments looks satisfactory, placing some K-wires through the plate holes can stabilize the reduction.

The quality of the reduction and the height of the plate can now be checked by the image intensifier. Having placed one screw in the center of the oval hole allows to slide the plate up or down by about 5 mm without removing it.

Radiographic images are obtained in different degrees of internal and external rotation.

The following step is placing the proximal screws. All the available holes should be exploited using locking screws, which should reach the subchondral bone mainly in the calcar region and in the upper part of the humeral head, where the bone density is higher.

The final step is the distal screw placement. In young patients the cortical screws' holding power is strong enough to ensure stability. If a plastic plate is used and the possible future removal of the screws is therefore free of risks, it is advisable to select locking screws for all of the holes except for the oval one.

The bone sutures if necessary can be tightened to the plate holes. The fixation should be stable when moving the shoulder in all planes in order to allow an early rehabilitation (Fig. 7.1d).

The length of the head screws should be closely checked by the image intensifier both in the anteroposterior view in different rotation angles and in the axillary view.

7.4.3.2 Three- or Four-Part Fracture with Valgus Deviation (Fig. 7.2)

These are very complex, mainly four-part fractures in which the humeral head is separated from the tuberosities and the epiphyseal cancellous bone is crushed between the head displaced in valgus and the metadiaphysis (Fig. 7.2a).

In order to obtain the fracture reduction, the head should be levered up with delicate movements acting on the calcar as a hinge, which is often comminuted and weak.

After removing the fracture hematoma, the greater and the lesser tuberosities which stay over the epiphysis deviated in valgus are identified. As described above, the fragments have to be carefully prepared and bone sutures applied. An incision of the rotator cuff between the fragments of the greater tuberosity is necessary in order to expose the humeral head and push it in varus (Fig. 7.2a part). Several authors suggest to open the rotator interval rather than the cuff. Controlling the head reduction through the rotator interval in our opinion is more difficult and the surgeon's manipulations therefore more aggressive, so this is advisable only in case that the greater tuberosity is a single large fragment separated from the lesser tuberosity. On the other side, a limited section of the supraspinatus allows to avoid surgical lesions of the pulley and of the richly vascularized area of the long head of the biceps, gaining a direct lateral view of the epiphysis and the diaphysis, which makes the reduction easier.

After placing the Lambotte forceps as described above, it is possible to proceed to the reduction, which requires a combined action. While the assistant tractions the shaft acting on the Lambotte forceps, the surgeon by a straight retractor gently elevates the head (Fig. 7.2b).

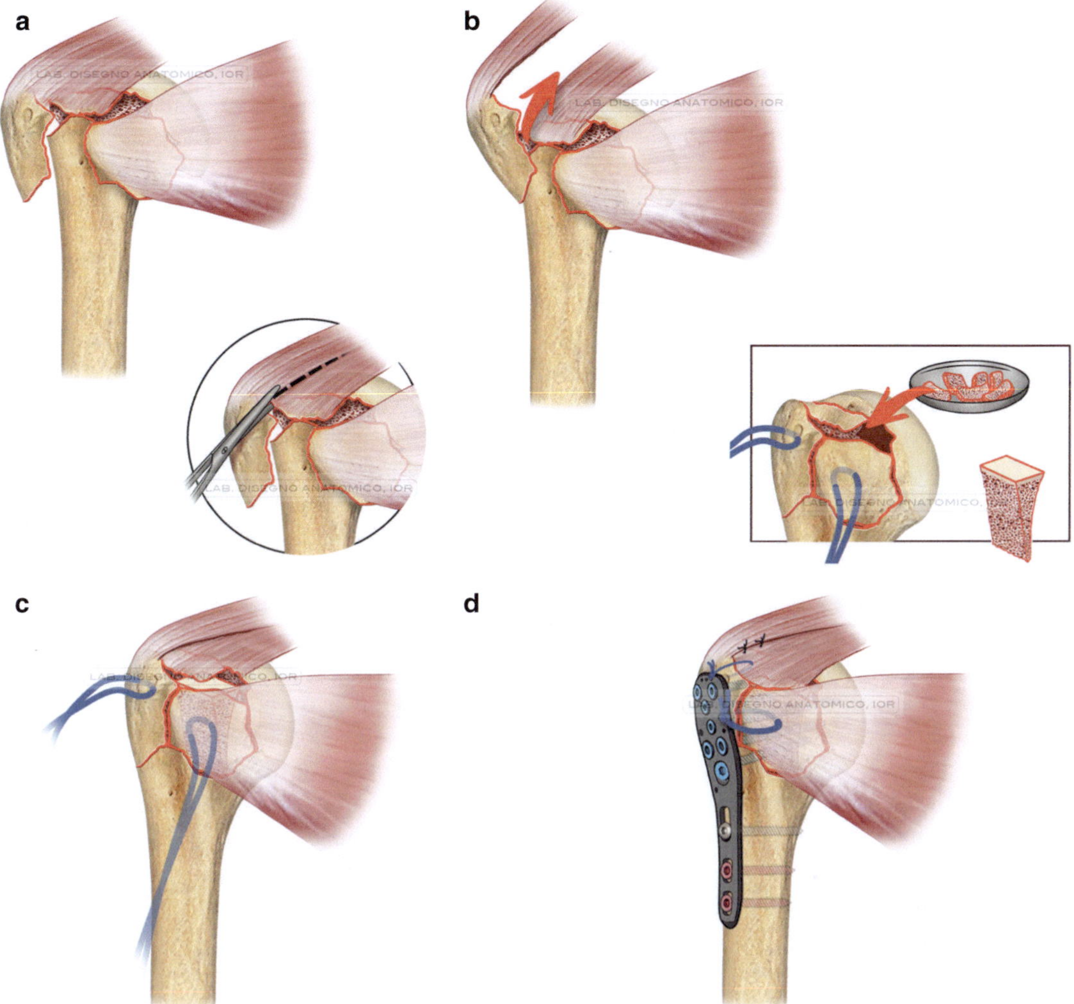

Fig. 7.2 Graphical representation of three- or four-part fracture with valgus deviation. The DiPhos PEEK Lima Corporate plate is represented (Anatomical School of Anatomical Imaging, University of Bologna, Italy). In some cases of complex fractures (**a**) the plate can be fixed to the humeral head first (**b**) and than a pre-countor plate is used to reduced the humeral head to the dyaphisis (**c**)

The bone loss in this area often prevents the maintenance of the reduction and needs augmentation. No type of graft has proven superior to others in this setting; anyway its application is necessary [33].

The graft should be mechanically strong to support the head, correctly sized in order to get stuck in the medullary canal without sinking, easy to pass through by the screws which have to reach the humeral head, and easy to remove in case of late failure. The type of graft that best fulfills these requirements is a homologous cancellous bone wedge, to be adapted to the patient's anatomy (Fig. 7.2b part).

The graft has to be introduced in the upper part of the medullary canal while adduction of the arm. Maneuvering the shaft below the head and adapting the size and shape of the graft allow to keep the head in the correct degree of varus (the graft can be impacted inside the canal if too proud or trimmed by a Luer or a saw if too thick). Additional small cancellous homologous grafts can be placed around the wedge for a better filling.

If the tuberosities are mechanically strong, the bone sutures can be tractioned in order to place them between the head and the shaft, overlaying the graft (Fig. 7.2c). Only at this point can the fracture be provisionally stabilized by the smaller possible number of K-wires.

These steps are quite delicate in the more comminuted fractures. If the bone sutures fail or the K-wires create additional fractures in the tuberosities or in the head, there is a high risk to have to shift to a hemiarthroplasty. It is therefore recommended to use the plate for obtaining a gradual reduction exploiting its strength and anatomic shape, as described above. Hertel [5] well describes the principles of this reduction; in his paper he suggests the use of a simple one-third tubular plate with cancellous bone screws. Nowadays the new plates have added the great advantage of the polyaxial locking screws, while the anatomic contour proves extremely useful for the reduction acting like a template.

Once the plate is fixed by one cortex screw in the oval hole, the bone sutures are provisionally knotted to the plate, some K-wires or proximal screws are inserted, and image intensifier images are obtained before definitively fixing the fracture (Fig. 7.2d).

The cuff incision has to be closed by resorbable sutures, even though tightening the tuberosities to the plate often pulls the edges so close as to make it unnecessary. It is not always possible to close the rotator interval, if it was opened and if the fracture reduction is not perfect.

7.4.3.3 Three- or Four-Part Fracture with Varus Deviation

This fracture pattern often occurs in younger patients. The comminution of the tuberosities is less severe; there is a better bone stock and usually a better calcar length.

The reduction however is not easier, and there is always a risk that the surgical manipulation can make the fracture more complex.

Once the fragments have been identified and the bone sutures prepared, it is useful to expose by a delicate dissection the lower part of the subscapularis to get access to the calcar. A smooth retractor can gently push the head to place it in valgus. Unfortunately this procedure can induce two risks:

- The axillary nerve lies very close and its course may have been modified by the fracture.
- The anterior circumflex artery and its ascending branch which have an important role in the head vascularization can be damaged.

It is therefore advisable to try to use the plate for obtaining the fracture reduction (Fig. 7.3).

The surgeon should try to set the tuberosities on the sides of the head deviated in varus by gentle traction on the bone sutures and to connect them to the head by K-wires (Fig. 7.3a).

The plate is then placed on the aligned fragments and provisionally fixed with other K-wires through its dedicated holes. If the anatomy reconstruction looks macroscopically and radioscopically acceptable, the fixation is performed placing the proximal screws (Fig. 7.3b), then the plate can be used like a joystick in order to move the proximal humerus in valgus and align it with the shaft. The fixation goes on with a cortex screw in the oval hole before obtaining new images with the image intensifier. The reduction can then be refined with additional bone sutures, possibly loosening and then tightening again some screws for the corrections before completing the fixation (Fig. 7.3c).

7.5 Important Tips

The long head of the biceps is a key structure in proximal humerus fractures. It is first of all an important landmark for anatomy comprehension during surgery. Locating it distally and following it proximally help find the lesser tuberosity and the rotator interval. Its bony groove is a crucial area for the vascular supply of the bony fragments and should be respected as much as possible. Restoring the continuity of the bicipital groove is extremely helpful for assessing the fracture reduction before radioscopic checking.

The surgical manipulation should not be extended beyond the medial edge of the long head of the biceps to minimize the risks of lesion of the anterior circumflex artery and of its branches, even though recent clinical evidences and angiographic studies suggest a major role of

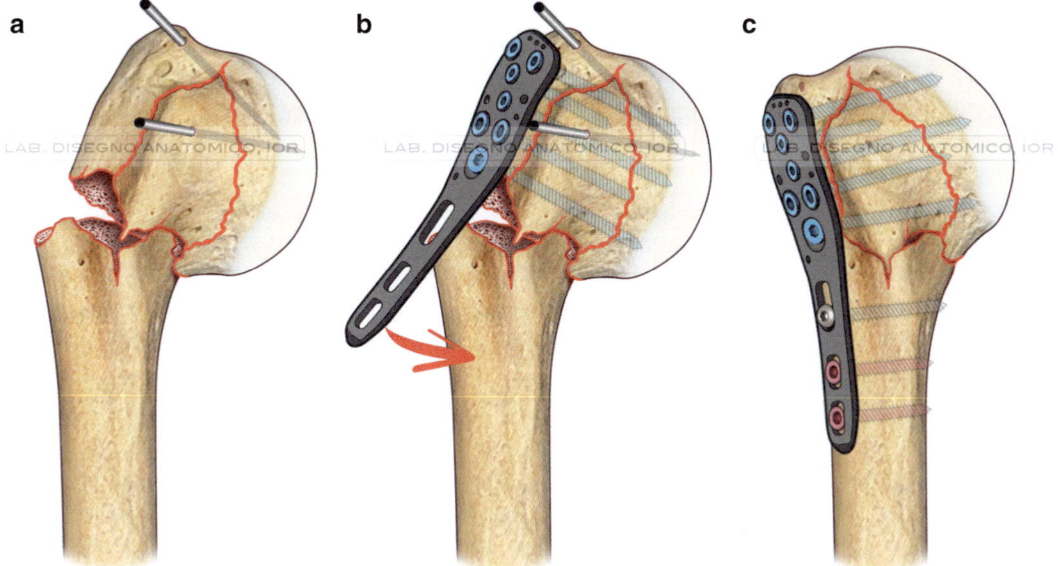

Fig. 7.3 In some cases of complex fractures (**a**) the plate can be fixed to the humeral head first (**b**) and than a precountor plate is used to reduced the humeral head to the dyaphisis (**c**). Graphical representation of three- or four-part fracture with varus deviation. The DiPhos PEEK Lima Corporate plate is represented (Anatomical School of Anatomical Imaging, University of Bologna, Italy)

the posterior circumflex artery in the vascular supply of the humeral head, in contrast with what was thought [34].

At the end of the surgery, the long head of the biceps can be left in place if undamaged (the sharp edges of the bony fragments often cause severe damage) and if its bony bed has a smooth continuity. If this is not the case, a proximal tenotomy and possibly a soft tissue tenodesis (depending on the patient's age) are advisable.

The good balance between the quality of the fracture reduction and the soft tissue damage to achieve it is the key point of the operation. The clinical results after conservative treatment of borderline fractures show that even non-perfectly reduced fractures can allow a satisfactory functional result. This balance is however quite hard to define in the form of guidelines. This is why these fractures are better treated not in emergency, not by unexpert surgeons, and not with insufficient radiographic pictures. It is better to take the time to obtain an accurate planning and to have an adequate surgical team available and the best surgical instrumentation (dedicated plates, bone grafts, and a shoulder prosthesis).

Codman realized the importance of the rotator cuff tendons in keeping proximal humerus fractures in mutual apposition. He emphasized "how tenaciously the short rotators with their periosteal prolongations cling to all the fragments, and tend to hold them together." Plate fixation of these fractures should be intended not as a strong construct depending on the holding power of the screws in bone, but rather as a solid *bridge/scaffold* connecting the various bony fragments to the plate and the plate to the humeral shaft. The tension of the tendons counterbalanced by the scapular glenoid will keep the fragments "loaded."

The passive glenohumeral arc of motion obtained is a valuable help in understanding if the reduction is acceptable, even when the radiographic aspects are not perfect. It is obvious that at follow-up, the joint mobility will not be superior to the intraoperative one. A stable fixation with a complete passive range of motion is the best starting point to expect a good functional result, avoiding to look for the absolutely perfect radiographic alignment.

When ORIF is chosen, careful attention has to be paid to the correct height of the plate; in fact if too distal it will not adequately support the tuberosities, while if too proximal it will be responsible for impingement. With each plate there are little tricks to know in order to obtain a correct position, and even the most expert surgeon should know and follow them.

The best possible anatomic reduction, the respect of the soft tissues, a stable fixation, filling the bone defects, and achieving a satisfactory contact between the head, tuberosities, and shaft are the key to limit at a minimum failures and complications of these fractures.

7.6 Postoperative Treatment

At the end of surgery the arm is protected in a sling with the shoulder in adduction and internal rotation.

If the fixation is stable and the patient is reliable, passive mobilization (with a CPM machine) and self-assisted mobilization begin in the first postoperative day. Pain relief is guaranteed by regional block under the supervision of the anesthesiologists until the patient's discharge.

The patient is encouraged to perform flexion and abduction movements with gradual increase, in the pain-free range. The patient is also invited to perform easy activities of daily living, like taking care of his/her personal hygiene, eating, and dressing, starting between days 7 and 14 post-op.

After the first radiographic control at 1 month from surgery, the sling is dismissed and the true rehabilitation program is started, with gentle manipulation for progressive recovery of joint motion and active assisted rehabilitation, best if possible in pool with warm water (hydrotherapy).

After 3 months, rehabilitation proceeds with increasingly heavier tasks, aiming at the best possible functional recovery.

7.7 Our Experience: Complications

Proximal humerus fractures, especially three-part and four-part fractures, still represent a challenge for orthopedic surgeons, trying to obtain an anatomic and stable reduction allowing a satisfactory and early functional recovery. There are a number of complications related to this type of fractures, first of all because people over 75 years are those more exposed to this risk.

Several authors stress the direct relationship between the severity of fracture and the risk of avascular necrosis (AVN). Thanasas [31] indicates a risk of AVN in these fractures treated by ORIF with PHILOS plate of 7.9 % that rises at 14.5 % when considering four-part fractures only. This figure, which may look high, should be considered in light of previous studies by Lee and Hansen [35] and Leyshon [36], who recorded an incidence of AVN with plates used before the advent of locking plates between 21 and 75 %. Humeral head necrosis is strictly related to several factors, well described by Hertel et al. [16]: the number of fragments and degree of displacement, mainly of the tuberosities; the "medial hinge"; and a calcar shorter than 8 mm. Angiographic studies indicate the important role of the retrograde blood supply by the anterior circumflex artery, penetrating the head in correspondence of the greater and lesser tuberosities after running just close to the calcar. Other vessels contributing to the head vascularization are the posterior circumflex artery and the small arteries running close to the rotator cuff. Hertel in his paper maintains that too much importance is attributed to the anterior circumflex artery. By a Doppler examination in a stable microenvironment (good cancellous bone bleeding and fragments not too displaced), he has shown that from the posterior circumflex artery, a sufficient number of vessels are generated to vascularize the whole head of the humerus. In any case AVN is undoubtedly difficult to predict and is barely related with pain and function of the fractured humerus [37, 38].

Another important complication related to plate fixation is the incorrect selection of the length of the head screws that occurs with an incidence from 2 to 17.9 % according to Thanasas et al. [31]. Lesions of the glenoid surface secondary to perforation of the head by one or more screws are strictly consequent and require an immediate reoperation to remove the hardware [39]. One more possible side effect related to the plate is its incorrect position, causing secondary subacromial impingement during shoulder abduction or secondary loss of fracture alignment in varus. Voigt suggests that the ideal position of the plate should be 5–8 mm below the greater tuberosity [39].

The use of locking plates in case of severe osteoporosis, especially if in the wrong position, can lead to screw cutout in 2.6 % of the implants. Charalambous et al. [40] hypothesized that the cause of cutout could be an incorrect position of the screw; however, other studies have shown that this complication can happen also when the screws are well placed. In any case it is stressed in the literature how a correct fracture reduction which is maintained at follow-up and a good reconstruction of the tuberosities are related to a better functional outcome and a superior result in the Constant score [40, 41].

Finally, two rare complications have to be mentioned, that is to say nonunion (1.6 %) and plate breakage (0.7 %). The latter event can be mainly due to a bad fracture reduction with a too rigid fixation, stressed by loads that overcome its mechanical resistance [35].

The clinical results achieved by patients who received ORIF for three-part and four-part fractures have been good, even though the functional scores' increase in time is in relationship with age and with complexity of the original fracture [38]. This point gives even more value to the opinion that this technique of fixation has a high effectiveness but requires the respect of a number of points. First of all a correct preoperative planning should be obtained preferably with CT scan with tridimensional rendering. During surgery the length of the screws should be always carefully checked to avoid the risk of humeral head perforation and glenoid cartilage lesion. The tuberosities should be reduced with meticulous attention so as to ensure a synergistic action between plate and bone sutures. The plate position should be accurately chosen even accepting a slight varus misalignment and supporting the inferior medial part with screws in order to prevent successive head collapse. In severely osteoporotic patients with valgus displacement of the humeral head, the use of a graft to strengthen the construct is recommended. All of these points allow to minimize the risk of surgical revisions that can mean an evolution toward secondary arthroplasty, whose results are well known to be disappointing [42, 43].

In our department a model of PEEK plate (DiPhos, Lima Corporate), developed in collaboration with the manufacturer and with a patent about self-threading titanium screws, is used in proximal humeral fractures since 2010.

The preliminary results of our case series are briefly summarized:

1. 90 DiPhos H plates (70 % F.) April 2010–May 2012
2. Mean age 60 years (36–84)
3. Mean FU 22 months (10–36)
4. Pattern of fractures (AO): 4 A2; 6 A3; 14 B1; 22 B2; 16 B3; 6 C1; 12 C2; 10 C3
5. Surgery: 87 deltopectoral approaches, 3 transdeltoid approaches, 10 % bone graft from donor
6. Intra-op complication 0.9 % (one case): plate breakage while screwing oval hole (first plate design)
7. Post-op complications 2.7 % (three cases): one humeral head necrosis, two plate-acromion impingement
8. Five plates removal at FU: three for post-op complications, two for patient request

Radiolucency of the plate, polyaxial direction of the locking screws, an elastic modulus quite similar to cortical bone, excellent biocompatibility, and an extreme easiness of hardware removal are the main qualifying points of this plastic fixation device.

At the present time the results in terms of complications are similar to those reported in the literature about locking plate fixation, while short-term results in terms of failures are superior. We do not expect that this new plate can lead to a revolution in ORIF technique. In our experience this plate shares the well-known positive features of the other locking plates, moreover:

- Radiolucency is a real advantage during intra-operative fluoroscopic checking.
- Hardware removal is easy and free of complications.

We therefore feel confident in recommending its use.

References

1. Palvanen M, Kannus P, Niemi S, Parkkari J (2006) Update in the epidemiology of proximal humeral fractures. Clin Orthop Relat Res 442:87–92
2. Obrant KJ, Bengnér U, Johnell O, Nilsson BE, Sernbo I (1989) Increasing age-adjusted risk of fragility fractures: a sign of increasing osteoporosis in successive generations? Calcif Tissue Int 44:157–167
3. Neer CS 2nd (1970) Displaced proximal humeral fractures. Treatment of three-four part displacement. J Bone Joint Surg Am 52(6):1090–1103
4. Rose SH, Melton LJ 3rd, Morrey BF, Ilstrup DM, Riggs BL (1982) Epidemiologic features of humeral fractures. Clin Orthop 168:24–30
5. Hertel R (2005) Fracture of the proximal humerus in osteoporotic bone. Osteoporos Int 16:S65–S72
6. Stableforth PG (1984) Four-part fractures of the neck of the humerus. J Bone Joint Surg Br 66:104
7. Edwards SL, Wilson NA, Zhang LQ, Flores S, Merk BR (2006) Two-part surgical neck fractures of the proximal part of the humerus. A biomechanical evaluation of two fixation techniques. J Bone Joint Surg Am 88(10):2258–2264
8. Seide K, Triebe J, Faschingbauer M, Schulz AP, Püschel K, Mehrtens G, Jürgens C (2007) Locked vs. unlocked plate osteosynthesis of the proximal humerus - a biomechanical study. Clin Biomech (Bristol, Avon) 22(2):176–182. Epub 2006 Nov 28
9. Kollig E, Kutscha-Lissberg F, Roetman B, Mielke E, Muhr G, Hahn MP (2003) [Primary hemiarthroplasty after complex fracture of the humeral head: functional late results]. Zentralbl Chir 128:125–130
10. Lill H, Josten C (2001) Conservative or operative treatment of humeral head fractures in the elderly. Chirurg 72:1224–1234
11. Misra A, Kapur R, Maffulli N (2001) Complex proximal humeral fractures in adults–a systematic review of management. Injury 32(5):363–372
12. Siffri PC, Peindl R, Coley ER, Connor PM, Kellam JF (2006) Biomechanical analysis of blade-plate versus locking-plate fixation for a proximal humerus fracture: a comparison with use of cadaveric and synthetic humeri. J Orthop Trauma 20(8):547–554
13. Brorson S, Rasmussen JV, Olsen BS, Frich LH, Jensen SL, Hróbjartsson A (2013) Reverse shoulder arthroplasty in acute fractures of the proximal humerus: a systematic review. Int J Shoulder Surg 7(2):70–78
14. Codman EA (1934) Fractures in relation to the subacromial bursa. In: Codman EA (ed) The shoulder, rupture of the supraspinatus tendon and other lesions in or about the subacromial bursa. Krieger Publishing, Malabar, pp 313–331
15. Sidor ML, Zuckerman JD, Lyon T et al (1993) The Neer classification system for proximal humerus fractures: an assessment of interobserver reliability and intraobserver reproducibility. J Bone Joint Surg Am 75-A:1745–1755
16. Hertel R, Hempfing A, Stiehler M, Leunig M (2004) Predictors of humeral head ischemia after intracapsular fracture of the proximal humerus. J Shoulder Elbow Surg 13(4):427–433
17. Müller ME, Allögover M, Schneider R (1991) Appendix A: the comprehensive classification of fractures of long bones. In: Manual of internal fixation: techniques recommended by AO-ASIF group, 3rd edn. Springer, Berlin, pp 118–125
18. Siebenrock KA, Gerber C (1993) The reproducibility of classification of fractures of the proximal end of the humerus. J Bone Joint Surg Am 75-A:1751–1755
19. Brien H, Noftall F, MacMaster S, Cummings T, Landells C, Rockwood P (1995) Neer's classification system: a critical appraisal. J Trauma 38(2):257–260
20. Schlegel TF, Hawkins RJ (1994) Displaced proximal humeral fractures: evaluation and treatment. J Am Acad Orthop Surg 2(1):54–78
21. Hessmann M, Baumgaertel F, Gehling H, Klingelhoeffer I, Gotzen L (1999) Plate fixation of proximal humeral fractures with indirect reduction: surgical technique and results utilizing three shoulder scores. Injury 30(7):453–462
22. Hintermann B, Trouillier HH, Schäfer D (2000) Rigid internal fixation of fractures of the proximal humerus in older patients. J Bone Joint Surg Br 82(8): 1107–1112
23. Kralinger F et al (2004) Outcome after primary hemiarthroplasty for fracture of the head of the humerus. A retrospective multicentre study of 167 patients. J Bone Joint Surg Br 86(2):217–219
24. Walsh S, Reindl R, Harvey E, Berry G, Beckman L, Steffen T (2006) Biomechanical comparison of a unique locking plate versus a standard plate for internal fixation of proximal humerus fractures in a cadaveric model. Clin Biomech (Bristol, Avon) 21:1027–1031
25. Sproul RC, Iyengar JJ, Devcic Z, Feeley BT (2011) A systematic review of locking plate fixation of proximal humerus fractures. Injury 42(4):408–413
26. Ricchetti ET, Warrender WJ, Abboud JA (2010) Use of locking plates in the treatment of proximal humerus fractures. J Shoulder Elbow Surg 19(2 Suppl):66–75
27. Lescheid J, Zdero R, Shah S, Kuzyk PR, Schemitsch EH (2010) The biomechanics of locked plating for repairing proximal humerus fractures with or without medial cortical support. J Trauma 69(5):1235–1242
28. Gardner MJ, Weil Y, Barker JU, Kelly BT, Helfet DL, Lorich DG (2007) The importance of medial support in locked plating of proximal humerus fractures. J Orthop Trauma 21(3):185–191
29. Osterhoff G, Ossendorf C, Wanner GA, Simmen HP, Werner CM (2011) The calcar screw in angular stable plate fixation of proximal humeral fractures–a case study. Orthop Surg Res 6:50
30. Marti A (2000) Cobalt-base alloys used in bone surgery. Injury 31(Suppl 4):18–21
31. Thanasas C, Kontakis G, Angoules A, Limb D, Giannoudis P (2009) Treatment of proximal humerus

fractures with locking plates: a systematic review. J Shoulder Elbow Surg 18(6):837–844
32. Hepp P, Theopold J, Voigt C, Engel T, Josten C, Lill H (2008) The surgical approach for locking plate osteosynthesis of displaced proximal humeral fractures influences the functional outcome. J Shoulder Elbow Surg 17(1):21–28
33. Namdari S, Voleti PB, Mehta S (2012) Evaluation of the osteoporotic proximal humeral fracture and strategies for structural augmentation during surgical treatment. J Shoulder Elbow Surg 21(12): 1787–1795
34. Hettrich CM, Boraiah S, Dyke JP, Neviaser A, Helfet DL, Lorich DG (2010) Quantitative assessment of the vascularity of the proximal part of the humerus. J Bone Joint Surg Am 92(4):943–948
35. Lee CK, Hansen HR (1981) Post-traumatic avascular necrosis of the humeral head in displaced proximal humeral fractures. J Trauma 21:788–791
36. Leyshon RL (1984) Closed treatment of fractures of the proximal humerus. Acta Orthop Scand 55:48–51
37. Jost B, Spross C, Grehn H, Gerber C (2013) Locking plate fixation of fractures of the proximal humerus: analysis of complications, revision strategies and outcome. J Shoulder Elbow Surg 22(4):542–549
38. Inauen C, Platz A, Meier C, Zingg U, Rufibach K, Spross C, Dietrich M (2013) Quality of life after osteosynthesis of fractures of the proximal humerus. J Orthop Trauma 27(4):e74–e80
39. Voigt C, Woltmann A, Partenheimer A, Lill H (2007) Management of complications after angularly stable locking proximal humerus plate fixation. Chirurg 78:40–46. Farmer KW, Wright TW (2010) Three- and four-part proximal humerus fractures: open reduction and internal fixation versus arthroplasty. J Hand Surg 35(11):1881–1884
40. Charalambous CP, Siddique I, Valluripalli K, Kovacevic M, Panose P, Srinivasan M, Marynissen H (2007) Proximal humeral internal locking system (PHILOS) for the treatment of proximal humeral fractures. Arch Orthop Trauma Surg 127:205–210
41. Kettler M, Biberthaler P, Braunstein V, Zeiler C, Kroetz M, Mutschler W (2006) Treatment of proximal humeral fractures with the PHILOS angular stable plate: presentation of 225 cases of dislocated fractures. Unfallchirurg 109:1032–1040
42. Tanner MW, Cofield RH (1983) Prosthetic arthroplasty for fractures and fracture-dislocations of the proximal humerus. Clin Orthop Relat Res 179: 116–128
43. Frangen TM, Dudda M, Martin D, Arens S, Greif S, Muhr G, Kalicke T (2007) Proximal humeral fractures with angle-stable plate osteosynthesis everything better now? Zentralbl Chir 132:60–69

8 Intramedullary Nail for Proximal Humerus Fractures: An Old Concept Revisited

Pascal Boileau, Thomas d'Ollonne, Philippe Clavert, and Armodios M. Hatzidakis

8.1 Introduction

Proximal humerus fractures commonly occur in elderly patients (mainly women) with decreased bone mineral density [1–4]. Approximately 15–20 % of such fractures are displaced or unstable and require surgical management [5, 6]. Optimal treatment for displaced or unstable 2-, 3-, and 4-part proximal humerus fractures remains controversial [7–12]. Traditionally, complex fracture-dislocations with detachment and devascularization of the head fragment are treated with humeral head replacement and tuberosity reconstruction; in elderly patients (>70 years old) with osteopenic bone, a reverse shoulder arthroplasty can even be indicated. If the head fragment is viable, reduction and internal fixation is the treatment of choice [4, 11, 13]. Various devices have been proposed for fixation, including pins, locked plates, and intramedullary (IM) nails. Although no stabilization device has attained definitive superiority yet, most experts agree that minimal soft tissue dissection and adequate fixation strength should be the goals of any internal fixation device [1]. Fixed-angle locked plates have become quite popular [2–4, 14]. However, several recent publications have included rates of complications, including hardware failure, screw penetration, and fracture redisplacement [5, 6, 14–17].

Intramedullary fixation with a locked nail is an attractive option because it provides several theoretical advantages compared to locked-plate fixation: (1) it is less invasive, requiring less soft tissue dissection and thus preserving periosteal blood supply and retaining surrounding soft tissue attachments; (2) it improves construct stability even in cases of comminuted fractures and osteopenic bone while keeping some elasticity (whereas locked plates are too rigid) [7–12, 18–23]; and (3) for simpler fracture types, operating time can be considerably shortened when a percutaneous, guided locking technique is used. Although the concept of IM nailing has been

P. Boileau, MD (✉) • T. d'Ollonne
Department of Orthopaedics and Sports Traumatology, L'Archet 2 Hospital, 151 route de St Antoine de Ginestière, Nice 06200, France

Department of Orthopaedic Surgery and Sports Traumatology, University of Nice Sophia-Antipolis, Hôpital de L'Archet, 151, Route de St. Antoine de Ginestière, Nice 06202, France
e-mail: boileau.p@chu-nice.fr

P. Clavert
Service de Chirurgie Orthopédique, Centre de Chirurgie Orthopédique et de la Main, Avenue Baumann, Illkirch, 67400, France

Department of Orthopaedic Surgery and Sports Traumatology, University of Nice Sophia-Antipolis, Hôpital de L'Archet, 151, Route de St. Antoine de Ginestière, Nice 06202, France

A.M. Hatzidakis
Department of Orthopedics, Western Orthopaedics, 1830 Franklin St, Denver, CO 80218, USA

Department of Orthopaedic Surgery and Sports Traumatology, University of Nice Sophia-Antipolis, Hôpital de L'Archet, 151, Route de St. Antoine de Ginestière, Nice 06202, France

F. Castoldi et al. (eds.), *Simple and Complex Fractures of the Humerus*, DOI 10.1007/978-88-470-5307-6_8, © Springer-Verlag Italia 2015

attractive to us for many years, none of the existing devices have met our expectations. This was the main impetus for our development of an entirely new IM nailing system.

The Aequalis IM nail (Tornier, Minneapolis, USA) is a new stabilization device for proximal humeral fractures, designed specifically to optimize tuberosity-fragment fixation and provide stable support for the humeral head, improving proximal humeral reconstruction and fixation in osteopenic bone. The objectives of this paper are to (1) analyze common complications related to traditional IM nailing of proximal humerus fractures and their causes; (2) describe the concept, design, and rationale of the Aequalis IM nail; (3) provide some tips on using this nail, based on fracture type (2-, 3-, or 4-part); and (4) report the clinical and radiographic results of a prospective, consecutive series of patients treated using this new device.

8.2 Complications and Technologic Problems Observed with Existing IM Nails for Proximal Humerus Fractures

Although published reports on using IM nails for displaced proximal humerus fractures are satisfactory [4, 9, 11, 13, 24–33], some recent studies have reported a high complication rate of 40 % and a high revision rate of up to 45 % [1, 34–38]. Based on our own experience, most of the complications and problems observed with existing IM nails are related to inadequate design of the nail itself, the orientation and locking mechanism of its proximal and distal screws, or the accompanying instrumentation.

8.3 Specific Complications and Problems in Detail

8.3.1 Rotator Cuff Tears (and Shoulder Pain)

Rotator cuff tears are visible when surgeon pierces the rotator cuff tendons through a lateral entry portal, which is unavoidable with a proximally bent IM nail (Fig. 8.1). The bent design, historically borrowed from trochanteric-entry femoral nails, is not only unnecessary but also flawed from an anatomic standpoint. As demonstrated in Fig. 8.2, which summarizes some of our anatomic work, the humeral IM axis is aligned with the top of the humeral head fragment, passing through what we have called the "hinge point" [2–4, 39]. A straight nail would ideally align with this point and the IM axis. In addition, a straight and low- profile nail can be inserted through the muscular, not the tendinous, part of the supraspinatus and the superior

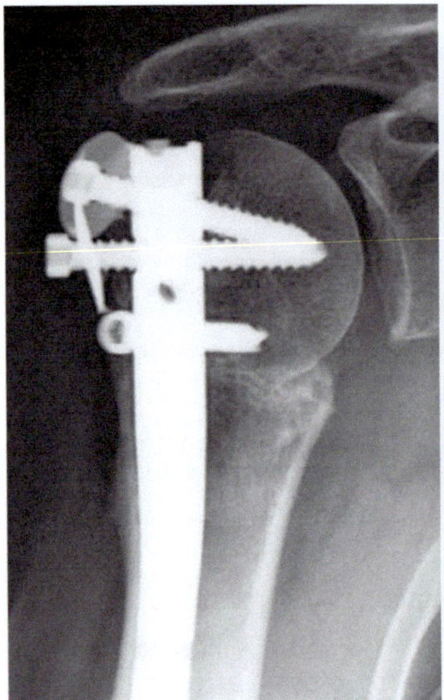

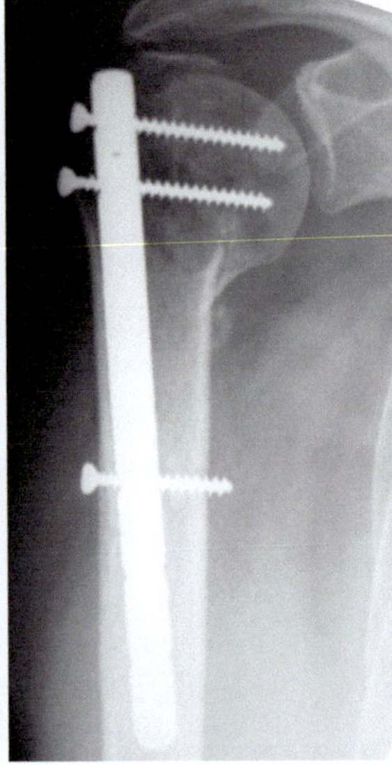

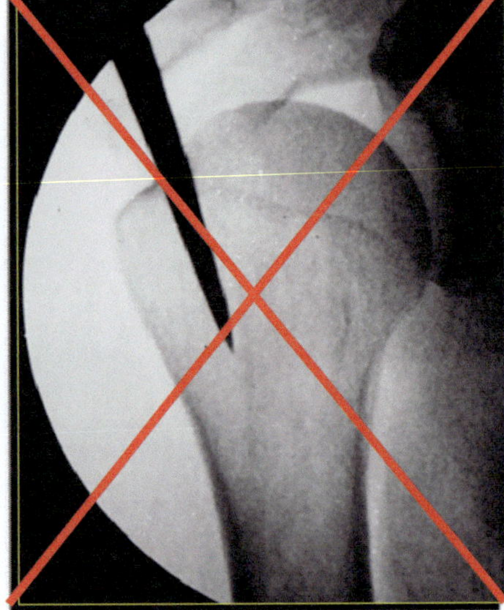

Fig. 8.1 Lateral entry of humeral nail leads to rotator cuff tear and greater tuberosity fracture with posterior migration

part of the humeral head—not the greater tuberosity (GT). This entry path has virtually no clinical consequences as proven by our experience and the literature, since humeral cartilage at that level does not come in contact with the glenoid. One must admit that it is illogical to repair the rotator cuff tears of some patients arthroscopically on the one hand, while on the other hand destroying

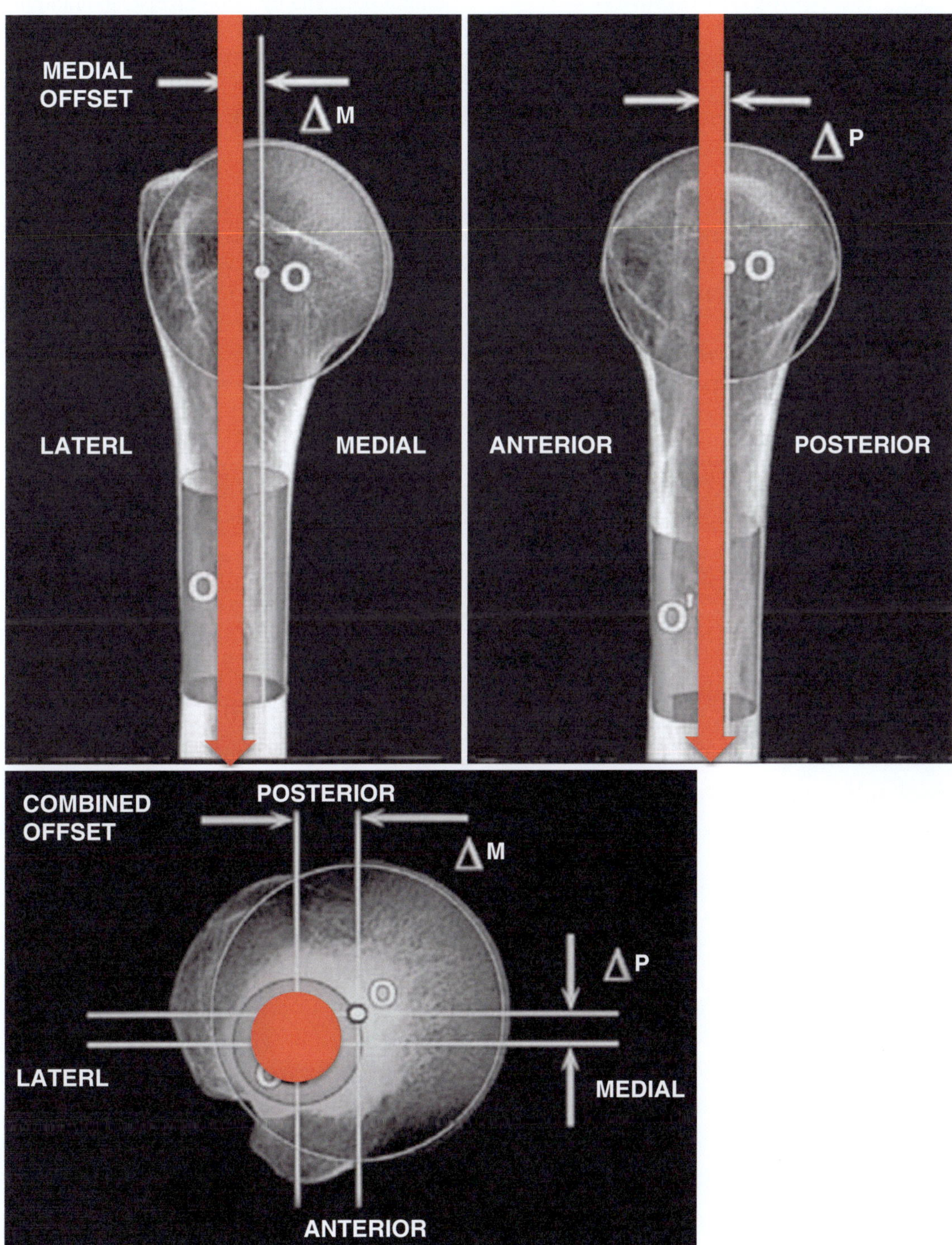

Fig. 8.2 The axis of the proximal humerus is aligned with the top of the humeral head fragment, passing through the "hinge point" [39]. Entry portal for a straight nail is 5 mm posterior to the bicipital groove and 5 mm medial the GT. Δ*M* medial offset, Δ*P* posterior offset

the rotator cuffs of other patients with an inadequately designed humeral nail.

8.3.2 Iatrogenic GT Fractures

These fractures are also related to a lateral entry point with bent and large-diameter nails (Fig. 8.1). The same is true for *fracture malreduction*—varus malalignment is frequent.

8.3.3 Acromial Impingement Secondary to Protrusion of the Proximal End of the Nail

This occurrence is related to (1) lateral entry with a bent nail (once again!) and (2) improper seating of the nail (Fig. 8.3) when using poor insertion jigs (which do not allow clear visualization of the nail's proximal end on the image intensifier). This complication can be avoided by proper seating of a straight nail below the subchondral bone and by using precise and radiolucent instrumentation.

8.3.4 Surgical Neck Nonunions

They are related to the unsuitable design of some nails, which are too long and too large distally, leading to premature "locking" through interference inside the distal medullary canal with distraction at the fracture site (Fig. 8.4). This complication can be easily avoided by using a straight, short, and small-diameter—i.e., a low-profile—IM nail with a fluted and smooth tip.

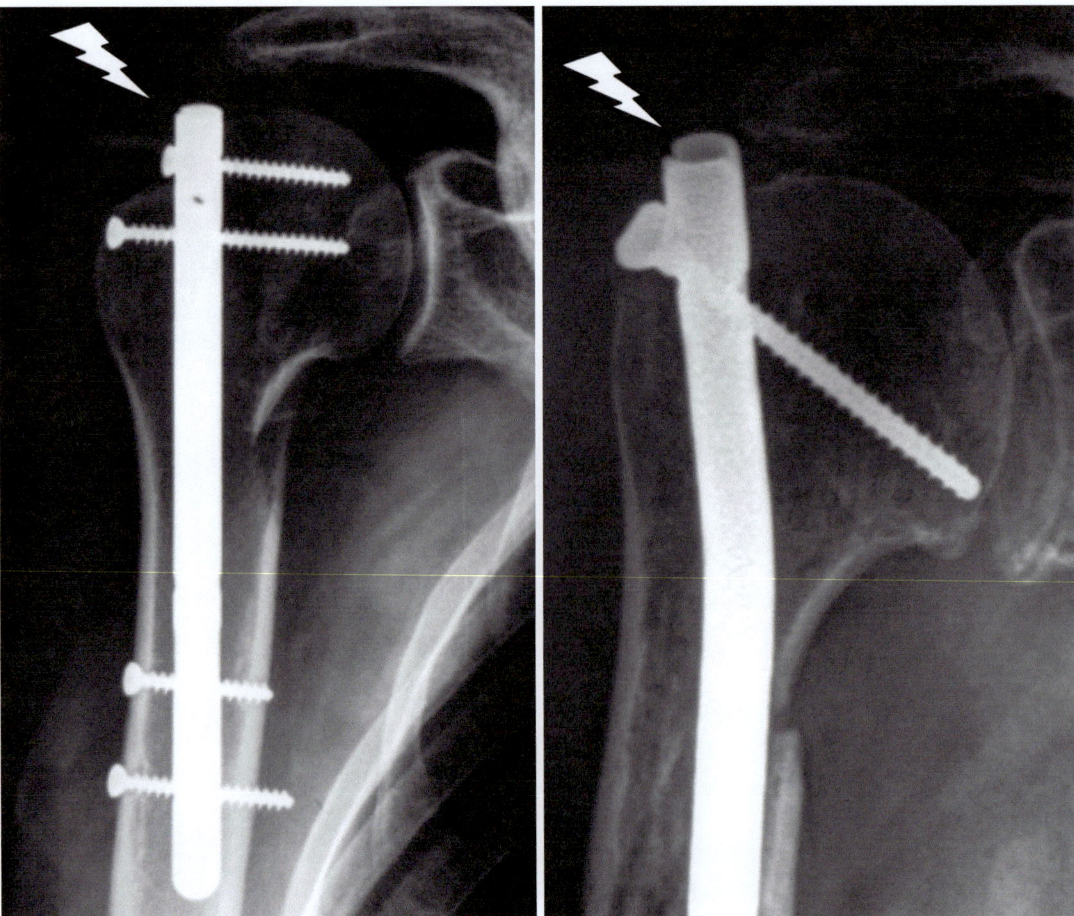

Fig. 8.3 Acromial impingement can be secondary to protrusion of a straight nail and/or lateral entry portal with a curved nail

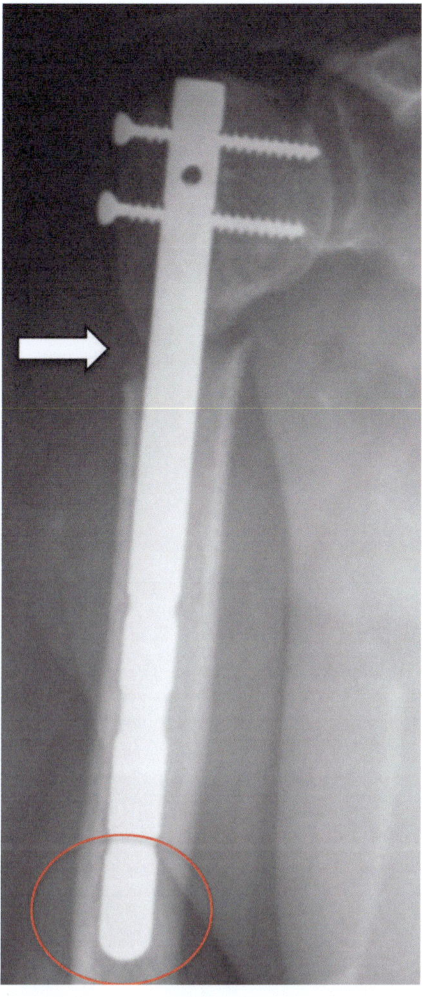

Fig. 8.4 Surgical neck nonunion due to distal locking of a too long and too big nail. *Arrow* denotes distraction at fracture site, *circle* denotes early cortical contact

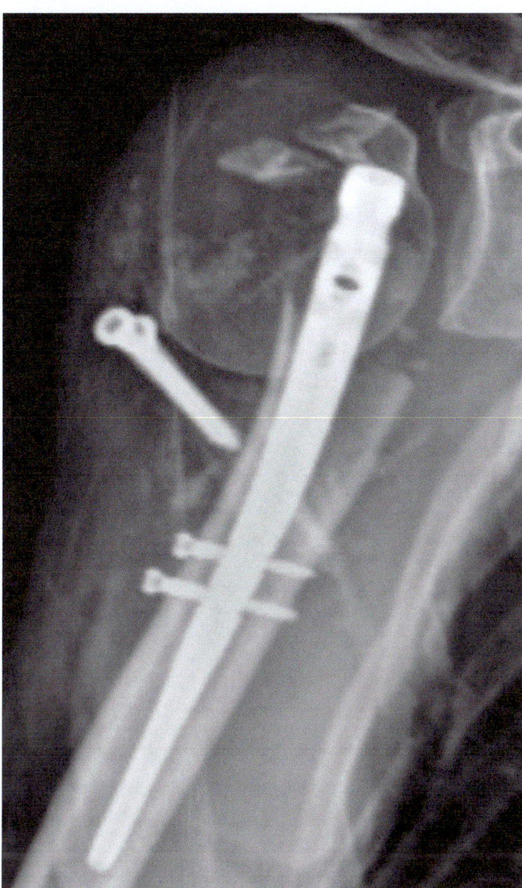

Fig. 8.5 Loss of reduction and fixation and proximal screw loosening/back out related to the absence of locking mechanism for proximal screws (bone-based fixation)

8.3.5 Failures of Proximal Fixation

Failures of proximal fixation (i.e., loss of tuberosity reduction and proximal screw loosening/back out) represent the number-one complication encountered with IM nailing of proximal humerus fractures. Based on our experience, failure of tuberosity and proximal screw fixation is due to two main factors: (1) absence of (or poor) locking mechanism for proximal screws in some nails (e.g., Polarus), what can be called *bone-based fixation*, and (2) poor proximal screw orientation in all existing nails, what can be referred to as *humeral head-based* (*lateromedial*) *orientation and fixation*:

- The ability of any screw to hold in osteopenic bone is limited [5, 6, 34, 37, 40], and secure fixation of the proximal screws should rely on a *locking mechanism within the nail* (via threaded holes). Such a *nail-based fixation is superior to any bone-based fixation* (Fig. 8.5). Reduction and fixation of both tuberosities provides additional support for the head—the so-called box theory [7–12].
- *Humeral head-based screw orientation and fixation* is a flawed biomechanical concept. Unfortunately, in all proximal humeral nails and other methods of fixation alike available today, the proximal screws are oriented toward the humeral head. Again, this error arises from the fact that surgeons have tried to apply to the shoulder what they had learned about the hip, although the two are *not* the same (Fig. 8.6). While it is logical to orient the proximal screws into the femoral head for a femoral neck fracture, since the goal is to counteract

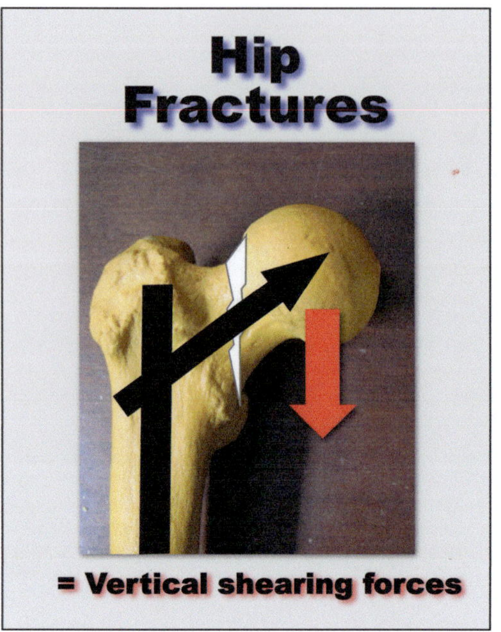

≠

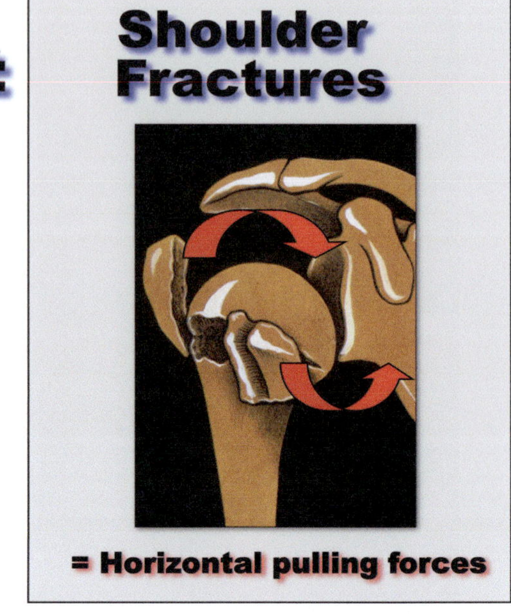

Fig. 8.6 While it is logical to orient screws in the femoral head to resist to vertical shearing forces (*arrow*) in proximal femur fractures, it is not logical to do so in proximal humerus where displacement of the bone fragments is horizontal, due to pulling forces on greater tuberosity and lesser tuberosity (*arrows*) by the rotator cuff muscles

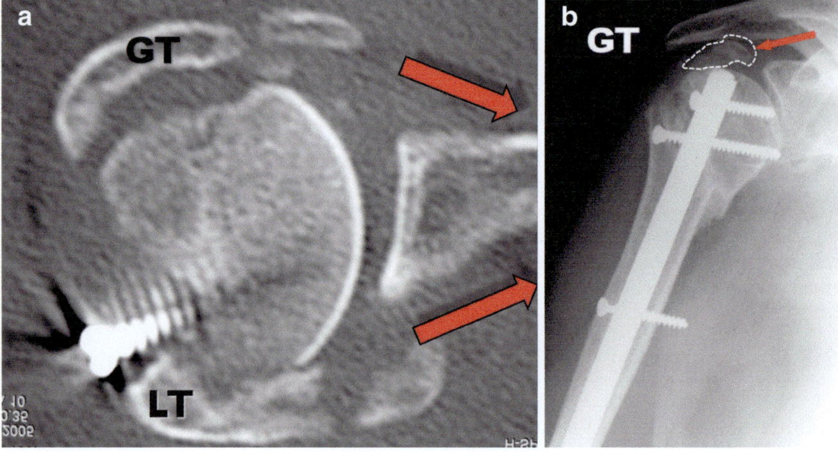

Fig. 8.7 Tuberosity migration related to poor (humeral head) orientation of proximal screws, which are parallel to the main vertical fracture line, splitting both tuberosities. (**a**) *GT* greater tuberosity, *LT* lesser tuberosity. *Arrows* denotes horizontal pulling forces on tuberosities. (**b**) Displaced greater tuberosity

vertical shearing forces, it is illogical to do the same in a 3- or 4-part proximal humerus fracture, in which the deforming forces are oriented mainly in the *horizontal* plane.

In a recent CT scan-based study of 4-part proximal humerus fractures, we demonstrated that the main vertical fracture plane separating the tuberosities is located *posterior to the bicipital groove,* and that the *principal displacement of such fractures occurs in the transverse (horizontal) plane* [4, 11, 13, 41]. In unstable 3- and 4-part fractures, displacement occurs because of the pull of the rotator cuff muscles on their attached tuberosities in the transverse plane, widening the gap created by the fracture plane posterior to the bicipital groove. The GT is pulled posteromedially by the infraspinatus and teres minor muscles, while the lesser tuberosity (LT) is pulled anteromedially by the subscapularis muscle (Fig. 8.7).

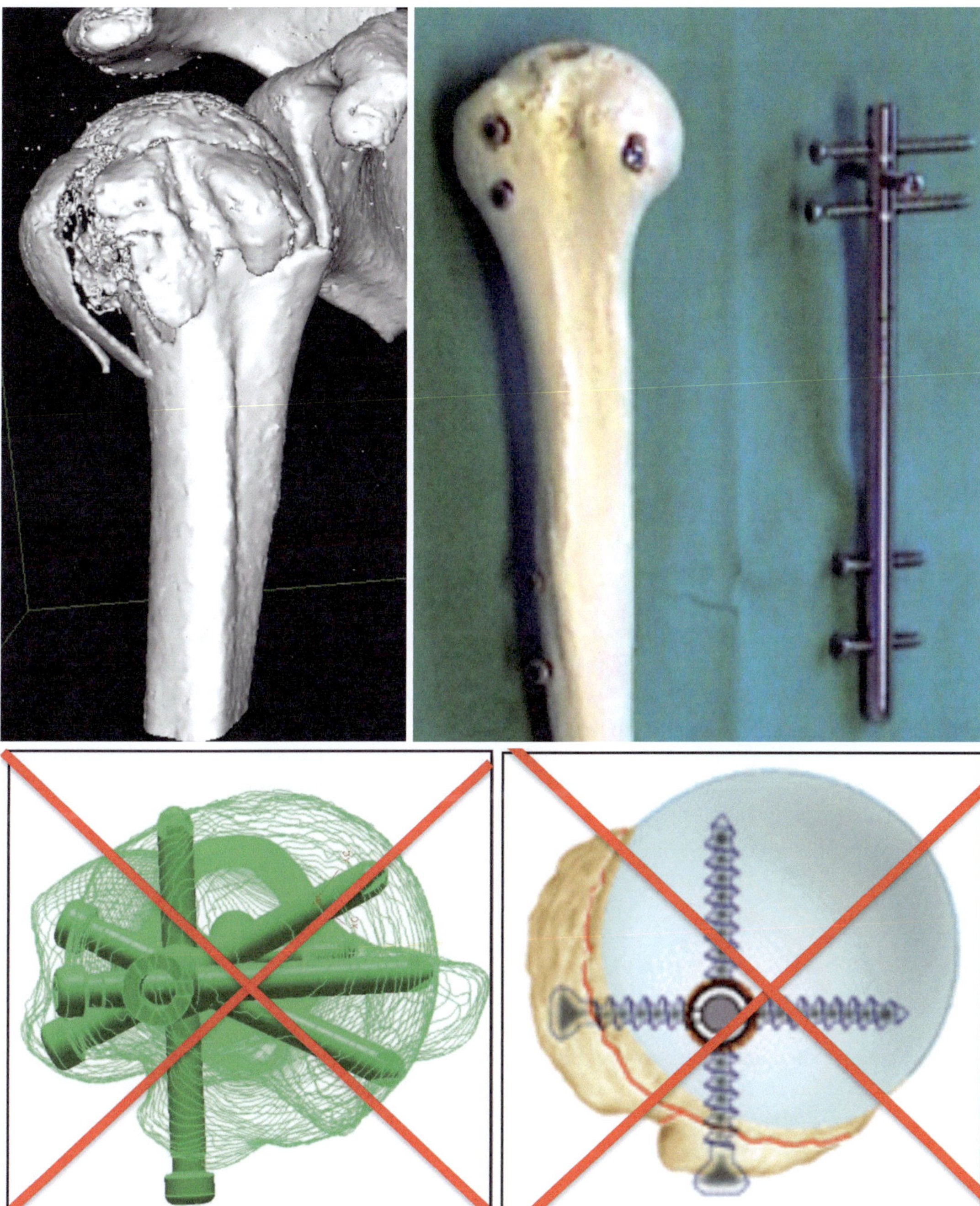

Fig. 8.8 In 2- and 3-part fractures, the main vertical fracture line is located behind the bicipital groove; proximal screw orientation must be perpendicular to this line (i.e., tuberosity oriented) and not parallel to it (i.e., humeral head oriented)

It follows that orienting the proximal screws from lateral to medial leads to their placement too closed and too parallel to the vertical fracture plane separating the tuberosities (Fig. 8.8). Such screws cannot counteract the pulling forces of the rotator cuff muscles. Moreover, this goes against one of the fundamental biomechanical principles espoused by the AO/ASIF [2–4, 42]: "any screw should be oriented as perpendicular to the fracture line

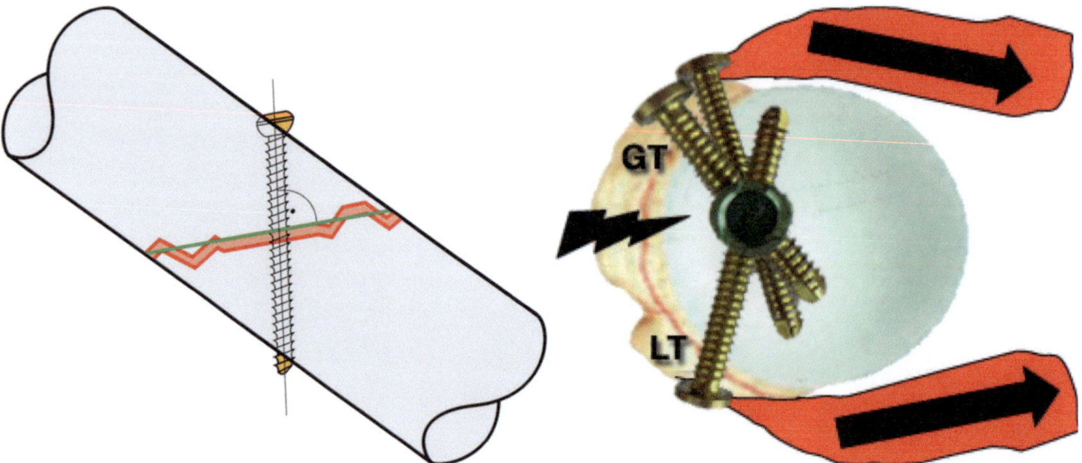

Fig. 8.9 According to a basic biomechanical principle, screws should be oriented perpendicular to the fracture line. With the Aequalis IM nail, the proximal screws are tuberosity oriented (i.e., *perpendicular* to the main fracture line) and captured inside the nail (nail-based fixation) in order to resist to pulling forces of infraspinatus and teres minor muscles on greater tuberosity (*GT*) and subscapularis muscle on lesser tuberosity (*LT*)

as possible" (Fig. 8.9). Therefore, to comply with this principle as well as resist the deforming forces, the proximal screws of any nail (or plate) should be placed in a posteroanterior direction to fix the GT and an anteroposterior direction to fix the LT. In other words, optimal proximal screw orientation must be tuberosity based (i.e., sagittal) and not humeral head based (i.e., coronal).

8.3.6 Proximal Screw Penetration of the Articular Cartilage

This is another potentially disastrous complication seen with IM nails (and locked plates) [5, 6, 16, 43, 44], leading to chondrolysis and early degenerative changes due to glenoid erosion (Fig. 8.10). Again, screw placement into the tuberosities rather than in the humeral head avoids the risk of this complication altogether.

8.3.7 Injury to Anatomic Structures

Injury to anatomic structures (axillary nerve, long head of the biceps) with proximal screws is possible. Injury to the axillary nerve occurs when laterally placed proximal screws are too low. Prince et al. [7–12, 45], comparing several different interlocking nails, concluded that proximal and lateral screws should be aimed horizontally, not obliquely, and placed within 4–5 cm of the acromion. Injury to the long head of the biceps (LHB) and bicipital groove can occur when rotation of the nail is not accurately controlled.

8.3.8 Nail Toggling and Fracture Malreduction

Fracture comminution and poor bone quality are not uncommon in elderly patients. This can lead to loss of fracture reduction and fixation. Varus bending represents a frequent physiological displacement of proximal humerus fractures. Varus deformity can interfere with shoulder elevation and should therefore be corrected during surgery and counteracted with the inserted fixation device (Fig. 8.11).

8.3.9 Nail Malrotation and Surgical Neck Malunions

They are related to the neglect of nail and fracture rotation. The most commonly committed error is fracture fixation with the arm in internal rotation, which leads to an internal rotation malunion.

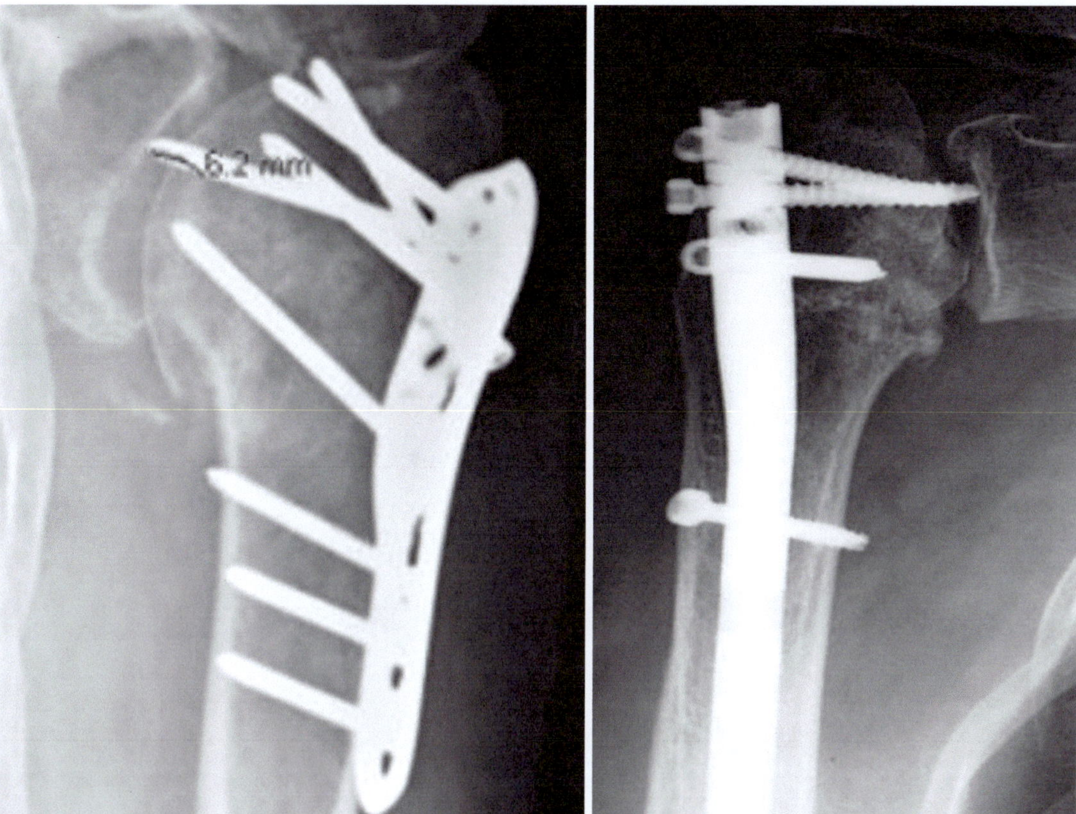

Fig. 8.10 Humeral head screw penetration leads to glenoid erosion in case of secondary bone impaction or necrosis; it can be seen with both proximal humeral plates and nails whose proximal screws are oriented toward humeral head

8.4 Concept, Design, and Rationale of the Aequalis IM Nail

The Aequalis IM nail has been *designed specifically to optimize tuberosity-fragment fixation and provide stable support for the humeral head*, improving proximal humeral reconstruction and fixation in osteopenic bone (Fig. 8.12). The nail's design and optimal screw orientation have been chosen after extensive study of the three-dimensional morphology and geometry of the proximal humerus [4, 11, 13, 39] and after revisiting the pathophysiology of displaced, unstable 2-, 3-, and 4-part fractures [1, 7, 39, 46].

8.5 Nail Design

As was shown in the previous section, the concept and design of all existing nails are poorly adapted to proximal humeral anatomy and not adapted at all to the common fracture patterns or poor bone quality that surgeons routinely encounter. Those nails are too long, too large, often bent, not centered, and with poorly oriented and poorly fixed proximal screws [9, 24–34, 37, 40].

In addition to being straight and cannulated, the Aequalis IM nail is of a low profile: its proximal *diameter* is 9 mm and distal diameter 8 mm, while its *length* is 130 mm (instead of 150 mm for most other nails). It is made of titanium alloy, the modulus of elasticity of which is close to that of bone. Since tuberosity orientation is different on each side, two nails exist: a green one for the right shoulder and a blue one for the left shoulder (Fig. 8.13).

As explained earlier, a straight nail design is preferable to a bent one for at least three reasons: (1) it avoids passage through the rotator cuff tendons and GT; (2) it allows alignment of the epiphyseal fragment with the diaphysis; and (3) it gives structural support to the humeral head fragment (acting as a strut/peg), since the IM axis is actually in line

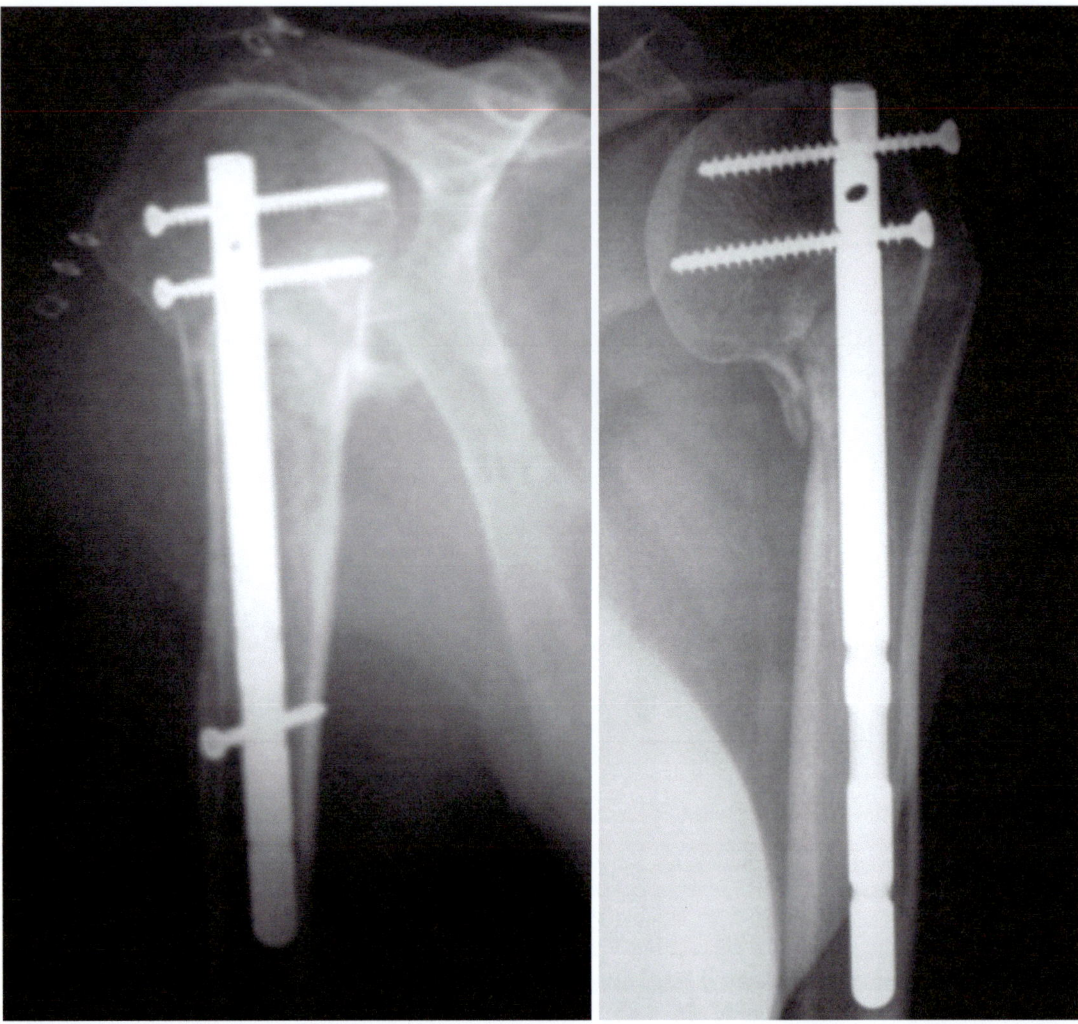

Fig. 8.11 Nail toggling and fracture malreduction or malunion because of poor centering of the nail (in valgus or varus)

with the top of the humeral head—the so-called hinge point [7, 39]. A cannulated nail allows percutaneous technique, while a short nail avoids unexpected distal locking of the device, thus preventing fracture distraction and surgical neck nonunion.

8.6 Proximal Locking Screws

In contrast to all previous devices, the proximal locking screws of the Aequalis nail are oriented to fix *not* the humeral head fragment but the two tuberosities. Reduction and fixation of both tuberosities indirectly provides additional head support—the so-called box theory [7, 41].

Four cannulated, yellow, 5 mm, proximal locking screws exist: two posterior locking screws for the GT, one anterior locking screw for the LT, and one (optional) lateral locked screw for the lower part of the humeral head (at the surgical neck level (Fig. 8.13). The screws are self-tapping (to easily engage the bone), with flat heads (to provide stronger fixation) and low profile (to avoid impingement with surrounding tissues). The design of the screw-hole pattern allows optimal screw positioning and prevents damage to anatomic structures, such as the axillary nerve, bicipital groove, or long head of the biceps tendon. The lowest proximal screw is at a safe distance from the axillary nerve: in 20 cadaver tests, the shortest distance from this screw to the nerve was 6 mm [46].

Rigidity of fixation of the proximal screws is not provided by purchase inside the osteopenic bone, but by *locking within the nail* itself, thanks to a poly-

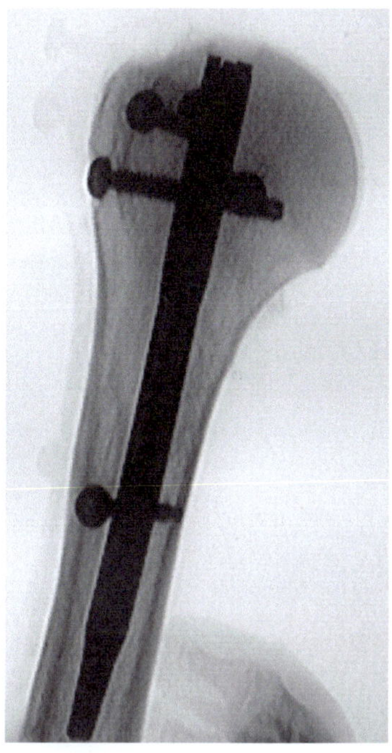
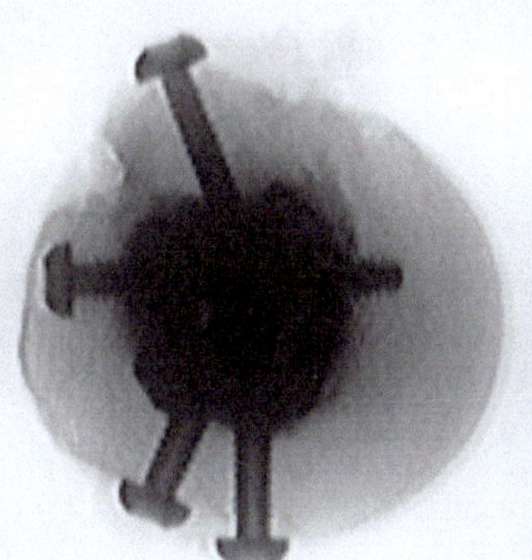
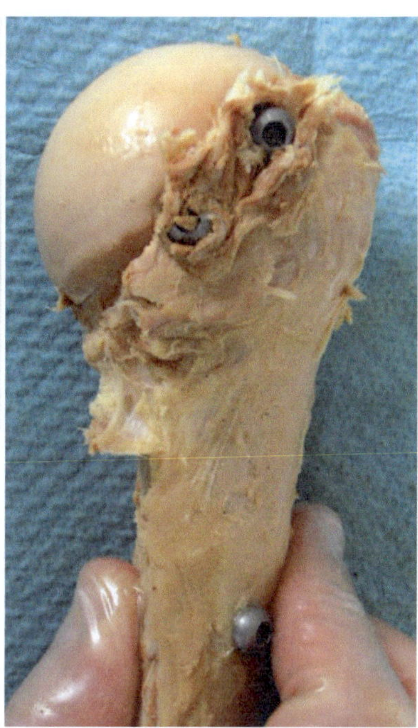

Fig. 8.12 Aequalis IM nail's concept: straight nail provides head support; proximal screw orientation provides tuberosity-based fixation; catching the nail with short screws is enough to provide secure bone-fragment fixation (nail-based fixation); and distal divergent screws provide nail centering and stabilization

ethylene bushing located inside the nail's proximal part. From a practical standpoint, this eliminates the need to look for purchase in the opposing cancellous bone with long screws; short screws stabilized by the nail itself provide sufficiently strong tuberosity fixation. In other words, with the Aequalis nail, catching the nail with short screws is enough to provide secure bone-fragment fixation.

Another important advantage of the proximal locking screw configuration of the Aequalis nail is that if the humeral head fragment necroses secondarily, the screws cannot erode the glenoid, as they are shorter and oriented in the sagittal plane. Moreover, anatomic reduction and healing of the tuberosities, together with the absence of screws directed into the humeral head, will facilitate secondary humeral arthroplasty if it should become necessary.

8.7 Distal Divergent Screws

Nail toggling movements are an issue with existing humeral nails. This could be even more of an issue with our shorter nail. However, diverging distal screws can eliminate such toggling and, in addition, allow automatic centering of the nail within the medullary canal. The nail has *two violet, 4.5 mm, divergent distal screws* (Fig. 8.13).

Distal locking of the nail protects the fracture against derotation or collapse and prevents migration of the implant itself. The Aequalis IM nail has the capacity to lock statically (if one uses the more distal, round hole) or dynamically (if one uses only the more proximal, oblong hole).

8.8 Radiolucent and Accurate Instrumentation

A radiolucent targeting guide facilitates accurate insertion and positioning of the nail and screws, with easy fluoroscopic visualization. A version rod, aligned with the forearm, helps achieve accurate rotational alignment of the proximal (epiphyseal) bone fragment in reference to the diaphysis (Fig. 8.14).

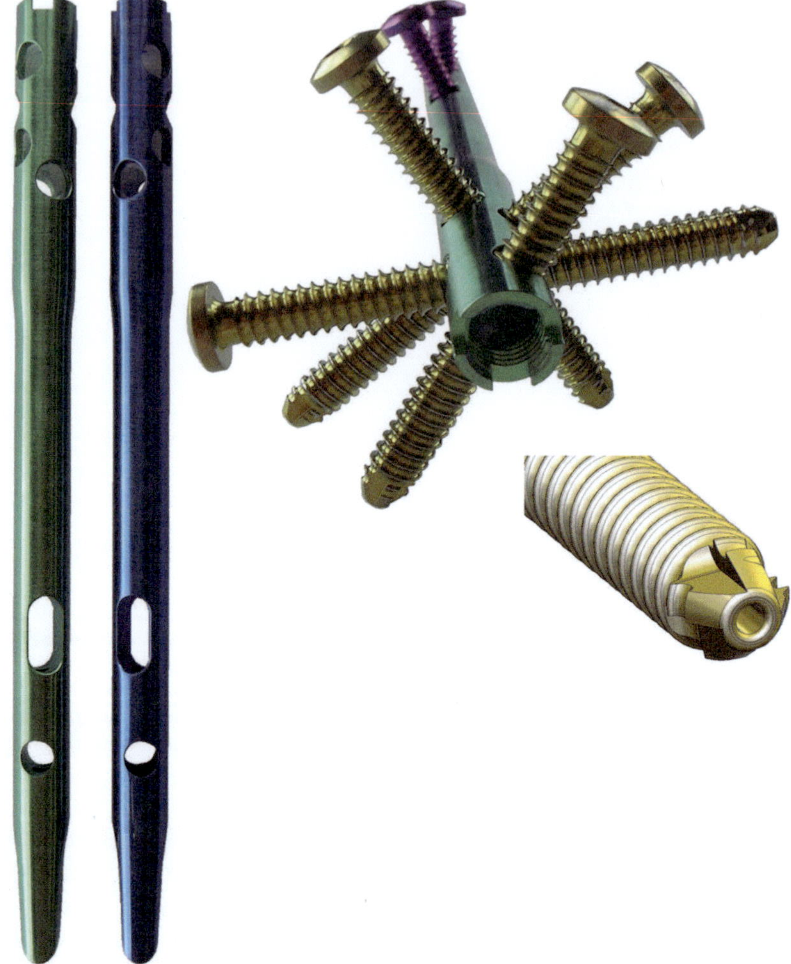

Fig. 8.13 The Aequalis IM nail is short, low profile, and cannulated; there are two nails to allow tuberosity-based fixation: a *green* one for the right shoulder and a *blue* one for the left shoulder; the proximal (*yellow*) screws are tuberosity oriented and self-tapped; the distal (*violet*) screws are 20° divergent for self-centering

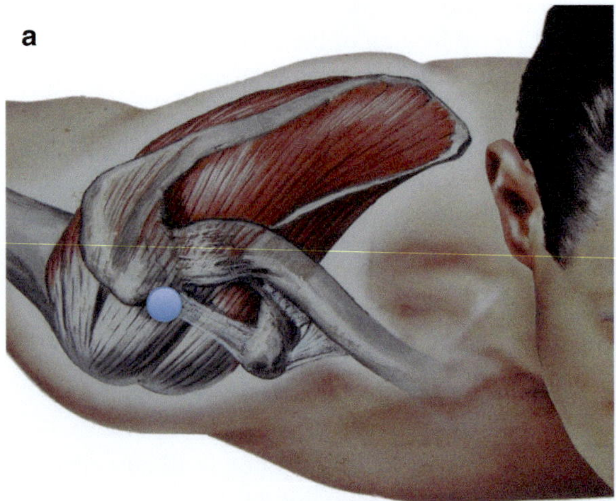

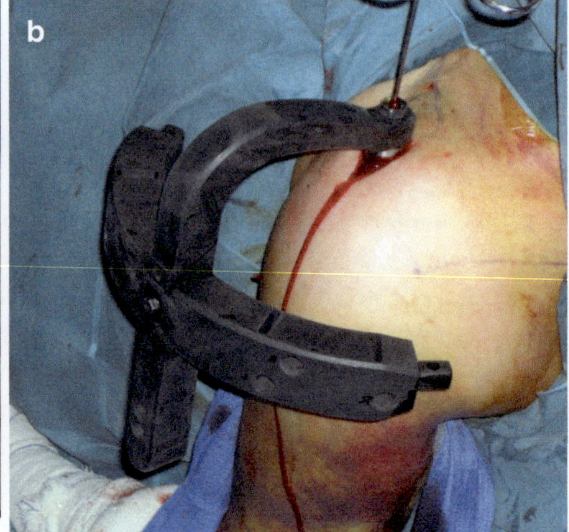

Fig. 8.14 Entry portal for the nail must be anterior to the acromion, allowing to pass through the supraspinatus muscle fibers (and not the tendon) and through the cartilage. For simple two-part fractures, percutaneous approach with fluoroscopic control is possible

8.9 Surgical Technique: Pearls and Pitfalls

The patient is placed in the beach-chair position with the elbow flexed at 90°. An image intensifier is used for obtaining anteroposterior (AP) and axillary intraoperative views.

Each type of proximal humerus fracture (2-, 3-, or 4-part) has its own pathophysiology and complications; the surgical technique must therefore vary accordingly. Three-dimensional CT scan images reveal the exact fracture geometry and allow accurate preoperative planning.

Three surgical approaches are possible depending on the fracture type and the surgeon's preference:

- *The percutaneous approach*, in which the deltoid muscle and supraspinatus are bluntly split through a superior, 1 cm incision
- *The superior transdeltoid approach*, in which the anterior head of the deltoid is detached from the anterior acromion with the tip of the acromion to expose the rotator cuff
- *The anterior deltoid approach*, in which the anterior deltoid muscle is retracted to expose the rotator cuff

The straight nail must be inserted medially either through the *supraspinatus muscle fibers or* through the *rotator interval* (Fig. 8.14). The entry portal of the nail is created with an awl and enlarged with a 9 mm hand reamer under fluoroscopic control. If the bicipital groove is fractured, the LHB must be tenodesed.

8.10 Two-Part (Surgical Neck) Fractures

In two-part (surgical neck) fractures, the epiphysis is correctly oriented and has a fixed position, because the internal rotator and external rotator muscles are still attached and balanced. The diaphysis, however, is medially displaced (due to the medial pull of the pectoralis major, latissimus dorsi, and teres major) and in internal rotation (because the forearm is usually held against the belly).

Two main complications are specifically encountered with 2-part (surgical neck) fractures and must be anticipated:

- *A rotational malunion* when the nail is locked proximally and distally with the arm in internal rotation; this leads to decreased humeral retroversion and, consequently, external rotation.
- *A surgical neck nonunion* in cases of persistent distraction at the fracture site.

With the Aequalis IM nail and instrumentation, these two complications can be avoided by:

- Aligning the version rod with the forearm
- Retrograde hammering after distal locking, which impacts the surgical neck fracture site, preventing nonunion

The "retrograde" (percutaneous) technique is used in 2-part (surgical neck) fractures (Fig. 8.15). After creation of the entry point, the 2.2 mm guidewire is inserted, and its position is confirmed fluoroscopically. After obtaining the reduction by manual manipulation, the guidewire is passed across the fracture. The nail is then inserted along the guidewire and pushed far distally—farther than for a 3- or 4-part fracture. The surgeon should ensure that (1) the nail is placed low enough so that its proximal tip is 10 mm lower than the highest part of the humeral head and (2) rotation is correct by aligning the version rod with the forearm. The nail is *first locked distally*, using only the more distal screw (static screw, in the round hole). The nail is then "pulled back up" with retrograde hammering to ensure impaction at the fracture site. If impaction and rotation are both satisfactory, then the nail can be locked proximally. Usually, one proximal locking screw (in the GT) provides enough stability to the construct.

8.11 Three-Part (Greater Tuberosity) Fractures

In three-part (GT) fractures, the head fragment is internally rotated due to traction by the subscapularis muscle and the absence of the counteracting force of the infraspinatus and teres minor due to the avulsed GT [47]. Additionally, the diaphysis is displaced medially and anteriorly. Therefore, the main goal must be to derotate the head fragment and anatomically reduce and fix the GT.

The "derotation" (transdeltoid) technique is used for 3-part fractures with avulsion of the GT (Fig. 8.16). The guidewire is inserted and its position is confirmed by C-arm. After obtaining fracture reduction by manual manipulation, the guidewire is passed across the fracture; then, the nail is inserted along the guidewire. The head fragment, which is in excessive internal rotation, is derotated either using a suture placed in the subscapularis or with a bone hook inserted through the incision. First, the version rod is placed in internal rotation and the anterior screw is inserted in the LT. With the LT and head now captured by the nail construct, the epiphyseal fragment is derotated (i.e., rotated externally) with the help of the external jig. At this point, the GT is manipulated using either a hook or a suture placed in the infraspinatus, and once anatomically reduced, it is fixed with its two screws.

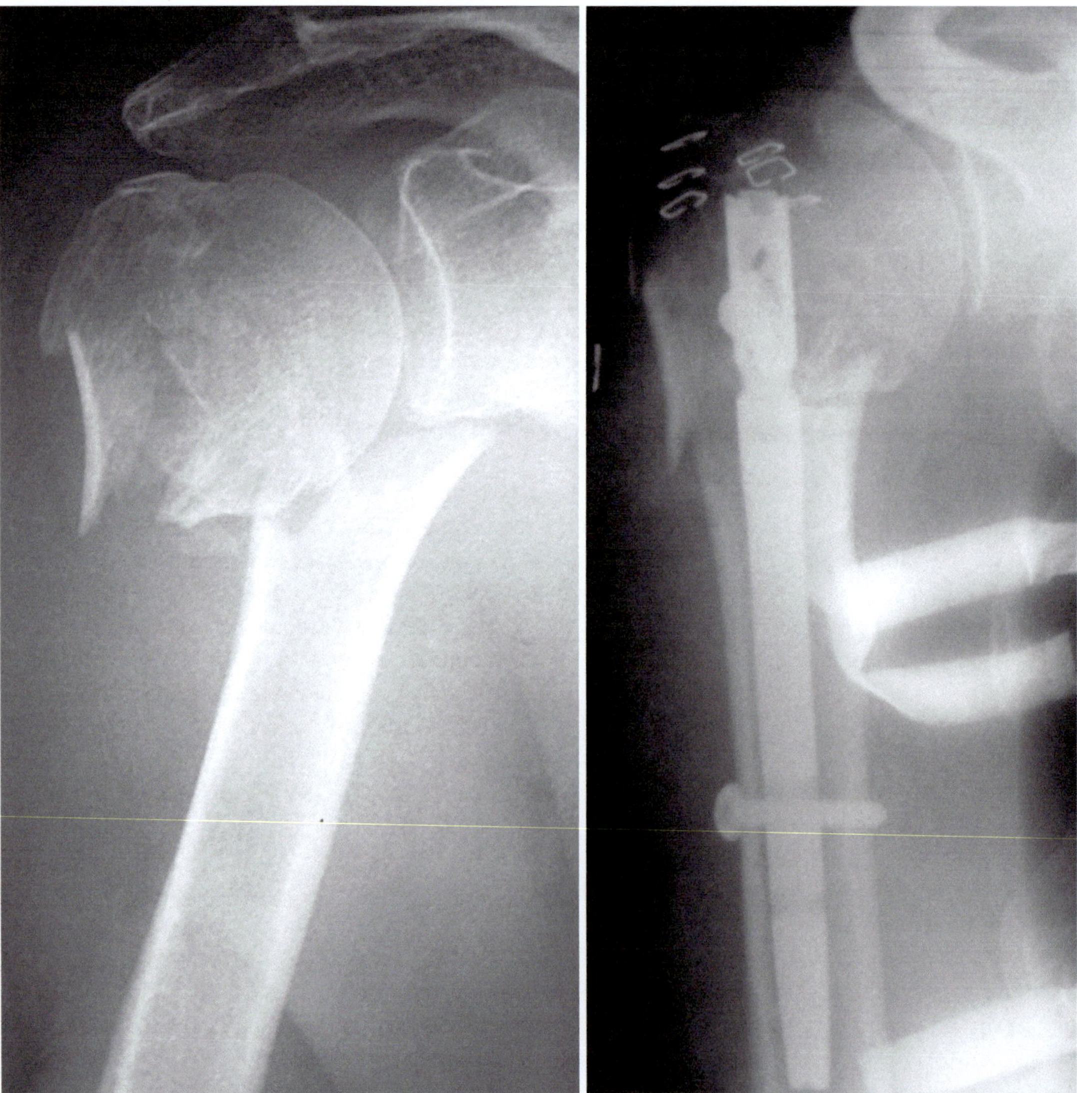

Fig. 8.15 Two-part displaced proximal humerus fracture fixed with Aequalis IM nail (notice the absence of screws oriented in the humeral head). Intraoperative retrograde hammering and version rod alignment. Active elevation at 3 months post-op

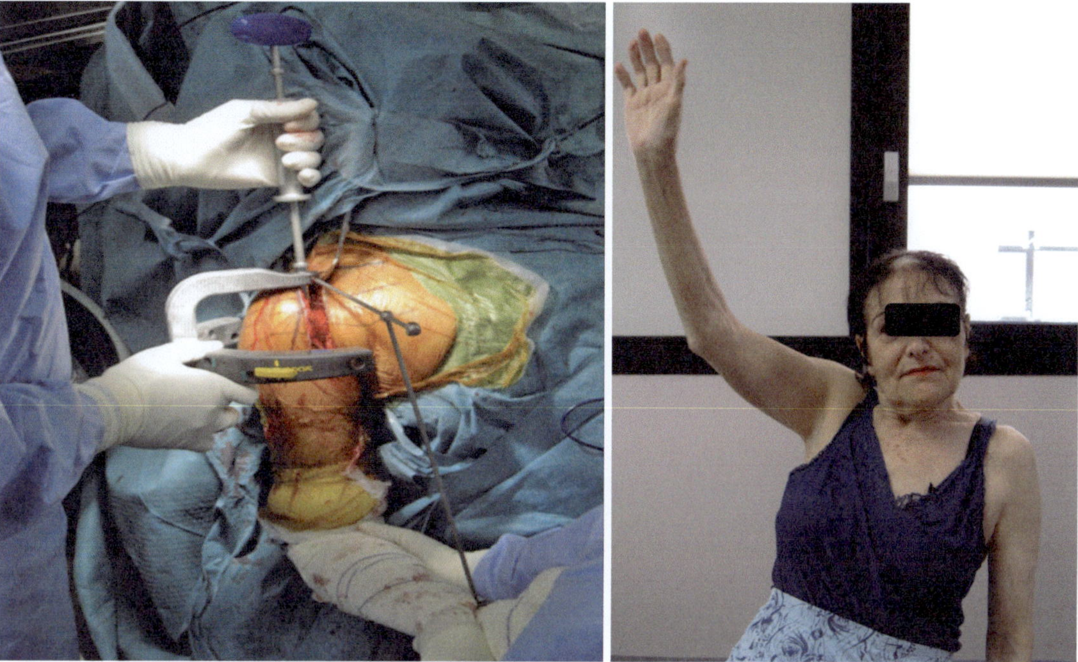

Fig. 8.15 (continued)

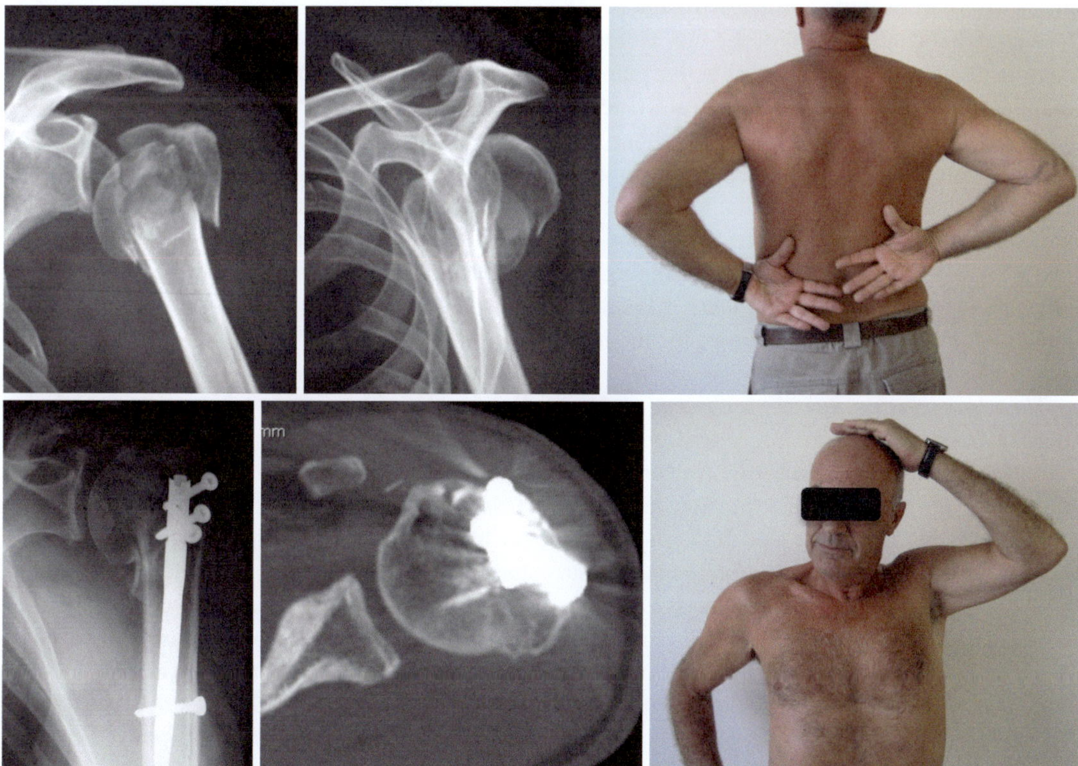

Fig. 8.16 Three-part displaced head-splitting fracture. Open reduction and fixation with Aequalis IM nail; post-op AP view shows healing and humeral reconstruction and CT scan demonstrates the absence of locking screws oriented in the humeral head

Since the GT is anatomically reduced and fixed, the two-part surgical neck fracture can now be viewed. This surgical neck fracture is then reduced by aligning the version rod to the forearm, which is placed in neutral rotation. Finally, compression at the fracture site is given by impacting the elbow, and the two distal screws are inserted.

8.12 Valgus Impacted Four-Part Fractures

In valgus impacted 4-part fractures, the tuberosities are split and retracted medially while the head fragment is collapsed [48, 49]. The blood supply is preserved with a medial soft tissue hinge [50, 51]. The main complication, encountered specifically with fractures involving the GT, is posterior migration of the GT with definitive loss of active external rotation.

The GT is, in our opinion, the key piece of the puzzle in 4-part proximal humerus fractures [7]. Posteromedial displacement of the GT with malunion leads to a definitive loss of active external rotation; this will compromise many activities of daily living such as eating, hair washing and combing, and holding a phone, among others. The main goal must therefore be to elevate the humeral head in order to reduce and fix the GT (and LT) in an anatomic position. Bringing the tuberosities together and fixing them "closes the door" and provides indirect support for the head (Fig. 8.17 and 8.18).

The "peg-closing book" technique (via a superior transdeltoid or deltopectoral approach) is used in valgus impacted 4-part fractures. One suture is placed on the infraspinatus tendon to manipulate the GT fragment and another is placed on the subscapularis tendon to manipulate the LT fragment. The biceps tendon is routinely tenodesed and its intra-articular portion resected after medial opening of the rotator interval. The vertical fracture plane is identified posterior to the bicipital groove. An elevator is inserted between the tuberosity fragments, and the head is elevated to its anatomic position, as indicated by the GT. It is important to keep the medial hinge intact and not to over-reduce the humeral head fragment. The entry portal of the nail is carefully created on the articular fragment, so as not to fragment it further. Alternatively, the nail can be inserted directly inside the medullary canal, passing lateral to the head fragment. The nail is first locked distally with the two distal screws, then it is used to support the head fragment. Next, the displaced GT is reduced using the stay sutures in the infraspinatus and placing the arm in external rotation. The GT in most cases regains its anatomic position when the articular fragment is elevated and the *arm is rotated externally*. The two posterior locking screws are then used to fix the GT to the nail. Similarly, the LT fragment is reduced using the subscapularis stay suture then fixed with its screw. In cases of osteopenic bone, it is recommended that this fixation be augmented with transverse cerclage and longitudinal tension-band sutures [52]. Finally, the anterior deltoid muscle is meticulously reattached to the acromion.

8.13 Varus Impacted Four-Part Fractures

Varus-type 4-part fractures are more difficult to reduce, and their open reduction and internal fixation should be approached with caution [14]. When the Aequalis nail is used, its entry portal must be *as medial as possible*.

8.14 Postoperative Management

A sling in *neutral rotation* is worn for 3–4 weeks. This position is the most relaxing position to keep the balance between the external and internal rotator cuff muscles. Pendular shoulder exercises as well as mobilization of the elbow, wrist, and fingers are started immediately. External rotation of the shoulder with the arm at the side and internal rotation with the hand in the back by a physiotherapist are prohibited for 6–8 weeks postoperatively. Active-assisted range of motion (ROM) exercises of the shoulder are allowed 4–6 weeks postoperatively. Swimming is recommended.

8.15 Early Clinical Experience with the Aequalis IM Nail

We have so far treated 24 patients with a mean age of 64 years (range, 27–83 years) for displaced and unstable fractures using the Aequalis IM nail. A fracture was considered to be displaced if it involved translation of more than 1 cm or an angulation of more than 45° in at least one view of the radiographic trauma series. On radiographs and CT scan, the fractures were classified using the Neer system: 9 were 2-part surgical neck fractures, 4 were 3-part fractures, and 11 were 4-part fractures. The fracture was secondary to low-energy falls in 20 patients (83 %). Nine patients (37 %) had severe osteoporosis. The time between injury and surgery averaged 8 days (range, 1–25 days). The approach was percutaneous in 5

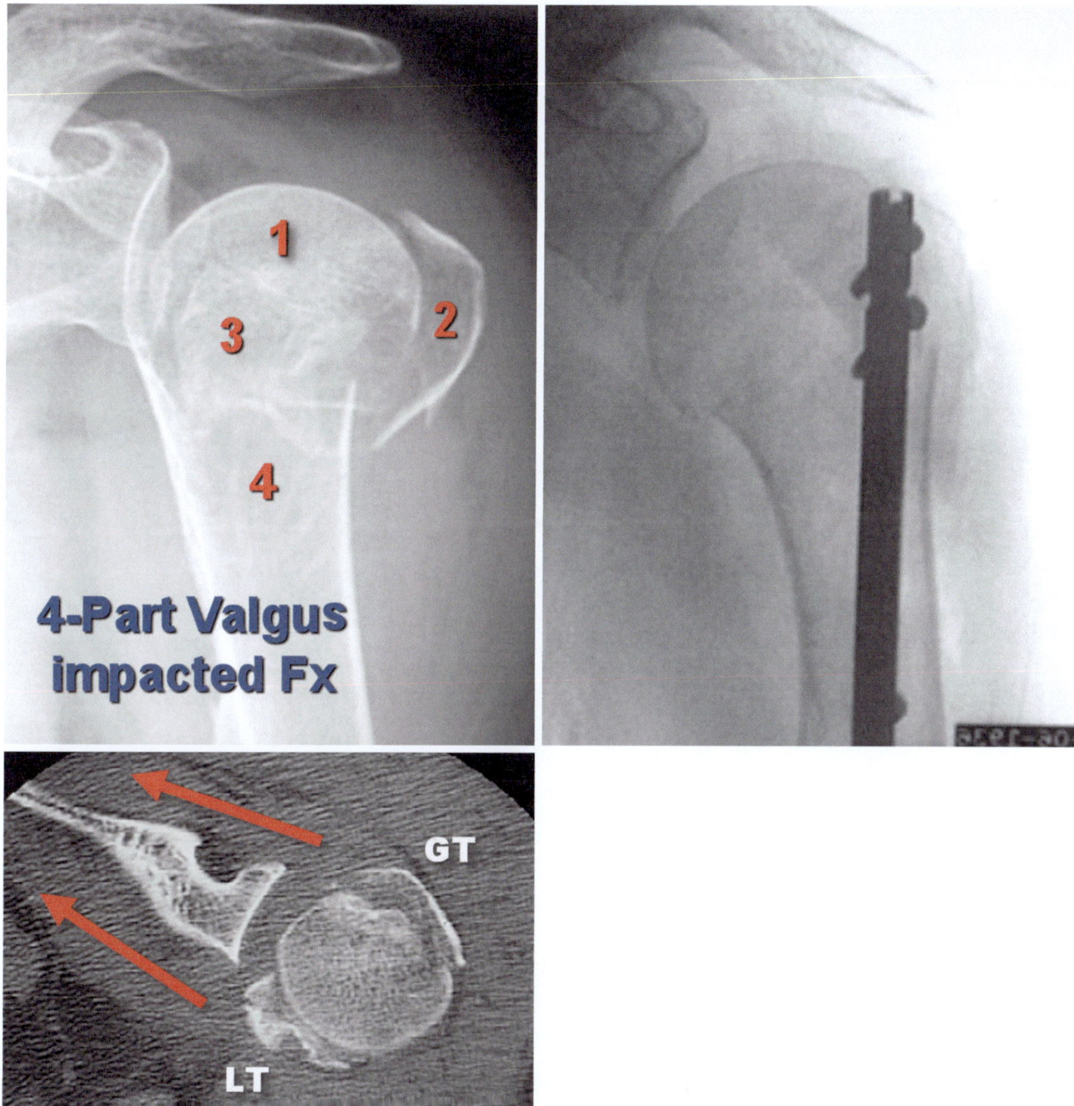

Fig. 8.17 (**a**) Four-part valgus impacted proximal humerus fracture with medial displacement of both tuberosities in a 67-year-old woman treated with IM nailing; proximal screws are oriented perpendicular to the tuberosities (tuberosity-based fixation). Notice the absence of screw oriented toward the humeral head. *Arrows* indicates horizontal pulling forces. (*GT*) greater tuberosity, (*LT*) lesser tuberosity, (*1*) humeral head, (*2*) greater tuberosity, (*3*) lesser tuberosity, (*4*) humeral shaft. (**b**) Functional result with 1-year FU

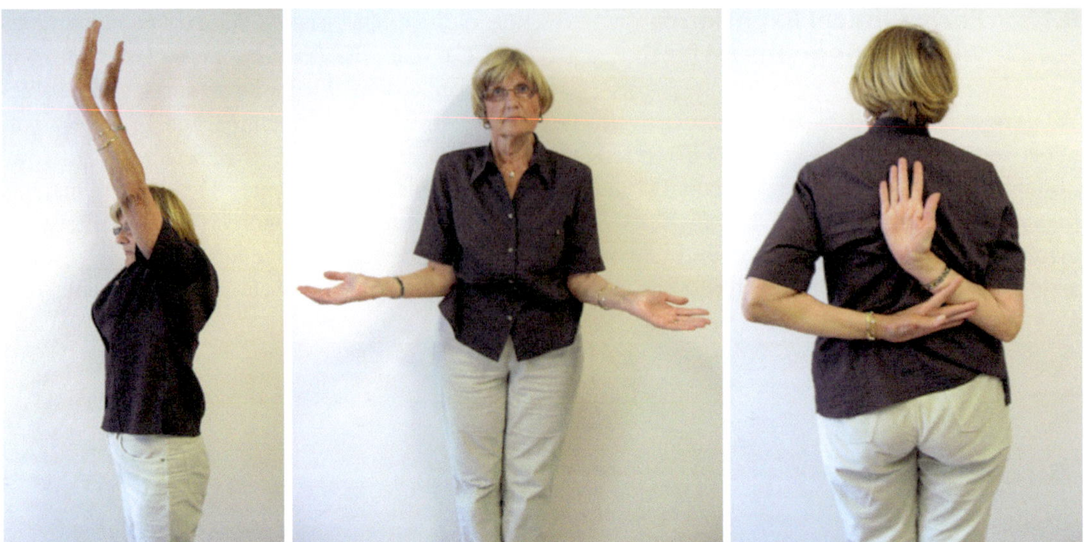

Fig. 8.17 (continued)

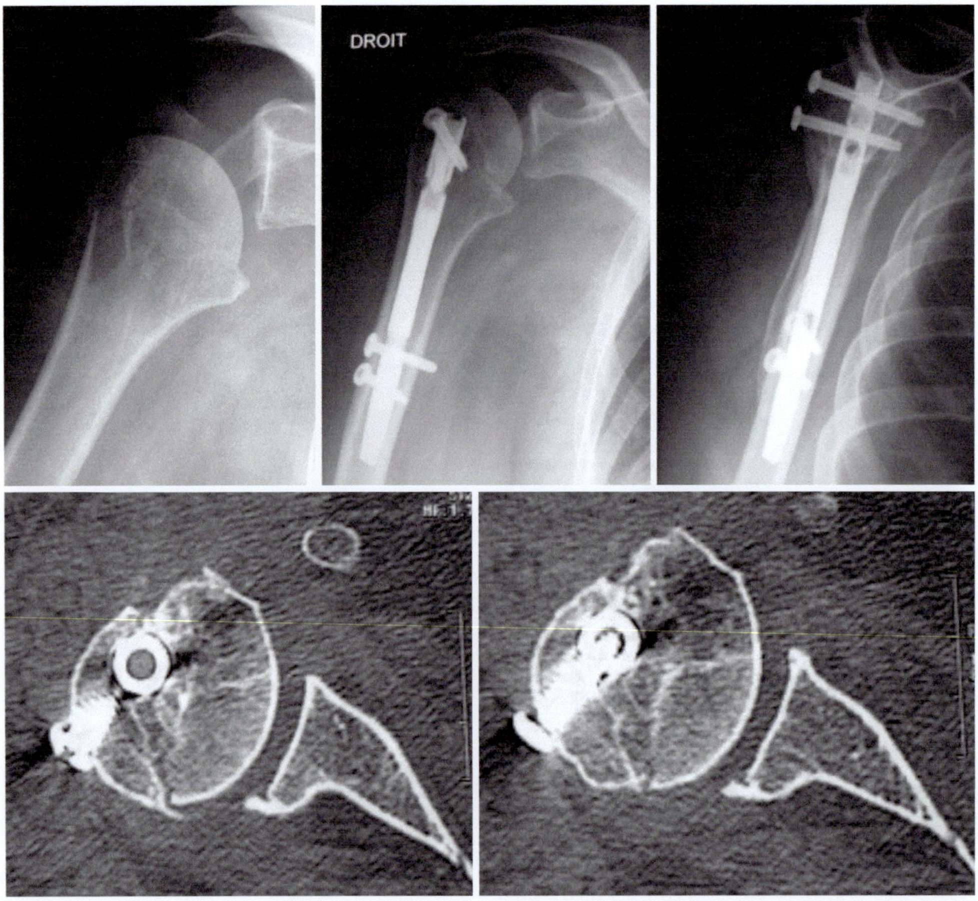

Fig. 8.18 (**a**) Four-part valgus impacted proximal humerus fracture in a 54-year-old woman; tuberosity-based screw orientation with Aequalis IM nail allows to resist to horizontal pulling forces of rotator muscles, while nail-based fixation is superior to any bone-based fixation, especially in osteopenic bone. (**b**) Good active mobility and no humeral head necrosis at 1 year, despite excessive elevation of the humeral head and loss of the medial hinge

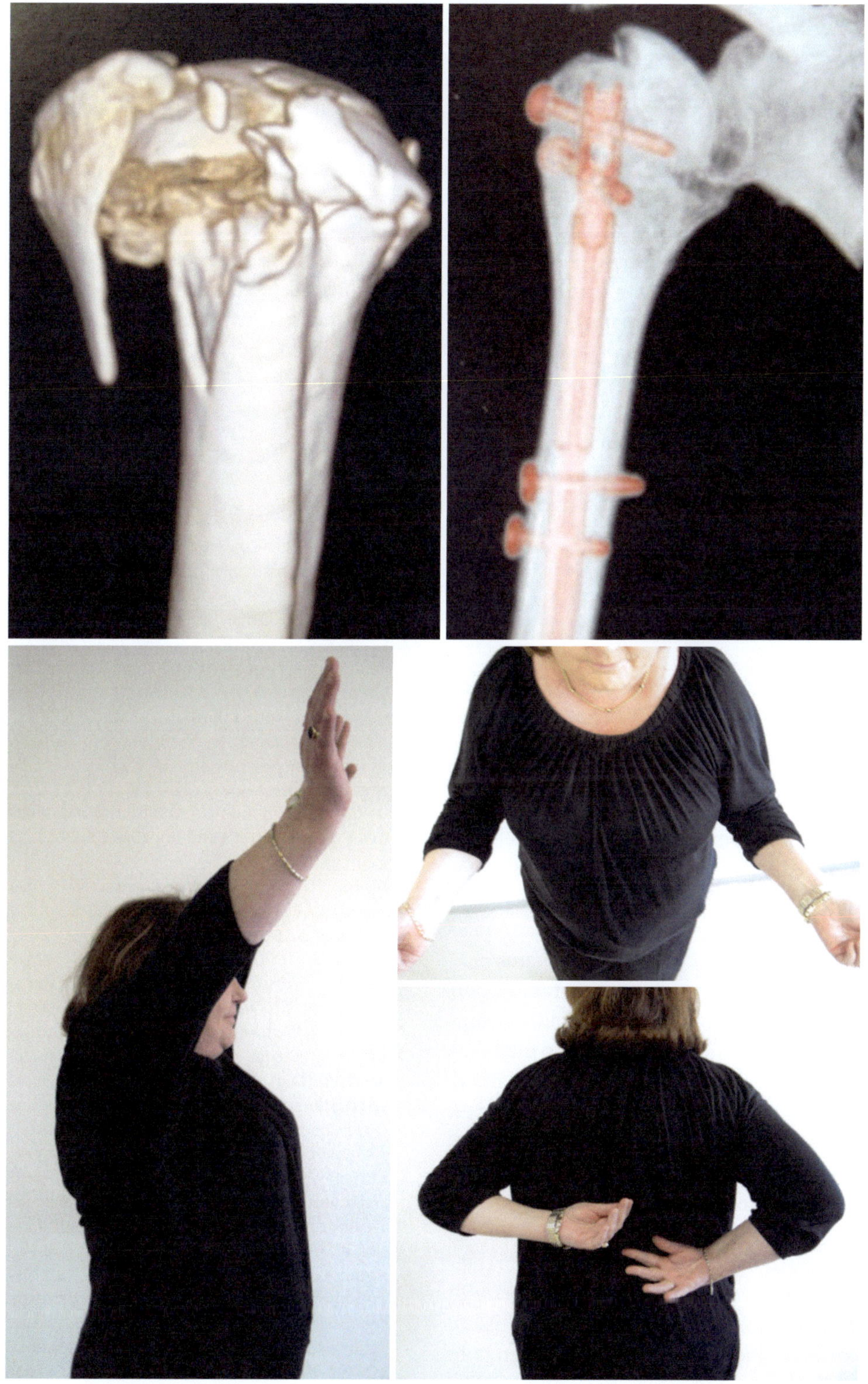

Fig. 8.18 (continued)

cases, transdeltoid in 13, and deltopectoral in 3. Follow-up was carried out at 4 weeks, 3, 6, and 12 months postoperatively and yearly thereafter. Patient follow-up averaged 9 months (range, 6–18 months).

No patient required further surgical intervention. All fractures healed and all patients recovered enough motion to perform daily activities independently. Postoperative outcomes as measured by Constant score averaged 69 points (95 % CI 49–83): pain 12.5 points, activity 15 points, mobility 28 points, and strength 13.5 points. The mean adjusted CS score was 81 % and the mean SSV score was 80 %. Active elevation was 132° (120–150), external rotation 37° (10–60), and internal rotation L3 (sacrum–D12). There was no tuberosity migration and no nonunion. Varus deformity was seen in 4 shoulders (16 %). Partial necrosis of the humeral head developed in one patient.

Conclusion

Proximal humeral fracture reduction and fixation remains a surgical challenge. The Aequalis IM nail is based on a new concept: the anatomic reduction and secure fixation of the greater tuberosity, which is the key piece of the puzzle in proximal humerus fractures. Loss of reduction and fixation of the greater tuberosity leads to definitive retraction and atrophy of the two single external rotator muscles of the shoulder (i.e., infraspinatus and teres minor). This loss of external rotator cuff muscles and tendons leads to a definitive pseudoparalyzed and stiff shoulder for which surgical options are limited. By contrast, posttraumatic humeral head necrosis is well tolerated since the greater tuberosity has healed in an anatomic position and there is no screw penetration or glenoid erosion. Thus, all efforts of the surgeon should *not* be directed toward the humeral head, but to the greater tuberosity fixation and reduction. Contrary to a common belief, humeral head fixation is *not* the problem since it becomes stable when both tuberosities are reduced and fixed. The Aequalis IM nail has been designed specifically to optimize tuberosity-fragment fixation and provide stable support for the humeral head, improving proximal humerus reconstruction and fixation in osteopenic bone. In addition, specific surgical techniques have been developed for reduction and fixation of each fracture type (2-, 3-, or 4-part). The design of this nail and these specific techniques have been created to avoid the common complications and problems related to IM nailing of proximal humeral fractures. Our early clinical experience is encouraging and lives up to the biomechanical and surgical concepts.

References

1. Krishnan SG, Lin KC, Burkhead WZ (2007) Pins, plates, and prostheses: current concepts in treatment of fractures of the proximal humerus. Curr Opin Orthop 18:380–385. doi:10.1097/BCO.0b013e32816aa3b7
2. Court-Brown CM, Garg A, McQueen MM (2001) The epidemiology of proximal humeral fractures. Acta Orthop 72:365–371. doi:10.1080/000164701753542023
3. Gerber C, Werner CML, Vienne P (2004) Internal fixation of complex fractures of the proximal humerus. J Bone Joint Surg Br 86:848–855
4. Sperling JW, Cuomo F, Hill JD et al (2007) The difficult proximal humerus fracture: tips and techniques to avoid complications and improve results. Instr Course Lect 56:45–57
5. Neer CS (1970) Displaced proximal humeral fractures. I. Classification and evaluation. J Bone Joint Surg Am 52:1077–1089
6. Neer CS (1970) Displaced proximal humeral fractures. II. Treatment of three-part and four-part displacement. J Bone Joint Surg Am 52:1090–1103
7. Boileau P, Pennington SD (2008) Common pitfalls in the management of proximal humeral fractures: how to avoid them. In: Boileau P, Walch G, Molé D et al (eds) Shoulder concepts 2008: proximal humeral fractures and fracture sequelae. Sauramps médical, Montpellier, pp 303–323
8. Drosdowech DS, Faber KJ, Athwal GS (2008) Open reduction and internal fixation of proximal humerus fractures. Orthop Clin North Am 39:429–39– vi. doi:10.1016/j.ocl.2008.06.003
9. Gradl G, Dietze A, Arndt D et al (2007) Angular and sliding stable antegrade nailing (Targon PH) for the treatment of proximal humeral fractures. Arch Orthop Trauma Surg 127:937–944. doi:10.1007/s00402-007-0425-5
10. Misra A, Kapur R, Maffulli N (2001) Complex proximal humeral fractures in adults—a systematic review of management. Injury 32(5):363–72

11. Lanting B, MacDermid J, Drosdowech D, Faber KJ (2008) Proximal humeral fractures: a systematic review of treatment modalities. J Shoulder Elbow Surg 17:42–54. doi:10.1016/j.jse.2007.03.016
12. Nho SJ (2007) Management of proximal humeral fractures based on current literature. J Bone Joint Surg Am 89:44. doi:10.2106/JBJS.G.00648
13. Petit CJ, Millett PJ, Endres NK et al (2010) Management of proximal humeral fractures: surgeons don't agree. J Shoulder Elbow Surg 19:446–451. doi:10.1016/j.jse.2009.06.012
14. Solberg BD, Moon CS, Franco DP, Paiement GD (2009) Surgical treatment of three and four-part proximal humeral fractures. J Bone Joint Surg Am 91:1689. doi:10.2106/JBJS.H.00133
15. Brunner F, Sommer C, Bahrs C et al (2009) Open reduction and internal fixation of proximal humerus fractures using a proximal humeral locked plate: a prospective multicenter analysis. J Orthop Trauma 23:163–172. doi:10.1097/BOT.0b013e3181920e5b
16. Owsley KC, Gorczyca JT (2008) Fracture displacement and screw cutout after open reduction and locked plate fixation of proximal humeral fractures. J Bone Joint Surg Am 90(2):233–240
17. Südkamp N, Bayer J, Hepp P et al (2009) Open reduction and internal fixation of proximal humeral fractures with use of the locking proximal humerus plate. Results of a prospective, multicenter, observational study. J Bone Joint Surg Am 91:1320–1328. doi:10.2106/JBJS.H.00006
18. Füchtmeier B, May R, Hente R et al (2007) Proximal humerus fractures: a comparative biomechanical analysis of intra and extramedullary implants. Arch Orthop Trauma Surg 127:441–447. doi:10.1007/s00402-007-0319-6
19. Edwards SL, Wilson NA, Zhang L, Flores S (2006) Two-part surgical neck fractures of the proximal part of the humerus. A biomechanical evaluation of two fixation techniques. J Bone Joint Surg Am 88(10):2258–2264
20. Hatzidakis AM (2008) Intramedullary nails/rods for proximal humerus fracture: design, technology and biomechanics. In: Boileau P, Walch G, Molé D et al (eds) Shoulder concepts 2008: proximal humeral fractures & fracture sequelae. Sauramps médical, Montpellier, pp 85–92
21. Hessmann MH, Hansen WSM, Krummenauer F et al (2005) Locked plate fixation and intramedullary nailing for proximal humerus fractures: a biomechanical evaluation. J Trauma 58:1194–1201
22. Kitson J, Booth G, Day R (2007) A biomechanical comparison of locking plate and locking nail implants used for fractures of the proximal humerus. J Shoulder Elbow Surg 16:362–366. doi:10.1016/j.jse.2006.01.019
23. McCormack RG, Brien D, Buckley RE et al (2000) Fixation of fractures of the shaft of the humerus by dynamic compression plate or intramedullary nail. A prospective, randomised trial. J Bone Joint Surg Br 82:336–339
24. Agel J, Jones CB, Sanzone AG et al (2004) Treatment of proximal humeral fractures with Polarus nail fixation. J Shoulder Elbow Surg 13:191–195. doi:10.1016/S1058274603003100
25. Bong MR, Kummer FJ, Koval KJ, Egol KA (2007) Intramedullary nailing of the lower extremity: biomechanics and biology. J Am Acad Orthop Surg 15:97–106
26. Cuny C, Pfeffer F, Irrazi M et al (2002) A new locking nail for proximal humerus fractures: the Telegraph nail, technique and preliminary results. Rev Chir Orthop Reparatrice Appar Mot 88:62–67
27. Kazakos K, Lyras DN, Galanis V et al (2007) Internal fixation of proximal humerus fractures using the Polarus intramedullary nail. Arch Orthop Trauma Surg 127:503–508. doi:10.1007/s00402-007-0390-z
28. Koike Y, Komatsuda T, Sato K (2008) Internal fixation of proximal humeral fractures with a Polarus humeral nail. J Orthop Traumatol 9:135–139. doi:10.1007/s10195-008-0019-1
29. Lin J (2006) Effectiveness of locked nailing for displaced three-part proximal humeral fractures. J Trauma 61:363–374. doi:10.1097/01.ta.0000224148.73016.30
30. Mittlmeier TWF, Stedtfeld H-W, Ewert A et al (2003) Stabilization of proximal humeral fractures with an angular and sliding stable antegrade locking nail (Targon PH). J Bone Joint Surg Am 85-A(Suppl 4):136–146
31. Parsons M, O'Brien RJ, Hughes JS (2005) Locked intramedullary nailing for displaced and unstable proximal humerus fractures. Tech Shoulder Elbow Surg 6:75
32. Rajasekhar C, Ray PS, Bhamra MS (2001) Fixation of proximal humeral fractures with the Polarus nail. J Shoulder Elbow Surg 10:7–10
33. Sosef N, Stobbe I, Hogervorst M et al (2007) The Polarus intramedullary nail for proximal humeral fractures: outcome in 28 patients followed for 1 year. Acta Orthop 78:436–441. doi:10.1080/17453670710014040
34. Bernard J, Charalambides C, Aderinto J, Mok D (2000) Early failure of intramedullary nailing for proximal humeral fractures. Injury 31:789–792
35. Cuomo F, Flatow EL, Maday MG et al (1992) Open reduction and internal fixation of two- and three-part displaced surgical neck fractures of the proximal humerus. J Shoulder Elbow Surg 1:287–295. doi:10.1016/S1058-2746(09)80055-4
36. Smith AM, Mardones RM, Sperling JW (2007) Early complications of operatively treated proximal humeral fractures. J Shoulder Elbow Surg 16:14–24
37. Broek CM, Besselaar M, Coenen JMF, Vegt PA (2006) Displaced proximal humeral fractures: intramedullary nailing versus conservative treatment. Arch Orthop Trauma Surg 127:459–463. doi:10.1007/s00402-006-0250-2
38. Young AA, Hughes JS (2008) Locked intramedullary nailing for treatment of displaced proximal humerus fractures. Orthop Clin North Am 39:417–428. doi:10.1016/j.ocl.2008.05.001, v–vi

39. Boileau P, Walch G (1997) The three-dimensional geometry of the proximal humerus. Implications for surgical technique and prosthetic design. J Bone Joint Surg Br 79:857–865
40. Boileau P, Krishnan SG, Tinsi L et al (2002) Tuberosity malposition and migration: reasons for poor outcomes after hemiarthroplasty for displaced fractures of the proximal humerus. J Shoulder Elbow Surg 11:401–412
41. d'Ollonne T, Challali M, Bronsard N, Boileau P (2012) Tridimensional geometry of proximal humeral fractures; three and four-part concept revisited. In: Boileau P (ed) Shoulder concepts 2012: arthroscopy, arthroplasty & fractures. Sauramps médical, Montpellier, pp 283–293
42. Muller ME, Allgower M, Schneider R, Willenegger H (1979) Manual of internal fixation, 2nd edn. Springer: Heidelberg
43. Bigorre N, Talha A, Cronier P, Hubert L (2009) A prospective study of a new locking plate for proximal humeral fracture. Injury 40(2):192–196
44. Meier RA, Messmer P, Regazzoni P et al (2006) Unexpected high complication rate following internal fixation of unstable proximal humerus fractures with an angled blade plate. J Orthop Trauma 20:253–260
45. Prince EJ, Breien KM, Fehringer EV, Mormino MA (2004) The relationship of proximal locking screws to the axillary nerve during antegrade humeral nail insertion of four commercially available implants. J Orthop Trauma 18:585
46. Clavert P, Adam P, Bevort A et al (2010) Pitfalls and complications with locking plate for proximal humerus fracture. J Shoulder Elbow Surg 19:489–494. doi:10.1016/j.jse.2009.09.005
47. Hawkins RJ, Bell RH, Gurr K (1986) The three-part fracture of the proximal part of the humerus. Operative treatment. J Bone Joint Surg Am 68:1410–1414
48. Resch H, Beck E, Bayley I (1995) Reconstruction of the valgus-impacted humeral head fracture. J Shoulder Elbow Surg 4:73–80
49. Robinson CM, Page RS (2003) Severely impacted valgus proximal humeral fractures. Results of operative treatment. J Bone Joint Surg Am 85-A:1647–1655
50. Bogner R, Hübner C, Matis N et al (2008) Minimally-invasive treatment of three- and four-part fractures of the proximal humerus in elderly patients. J Bone Joint Surg Br 90-B:1602–1607. doi:10.1302/0301-620X.90B12.20269
51. Hertel R, Hempfing A, Stiehler M, Leunig M (2004) Predictors of humeral head ischemia after intracapsular fracture of the proximal humerus. J Shoulder Elbow Surg 13:427–433. doi:10.1016/S1058274604000795
52. Park J-Y, An J-W, Oh J-H (2006) Open intramedullary nailing with tension band and locking sutures for proximal humeral fracture: Hot air balloon technique. J Shoulder Elbow Surg 15:594–601. doi:10.1016/j.jse.2006.01.001

9 Anatomic Shoulder Arthroplasty for Fracture: Indications and Technique

Filippo Castoldi, Andrea Cimino, and Raffaele Garofalo

9.1 Introduction

Hemiarthroplasty is the procedure of choice for certain 3- and 4-part fractures, fracture-dislocations, and head-splitting fractures of the proximal humerus. It is a difficult procedure that requires experience in trauma and joint replacement surgery. The main difficulties arise from the management of the tuberosities and restoring of the correct version and length. The results are highly variable and sometimes unpredictable, related to effective pain control and restoration of normal function [1].

In particular, the main difficulty is the proper healing of the tuberosities which can be reabsorbed due to the poor quality of the bone and vascularization or migration and healing in an incorrect place.

F. Castoldi
Department of Orthopaedics and Traumatology, 2nd University Clinic, CTO Hospital Turin, Largo Turati 62, Turin 10128, Italy
e-mail: filippo.castoldi@unito.it

A. Cimino (✉) • R. Garofalo
Department of Orthopaedics and Traumatology, Mauriziano-Umberto I Hospital, Largo Turati 62, Turin 10128, Italy
e-mail: andreacimino87@gmail.com

9.2 Indications and Preoperative Planning

As already described in the chapter regarding the understanding of the fracture, one of the treatment cornerstones is the correct indication. This comes from the overall understanding of the type of both fracture and patient that we have to deal with concerning age, functional requirements, compliance, dominant side, and quality of the tissues [2–4].

9.2.1 Age

The age of the patient plays a vital role in our decision to treat. The patient under the age of 60 with high expectations is the ideal candidate for a hemiarthroplasty. This consideration should be made also on the basis of his ability to follow a demanding rehabilitation protocol completely different from that required when a reverse prosthesis is implanted.

Between 60s and 70s, the decision is related to the biologic age of the patient, to his general health, and to the presence of functional disorders prior to the trauma.

Above the age of 70, the patient's characteristics and the quality of the bone would be often in favor of the placement of a reverse prosthesis.

F. Castoldi et al. (eds.), *Simple and Complex Fractures of the Humerus*,
DOI 10.1007/978-88-470-5307-6_9, © Springer-Verlag Italia 2015

9.2.2 Bone Quality

The quality of the bone affects (all) procedures: a poor quality of the bone with comminution of the tuberosity and a thin cortical can make the procedure extremely complex. The bone quality can be evaluated with standard X-ray picture and CT scan, but definitive assessment is still intraoperative. Therefore, it is recommended to have many different solutions available in the operating theater before operation, to solve any problem identified during the procedure [5].

9.2.3 Fracture Pattern

Three- and four-part fractures, fracture-dislocations, head-splitting fractures of the proximal humerus, impacted fractures of the humeral head with involvement of more than 50 % of the articular surface, and a very unstable calcar are the most frequent injury patterns we have to deal with. For details we refer to the chapter "Understanding the Fracture."

9.2.4 Rotator Cuff

The rotator cuff integrity can be assessed only intraoperatively. You can have an idea of the cuff condition, prior to surgery, inquiring the shoulder level of functional impairment before the injury and knowing that CT image that can sometimes highlight an atrophy of the rotator muscles.

9.2.5 Surgeon Experience

The surgeon experience plays an important role. As previously said, implanting a prosthesis in case of proximal humerus fracture is a complex procedure requiring extensive knowledge of technical and anatomic details.

Our specific relative indications for hemiarthroplasty in proximal humerus fracture are as follows:

- Age <70
- Fracture pattern: 3- and 4-part fractures, fracture-dislocations, head-splitting fractures of the proximal humerus, head ischemia based on Hertel criteria
- Good bone quality
- Non-comminuted tuberosities
- Patient with good compliance
- No cuff deficiency

9.2.6 X-rays

An AP view and an axillary view are mandatory. A CT is needed to better understand the nature of the fracture fragments, to identify their management and reduction, and also to have a perfect view of the glenoid.

9.3 Surgical Technique

9.3.1 Positioning/Exposure

The patient is placed in a beach-chair position on the edge of the operating table, taking care of leg position. The whole scapula must be visible and the arm must be freely movable.

The deltopectoral is the best approach for this surgical procedure. The skin incision goes straight from the lateral edge of the coracoid to the insertion of the deltoid muscle, paralleling the cephalic vein. You need to retract the pectoralis major medially and the deltoid laterally, splitting the two muscles apart (Fig. 9.1).

The subcutaneous tissues are divided and the deltopectoral interval is entered; the cephalic vein may be retracted either medially or laterally. Sometimes it could be difficult to identify the deltopectoral groove because of hematoma or poor quality of the muscles. It is easier to find the groove between the deltoid and the pectoralis, proximally near the clavicle where there is a natural fat space.

Bursectomy is often an important step: hematoma and bursa must be removed to gain a good view of the fracture anatomy.

It is necessary to identify the superior margin of the pectoralis major, which is an important anatomic landmark in verifying the height of the future implant, to correctly access the surgical site (Fig. 9.2). The clavipectoral fascia is opened

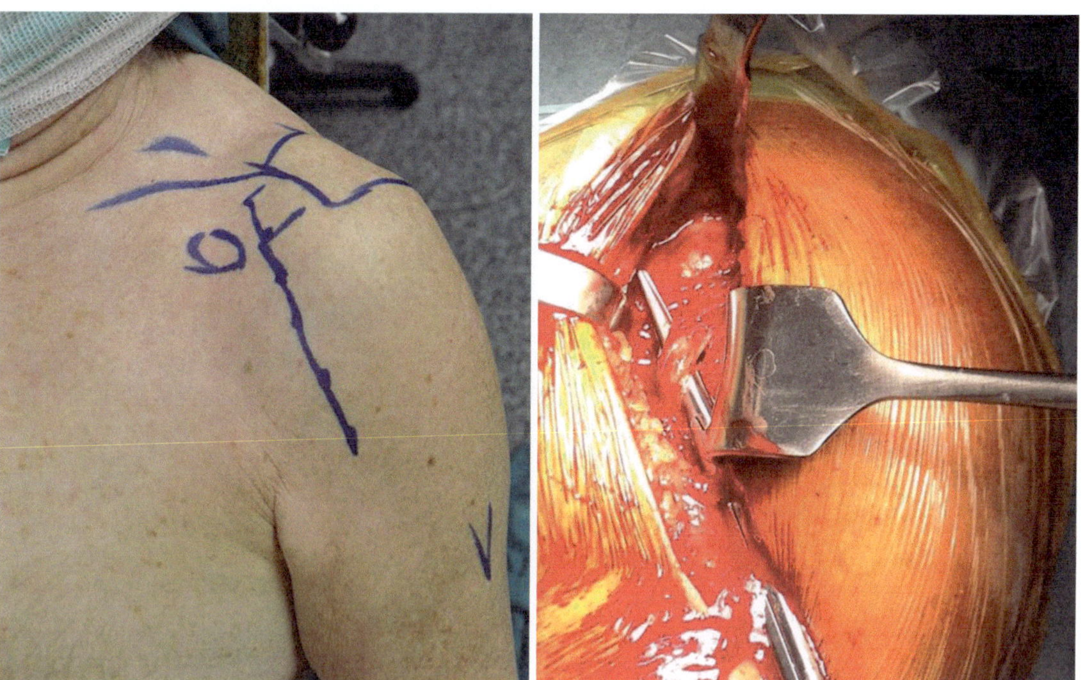

Fig. 9.1 Deltopectoral approach. Main landmarks: coracoid process, acromion, and distal deltoid insertion. Vision from this approach is optimal

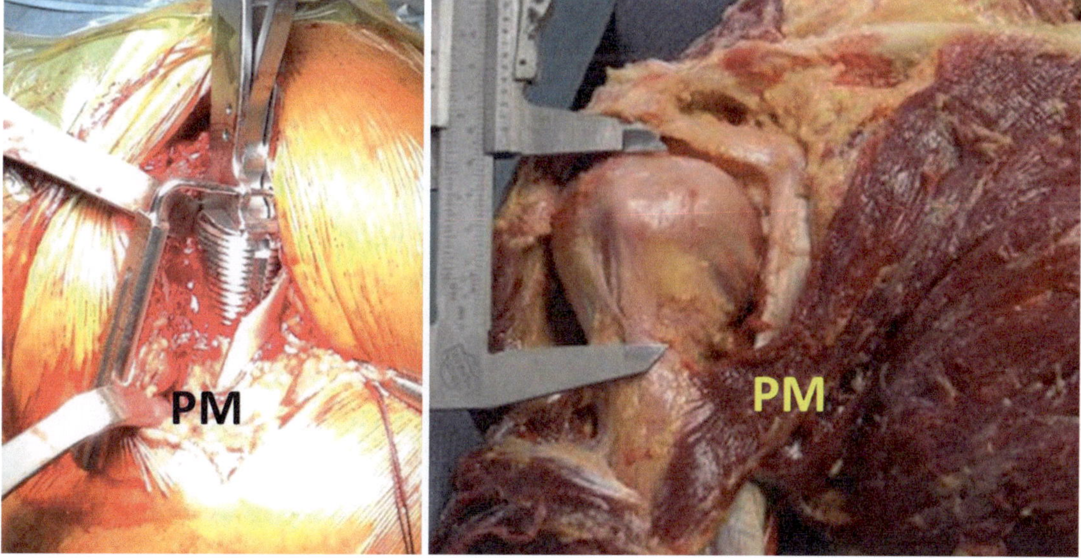

Fig. 9.2 It is very important to identify the top margin of the pectoralis major muscle (*PM*) that allows to define the height of the implant. To the left there is a ruler that measures the height of the rasp in relation to the tendon

and a self-retaining retractor is placed between the conjoined tendon and deltoid. It is easy to identify the long head of the biceps that is an excellent landmark to find the interval between the tuberosities. Tenotomy is performed (Fig. 9.3). The arm is then placed into abduction and internal rotation, and the greater and lesser tuberosities are identified. It is essential to

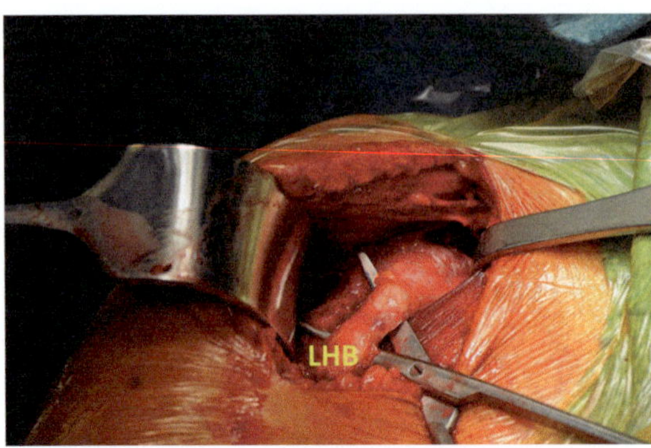

Fig. 9.3 Identify the tendon of the long head of the biceps (*LHB*). Frequently you perform a tenotomy

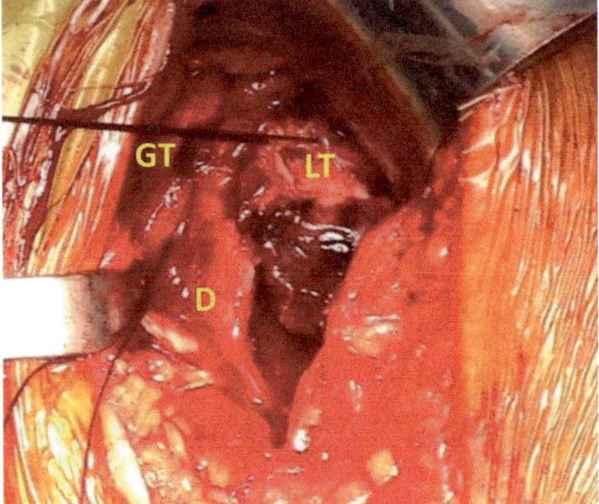

Fig. 9.4 Two no. 2 nonabsorbable sutures are placed in Mason-Allen-type stitches at the bone-tendon junction through the subscapularis and infraspinatus in order to manage the tuberosities (*GT* greater tuberosities, *LT* lesser tuberosities, *D* diaphysis)

preserve them with all the bone. Two no. 2 nonabsorbable sutures are placed in Mason-Allen-type stitches at the bone-tendon junction through the subscapularis and infraspinatus in order to manage the tuberosities (Fig. 9.4). It is helpful to release both tendons (subscapularis, infraspinatus) to obtain free fragments that can be easily placed around the implant.

The rotator interval is opened till the glenoid to release the coracohumeral ligament to expose the humeral head and the glenoid.

With the tuberosities retracted, the head fragment is removed; in order to measure the head size, it should be better to remove it in one piece (Fig. 9.5).

At this point the inspection of the glenoid can be easily done in order to assess its integrity and the good condition of the cartilage.

9.3.2 Humeral Preparation

The arm is left along the trunk and externally rotated, and the humeral shaft is exposed.

Since the metaphysis is typically "absent" due to the fracture, the humeral shaft is prepared with hand reamers until there is a gentle cortical resistance. A humeral trial is then placed. During this step, the surgeon must check carefully the fit of the diaphysis and the version and the depth of the implant. The fit is obtained evaluating the relationship between the stem and the canal; the retroversion is identified with anatomic references according to the used system (the alignment rod into the appropriate retroversion hole, referring to the forearm and to the condyles) (Fig. 9.6); the appropriate depth of the implant is measured referring to anatomic landmarks: the calcar and the distance between the tip of the humeral head and the upper margin of the pectoralis major [5.5 cm; (Fig. 9.7)].

It is important to measure the resected humeral head to decide the correct size (diameter and height) of the implant. In order to decide which size is best, it is important to remember that undersizing the head avoids the overstuffing that might lead to complications such as glenoiditis and tendon impingement (Fig. 9.8). The selected humeral trial head is placed.

You need to mobilize the tuberosities in order to approximate them around the prosthesis and the humeral shaft: the primary goal is the maximum contact between stem and shaft to restore their anatomic position (Fig. 9.9). The V-shaped fracture in the diaphysis represents a very important landmark for the reduction of the greater tuberosity (Fig. 9.10) [6]. The initial reduction of the greater tuberosity allows testing of both height and retroversion of the implant. With the tuberosities reduced, it is possible to define the

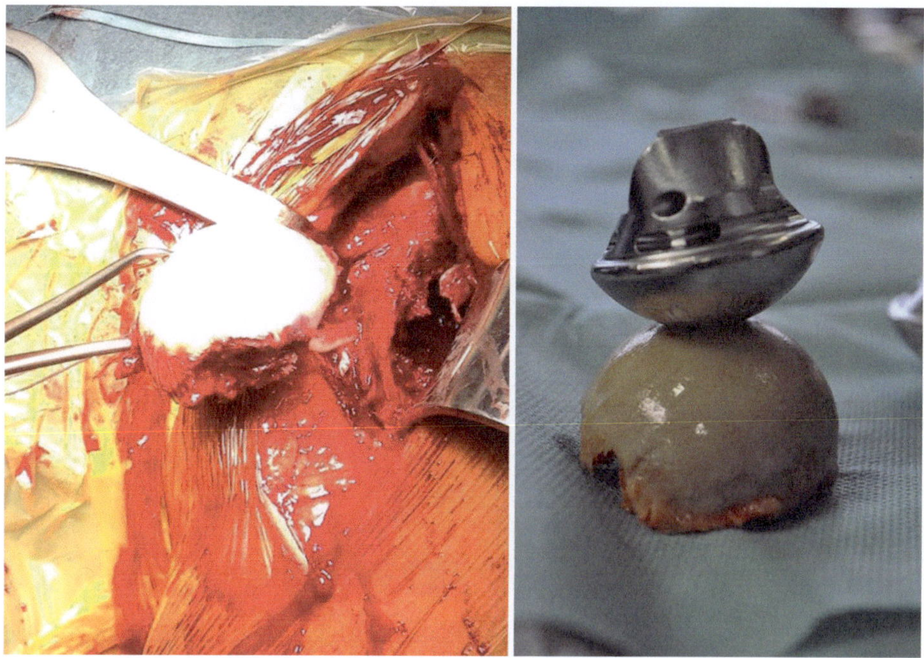

Fig. 9.5 Removal of the head if possible in one piece to allow a correct measurement

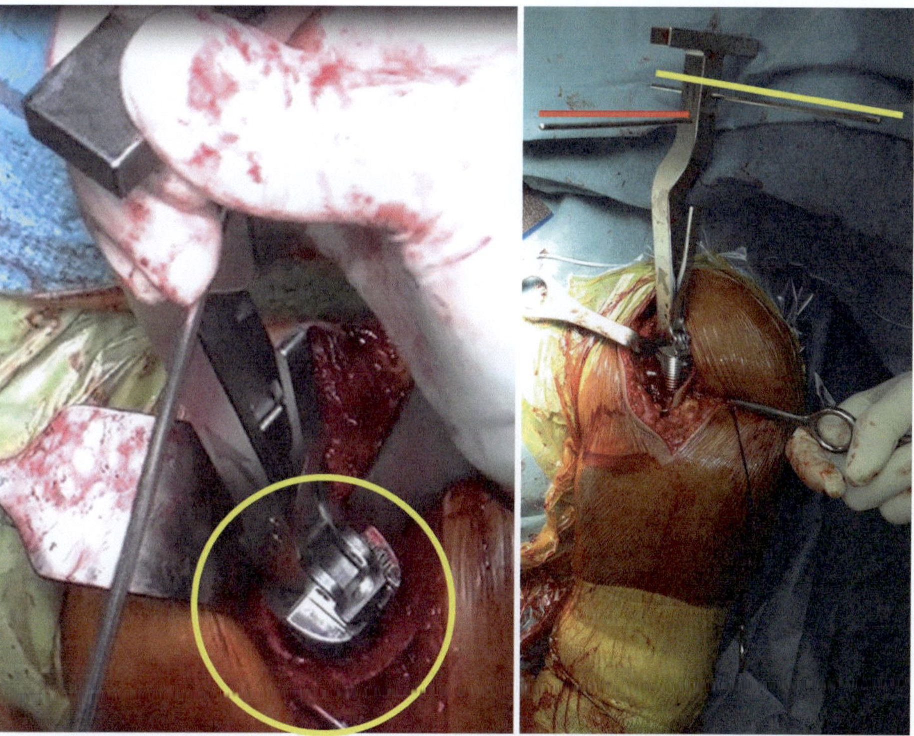

Fig. 9.6 *Left:* evaluation of the (*yellow circle*) refers to the filling of the rasp in the diaphysis. *Right*: evaluation of the orientation of the stem with the alignment rod: transepicondylar axis, *yellow*; forearm axis, *red*

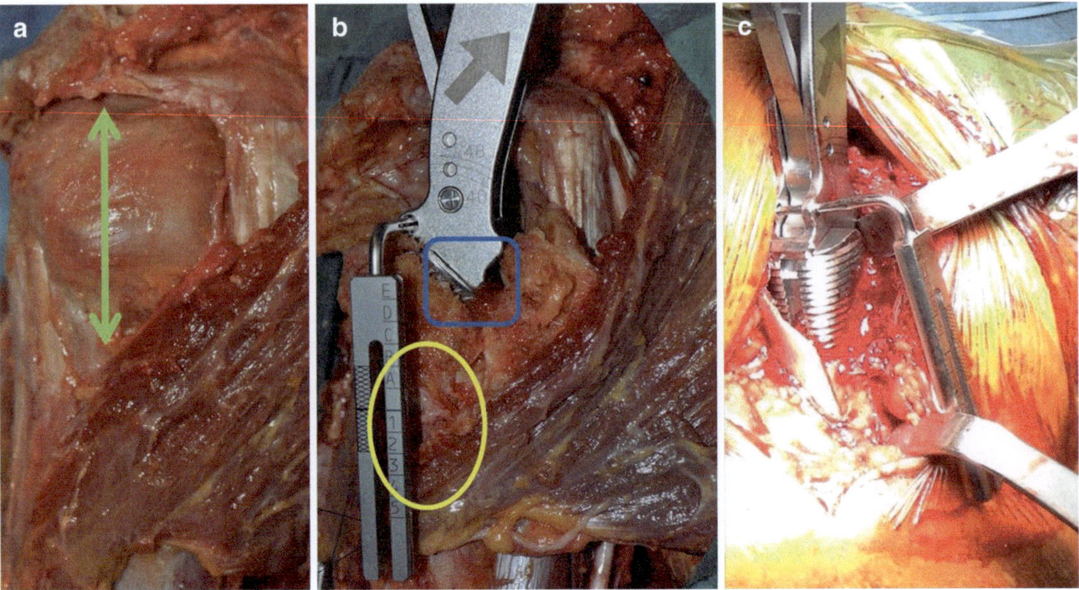

Fig. 9.7 (**a**) The distance between the tip of the humeral head and the upper border of the pectoralis major (*green arrows*). (**b**) The appropriate depth of the implant is measured referring to anatomic landmarks: the calcar (*blue circle*) and the distance between the tip of the humeral head and the upper margin of the pectoralis major (5.5 cm) (*yellow circle*). (**c**) The same ruler intraoperatively

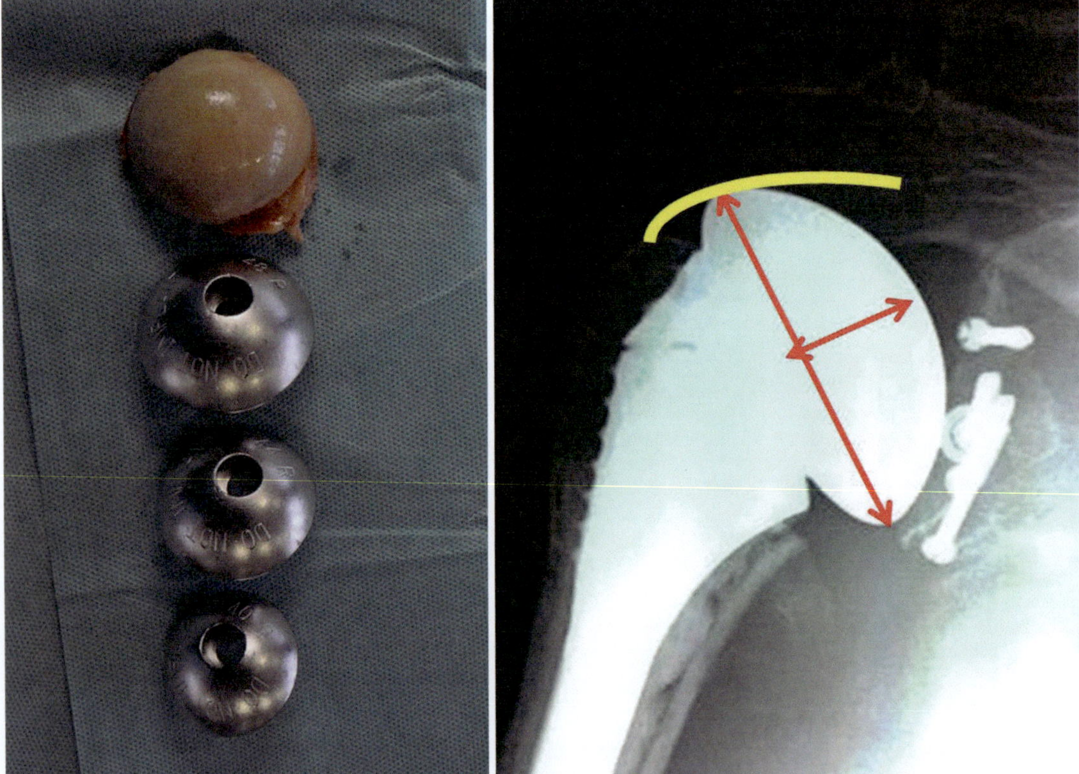

Fig. 9.8 Measurement of the humeral head: undersizing the head. *Right*: *yellow* tendon impingement of a humeral head oversized. *red arrows*: size(diameter and hight)

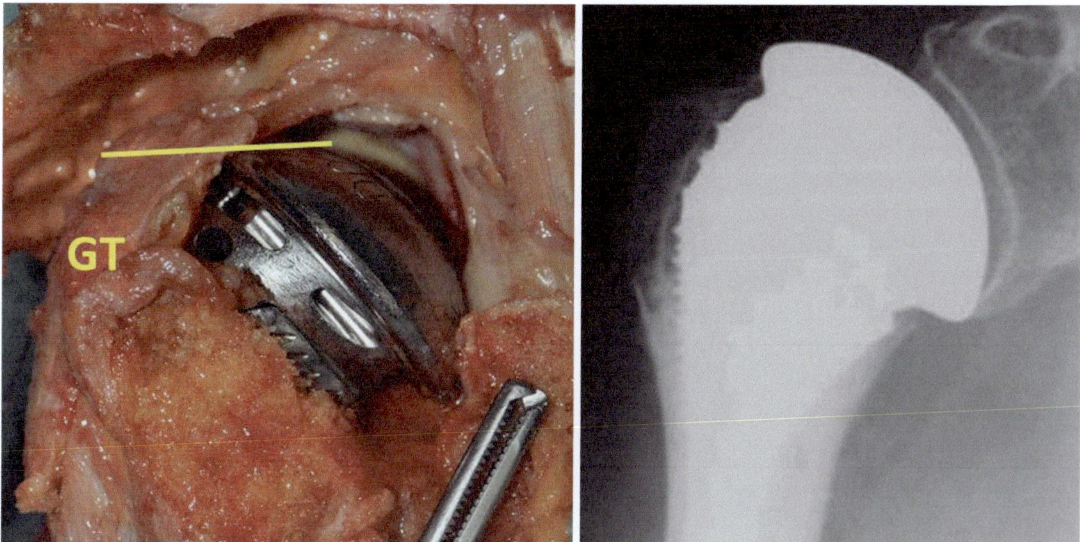

Fig. 9.9 *Left*: *yellow line* refers to level of gt and contact with the implant (*GT*). *Right*: post-op X-ray control demonstrating the perfect restoration of the anatomy

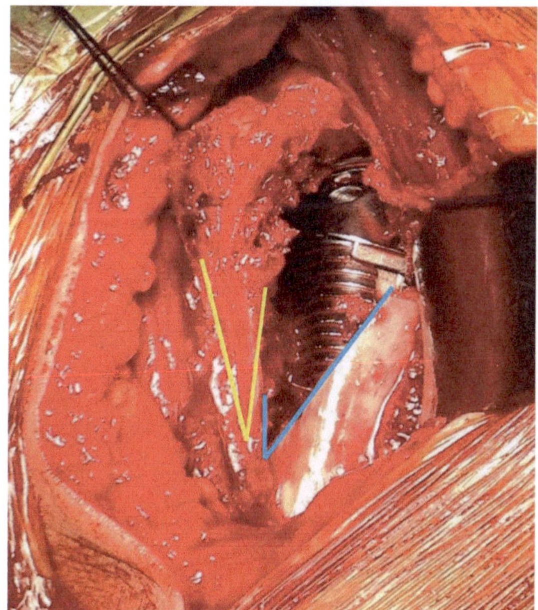

Fig. 9.10 The V-shaped fracture in the diaphysis (*blue line*) represents a very important landmark for the reduction of the greater tuberosity (*yellow line*)

correct position of the sutures that are supposed to anchor the tuberosities to the diaphysis and drill the holes for passing them (Fig. 9.11). The sutures must close the fragments around the implant stabilizing them and neutralizing the traction forces of the tendons (Fig. 9.12).

This calibration phase of the tuberosity reduction represents the key moment of the procedure: it may take time and it has to be done very precisely (Fig. 9.13) [7].

There is no known suture system that guarantees a reliable suture and an appropriate stability of the tuberosity: we consider of great importance the positioning of four circular sutures that span the two tuberosities and of two sutures anchored to the shaft that can neutralize the tension of the tendons.

Usually a conflict between the supraspinatus tendon and the prosthetic head and an incorrect reduction of the tuberosities can compromise their healing and the functional recovery of the shoulder.

A cement restrictor is then placed and the humeral canal cleaned and dried with pulsatile lavage. The cementation is performed with the definitive implant: it is essential to remove all the cement from the metaphyseal region and between the tuberosities. The height and the direction of the prosthesis are set as previously noted.

After all sutures are tied, trial motion is tested to ensure stable fixation of the tuberosities to the shaft (no movements are allowed between all the structures) and to rule out any abnormal

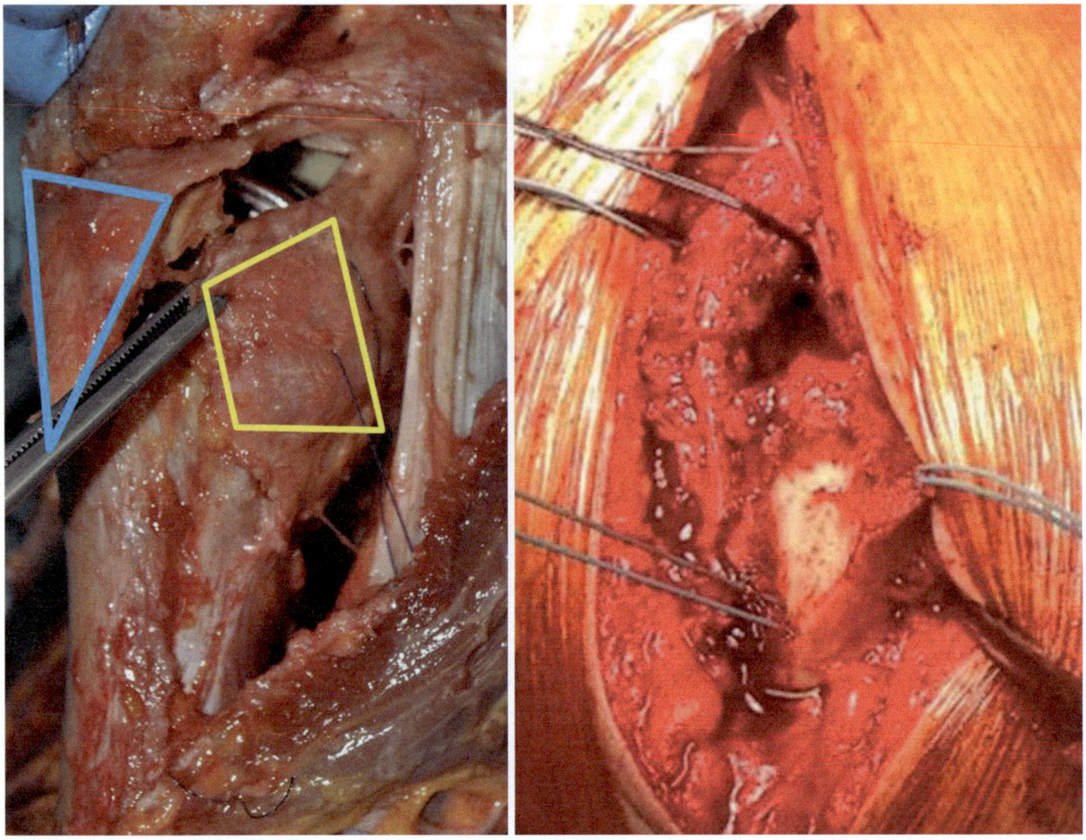

Fig. 9.11 With the greater (*blue*) and lesser (*yellow*) tuberosities reduced, it is possible to define the correct position of the sutures anchoring the tuberosities to the diaphysis and drill the holes for passing them. *Right*: sutures passing the diaphysis

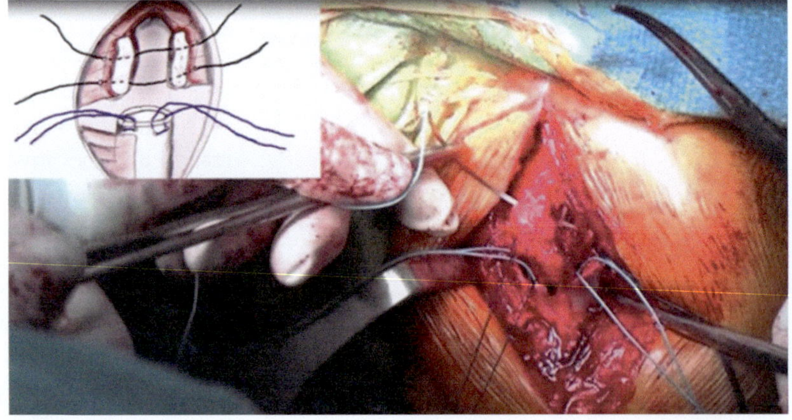

Fig. 9.12 The sutures close the fragments around the implant. Sutures passing in the supra- and infraspinatus tendons. The blue sutures come out from the canal, neutralizing the traction forces of the tendons

impingement of the implant prior to closure. The deltopectoral interval is then closed with no. 2 absorbable braided suture, followed by closure of the subcutaneous tissue with interrupted no. 0 absorbable sutures and a running no. 2/0 absorbable suture. The skin edges are re-approximated with staples and a sterile dressing applied (Fig. 9.14).

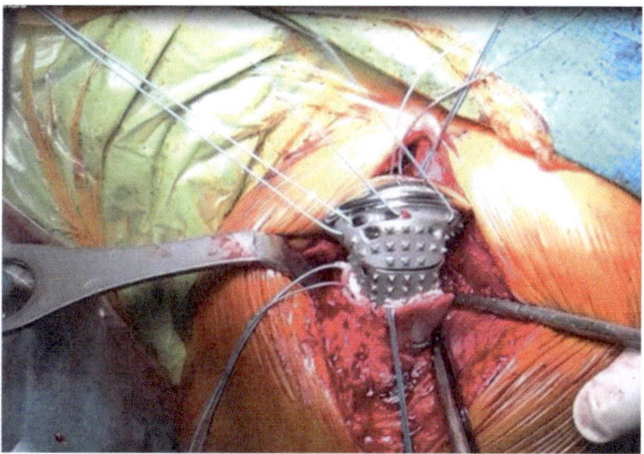

Fig. 9.13 In some cases the implant has holes to pass the sutures and ensure the tuberosities. It is mandatory to have the sutures well organized

9.4 Postoperative Management

Postoperatively, patients are immobilized for 6 weeks in a sling, which is only removed to bathe and perform physical therapy. Patients are immediately started on gentle elbow, wrist, and hand range of motion and scapular stabilization exercises. For the first 4 weeks, we allow supine passive elevation to 90° and external rotation to 30° with the arm at the side. Four to six weeks after surgery, patients are advanced to full supine passive elevation and only 30° of external rotation with the arm at the side. From the seventh week, full active forward elevation is

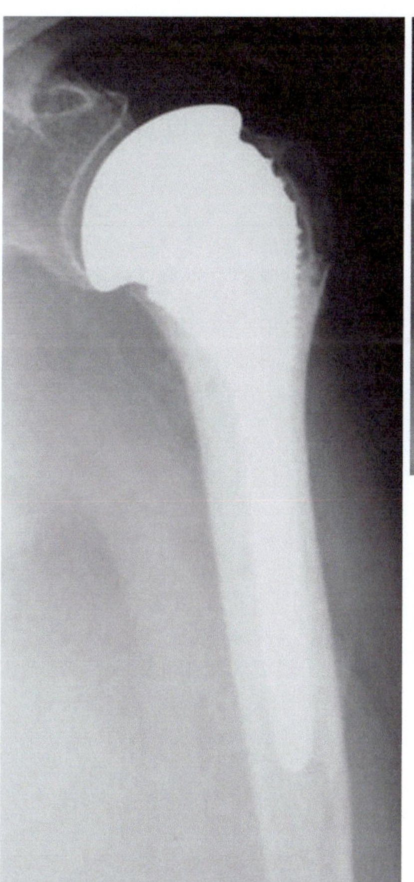

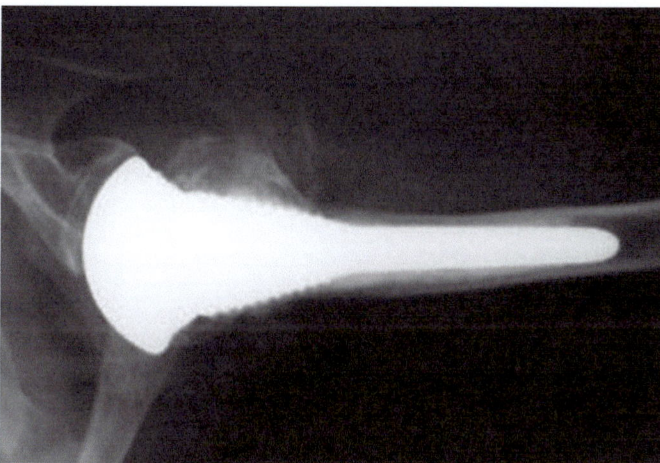

Fig. 9.14 Post-op X-ray control

allowed and external and internal rotations are started. Resistance exercises begin at the tenth week [8].

References

1. Konrad GG, Mehlhorn A, Kühle J, Strohm PC, Südkamp NP (2008) Proximal humerus fractures – current treatment options. Acta Chir Orthop Traumatol Cech 75(6):413–421
2. Solberg BD, Moon CN, Franco DP, Paiement GD (2009) Surgical treatment of three and four-part proximal humeral fractures. J Bone Joint Surg Am 91(7): 1689–1697
3. Kontakis G, Tosounidis T, Galanakis I, Megas P (2008) Prosthetic replacement for proximal humeral fractures. Injury 39(12):1345–1358
4. Kontakis G, Koutras C, Tosounidis T, Giannoudis P (2008) Early management of proximal humeral fractures with hemiarthroplasty: a systematic review. J Bone Joint Surg Br 90(11):1407–1413
5. Smith AM, Mardones RM, Sperling JW, Cofield RH (2007) Early complications of operatively treated proximal humeral fractures. J Shoulder Elbow Surg 16(1):14–24
6. Besch L, Daniels-Wredenhagen M, Mueller M, Varoga D, Hilgert RE, Seekamp A (2009) Hemiarthroplasty of the shoulder after four-part fracture of the humeral head: a long-term analysis of 34 cases. J Trauma 66(1):211–214
7. Sirveaux F, Roche O, Molé D (2010) Shoulder arthroplasty for acute proximal humerus fracture. Orthop Traumatol Surg Res 96(6):683–694
8. Bastian JD, Hertel R (2009) Osteosynthesis and hemiarthroplasty of fractures of the proximal humerus: outcomes in a consecutive case series. J Shoulder Elbow Surg 18(2):216–219

10 Reverse Total Shoulder Arthroplasty for Fracture: Indications and Technique

Brody A. Flanagin, Raffaele Garofalo, and Sumant G. Krishnan

10.1 Introduction

Proximal humeral fractures represent the third most frequent fracture of the appendicular skeleton in elderly patients [1]. The incidence of proximal humerus fractures associated with osteoporosis in elderly persons has been increasing as the elderly population expands [2]. The majority of proximal humerus fractures in the elderly will result in minimal displacement and are treated nonoperatively. However, displaced and/or unstable fractures often require operative intervention, and there currently exists no consensus regarding the ideal management of these fractures. In addition to fracture geometry, many patient factors, including age, general medical condition, activity level, bone quality, and ability to comply with postoperative rehabilitation, are taken into account when deciding on operative treatment of choice.

Several techniques, including open reduction and internal fixation (ORIF) and hemiarthroplasty, have been described for operative treatment of proximal humerus fractures in the elderly. Although the advent of locking plate technology offers the advantage of improved mechanical fixation in weaker bone, achieving adequate stability to maintain reduction and prevent tuberosity displacement is challenging in elderly patients. Furthermore, the results of ORIF of proximal humerus fractures in elderly patients have been somewhat inconsistent and prone to high rates of complications and worse functional outcomes [3, 4]. Hemiarthroplasty has been suggested as a treatment for patients with 3- or 4-part fractures, fracture dislocations, head-splitting fractures, and impacted fractures of the humeral head with involvement of more than 50 % of the articular surface [5]. However, hemiarthroplasty represents a technically difficult option, with particular attention required to achieve adequate restoration of humeral length and version along with anatomic, stable tuberosity reconstruction. Similar to plate osteosynthesis, results of hemiarthroplasty for proximal humerus fractures have been variable, with overall more dependable relief of pain than restoration of adequate range of motion and function [5–7]. In particular, tuberosity nonunion or malunion after hemiarthroplasty has been identified as a significant risk factor for superior migration of the prosthesis, stiffness or weakness, persistent pain, and worse functional results [5, 7]

Although reverse total shoulder arthroplasty (TSA) was originally designed for surgical management of the arthritic, rotator cuff-deficient shoulder, the indications have expanded significantly and now include acute proximal humerus

B.A. Flanagin • S.G. Krishnan, MD (✉)
The Shoulder Center, Baylor University Medical Center, 3900 Junius Street, Suite 740, Dallas, TX 75246, USA
e-mail: brodya.flanagin@baylorhealth.edu; skrishnan@baylorhealth.edu

R. Garofalo
Shoulder Service, Miulli Hospital, 70025 Acquaviva delle fonti, Bari, Italy
e-mail: raffaelegarofalo@gmail.com

F. Castoldi et al. (eds.), *Simple and Complex Fractures of the Humerus*, DOI 10.1007/978-88-470-5307-6_10, © Springer-Verlag Italia 2015

fractures in the elderly. Initial short-term studies have shown promising outcomes, especially when compared to hemiarthroplasty [8–12]. Herein we describe our comprehensive treatment algorithm (indications, preoperative planning, surgical technique, and postoperative management) for the use of reverse TSA in the treatment of acute proximal humerus fractures.

10.2 Indications and Preoperative Planning

This stage is the most critical part of the surgical procedure. We routinely evaluate four criteria when deciding which treatment to offer patients with a proximal humerus fracture.

10.2.1 Age

One of the most important considerations in selecting a method of treatment in proximal humeral fractures is the chronological and physiological age of the patient. Most female patients, by the sixth decade of life, have some degree of osteoporosis and many have impaired neuromuscular control as well. These factors may compromise osteosynthesis and lead to poor results by increasing the risk of fixation failure, postoperative fracture displacement, nonunion, and/or avascular necrosis. Fractures in patients aged 65 years or less appear to be more amenable to humeral head preservation techniques. Moreover, patients older than 75 may have an increased chance of tuberosity-related complications and poor functional outcomes after hemiarthroplasty for acute 3- and 4-part proximal humerus fracture [13].

10.2.2 Bone Quality

Similar to age, a patient's bone quality can affect the success of any humeral head preserving fixation technique. Recent studies have demonstrated that the cortical thickness of the proximal humeral diaphysis is a reliable predictor of bone quality in the proximal humerus [14, 15]. Despite the improved strength of fixation in osteoporotic bone afforded by locking plate technology, successful treatment after ORIF depends to a certain degree on overall bone quality, which may lead to a higher risk of complications in geriatric patient population [3, 4].

10.2.3 Fracture Pattern

Hertel et al. investigated perfusion of the humeral head after an intracapsular fracture and were able to prospectively correlate radiographic fracture morphology with intraoperative humeral head vascularity [16]. Radiographic criteria predictive of humeral head ischemia include metaphyseal head extension of the fracture less than 8 mm, disruption of the medial hinge >2 mm, and basic fracture pattern (i.e., fracture through the anatomic neck). When these three radiographic findings were present preoperatively, there was a 97 % positive predictive value for humeral head ischemia. Furthermore, even when the humeral head is vascular and amenable to preservation, the ability to maintain adequate fracture stability is necessary for successful fracture healing. The medial calcar of the humerus must be intact or restored at the time of surgery for a "stable" reduction [17]. Comminution in this region increases the risk of a varus fracture malreduction.

10.2.4 Timing of Surgery

The delay between injury and definitive surgery is yet another variable that may affect functional outcomes following surgical management of proximal humeral fractures. For example, a fracture amenable to percutaneous fixation techniques may become impossible to reduce closed and pin percutaneously after 7–10 days or when early callus has formed. It is also clear that the outcomes following early arthroplasty for proximal humeral fractures are significantly improved compared to arthroplasty more than 4 weeks after injury [5, 16, 19]. We believe that optimal surgical timing for shoulder fracture arthroplasty is 6–14 days after injury to allow for partial resolution of the soft tissue swelling (assuming no acute neurovascular injury or other situation necessitating an earlier intervention).

As experience with reverse shoulder arthroplasty increases, the indications for utilizing this prosthesis in the initial treatment of proximal humerus fractures have become better defined. In part based on the above criteria, our specific relative indications for the use of reverse TSA in the treatment of proximal humerus fractures are as follows:

- Age >70
- Fracture pattern: ischemic head based on Hertel criteria
- Poor bone quality with inability to reconstruct tuberosities
- Previous known cuff deficiency
- Ipsilateral lower extremity fracture that requires upper extremity weight bearing (on the fractured shoulder) for mobilization
- Greater than 4 weeks after injury (chronic fracture sequelae)

In addition, Visser et al. prospectively performed an electromyographic investigation of 143 consecutive proximal humerus fractures treated either conservatively or operatively [20]. They found nerve lesions to be far more frequent in displaced fractures with an overall 67 % incidence of acute neurological injury after proximal humerus fracture. While a combination of nerve lesions was frequently seen, the most common isolated peripheral nerves involved were the axillary (58 %) and suprascapular (48 %) nerves. While we prefer an anterosuperior approach for primary reverse TSA for cuff arthropathy, based on the findings of Visser et al., we perform all cases of reverse TSA for acute proximal humerus fracture through a deltopectoral approach to avoid further trauma to the deltoid.

Furthermore, restoration of humeral length with anatomic tuberosity reconstruction around the prosthesis and to the humeral shaft is necessary to optimize functional results following reversed shoulder arthroplasty. As we have previously described in performing hemiarthroplasty for proximal humerus fractures, we preoperatively calculate the appropriate height of the humeral implant based on comparison to the contralateral limb for all cases where we perform reverse TSA for proximal humerus fracture [21]. Using scaled radiographs of both humeri, the ipsilateral humerus is measured from the medial epicondyle to the fracture, and the contralateral humerus is measured from the medial epicondyle to the top of the greater tuberosity. The difference between these two measurements is the height at which the metaphysis of the reverse prosthesis should be placed above the lateral aspect of the fracture. This number is recorded and marked on the prosthetic implant at the time of surgery. The length of the greater tuberosity fracture fragment is then measured radiographically and recorded for later comparison to the intraoperative measurement of the greater tuberosity fracture fragment.

10.3 Surgical Technique

10.3.1 Positioning/Exposure

The patient is placed in a semisupine position on a standard operating room table with the head elevated between 20° and 30° and the scapula supported. A 3-in. modified deltopectoral incision is utilized beginning just inferior to the base of the coracoid process and paralleling the cephalic vein. The subcutaneous tissues are divided and the deltopectoral interval entered, taking the cephalic vein medial with the pectoralis major. Once the deltopectoral interval is opened, a small Hohmann retractor is placed just above the coracoid process/coracoacromial (CA) ligament; a second modified bent Hohmann retractor is placed lateral to this under the deltoid and on top of the acromion. The clavipectoral fascia is opened and a self-retaining retractor is placed between the conjoined tendon and deltoid. The biceps tendon is identified within the intertubercular groove and a tenotomy is performed. The arm is then placed into abduction and internal rotation and the greater and lesser tuberosities identified with the aid of a blunt elevator and/or osteotome depending on the chronicity of the fracture. The humeral head fragment is removed. Four no. 5 nonabsorbable sutures are then placed

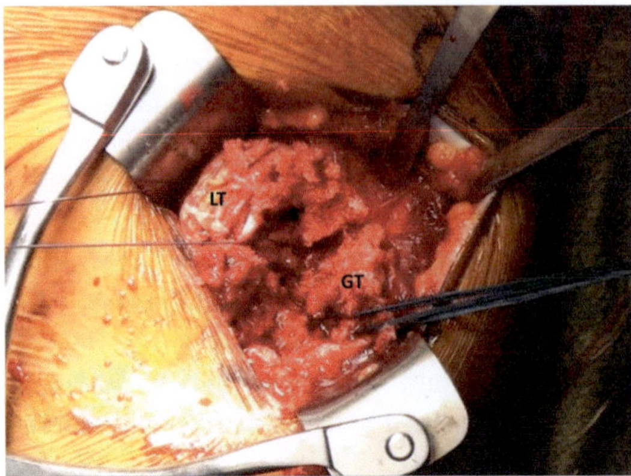

Fig. 10.1 Four nonabsorbable and one temporary stay suture placed at the bone-tendon junction of the greater (*GT*) and lesser (*LT*) tuberosities, respectively

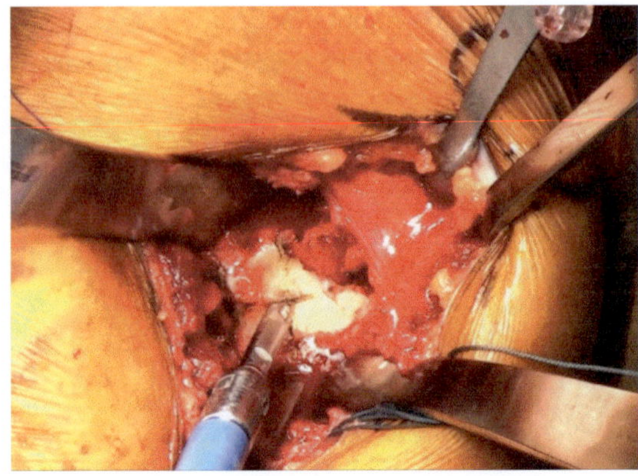

Fig. 10.2 Preferred starting point for drilling of the central hole in the glenoid

in a mattress-type fashion around the greater tuberosity at the bone-tendon junction (two in the infraspinatus and two teres minor). One temporary stay suture is then placed at the bone-tendon junction between the subscapularis and lesser tuberosity (Fig. 10.1). The rotator cuff is sharply divided in line between the tuberosities to the level of the glenoid. Three retractors are then sequentially placed around the glenoid: a small Darrach retractor posteroinferiorly, a glenoid neck retractor anteriorly, and a Hohmann retractor posterosuperiorly. The biceps insertion is exposed and any remaining labrum is excised circumferentially around the glenoid rim. In addition, we release roughly 1–2 mm of the long head of the triceps insertion along the 5–7 o'clock position of the glenoid.

10.3.2 Glenoid Preparation

We prefer to perform all glenoid arthroplasty prior to performing humeral arthroplasty. We place the arm in a posterior and inferior position, thereby moving the humerus out of the surgical window in order to adequately access the glenoid. Placement of the patient in the semisupine position with the head of bed elevated 20–30° as previously described allows for gravity to assist the exposure by aiding to place the arm in a posterior position. The center of the glenoid articular surface is first marked with a Bovie. Our preferred starting point for placement of the baseplate peg is just posterior and inferior to the native center of the glenoid (Fig. 10.2). After the center hole is drilled, a curette is used to confirm that the drill has not perforated the glenoid vault either anteriorly or posteriorly. The glenoid is sequentially reamed up to the size of the glenosphere. After each reamer is engaged within the center hold of the glenoid, we drop our hand approximately 10–15° to allow for inferior tilt of the baseplate/glenosphere. We prefer to ream the glenoid minimally so as to create a smooth, flat surface on which the baseplate will sit while preserving the structural stability of the subchondral bone. An enlarging drill is then used to finish the preparation for the central post and the baseplate is impacted into place. Our preference is to "match" the size of the baseplate and glenosphere to each individual patient based on height and weight. With the particular implant system, we prefer for reverse arthroplasty, there are two different-sized baseplates available. As a general rule, we implant the smaller baseplate in women and the larger baseplate in men. Similarly, each baseplate is also available with either a "short" or "long" central post. We prefer to use a long central post in all fracture patients in an effort to maximize the stability between the glenoid and baseplate. We place two compression screws (anterior and posterior) followed by two locking screws (superior and inferior) through the baseplate. The posterior screw captures the lateral pillar of the scapula, the anterior screw the scapular spine, the superior screw the coracoid base, and the inferior screw parallels the central post of the baseplate along the glenoid neck. We feel this represents the four most important points of fixation for the baseplate screws within the native scapula. The baseplate is then exposed circumferentially in order to allow for appropriate engagement of the morse taper and countersunk screw of the particular medial center of rotation glenosphere we utilize for reverse TSA. The glenosphere is then impacted onto the baseplate and locked into place.

10.3.3 Humeral Preparation

The humeral shaft is exposed with an osteotome anteriorly and posteriorly. Since the metaphysis is typically "absent" due to the fracture, the humeral shaft is prepared with hand reamers until there is gentle cortical resistance. A humeral trial is then placed. Appropriate height of the humeral implant and length of the greater tuberosity fracture fragment is calculated preoperatively as noted above (see Sect. 10.2) based on comparison to the contralateral limb. This measurement is confirmed intraoperatively (Fig. 10.3). It should be noted that if the radiographic measurement of length of the greater tuberosity fragment performed preoperatively is not equal to that measured intraoperatively, the latter number should supersede the former. Humeral version is then set by placing the arm in a neutral position at the side and pointing the humeral component/tray toward the glenoid (Fig. 10.4). Two drill holes are then placed on either side of the bicipital groove and a single heavy nonabsorbable suture is placed through each for final vertical, tension-band fixation of the tuberosities. A cement restrictor is then placed at a distance equal to two canal diameters distal to the tip of the prosthesis and the humeral canal cleaned and dried with pulsatile lavage and an epinephrine soaked sponge. We then cement the humeral canal using a third-generation technique utilizing a ventilation tube to remove all blood and minimize embolic phenomenon within the endosteal vessels of the humeral shaft. The proximal 1–2 cm of cement is removed and the final humeral implant is manually placed down the shaft of the humerus. The height and version of the prosthesis are set as noted previously. Once the cement is cured, we place a constrained polyethylene trial onto the humeral component and the prosthesis is gently reduced to confirm adequate positioning and stability. The humeral component is then dislocated, and the final constrained polyethylene liner is impacted in place. The four nonabsorbable sutures previously placed at the greater tuberosity at the bone-tendon junction are then cerclaged around the humeral

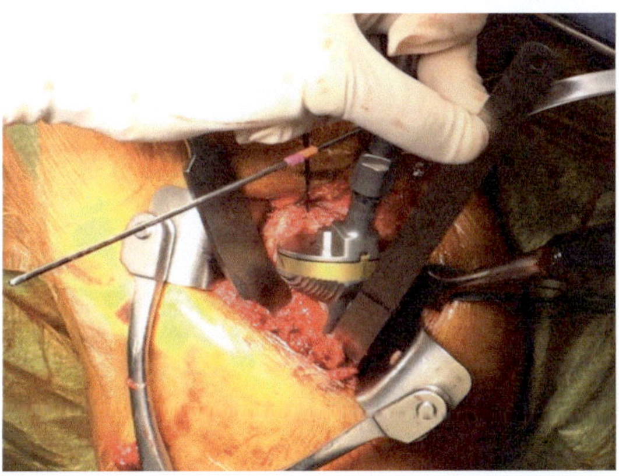

Fig. 10.3 Appropriate height of the humeral trial marked with a simple metal ruler based on the preoperative calculation of the distance from the fracture to the top of the lateral aspect of the humeral component

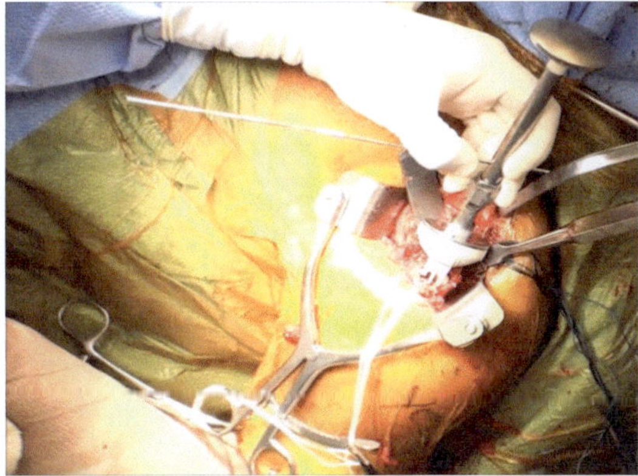

Fig. 10.4 Appropriate version of implant noted with arm held in the neutral position and pointing the humeral component toward the glenoid

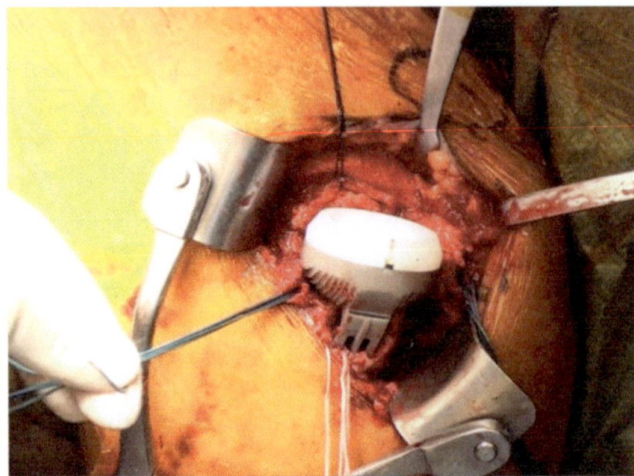

Fig. 10.5 The four nonabsorbable sutures previously placed at the greater tuberosity at the bone-tendon junction are cerclaged around the humeral stem prior to reduction of the final humeral component

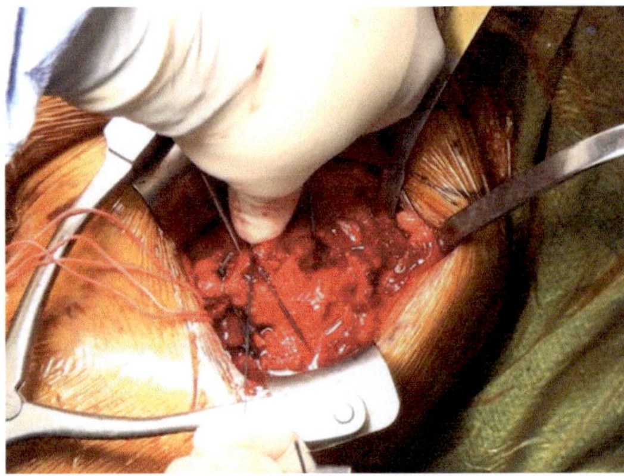

Fig. 10.6 The four nonabsorbable sutures previously placed through the greater tuberosity at the bone-tendon junction are used to affix the tuberosities to one another around the prosthesis in the horizontal plane

stem prior to gentle reduction of the final humeral component (Fig. 10.5).

The greater tuberosity is then reduced and held in its anatomic position with a pointed awl. Two of the four nonabsorbable sutures previously placed around the greater tuberosity at the bone-tendon junction and cerclaged around the prosthesis are tied. The two remaining sutures are then placed through the lesser tuberosity bone-tendon junction and tied with the lesser tuberosity held in an anatomic position with the pointed awl (Fig. 10.6). This affixes the tuberosities to one another around the prosthesis in the horizontal plane. The two nonabsorbable sutures previously placed through bone tunnels on either side of the intertubercular groove are not passed through the rotator cuff (one anterior to posterior and the other from posterior to anterior), thereby creating a figure-of-eight vertical tension-band fixation of the tuberosities to the shaft (Fig. 10.7). After all sutures are tied, trial motion is demonstrated to ensure stable fixation of the tuberosities to the shaft and to rule out any abnormal impingement of the implant prior to closure. The deltopectoral interval is then closed with no. 2 absorbable braided suture, followed by closure of the subcutaneous tissue with interrupted 0 absorbable sutures and a running 2/0 absorbable suture. The skin edges are re-approximated with staples and a sterile dressing applied. The ipsilateral extremity is then placed into a simple Velpeau arm sling with the arm resting at the side prior to extubation.

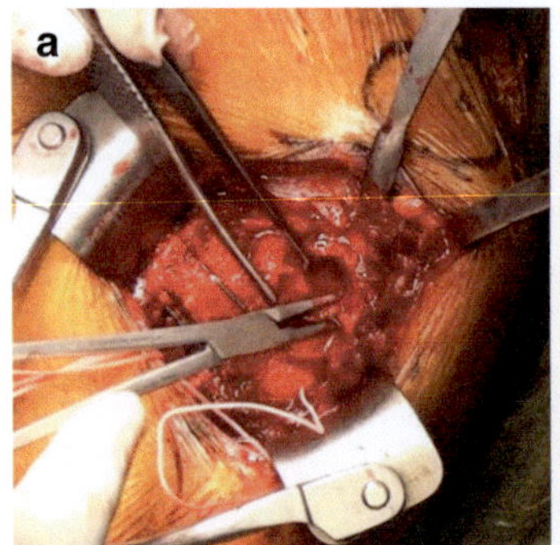

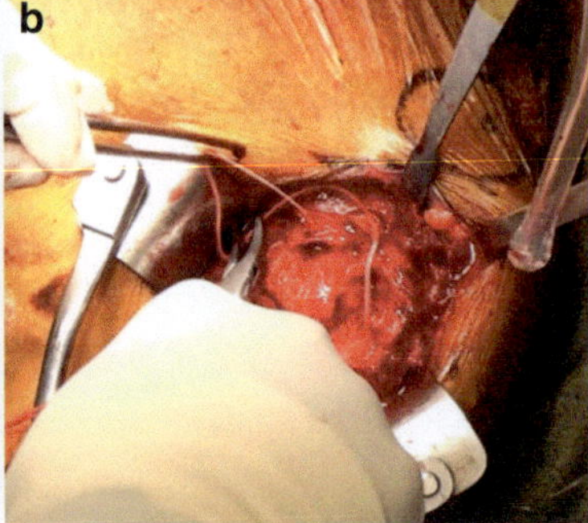

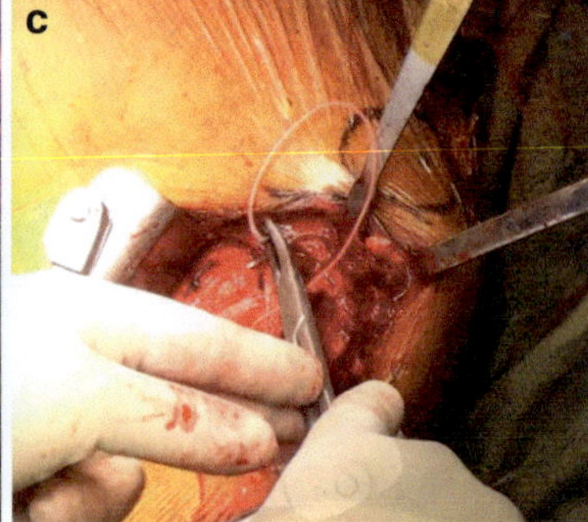

Fig. 10.7 Vertical tension-band fixation of the tuberosities to the shaft. One limb of the nonabsorbable suture previously placed through a drill hole posterior to the bicipital groove is passed from posterosuperior cuff (**a**) through anterosuperior cuff (**b**) and out through anteroinferior cuff (**c**) before tying. This is repeated in the opposite direction for the suture placed anterior to the bicipital groove, thereby bringing the tuberosities into apposition with the humeral shaft

10.4 Postoperative Management

Postoperatively, patients are immobilized in a sling for 6 weeks, which is only removed to bathe and perform physical therapy. Patients are immediately started on gentle elbow, wrist, and hand range of motion and scapular stabilization exercises. For the first 4 weeks, we allow supine passive elevation to 90° and external rotation to 30° with the arm at the side. From 4 to 6 weeks after surgery, patients are advanced to full supine passive elevation and still only 30° of external rotation with the arm at the side. At week 7 full active forward elevation, external rotation, and internal rotation are begun. Resistance exercises begin at week 10. We advise all patients that full recovery after reverse total shoulder arthroplasty for fracture can take up to 18 months from the date of the original injury.

10.5 Results

Short-term outcomes following reverse TSA for acute proximal humerus fracture in elderly patients appear to be satisfactory in terms of pain relief, range of motion, and functional outcomes [8, 9]. Moreover, several comparative studies of reverse TSA and hemiarthroplasty for acute proximal humerus fractures have all demonstrated improved results with the reverse prosthesis [10–12]. Recent evidence also suggests there may be an association between the use of either a conventional or fracture-specific stem and final range of motion and functional outcomes [22]. Overall complication rates after reverse TSA for acute proximal humerus fractures appear to be similar to those reported for other treatment alternatives [8, 9, 12].

References

1. Baron JA, Barrett JA, Karagas MR (1996) The epidemiology of peripheral fractures. Bone 18(3 Suppl): 209S–213S
2. Palvanen M, Kannus P, Niemi S et al (2006) Update in the epidemiology of proximal humeral fractures. Clin Orthop Relat Res 442:87–92
3. Owsley KC, Gorczyca JT (2008) Fracture displacement and screw cutout after open reduction and locked plate fixation of proximal humeral fractures. J Bone Joint Surg Am 90:233–240
4. Clavert P, Adam P, Bevort A et al (2010) Pitfalls and complications with locking plate for proximal humerus fracture. J Shoulder Elbow Surg 19:489–494
5. Mighell MA, Kolm GP, Collinge CA et al (2003) Outcomes of hemiarthroplasty for fractures of the proximal humerus. J Shoulder Elbow Surg 12:569–577
6. Antuna SA, Sperling JW, Cofield RH (2008) Shoulder hemiarthroplasty for acute fractures of the proximal humerus: a minimum five-year follow-up. J Shoulder Elbow Surg 17:202–209
7. Boileau P, Krishnan SG, Tinsi L et al (2002) Tuberosity malposition and migration: reasons for poor outcomes after hemiarthroplasty for displaced fractures of the proximal humerus. J Shoulder Elbow Surg 11:401–412
8. Lenarz C, Shishani Y, McCrum C et al (2011) Is reverse shoulder arthroplasty appropriate for the treatment of fractures in the older patient? Clin Orthop Relat Res 469:3324–3331
9. Klein M, Juschka M, Hinkenjann B et al (2008) Treatment of comminuted fractures of the proximal humerus in elderly patients with the Delta III reverse shoulder prosthesis. J Orthop Trauma 22:698–704
10. Garrigues GE, Johnston PS, Pepe MD et al (2012) Hemiarthroplasty versus reverse total shoulder arthroplasty for acute proximal humerus fractures in elderly patients. Orthopedics 35:703–708
11. Boyle MJ, Youn SM, Frampton CM et al (2013) Functional outcomes of reverse shoulder arthroplasty compared with hemiarthroplasty for acute proximal humeral fractures. J Shoulder Elbow Surg 22:32–37
12. Cuff D, Pupello D (2013) Hemiarthroplasty vs. reverse shoulder arthroplasty for the treatment of comminuted proximal humeral fractures in elderly patients. Abstract presented at annual American Shoulder and Elbow Surgeons Specialty Day Meeting, Chicago
13. Boileau P, Winter M, Cikes A et al (2013) Can surgeons predict what makes a good hemiarthroplasty for fracture? J Shoulder Elbow Surg. doi:10.1016/j.jse.2013.04.018
14. Tingart MJ, Apreleva M, von Stechow D et al (2003) The cortical thickness of the proximal humeral diaphysis predicts bone mineral density of the proximal humerus. J Bone Joint Surg Br 85:611–617
15. Mather J, MacDermid JC, Faber KJ et al (2013) Proximal humerus cortical bone thickness correlates with bone mineral density and can clinically rule out osteoporosis. J Shoulder Elbow Surg 22:732–738
16. Hertel R, Hempfing A, Stiehler M et al (2004) Predictors of humeral head ischemia after intracapsular fracture of the proximal humerus. J Shoulder Elbow Surg 13:427–433
17. Gardner MJ, Weil Y, Barker JU et al (2007) The importance of medial support in locked plating of proximal humerus fractures. J Orthop Trauma 21:185–191

18. Boileau P, Trojani C, Walch G et al (2001) Shoulder arthroplasty for the treatment of the sequelae of fractures of the proximal humerus. J Shoulder Elbow Surg. 2013;22(11):1495–1506. doi: 10.1016/j.jse.2013.04.018. Epub 2013 Jul 5
19. Mansat P, Guity MR, Bellumore Y et al (2004) Shoulder arthroplasty for late sequelae of proximal humeral fractures. J Shoulder Elbow Surg 13:305–312
20. Visser CP, Coene LN, Brand R et al (2001) Nerve lesions in proximal humeral fractures. J Shoulder Elbow Surg 10:421–427
21. Krishnan SG, Pennington SD, Burkhead WZ et al (2005) Shoulder arthroplasty for fracture: restoration of the "gothic arch". Tech Shoulder Elbow Surg 6:57–66
22. Lo EY, Feher L, Garofalo R et al (2014) Reverse total shoulder arthroplasty for acute proximal humerus fracture: is there a benefit in using a fracture-specific stem? Abstract accepted for presentation at the annual American Shoulder and Elbow Surgeons Specialty Day Meeting, New Orleans

11 Surgical Neck Fracture

Luigi Murena, Gianluca Canton, and Ettore Vulcano

11.1 Epidemiology

Surgical neck fractures are frequent, and they account for 12–28 % of proximal humeral fractures [1]. Elderly patients with osteoporotic bone are typically affected. In fact, this lesion has a unimodal age distribution, with 72 years being the average age of onset. Moreover, it is rarely seen under 50 years of age, presenting as high-energy trauma and mostly related to motor-vehicle accidents [1].

11.2 Radiographic Assessment and Classification

For surgical neck fractures, standard true antero-posterior (AP), lateral, and axillary radiographs obtained in the emergency department are sufficient for diagnosis and classification. A CT scan can be helpful if an articular or tuberosity fracture is suspected [2]. Proximal humeral fracture classification is a highly debated topic [3]. Several attempts have been made to update and improve the classical and often criticized classification systems, the Neer classification and AO/OTA classification, especially for complex fractures. However, surgical neck fractures are classified following the same rationale [3]. In fact, the Neer classification [4] of two-part surgical neck fractures identifies types A, B, and C for undisplaced, displaced, and comminuted fractures, respectively. Neer's criteria for displacement are 1 cm and/or 45° of angulation. The AO/OTA classification [5] considers surgical neck fractures as extra-articular (group A), identifying types 2 and 3 for undisplaced and displaced fractures respectively. Subgroups are also described based on fracture angulation (varus and valgus alignment) and comminution/fragmentation. Whatever classification system should be used, it appears clear that neck-shaft displacement, angulation, and comminution of fragments are the key elements that need to be considered in order to correctly assess these fractures as they represent the discriminants to define proper treatment and technique [3].

11.3 Treatment: Conservative or Surgical?

Conservative treatment is reported to be the treatment of choice for undisplaced and minimally displaced proximal humerus fractures, which account for 75–80 % of these lesions [1, 2]. For the remaining 20–25 %, 55 % of which are surgical neck fractures [6], current literature generally supports surgical treatment, but there is no consensus on the surgical technique which should be chosen [7–9]. Moreover, some authors report satisfying results with conservative treatment even

L. Murena (✉) • G. Canton • E. Vulcano (✉)
Orthopaedics and Traumatology, Ospedale di Circolo, Department of Biotechnologies and Life Sciences (DBSV), University of Insubria, Viale Borri 57, Varese, Italy
e-mail: luigi.murena@gmail.com; gcanton84@gmail.com; ettore.vulcano@hotmail.com

F. Castoldi et al. (eds.), *Simple and Complex Fractures of the Humerus*,
DOI 10.1007/978-88-470-5307-6_11, © Springer-Verlag Italia 2015

for displaced surgical neck fractures, and many authors have failed to demonstrate a clear clinical advantage for surgical treatment compared to the conservative option [7, 10]. Therefore, choosing the correct treatment for a surgical neck fracture can be challenging. Some authors help us to understand what the rationale is leading to the choice of a surgical treatment for surgical neck fractures. Court-Brown et al. [1] report that surgical treatment should be reserved only to fractures that are unlikely to heal with conservative treatment because of a lack of bone contact between fragments. Warner et al. [2] better clarify this statement, distinguishing between elderly low-demanding patients in which bone contact may be all that is necessary and young active patients in which 45° of angulation and displacement lesser than 50 % of the diaphyseal diameter are the limit of tolerance. Moreover they identify varus displacement, valgus displacement, comminution, and 100 % displacement as indications for surgical treatment. Nho et al. [9] recently proposed neck-shaft displacement greater than 66 % of diaphyseal diameter as an indication for surgical treatment. They also identified comminution and cortex thickness as crucial for the choice of the best surgical technique. It seems clear that the degree and characteristics of displacement are a cardinal element to consider, but age and functional demands are maybe the most important. Elderly and low-demanding patients seem to reach a satisfying subjective result once union occurs, despite possible malunion. Warner et al. [2] found the predictive factors for nonunion of these fractures to be severe osteopenia, very proximal fracture line, and substantial displacement. Therefore, in these patients surgical treatment could be considered as an attempt to avoid nonunion, thus obtaining bone contact and mechanical stability between fragments even in the presence of nonanatomic reduction. Indeed, a surgical neck nonunion is invalidating, and its treatment is challenging for both the surgeon and the patient (i.e., blood loss, longer operating times, longer rehabilitation, etc.) [11]. On the other hand, the goal for younger active patients must be complete functional recovery, and surgical treatment consisting of anatomic reduction and stable fixation should be chosen whenever this goal is not otherwise achievable [8, 9, 12]. Once surgical indication has been established, the best surgical modality has to be ruled out. As already stated, current literature is still controversial on this topic. Nho et al. [9] recently reviewed the current literature indications for the management of proximal humeral fractures, identifying closed reduction and percutaneous pinning (CRPP), locking plate fixation, and intramedullary nailing as the most suitable surgical alternatives for surgical neck fractures. To the best of our knowledge, few studies comparing two of these techniques are available in the literature [13, 14], and only one study compares all the three [12]; thus there is a lack of any evidence clearly supporting one technique over another. However, indications and contraindications for each technique can be identified, thereby addressing their proper use in each different case.

11.4 Closed Reduction and Percutaneous Pinning

According to several authors [15, 16], a two-part surgical neck fracture is the ideal indication for CRPP. Closed reducibility and patient compliance to pin management, and often prolonged immobilization, are required for successful treatment. Severe osteopenia and metaphyseal comminution have been reported as contraindications [9, 15, 16].

For CRPP techniques closed reduction is the first step. If proper reduction cannot be achieved with closed maneuvers, small incisions can be performed in order to allow for the positioning of bone elevators and hooks to manipulate fragments [15, 16]. The most used technique consists of the insertion of threaded 2.5-mm pins from the lateral shaft cortex in a distal to proximal direction, drilled under fluoroscopic control to the humeral head until reaching the subchondral bone. The orientation of wires into the head must be divergent, and wire tips must reach different areas of the head without concentrating them at one point only [15, 16]. Several studies report good functional outcome with this technique, especially for two-part fractures, with very low incidence of avascular necrosis of the humeral head [15, 16]. In fact, the greatest advantage of this technique is the absolute respect of humeral head vascularity [9, 12]. On the other hand, shoulder stiffness can be a complication of this treatment [7], mainly because of the long (4–6 weeks) period of pin permanence affecting the possibility of early mobilization [16]. Other complications associated with pin treatment have been described as pin tract infection, lateral pin migration with loss of reduction, medial pin migration with articular cartilage damage, and the possible but rarely described intrathoracic migration [8]. The supporters of this technique attribute the high failure rate to the use of smooth pins rather than threaded pins and to technical errors mainly represented by the convergence of pin tips in a small area, usually in the inferomedial quadrant of the humeral head [15, 16]. However, the use of threaded pins has only limited the incidence of these complications, which still remain a concern to many authors [8, 9]. Moreover, many anatomic studies demonstrate the close proximity of pin tracts to the axillary nerve and cephalic vein with this technique, thus reducing its safety [17]. An alternative technique of CRPP which is particularly suitable for surgical neck fractures is the palm tree technique [18, 19]. This technique consists of the use of smooth pins which are inserted from the lateral humeral shaft cortex at the level of the deltoid tuberosity. Pins are curved before insertion at 45° at the proximal end and gently curved along all their length to facilitate insertion. The wires are inserted in a divergent fashion achieving a 3-point stability in the cortex, shaft, and head [18, 19]. Some disadvantages of this technique have been reported, and these are partly comparable to the straight pins technique: convergence of wires, loss of reduction, pin tract infection, radial nerve lesion if the posterior cortex is accidentally violated, and humeral shaft fracture [19]. Some technical modifications can be made to the original technique which partly avoid the described complications. In the past years at our institution, a modified palm tree technique has been used to manage two-part proximal humeral fractures, with very satisfying long-term results and a very low incidence of complications limited to pin tract infections and minor malunions [unpublished data of the authors]. The modified technique we use for surgical neck fractures consists of the insertion of three K wires from three separated drill holes in the humeral shaft, the first and more proximal in the original position described by Kapandji, the second more distal in the interval between brachialis and biceps brachii muscles, and the third most distal anteriorly through the anterior muscles of the arm. This configuration assures a divergent orientation of wire tips in the humeral head, thereby leading to the maximal rotational and axial stability obtainable with respect to the intrinsic characteristics of the implant. Moreover, the risk of humeral shaft fracture is reduced because of the distribution of stresses to the shaft in three different points. The avoidance of a larger skin incision (a stab incision is enough) and a theoretical shorter surgical time are advantages of this technique. Recently the results of a modified palm tree technique with similar features were published in the literature, reporting comparably encouraging results in two- and also three-part fractures [20]. Because of its low invasivity, CRPP would be the ideal treatment for elderly patients with comorbidities, but osteopenia limits its use for the risk of pin migration and loss of reduction [8, 9, 15, 16]. On the other hand, CRPP would have the advantage of an elastic fixation, which is preferable in the osteopenic bone to limit fixation failure [21]. In our experience, the palm tree technique has also proven to be a successful treatment for these patients because of the use of pins without sharp ends significantly limiting the risk of medial migration and loss of reduction. Medial migration risk is much higher if the subchondral bone is violated during pin insertions, thus penetrating articular cartilage [20, 22]. Therefore, we have considered and still consider this technique to be the best choice in the elderly patient with a displaced surgical neck fracture without metaphyseal comminution, especially if affected by significant comorbidities.

11.5 Angular Stable Internal Fixation: Locking Plate or Nail?

Angular stable fixation is the most commonly used technique for surgical neck fractures [6–9]. Whatever implant is used, it provides a strong and relatively rigid fixation even in the osteopenic bone as biomechanical studies clearly demonstrate [23]. For its intrinsic stability, it is also suitable for fractures with metaphyseal comminution [9, 21, 23]. For the same reason it allows early mobilization with a faster return to daily living activities. As previously stated, there are limited studies comparing nails and plates for proximal humeral fractures, very few of which specifically evaluate surgical neck fractures [12–14]. The results of these studies are controversial, with clinical and radiographic outcome almost comparable between the two techniques. Some biomechanical studies have outlined a slight superiority of locking plates as far as rotational stability is concerned [23]. However, it is not clear whether this finding could have any clinical application [23]. Some studies were able to show a moderate superiority of plates in terms of functional recovery time and objective clinical outcome at the expense of a higher incidence of complications [14]. Other studies, however, showed no significant differences [12, 13]. Locking plates are usually implanted through a deltopectoral approach, which is more aggressive to soft tissues and thus presents a theoretically higher risk of vascular damage [8, 9]. This approach, together with the lateral position of the implant, could lead to excessive scarring, therefore affecting rehabilitation [8, 9]. On the other hand, the advantages of this implant reside in the highest biomechanical strength [23], the possibility to use cortical screws as reduction tools [24, 25], the higher possibilities for screw fixation in the proximal fragment, and the possibility to buttress the calcar region and fix medial metaphyseal fragments with dedicated inferomedial screws [26, 27]. Moreover, dedicated holes on most plates allow to reinforce the construct with sutures between the rotator cuff and the plate. The use of these sutures is necessary in cases of poor bone quality to obtain maximal stability and to minimize the risks of implant failure [22]. Intramedullary nails have the advantage of lesser soft tissues stripping due to the limited anterolateral deltoid-splitting approach required [6, 12], which also allows to recognize and treat concomitant lesions (i.e., rotator cuff tears, acromial spurs, etc.) which are present in up to 21 % of cases [6]. The main disadvantage is the violation of the rotator cuff, especially with curved nails entering the proximal fragment laterally at the level of the sulcus, leading to a high incidence (20–40 %) of shoulder pain [28]. The development of straight nails with an entry point at the top of the humeral head allowed for the supraspinatus tendon split to be performed more medially, where the well-vascularized tissue can be successfully repaired [6, 12, 29]. Park et al. [30] described an access through the rotator interval in order to avoid rotator cuff damage. The latter approach is not used often and is also associated to a theoretic risk of damage to the biceps tendon. Moreover, this technique limits the access to the correct entry point at the top of the humeral head which is the ideal entry point for proximal humeral fractures [6, 29, 30]. The entry point topic is of critical importance, because it allows to achieve and maintain the reduction of the proximal fracture fragment and restore head-shaft alignment [6, 28, 29]. Moreover, the entry point affects stability of the implant. In fact, the correct entry point is in the center of the humeral head in its cartilaginous portion where strong subchondral bone can be retrieved. In this condition, the stability of fixation of the proximal fragment relies not only on proximal screws but also on the nail-subchondral bone interface [29]. On the other hand, some fracture patterns do not allow to achieve this goal. Undisplaced or partial tuberosity fractures may become displaced if the nail entry point is too close to the fracture line (Fig. 11.1) [6, 29]. A final disadvantage is the lack of control of medial calcar fragments [12–14]. Minimally invasive plate osteosynthesis is the third choice that has been reported recently in the literature, with the first short-term reports showing promising results [24, 25]. It combines the structural advantages of plate fixation with the lesser

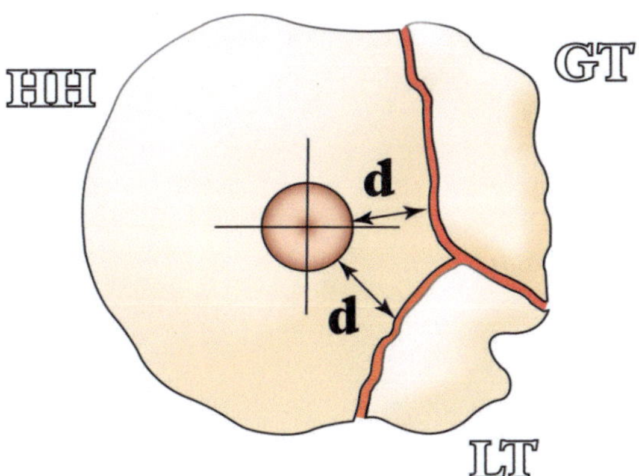

Fig. 11.1 Schematic drawing of the proximal humerus, axial view (*red line* tuberosity fracture, *orange circle* nail entry point, *HH* humeral head, *GT* greater tuberosity, *LT* lesser tuberosity): an adequate distance (*d*) between the tuberosity fracture line and the nail entry point is crucial to ensure implant stability and to avoid tuberosity fracture displacement

invasivity of the anterolateral deltoid-splitting approach. However, a limit to this technique is the missing possibility to implant buttressing inferomedial screws as the literature reports a high risk of axillary nerve lesion without isolation of the nerve itself [31]. Despite these differences, the literature shows how the failure of fixation can occur with both implants, and it is generally secondary to metaphyseal medial impaction and varus displacement of the proximal fragment [21, 22, 32]. Screw cutout has been reported in up to 19 % of cases for plate and screw fixation [14]. This common complication is usually the result of osteopenia rendering fixation of the proximal fragment inadequate together with the lack of bone contact in the calcar region due to fragmentation or non-reduction of that component of the fracture [26]. Technical errors may also represent causes of failure [21, 22]. Therefore, some authors have outlined some technical tips to limit the incidence of these complications [21, 22, 32, 33]:

- Screws should always be directed to the subchondral bone which represents the strongest bone in the humeral head, avoiding cartilage perforation with screws and drill.
- Reduction of varus displacement must be achieved because varus malreduction has been proven to be a risk factor to further varus and distal displacement.
- The proximal fragment should be secured to the implant with rotator cuff sutures, which are more reliable and stronger than screws in osteopenic bone.

As far as calcar region defects are concerned, there are more considerations to be made. These medial defects are usually the result of comminution or fragmentation at the calcar posteromedial region, which is the carrying portion of the surgical neck [32]. This region should be reduced and reconstructed if possible, thereby obtaining proper bone contact between the proximal and distal fragments and thus preventing impaction and varus displacement [21]. If comminution is present and there are no fixable medial fragments, the literature suggests the impaction of fragments with relative shortening to be a useful solution [34], and some authors attribute the possibility of gradual controlled impaction to be a possible advantage of nails implanted in a dynamic configuration [6]. A possible alternative is the use of buttressing inferomedial screws, which is obviously only applicable with plates implanted through an extensile approach (Fig. 11.2). [26, 27]. If fragmentation is present with medial fixable cortical fragments, there is a clear indication for plate fixation aimed at reconstructing and rigidly fixing the calcar region [21, 26, 27].

11.6 Authors' Preferred Method of Treatment

Functional demand, age, bone quality, and fracture characteristics such as type and entity of displacement, comminution, and associated shoulder injuries (i.e., rotator cuff tears) must be considered as a whole to define the best surgical treatment for surgical neck fractures. In the elderly and low-demanding patients who are often affected by arthritic or cuff-deficient shoulders, surgical intervention should aim to avoid a nonunion rather than to achieve anatomic reduction. In our opinion, in such cases a modified palm tree technique helps to achieve

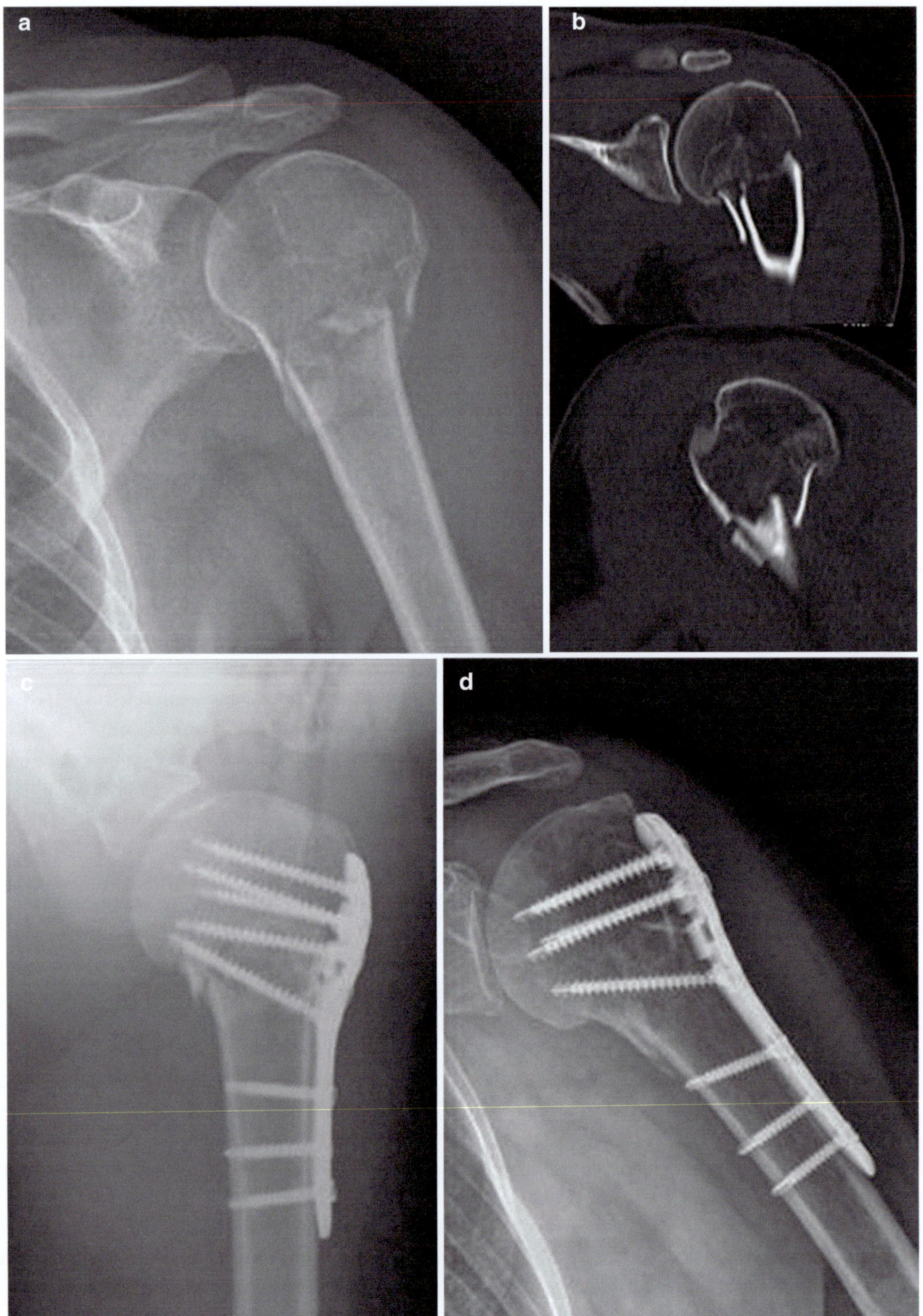

Fig. 11.2 Surgical neck fracture in a 50-year-old woman. (**a**, **b**) Preoperative radiograph and CT scans showing an inferomedial fragment detachment causing a calcar defect. (**c**) Reduction and fixation with angular stable plate through a deltopectoral approach: an inferomedial buttressing screw has been used. (**d**) Radiograph 6 months after surgery

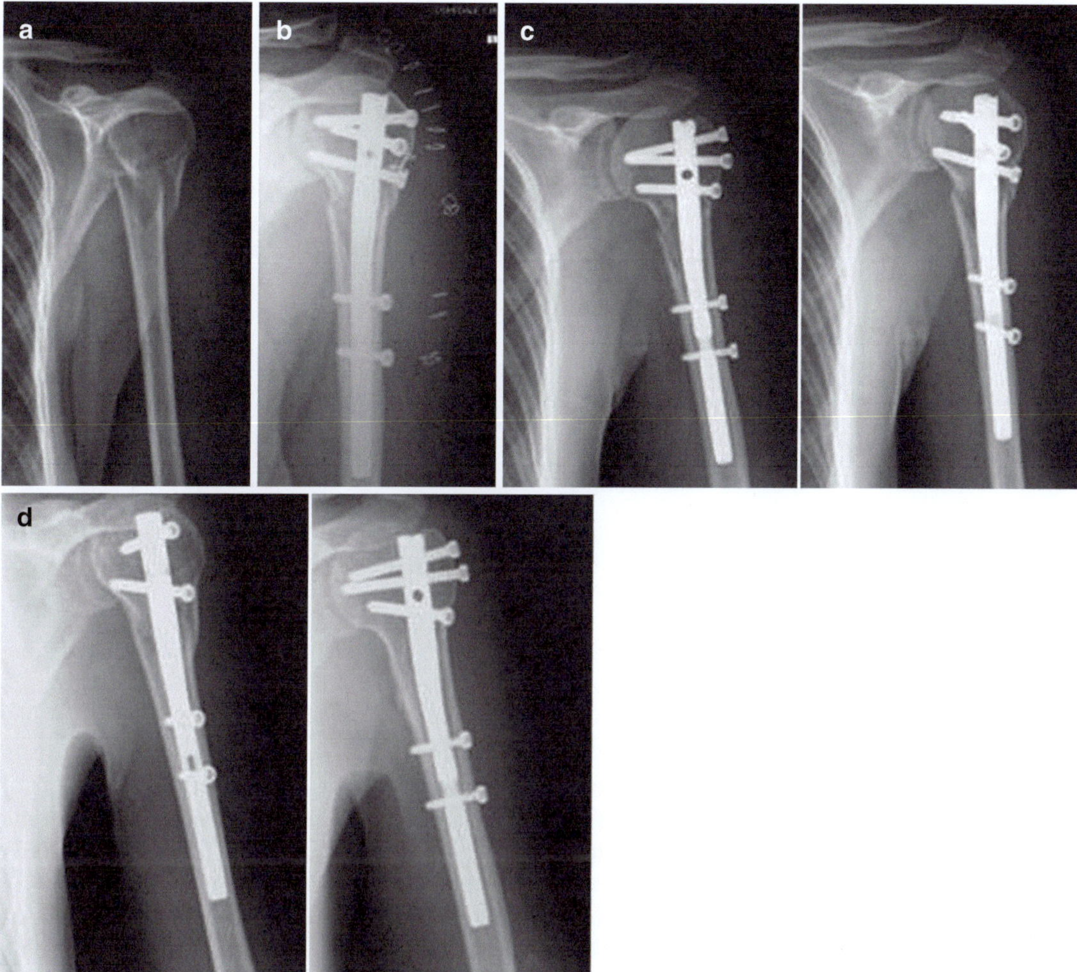

Fig. 11.3 Surgical neck fracture extending to the greater tuberosity in a 49-year-old woman: closed reduction and internal fixation with a nail. (**a**) preoperative radiograph; (**b**) immediate postoperative radiograph; (**c**) 1-month postoperative radiograph; (**d**) 4-month postoperative radiograph demonstrating fracture healing

fracture union despite possible malreductions. Advantages of the technique are an elastic fixation which is preferable in the osteopenic bone to limit fixation failure, limited blood loss, reduced surgical time, and the avoidance of general anesthesia. Furthermore, postoperative immobilization is tolerated better in elderly patients who are usually not very compliant to immediate post-op rehabilitation. Conversely, in younger and high-demanding patients, the aim of the intervention must be anatomic reduction, stable fixation, and early mobilization. An immediate post-op rehabilitation program that includes pendulum movements and passive mobilization on all planes prevents shoulder stiffness and a more prompt return to daily living activities. In these patients, the reduction and fixation with a locking plate or a nail represent the best option (Fig. 11.3). The use of minimally invasive techniques is encouraged whenever possible, especially because surgical neck fractures are their most suitable indication. To clarify, minimally invasive techniques in proximal humeral fractures do not refer to small skin incisions but to the absolute respect of vascularity, anatomic structures, and fracture site biology [35]. Therefore, both nails and plates can be implanted in this fashion, especially if an anterolateral deltoid-splitting

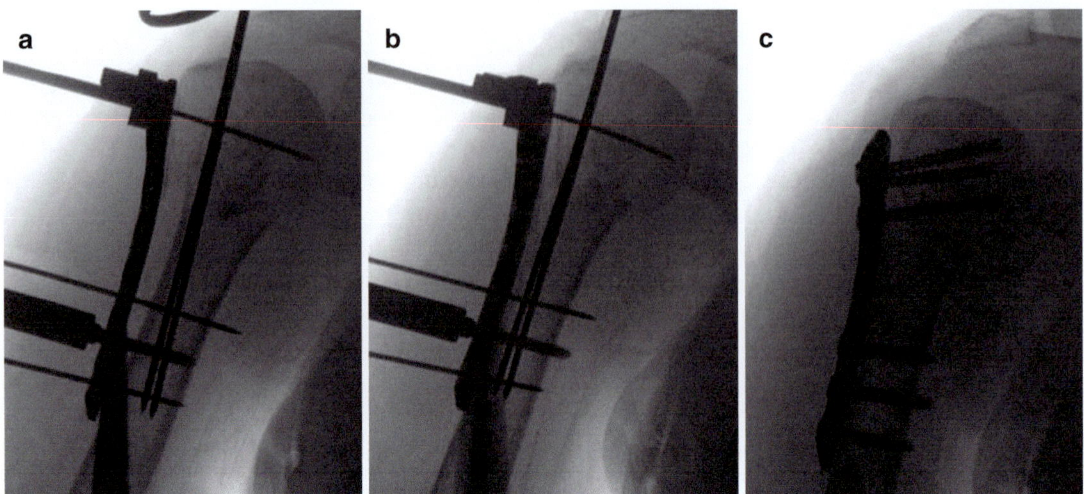

Fig. 11.4 Minimally invasive plate osteosynthesis through a deltoid splitting approach of a surgical neck fracture with medial diaphyseal displacement: note the use of a cortical screw to achieve reduction. (**a**) Cortical screw before tightening; (**b**) tightened cortical screw; (**c**) final result

approach is used. The latter is also a valuable solution in patients requiring a better cosmetic result. The extension of the approach can vary according to the characteristics of the fracture and of the implant used. The nail requires a more aggressive deltoid-splitting approach (i.e., partial subperiosteal elevation of the deltoid from the acromion) in order to reach the rotator cuff, which is crucial to guarantee optimal functional results. This is the only way to longitudinally split the supraspinatus medial to the footprint avoiding the risk to detach it from the greater tuberosity. Side-to-side stitches allow us to repair the approach accordingly. At the end of the procedure, the deltoid must be safely reinserted on the acromion with transosseous sutures to prevent iatrogenic lesions and undesirable functional results. In our opinion, if the deltoid is not detached from the acromion, the rotator cuff is poorly visualized, thus leading to over-retraction and consequent unrepairable iatrogenic damage to the muscle fibers. The nail should always be straight, and its entry point should be at the top of the humeral head in order to facilitate the reduction of the proximal fragment on the diaphysis. Wide proximal meta-diaphyseal canals are more prone to residual translation of the proximal fragment with respect to the diaphysis, although this does not generally affect the final outcome. Intramedullary nailing is relatively contraindicated in fractures extending to the tuberosities. Most fractures of the humerus neck with infraction of the tuberosity are not typically associated with displacement of the latter. Nonetheless, the risk of displacement of the tuberosity still exists. This is particularly true in older patients with poor bone quality in which the bone bridge between the entry point of the nail and the tuberosity fracture line could more easily collapse. Therefore, a CT scan could be useful for preoperative planning, not only to assess the head-tuberosity relationship but also to precisely locate the entry point with respect to the fracture line. The minimally invasive locking plate is indicated in young patients with optimal bone quality, valgus deformity, and/or medial translation of the diaphysis. In these cases cortical screws can be used to reduce the valgus deformity and the translation (Fig. 11.4). The plate may also be used instead of the nail to treat fractures extending to the tuberosity. Furthermore, the plate is less invasive than the nail as it spares the rotator cuff and does not require us to detach the deltoid from the acromion. The latter advantage may be lost in cases requiring the use of sutures between the plate and the cuff, where partial detachment of the deltoid from the acromion could be required. Such cases include

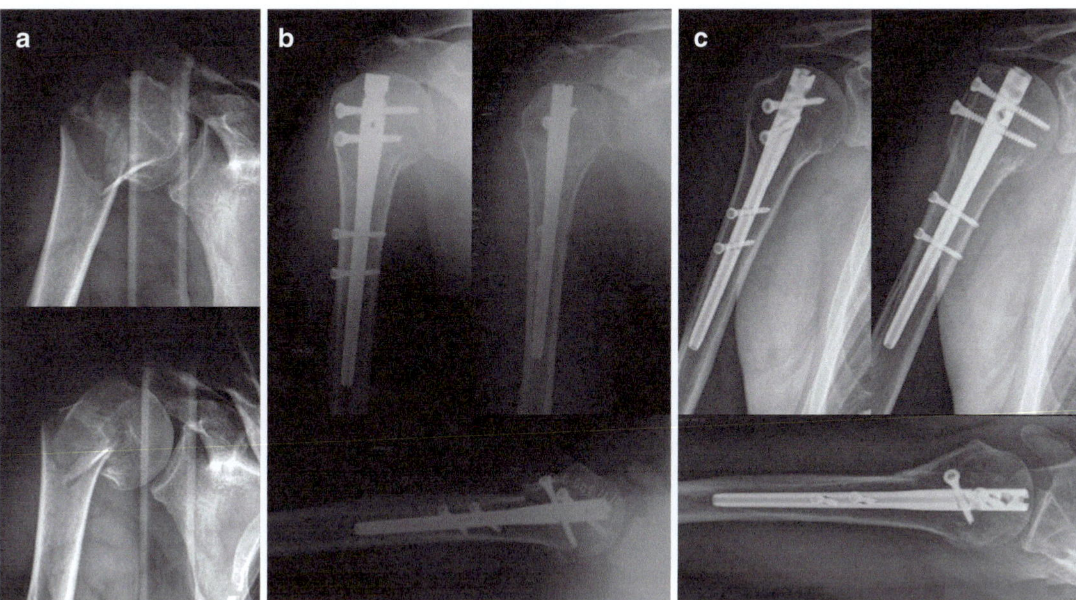

Fig. 11.5 Surgical neck fracture in a 57-year-old man. (**a**) Preoperative radiographs showing metaphyseal comminution. (**b**) Reduction and fixation with an angular stable nail: postoperative radiographs. (**c**) Radiographs 7 months after surgery

patients with a poor bone quality and fractures with metaphyseal comminution in which stabilization with inferomedial screws is not achievable as per the minimally invasive plate technical configuration. Patients affected by metaphyseal comminution may be better off if treated with a nail instead of a minimally invasive locking plate (Fig. 11.5). Intramedullary nailing has the advantage of providing mechanical stability of the proximal fragment with both the screws and the subchondral bone-nail interface [29, 36]. To maximize this effect while avoiding rotator cuff secondary damage and subacromial impingement by an overriding nail, the optimal depth of nail insertion should be 3–4 mm under the cartilage surface [6, 29]. In any case, both the nail and the plate allow us to optimally intervene on the rotator cuff through an anterolateral deltoid-splitting surgical approach should the surgeon suspect rotator cuff lesions. The use of a locking plate implanted through a traditional deltopectoral approach is our preferred choice in particular cases. These include complex lesions requiring significant reduction maneuvers, varus deformity associated with a significant bone loss requiring bone grafts, cases with a fixable medial calcar fragments, and a poor-quality bone requiring substantial use of osteosutures. The technique must be rigorous, and particular attention should be given to the soft tissue envelope. Periosteal elevation should be avoided. The transverse ligament above the bicipital groove and the anterior circumflex vessels must all be identified and respected in order to protect the ascending branch and the vascularization of the head. It is our belief that complex fractures always require osteosutures. Furthermore, the plate should be placed meticulously in terms of height and screw insertion so as to avoid subacromial impingement and violation of the articular surface. In conclusion, we recommend using a minimally invasive plate technique in young active patients, especially for valgus/medial translation deformity of the fracture. The bone quality should be optimal. Intramedullary nailing is the best option to treat comminuted metaphyseal fractures in older patients with fair bone quality. The abovementioned cases must be addressed through an anterolateral deltoid-splitting approach with minimal soft tissue manipulation. The remaining complex fractures and/or patients with poor bone quality may be treated with a locking plate through a traditional deltopectoral approach. Nonetheless, a rigorous surgical technique that is respectful of the vascularization and biology of the fracture is paramount. Finally, CRPP—especially the modified palm tree technique—may play a role in the elderly, low-demanding patients to prevent nonunions.

References

1. Court-Brown CM, Garg A, McQueen MM (2001) The translated two-part fracture of the proximal humerus. Epidemiology and outcome in the older patient. J Bone Joint Surg 83-B:799–804
2. Warner JJP, Costouros JG, Gerber C (2006) Fractures of the proximal humerus. In: Rockwood & Green's fractures in adults, 6th edn. Lippincott Williams & Wilkins, Philadelphia
3. Brorson S, Eckardt H, Audigé L, Rolauffs B, Bahrs C (2013) Translation between the Neer- and the AO/OTA-classification for proximal humeral fractures: do we need to be bilingual to interpret the scientific literature? BMC Res Notes 6:69
4. Neer CS (1970) Displaced proximal humeral fractures. I. Classification and evaluation. J Bone Joint Surg Am 52(6):1077–1089
5. Marsh JL, Slongo TF, Agel J, Broderick JS, Creevey W, DeCoster TA, Prokuski L, Sirkin MS, Ziran B, Henley B, Audigé L (2007) Fracture and dislocation classification compendium - 2007. Orthopaedic trauma association classification, database and outcomes committee. J Orthop Trauma 21(Suppl):S1–S133
6. Hatzidakis AM, Shevlin MJ, Fenton DL, Curran-Everett D, Nowinski RJ, Fehringer EV (2011) Angular-stable locked intramedullary nailing of two-part surgical neck fractures of the proximal part of the humerus. A multicenter retrospective observational study. J Bone Joint Surg Am 93:2172–2179
7. Handoll HHG, Ollivere BJ, Rollins KE (2012) Interventions for treating proximal humeral fractures in adults (Review). Cochrane Database Syst Rev (12):CD000434 10.1002/14651858
8. Maier D, Jager M, Strohm PC, Sudkamp NP (2012) Treatment of proximal humeral fractures – a review of current concepts enlightened by basic principles. Acta Chir Orthop Traumatol Cech 79(4):307–316
9. Nho SJ, Brophy RH, Barker JU, Cornell CN, MacGillivray JD (2007) Management of proximal humeral fractures based on current literature. J Bone Joint Surg Am 89:44–58. doi:10.2106/JBJS.G.00648
10. Olerud P, Ahrengart L, Soderqvist A, Saving J, Tidermark J (2010) Quality of life and functional outcome after a 2-part proximal humeral fracture: a prospective cohort study on 50 patients treated with a locking plate. J Shoulder Elbow Surg 19:814–822
11. Martinez AA, Bejarano C, Carbonel I, Iglesias D, Gil-Alvaroba J, Herrera A (2012) The treatment of proximal humerus nonunions in older patients with the reverse shoulder arthroplasty. Injury 43(Suppl 2):S3–S6. doi:10.1016/S0020-1383(13)70172-4
12. Urda A, Gonzalez A, Colino A, Lopiz Y, Garcıa-Fernandez C, Marco F (2012) Management of displaced surgical neck fractures of the humerus: health related quality of life, functional and radiographic results. Injury 43(S2):S12–S19
13. Lekic N, Montero NM, Takemoto RC, Davidovitch RI, Egol KA (2012) Treatment of two-part proximal humerus fractures: intramedullary nail compared to locked plating. HSS J 8:86–91. doi:10.1007/s11420-012-9274-z
14. Zhu Y, Lu Y, Shen J, Zhang J, Jiang C (2011) Locking intramedullary nails and locking plates in the treatment of two-part proximal humeral surgical neck fractures. A prospective randomized trial with a minimum of three years of follow-up. J Bone Joint Surg Am 93:159–168. doi:10.2106/JBJS.J.00155
15. Herscovici D Jr, Saunders DT, Johnson MP, Sanders R, Di Pasquale T (2001) Percutaneous fixation of proximal humeral fractures. J Bone Joint Surg Am 83-A(11):1695–1699
16. Harrison AK, Gruson KI, Zmintowski B, Keener J, Galatz L, Williams G, Parsons BO, Flatow EL (2012) Intermediate outcomes following percutaneous fixation of proximal humeral fractures. J Bone Joint Surg Am 94:1223–1228
17. Kaminemi S, Ankema H, Sanghavi S (2004) Anatomical considerations for percutaneous proximal humeral fracture fixation. Injury 35:1133–1136
18. Kapandji A (1989) Osteosynthesis using the "palm-tree" nail technique in fractures of the surgical neck of the humerus. Ann Chir Main 8(1):39–52
19. Le Bellec Y, Masmejean E, Cottias P, Alnot JY, Huten D (2002) Internal fixation of proximal humerus fracture by "palm tree" pinning. Rev Chir Orthop Reparatrice Appar Mot 88(4):342–348
20. El-Alfy BS (2011) Results of the percutaneous pinning of proximal humerus fractures with a modified palm tree technique. Int Orthop 35: 1343–1347
21. Resch H (2011) Proximal humeral fractures: current controversies. J Shoulder Elbow Surg 20:827–832
22. Ring D (2007) Current concepts in plate and screw fixation in osteoporotic proximal humerus fractures. Injury 38(S3):S59–S68
23. Edwards SL, Wilson NA, Zhang L, Flores S, Merk BR (2006) Two-part surgical neck fractures of the proximal part of the humerus. A biomechanical evaluation of two fixation techniques. J Bone Joint Surg 88-A:10
24. Aklin YP, Stoffel K, Sommer C (2013) A prospective analysis of the functional and radiological outcomes of minimally invasive plating in proximal humerus fractures. Injury 44:456–460
25. LaFlamme GY, Rouleau DM, Berry GK, Beaumont PH, Reindl R, Harvey EJ (2008)

Percutaneous humeral plating of fractures of the proximal humerus: results of a prospective multicenter clinical trial. J Orthop Trauma 22:3
26. Gardner MJ, Weil Y, Barker JU, Kelly BT, Helfet DL, Lorich DG (2007) The importance of medial support in locked plating of proximal humerus fractures. J Orthop Trauma 21:3
27. Jung W, Moon ES, Kim S, Kovacevic D, Kim M (2013) Does medial support decrease major complications of unstable proximal humerus fractures treated with locking plate? BMC Musculoskeletal Disorders 14:102
28. Nolan BM, Kippe MA, Wiater JM, Nowinski GP (2011) Surgical treatment of displaced proximal humerus fractures with a short intramedullary nail. J Shoulder Elbow Surg 20:1241–1247
29. Linhart W, Ueblacker P, Grobterlinden L, Kschowak P, Briem D, Janssen A, Hassunizadeh B, Schinke M, Windolf J, Rueger JM (2007) Antegrade nailing of humeral head fractures with captured interlocking screws. J Orthop Trauma 21:285–294
30. Park JY, Pandher DS, Chun JY, Lee ST (2008) Antegrade humeral nailing through the rotator cuff interval: a new entry portal. J Orthop Trauma 22:419–425
31. Stecco C, Gagliano G, Lancerotto L, Tiengo C, Macchi V, Porzionato A, De Caro R, Aldegheri R (2010) Surgical anatomy of the axillary nerve and its implication in the an antero-lateral deltoid splitting approaches to the shoulder. J Shoulder Elbow Surg 19:1166–1174
32. Osterhoff G, Hoch A, Wanner GA, Simmen H, Werner CML (2012) Calcar comminution as prognostic factor of clinical outcome after locking plate fixation of proximal humeral fractures. Injury 43:1651–1656
33. Robinson CM, Amin AK, Godley KC, Murray IR, White TO (2011) Modern perspectives of open reduction and plate fixation of proximal humerus fractures. J Orthop Trauma 25:618–629
34. Weeks CA, Begum F, Beaupre LA, Carey JP, Adeeb S, Bouliane MJ (2013) Locking plate fixation of proximal humeral fractures with impaction of the fracture site to restore medial column support: a biomechanical study. J Shoulder Elbow Surg. doi: 10.1016/j.jse.2013.02.003
35. Lill H (2010) Was ist eine minimalinvasive Operationstechnik zur Versorgung proximaler Humerusfrakturen? Unfallchirurg 113:1058
36. Sosef N, van Leerdam R, Ott P, Meylaerts S, Rhemrev S (2010) Minimal invasive fixation of proximal humeral fractures with an intramedullary nail: good results in elderly patients. Arch Orthop Trauma Surg 130:605–611

The Tuberosities

12

Paolo Baudi, Gabriele Campochiaro, Manuela Rebuzzi, Fabio Serafini, Giovanni Matino, and Fabio Catani

12.1 Introduction

Fractures of the greater and lesser tuberosities of the humerus are a rare clinical occurrence (20 and 2 % of all proximal humeral fractures, respectively). They often arise in association with a traumatic glenohumeral dislocation (10–30 % of cases) or as a result of a high-energy direct trauma [1]. Recent studies have reported that approximately 60 % of such fractures remain undiagnosed at initial clinical-radiological assessment [2]. Undisplaced fractures generally show good results if treated conservatively and with an appropriate rehabilitation program [3]. Most authors agree that surgery is indicated when the fracture is displaced with posterosuperior dislocation of fragments. In fact, these cases often develop acromial impingement, an alteration in the balance of forces between the rotator cuff muscles and the deltoid, with resulting articular impairment especially during abduction and pseudarthrosis [4, 5]. In view of the above, it is crucial to formulate an early diagnosis, in some cases by means of more specific radiological investigations such as ultrasound and computed tomography (CT), and to establish which lesions really deserve an operative approach. In the event of surgery, one will have to decide whether to perform open or arthroscopic reduction and what fixation devices need to be used, on the basis of the number and size of fragments, and the extent degree of displacement.

12.2 Greater Tuberosity

12.2.1 Epidemiology, Pathogenesis, and Classification

Isolated fractures of the greater tuberosity are reported to account for approximately 20 % of all proximal humeral fractures, a percentage that is probably an underestimation due to misdiagnosis on plain radiography, whereas the proportion of greater tuberosity fractures that are treated surgically is 5 % [1, 6–8].

In 10–30 % of cases, these fractures are associated with anterior glenohumeral dislocation [1, 9]: this means that a high proportion are also associated with partial or complete rotator cuff tears, instability of the long head of the biceps tendon, and injury to the anterior glenoid rim [10].

Isolated greater tuberosity fractures should be regarded as a distinct disease entity among fractures of the proximal epiphysis of the humerus. In 2005, Kim et al. [7] described the epidemiological features of these fractures, on the basis of a sample of 115 isolated greater tuberosity fractures

P. Baudi (✉) • G. Campochiaro • M. Rebuzzi
F. Serafini • G. Matino • F. Catani
Department of Orthopaedic Surgery,
University of Modena and Reggio Emilia,
Via del Pozzo, 71, Modena 41124, Italy
e-mail: baudispallaonline@gmail.com;
campochiaro.g@libero.it; manuela.rebuzzi@libero.it;
serafini.fab6@alice.it; giovamat3@yahoo.it;
fabio.catani@unimore.it

F. Castoldi et al. (eds.), *Simple and Complex Fractures of the Humerus*,
DOI 10.1007/978-88-470-5307-6_12, © Springer-Verlag Italia 2015

among a total of 610 proximal humeral fractures: the mean age of patients is 42.8 years versus 54.2, with a male predominance, and there is a stronger correlation with glenohumeral dislocation and therefore with higher-energy traumas. Moreover, isolated fractures of the greater tuberosity are considerably less likely to be associated with comorbidities, 13 % versus 35 %, as also reported by Chun et al. [6].

Historically, isolated greater tuberosity fractures have been described as avulsion fractures of the rotator cuff. However, in 2006, Bahrs et al. [9] found 25 % of inferior displacements of the greater tuberosity, in contrast with the avulsion dynamics which would pull the fragment posteriorly or posterosuperiorly. The mechanism of trauma therefore deserves close attention. First, this type of fracture may arise as a result of an injury to the shoulder which may be direct—as occurs in the majority of cases [9]—or indirect after a fall with outstretched hand and extended or flexed elbow or after a movement of shoulder abduction and external rotation that has sufficient energy to produce a fracture [9, 11]. With both mechanisms, the greater tuberosity may fracture as a result of avulsion of the rotator cuff or impact against the acromion. An additional, less common, cause is an epileptic seizure. When associated with anterior glenohumeral dislocation, the fracture is caused by impact against the anterior edge of the glenoid cavity, and often the reduction maneuver indirectly also reduces displacement of the tuberosity. The role played by osteoporosis in the mechanism of injury is still unclear [11].

The most commonly used classification systems for fractures of the proximal humeral epiphysis, namely, Neer [5] and AO, are of limited use in isolated greater tuberosity fractures, as these make up a very different clinical entity. According to the Neer classification, still the most commonly used, these fractures have the features of a two-part fracture when the displacement exceeds 1 cm or 45° angulation; this model has been found to have fair/moderate inter- and intraobserver reliability, in that interpretation is not always unequivocal on plain radiographs obtained in the emergency department, due to the risk of missing a three-part fracture especially in cases of valgus impacted fractures of the neck or missing the fracture because of calcifications or small mobile fragments [1]. Moreover, the Neer classification does not take into account the direction of the displacement, comminution, and associated rotator cuff injuries, which tend to be more likely and extensive with more severely displaced fragments. Over the past decade, many authors have agreed that the displacement values are inadequate and too large and lack correlation with the patients' functional characteristics and requirements [12, 13]. Platzer et al. in 2005 [3] examined 135 isolated greater tuberosity fractures with 1–5 mm displacement treated nonoperatively and assessed using the main clinical scores after a mean interval of 3.7 years and found 97 % of good to excellent results. However, to relate shoulder outcomes to the extent of displacement alone, without considering direction, number of fragments, associated rotator cuff injuries, and type of patient, appears to be reductive and nongeneralizable. Displacement remains nonetheless crucial, as beyond a certain, unpredictable degree rotator cuff injuries are inevitable. In the AO/ASIF classification, isolated fractures of the greater tuberosity are identified by the code 11A1.2. However, even this classification system is morphologic descriptive and not predictive of outcomes in the long term. In 2003, Gotzen et al. [14] proposed another, more detailed, topographic-morphologic classification for isolated greater tuberosity fractures. These fractures are defined by the letter G, which is combined with the morphologic criterion, indicated by the letter S, which ranges from 1 to 4 based on displacement severity, fragment instability and number/comminution. This classification considers a fracture to be displaced when it exceeds 25° of angulation or rotation or 5 mm of displacement. Only type G.S1 fractures are considered minimally displaced and stable with preserved soft tissue. The authors themselves state, however, that a new, more accurate and reproducible classification is warranted [15] which is capable of taking into account the pathogenetic mechanism and the site and type of displacement, as well as providing information on outcomes and treatment.

Parsons et al. [16] in 2005 came to the conclusion that the classification systems generally used for the proximal humeral epiphysis are still unreliable owing to the difficulty in accurately assessing greater tuberosity displacements on plain radiographs. In 2006, Bahrs et al. [9], in a study investigating a sample of 103 greater tuberosity fractures, half of which associated with glenohumeral dislocation, concluded that there was no correlation between mechanism of injury and fracture pattern and that in the event of associated dislocation, the fragments tended to be more numerous and larger. Larger patient series should therefore be studied to better understand the biomechanical mechanisms underlying this type of fracture and identify significant correlations with clinical outcomes.

12.2.2 Clinical and Imaging Diagnosis

Clinically, in the acute phase it is difficult to distinguish an isolated greater tuberosity fracture from a multipart fracture of the humeral epiphysis or acute rotator cuff disease: in either case patients report pain and reduction or absence of active mobilization and/or mobilization against resistance, especially during abduction and external rotation [17, 18]. The clinical diagnosis is more straightforward when the fracture is associated with dislocation, and in these cases an accurate neurovascular assessment is always mandatory. Nerve lesions, in particular to the axillary nerve and secondary trunk, occur in about one third of scapulohumeral dislocations with greater tuberosity fracture, with recovery in the majority of cases after several months. In most cases, electromyography (EMG) at 45 days, 3 months, and 6 months confirms low-grade neurapraxia or axonotmesis, related to stretch or external pressure during the initial trauma. Imaging diagnosis is first based on a radiographic trauma series: an AP view in neutral rotation (X-ray beam perpendicular to the scapular plane), a view of the "scapular Y" (beam parallel to the spine of the scapula), and an axillary view (supine position, at least 30° of abduction, with beam from a caudal position). If pain precludes the axillary view, this can be replaced with Velpeau axillary lateral view (with the patient standing, leaning backward 30° over the X-ray table, the beam passes through the shoulder from above). In a cadaver study, Parsons et al. [16] highlighted that the best measurement of the extent of posterosuperior displacement is obtained with an AP view in external rotation and an AP view with 15° caudal inclination. Therefore, in cases of suspected greater tuberosity fracture, it is advisable to add an AP projection with external rotation to the trauma series [1, 5, 16, 19]. CT in the coronal and sagittal plane and with 3D reconstructions may be used as a diagnostic supplement to better characterize the fracture: number of fragments, direction and extent of displacement, occult fracture lines, and intra-articular extension (three-part valgus impacted fractures), which bear an influence on the type of treatment and the choice of fixation device and technique [20]. CT as a first-line investigation may prove useful in obese patients or those unable to comply with plain radiography [1]. Published studies about the appropriateness of CT imaging are conflicting: while a recent study [21] found an improvement in interpretation reliability in terms of the number of fragments identified, assessment of associated lesser tuberosity displacement, and articular involvement, other papers reported limited reproducibility of the classification of fractures with the addition of CT [22]. In our department, we use CT with 3D reconstructions in cases with a surgical indication for radiography (to plan the arthroscopic or open procedure and the type of fixation), in cases where plain radiography cannot establish the extent of displacement and in cases of suspected valgus impacted fracture. Ultrasound and magnetic resonance imaging (MRI) performed in acute shoulder trauma to investigate suspected traumatic rupture of the rotator cuff proved to be useful for detecting occult tuberosity fractures when initial plain radiography had been negative. The true prevalence of occult greater tuberosity fracture is unknown. However, Zanetti et al. in a study of 24 patients undergoing MRI for suspected traumatic rotator cuff rupture found that a previously missed greater tuberosity fracture was detected in 9/24 subjects examined (38 %) [18]. Another study by Gumina et al. presented a cohort of 24 patients with a greater tuberosity fracture initially missed on plain radiography in the emergency department and subsequently detected on MRI; retrospective review of the radiograms revealed that subtle fracture lines could be seen in 75 % of patients. Moreover, 46 % of patients had a partial anterior or posterosuperior tear of the rotator cuff and only 12.5 % of all subjects had involvement of two tendons (supra- and infraspinatus) [17].

It is therefore crucial to obtain high-quality radiograms in appropriate projections to assess the greater tuberosity, that is, in AP view with external rotation of the arm. Ultrasound may play an important role to identify occult fractures in acute settings and provide concurrent assessment of the rotator cuff when radiography is positive. Speed of performance, relative inexpensiveness, and increasing availability in emergency departments make ultrasound particularly suited for diagnosing tuberosity fractures in emergency settings and monitoring the clinical course after conservative treatment. We use MRI only in the event that ultrasound shows a tear larger than 2–3 cm or involving more than one tendon, for the purpose of assessing tendon retraction and muscular atrophy.

12.2.3 Treatment

The treatment of greater tuberosity fractures is still controversial, as there is no consensus among the various authors. A correct and timely diagnosis in addition to an optimal choice of surgery is the keystone for good functional results.

A retrospective study with 3-year follow-up conducted by Mattyasovszky et al. [23] in 2011 reported on a series of 30 isolated greater tuberosity fractures treated both operatively and nonoperatively. They concluded that irrespective of treatment the results were good for slightly or moderately displaced fractures, as also reported by Gruson et al. in 2008 [1]. However, the numerous short- and long-term sequelae such as osteonecrosis, pseudarthrosis, subacromial impingement up to joint locking during abduction or external rotation, and consolidation defects with severe functional disability have led to consider the need for surgical treatment more frequently.

Over the years, indications for surgical treatment have in fact seen a progressive reduction of the tolerated extent of displacement. Neer [5] in 1970 recommended operative treatment for displacements greater than 1 cm. In the 1990s, Bigliani and Park [12, 24] lowered the indication to 5 mm and Resch [13] to 3 mm in young active patients, athletes, or heavy manual workers.

A correct assessment of the extent of—especially posterosuperior—displacement of the greater tuberosity is fundamental because, as demonstrated by Bono et al.'s biomechanical studies [4], beyond a certain threshold, it can alter the balance of forces between rotator cuff and deltoid, with up to 30 % increase in force requirement during abduction and external rotation and a decrease in the mean functional scores with higher displacement values.

Another key factor in addition to extent of displacement is its direction. There are three main displacements in a greater tuberosity fracture: inferior, which is rare and well tolerated even when greater than 3 mm; superior, which decreases the subacromial space causing impingement syndrome up to joint locking during abduction and which is usually the least well tolerated, with functional defects occurring with displacements as small as 3 mm; and posterior, which is well tolerated even up to 5 mm, may cause joint locking during external rotation, and may be associated with an anterosuperior tear of the rotator cuff.

In our experience, surgery is indicated for superior or posterosuperior displacements greater than 3 mm especially in young or active patients, athletes, or heavy laborers. Posterior displacements up to 5 mm may be tolerated, provided that the patient is carefully assessed for an associated anterosuperior rotator cuff tear.

In elderly patients with severe comorbidities and limited functional requirements, the tolerance can be increased to 1 cm, as illustrated by Gruson et al. [1].

12.2.3.1 Nonoperative Treatment

Where there is an indication for nonoperative treatment, we advise a period of immobilization with a shoulder sling at 10–15° of abduction and neutral rotation for 30 days followed by radiographic follow-up at 7 and 15 days to detect any secondary displacements. At 30 days we start passive mobilization of the shoulder which is continued for 10–15 days, if necessary with the help of mechanical aids, and then assisted active rehabilitation and strengthening. At 2 months we recommend a dynamic comparative ultrasound examination of the shoulders to highlight any rotator cuff tears. It is important to remember that nonoperative treatment is characterized by a higher frequency of shoulder rigidity due to adhesive capsulitis, which significantly complicates rehabilitation, usually a simple process, of an undisplaced greater tuberosity fracture.

12.2.3.2 Operative Treatment

Operative treatment of greater tuberosity fractures may be carried out both as open surgery and arthroscopically.

In open surgery the classic deltopectoral or transdeltoid access is used: the surgeon's experience and the size of the fragments will suggest the approach, remembering that visualization of large fragments may be limited in the deltoid split, where distal exposure is impaired by the axillary nerve.

Many open fixation techniques have been reported: screws +/– tension band, Kirschner wires, transosseous sutures and/or anchors, and plates. Irrespective of the fixation technique, it is fundamental to achieve an anatomic reduction.

The use of 1–2 cannulated screws + tension band is regarded as the gold standard for open surgery [11, 25, 26].

However, the choice of fixation procedure depends on fragment size and comminution. The presence of a single large fragment may allow for fixation with 1 or 2 screws with or without washer, in particular in conditions of poor bone stock: in this case we recommend that the fixation always be done with a screw combined with a tension band so as to reduce the traction forces on the rotator cuff and facilitate earlier mobilization [26] (Fig. 12.1). This type of fixation should be avoided in cases of a multifragmented fracture of the greater tuberosity and in patients with severe osteoporosis so as not to risk mobilization of the screw or fragmentation of the greater tuberosity during fixation.

Where there are several small or poor-quality fragments, fixation with transosseous nonabsorbable sutures should be preferred, through direct repair of the rotator cuff [1]. Even in this case various techniques have been adopted: Park et al. and Flatow et al. [11, 12] reported good results using transosseous sutures in a figure-of-eight pattern placing the fragments back into the fracture bed and thereby minimizing potential hardware mobilization problems.

Transosseous fixation can also be achieved by using small anchors: Bhatia et al. [27] reported excellent long-term results with a double row of suture anchors: the sutures arranged in this way buttress the fragments against the fracture surface. We currently prefer open surgery to fix these fractures with transosseous sutures using a new device (SharcFT®) that allows for the creation of transosseous tunnels even in conditions of poor bone stock [28] (Fig. 12.2).

Arthroscopic fixation is more recent and offers many advantages: considerably less trauma to soft tissue; possibility of having a comprehensive view of associated lesions, together with the opportunity to treat them; better visualization of the fixation obtained; and unscathed deltoid muscle [4, 10]. There are, however, also disadvantages: greater difficulty in obtaining a stable fixation, complex conversion to open surgery, higher cost, and longer learning curve [29].

The literature contains few case series concerning arthroscopic treatment of greater tuberosity fractures: Taverna et al. [30] reported excellent results with the described technique in which the posterior portal is placed superiorly and laterally to improve visualization of the tuberosity fragment. After debridement of the fracture site, the greater tuberosity is reduced and temporarily stabilized using K-wires, with subsequent definitive fixation using cannulated screws with the aid of fluoroscopy.

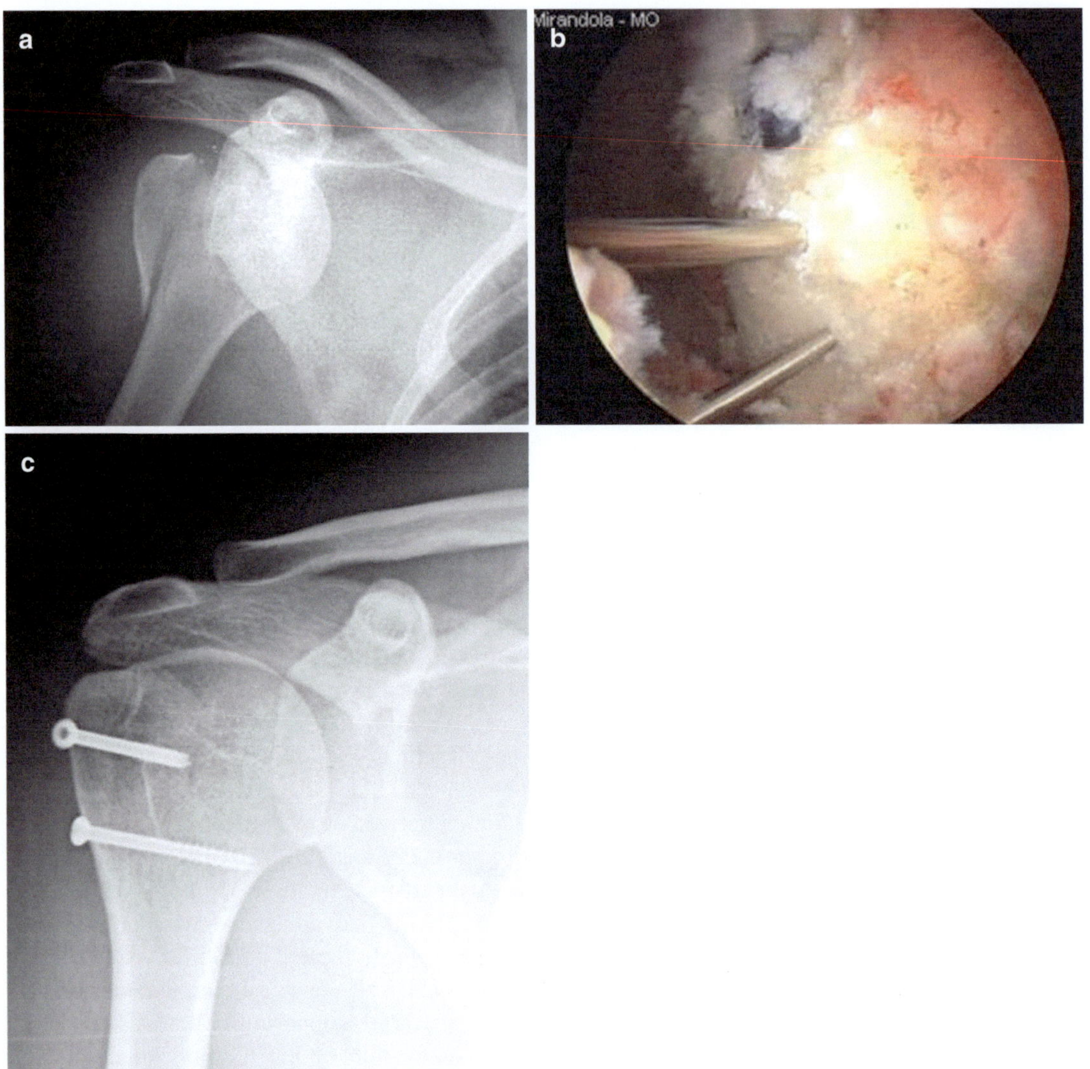

Fig. 12.1 (**a**) Single large fragment of greater tuberosity fracture: X-ray. (**b**) Arthroscopic treatment with two cannulated screws. (**c**) Postoperative X-ray

In the presence of multifragmented fractures, one often has to handle smaller fragments with the cuff inserted, predominantly supraspinatus or supra-infraspinatus. In such cases the fracture may be treated as a rotator cuff tear using the technique described by Bhatia et al. [27], which addresses the fixation of the tuberosity fragments indirectly by repairing the rotator cuff with anchors (Fig. 12.3).

Other authors such as Ji et al. [31, 32] and Song et al. [33] reported direct rotator cuff repair by using double-row and suture-bridge techniques to reduce and fix the tuberosity fragments, especially when comminuted, with good or excellent results. A 2012 cadaveric biomechanical study by Lin et al. [34] demonstrated that in greater tuberosity fractures, fixation techniques relying on anchors last longer than those relying on screws.

A fundamental aspect is the correct choice of indication for arthroscopic fixation: isolated greater tuberosity fractures or those associated

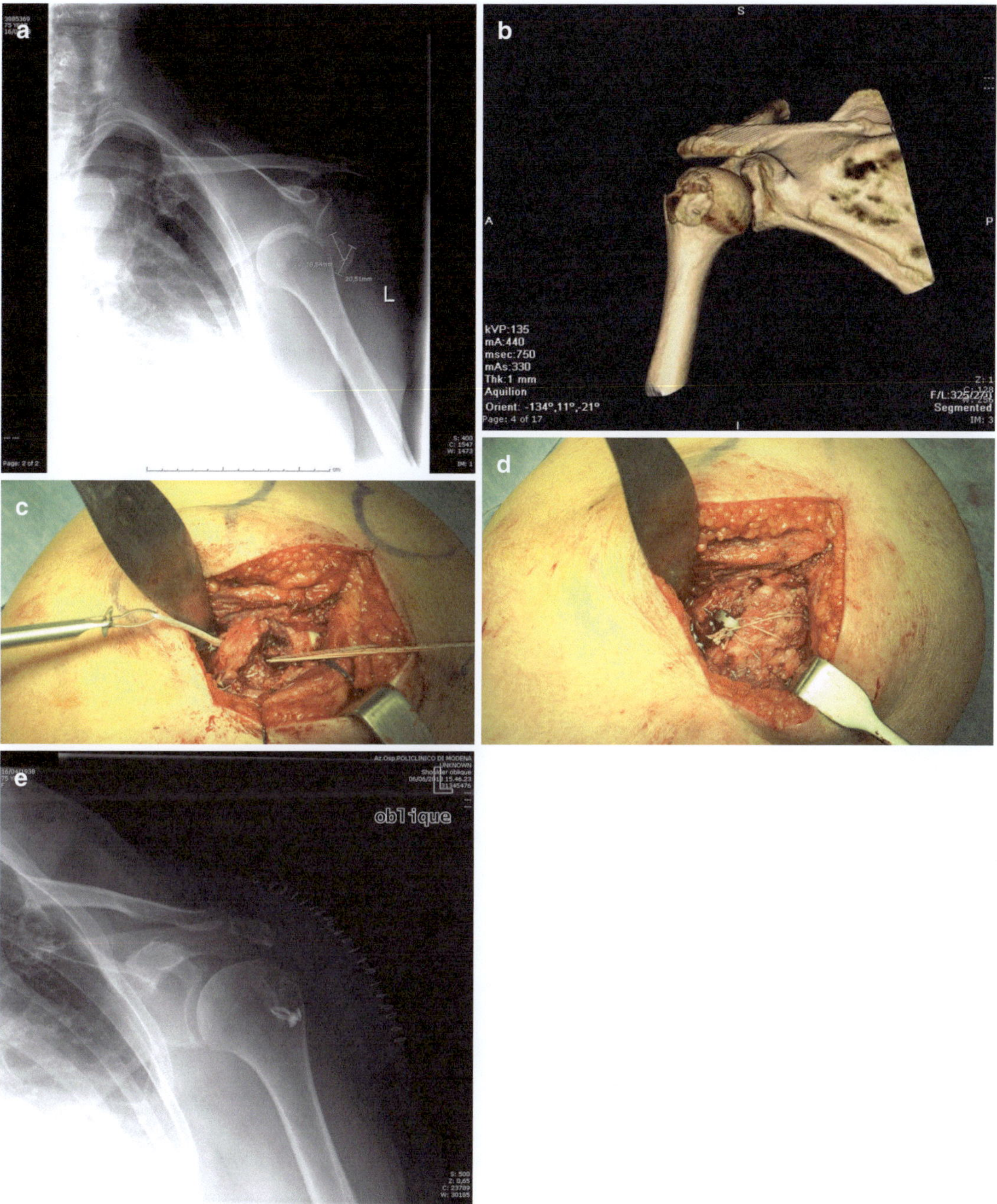

Fig. 12.2 (**a**) Several fragments of greater tuberosity fracture-dislocation: X-ray. (**b**) 3D-CT fracture view. (**c**) Open fixation with transosseous system, the SharcFT®. (**d**) Final suture configuration. (**e**) Postoperative X-ray

with reduced glenohumeral dislocation; single fragment of 2–3 cm with minimal displacement, preferably treated with 1–2 cannulated screws; and comminuted fractures or with a main fragment of 1–2 cm if displaced posterosuperiorly and associated with rotator cuff tears [1, 35] to be treated with double-row sutures of suture-bridge technique only if bone

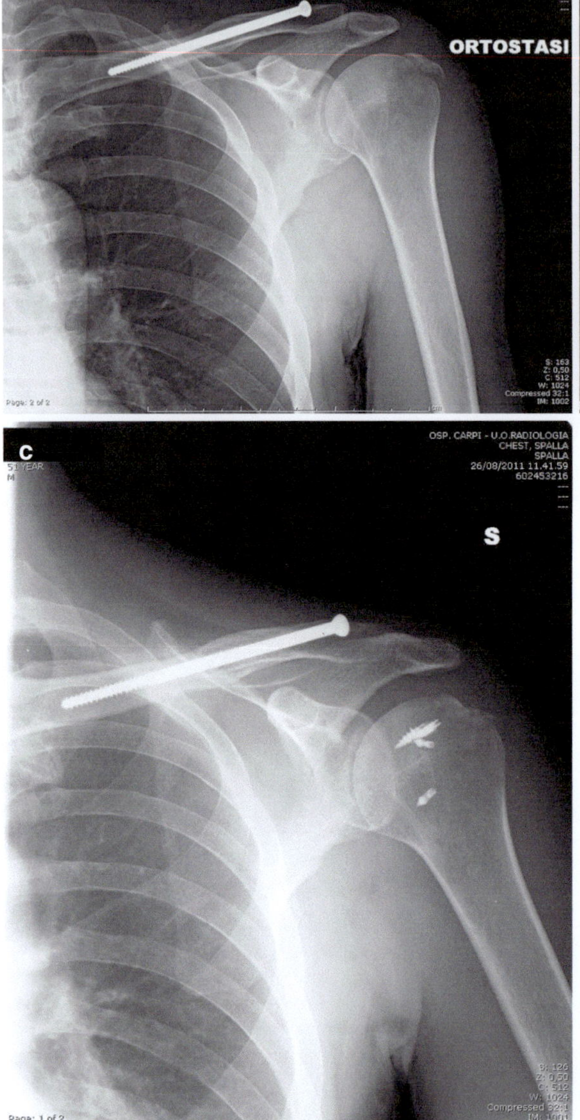

Fig. 12.3 (**a**) Several small fragments of greater tuberosity fracture: X-ray. (**b**) 3D-CT fracture view. (**c**) Arthroscopic indirectly fixation with transosseous equivalent technique (suture bridge) as a rotator cuff tear repair: postoperative X-ray

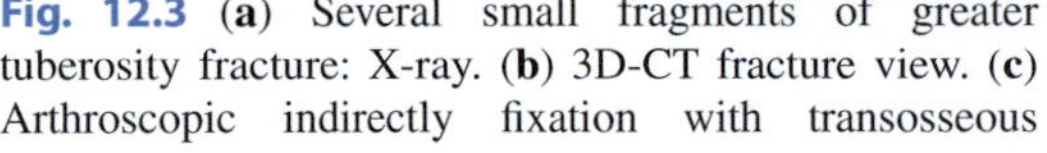

quality is good. Arthroscopic treatment also has some limitations: multifragmented fractures; fragments larger than 3 cm or than 2 cm but severely displaced, owing to the difficulty achieving a good anatomic reduction and a stable fixation; valgus impacted fractures; and presence of severe osteoporosis (where the transosseous system with SharcFT® device could overcome the problem).

As regards postoperative treatment of both open and arthroscopic fixation, we prefer to use a shoulder sling at 10–15° of abduction and neutral rotation for 4 weeks. Passive mobilization is allowed at 1 week even with the help of mechanical aids, whereas active mobilization is recommended at 4–6 weeks, alternating exercise on land and in water with a maximum of three sessions a week.

12.2.4 Conclusions

Greater tuberosity fractures form a distinct disease entity within the spectrum of fractures of the proximal humeral epiphysis. Current classifications are inadequate both for diagnostic interpretation and for providing the correct indication for treatment. The clinical and rehabilitation course after operative and nonoperative treatment is often more complex than expected or communicated to the patient. When indicated, arthroscopic fixation may play a crucial role in the technical result and the postoperative course.

12.3 Lesser Tuberosity

Fractures of the lesser tuberosity are even rarer than those affecting the greater tuberosity, accounting for approximately 2 % of all proximal humeral fractures [36].

From the point of view of demographics, pathological anatomy, etiology, and pathogenesis, we can distinguish two types of lesion: fractures-avulsions in the adolescent and fractures in the adult.

Fractures-avulsions of the adolescent are relatively rare but increasing in frequency: a recent review of the literature published in 2012 [37] reports on a study of 33 cases among patients aged 11–20 years, predominantly males, with a mean age of 13 years. The growing incidence reported by some authors [38] is related to the increasingly earlier and more intense engagement of adolescents in high-level contact or overhead sports. Another peculiarity of these lesions is the delay in diagnosis and treatment relative to the traumatic event. Vezeridis et al. [39] reported a mean time from trauma to diagnosis of 6.5 weeks, and Levine et al. [40] in a review of 32 cases confirmed a delay of over 6 months in 50 % of cases. The reported traumatic mechanisms are basically two: forced and resisted abduction-external rotation during a throwing action, a backward fall with extended and externally rotated shoulder. In both cases there is an eccentric contraction of the subscapularis which opposes the forced external rotation. The third mechanism, specific to sports like baseball or fishing, is related to repetitive abduction-external rotation that can cause microtraumatic detachment of the lesser tuberosity (little league shoulder). In terms of pathological anatomy, fracture-avulsion of the lesser tuberosity cannot be defined as either epiphyseal detachment or apophysitis in the rare cases of little league shoulder, since the ossification center of the lesser tuberosity fuses with the humeral head between the ages of 7 and 11 years. Because a relative weakness of the lesser tuberosity-head transition zone is thought to persist between the ages of 12 and 16–17 years, the lesion can be defined as a transitional fracture or a lesser tuberosity stress lesion.

The clinical examination of these patients reveals anterior shoulder pain which is put in relation to a precise traumatic event in some cases only; in the majority of patients, no precise traumatic event can be identified. For this reason, the first clinical suspicion is anterior instability, though careful assessment will reveal a limitation and weakness in internal rotation-retropulsion, positive belly-press test and lift-off test, and in some cases increased external rotation at ER1 (external rotation with elbow close to trunk). In cases in which the time from traumatic event to diagnosis exceeds 6–12 months, there may be an anterior bony mass due to exostotic callus formation.

Standard radiography often does not allow for a precise diagnosis with even the axillary view not permitting a diagnosis in over 50 % of patients [41] since the detached fragment is mostly cartilaginous. Only in patients undergoing assessment a long time after the traumatic event does the development of an exostosis visible on the axillary view allow the diagnosis.

MRI is specific and sensitive for this type of lesion and is therefore indicated in anterior shoulder pain in 11–17-year-old adolescents with a history of trauma during abduction-external rotation and backward fall during external rotation or in young athletes with repeated throwing action. In some cases MRI will allow visualization of the associated capsular detachment and/or medial displacement of the long head of the biceps.

Conservative treatment is reserved for cases in which the pathogenetic mechanism is repetitive throwing in abduction-external rotation (e.g., baseball) and in which investigations reveal an undisplaced stress lesion. Follow-up at 2 years shows complete recovery of function. Persistence of symptoms or imaging evidence of fragment displacement constitutes an indication for reduction and fixation [38].

Open surgical reduction and fixation via deltopectoral approach is instead warranted for all other posttraumatic cases to avoid short- and long-term sequelae. Goeminne and Debeer [37] report two severe sequelae in two patients aged 37 and 39 years who had sustained trauma as adolescents and required complex surgical procedures to restore function.

The lesser tuberosity fragment, which is usually small, can be reinserted through transosseous tunnels starting at the bicipital groove or with the aid of paracartilaginous medial anchors at the tendon-bone junction and lateral-row anchors (suture-bridge construct). In the event of biceps dislocation, tenodesis is performed within the bony groove.

Vezeridis et al. [39], in a series of eight patients treated between 2000 and 2010, report return to sport after an average of 4.5 months, with a mean limitation to external rotation of 13° in only 3/8 patients at 2-year follow-up.

Lesser tuberosity fractures in the adult may be isolated or associated with posterior glenohumeral dislocation; in either case they are relatively rare with an incidence ranging from 0.46 per 100,000 persons/year to 110 per 100,000 persons/year [42]. Given the peculiarity of fractures associated with posterior dislocation, these will not be discussed.

There are considerable variations in the reported age and sex of patients at risk of this type of fracture, but most of them are males aged 40–50 years. These fractures are caused by high-energy traumatic events such as a fall down the stairs or a fall from a horse or bicycle, which entail a forceful contraction of the subscapularis when the arm is forced into external rotation and extension. In cases associated with posterior dislocation, detachment of the lesser tuberosity appears as a propagation of the anterior osteochondral fracture of the humeral head. As with fractures-avulsions in adolescents, the clinical and radiological diagnosis is not always straightforward. Patients are mostly victims of high-energy traumas and therefore they are seen in the emergency department where, on the one hand, the intense pain of acute injury precludes a thorough clinical assessment and, on the other, it is difficult to obtain a correct axillary projection which would facilitate the diagnosis. In the AP view, these fractures appear as an altered bone profile medially to the bicipital groove or, where the groove is involved, an altered profile of the groove itself. Such radiographic changes associated with a history of a fall with extended or externally rotated arm, with intense pain and complete functional disability, should prompt the performance of an emergent CT scan.

In 20–30 % of cases, the diagnosis is not established immediately but only at subsequent follow-up visits, by means of MRI, performed to investigate persisting clinical signs of subscapularis injury (pseudoparalytic shoulder, limitation and pain during internal rotation and retropulsion, positive belly press, and increased external rotation), which shows detachment of the subscapularis with lesser tuberosity bone fragment, and subsequently CT which allows assessment of the size, involvement of the joint or bicipital groove, and retraction of the bone fragment. MRI enables evaluation of the displacement of the long head of the biceps, subscapularis muscle mass, and any associated lesions. Surgical treatment involves reinsertion of the bone fragment or, in the case of small fragments, reinsertion of the subscapularis alone. In our experience, these cases are ideally suited to arthroscopic treatment, which in practice entails reinsertion of the subscapularis with single-row or suture-bridge technique after removal of the small bone fragment, tenolysis of the subscapularis, and tenotomy-tenodesis of the long head of the biceps. If the fragment is larger than 1 cm and involves the cartilage surface or bicipital groove, then this requires open surgery by deltopectoral approach. Three possible techniques can be used to achieve release of the rotator interval, tenotomy with possible tenodesis of the long head of the biceps, and reinsertion of the bone fragment: transosseous sutures starting from the bicipital groove, 2-thread metal paracartilaginous anchors for cancellous bone and lateral-impact anchors for suture-bridge construct, and, more recently, fixation with the SharcFT® transosseous fixation system (Fig. 12.4). As in the case of greater tuberosity fractures, SharcFT® is placed in the

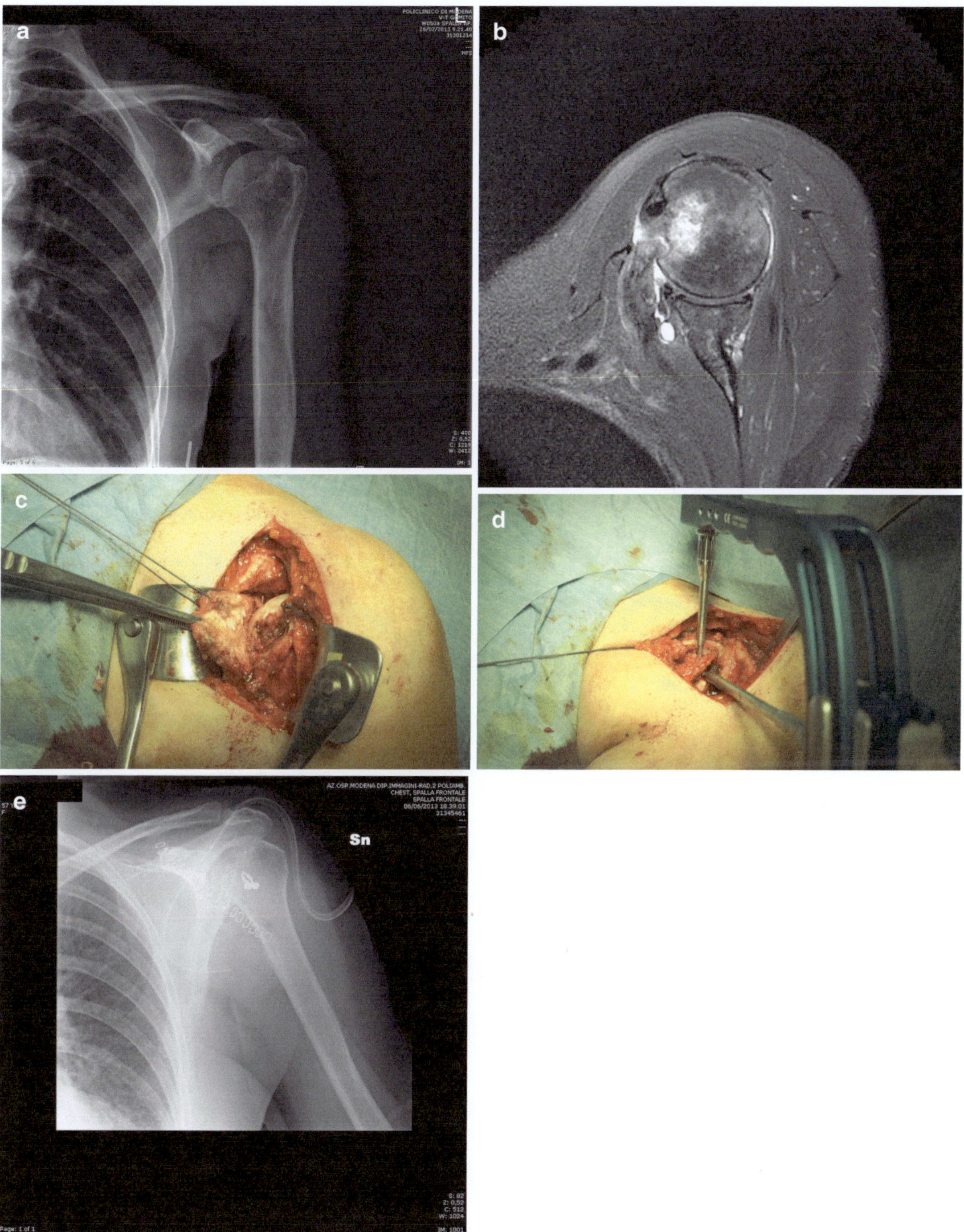

Fig. 12.4 (**a**) Lesser tuberosity fracture in adult: X-ray. (**b**) Axial CT fracture view. (**c**) Bicipital groove preparation as a bed for lesser tuberosity with subscapularis reduction and fixation. (**d**) Open fixation with transosseous system, the SharcFT®: tunnel creation by Compasso®, a dedicated instrumentation. (**e**) Postoperative X-ray

bicipital groove after having created one or more transosseous tunnels with paracartilaginous opening, transporting one or more high-resistance sutures inside the tunnel. U-knots are tied at the tendon-lesser tuberosity junction and the sutures are then pulled out through the dorsal hole of the device in order to close the tuberosity fixation system, thereby immediately achieving a high level of biomechanical stability, higher than provided by the traditional screw-washer systems of plain transosseous sutures. This allows for rapid referral for rehabilitation and complete functional recovery.

References

1. Gruson KI, Ruchelsman DE, Tejwani NC (2008) Isolated tuberosity fractures of the proximal humerus: current concepts. Injury 39:284–298
2. Ogawa K, Yoshida A, Ikegami H (2003) Isolated fractures of the greater tuberosity of the humerus: solutions to recognizing a frequently overlooked fracture. J Trauma 54:713–717
3. Platzer P, Kutscha-Lissberg F, Lehr S et al (2005) The influence of displacement on shoulder function in patients with minimally displaced fractures of the greater tuberosity. Injury 36:1185–1189
4. Bono CM, Renard R, Levine RG et al (2001) Effect of displacement of fractures of the greater tuberosity on the mechanics of the shoulder. J Bone Joint Surg Br 83:1056–1062
5. Neer CS II (1970) Displaced proximal humeral fractures. Part I. Classification and evaluation. J Bone Joint Surg Am 52:1077–1092
6. Chun JM, Groh GI, Rockwood CA Jr (1994) Two-part fractures of the proximal humerus. J Shoulder Elbow Surg 3:273–287
7. Kim E, Shin HK, Kim CH (2005) Characteristics of an isolated greater tuberosity fracture of the humerus. J Orthop Sci 10:441–444
8. Court-Brown CM, Garg A, McQueen MM (2001) The epidemiology of proximal humeral fractures. Acta Orthop Scand 72:365–371
9. Bahrs C, Lingenfelter E, Fischer F et al (2006) Mechanism of injury and morphology of the greater tuberosity fracture. J Shoulder Elbow Surg 15: 140–147
10. Kim SH, Ha KI (2000) Arthroscopic treatment of symptomatic shoulders with minimally displaced greater tuberosity fracture. Arthroscopy 16(7):695–700
11. Flatow EL, Cuomo F, Maday MG et al (1991) Open reduction and internal fixation of two-part displaced fractures of the greater tuberosity of the proximal part of the humerus. J Bone Joint Surg Am 73:1213–1218
12. Park TS, Choi IY, Kim Y et al (1997) A new suggestion for the treatment of minimally displaced fractures of the greater tuberosity of the proximal humerus. Bull Hosp Jt Dis 56(3):171–176
13. Resch H, Thoni H (1992) Dislocation fractures of the shoulder. Special status and therapeutic concepts. Orthopade 21(2):131–139 [article in German]
14. Gotzen L, Bahrs C, Leppek R et al (2003) Suggestion for a modular topographic-morphologic classification of proximal humeral fractures. Eur J Trauma 1:31–41
15. Bahrs C, Schmal H, Lingenfelter E et al (2008) Inter- and intraobserver reliability of the MTM-classification for proximal humeral fractures: a prospective study. BMC Musculoskelet Disord 9:21
16. Parsons BO, Klepps SJ, Miller S et al (2005) Reliability and reproducibility of radiographs of greater tuberosity displacement. J Bone Joint Surg Am 87(1):58–65
17. Gumina S, Carbone S, Postacchini F (2008) Occult fractures of the greater tuberosity of the humerus. Int Orthop 33:171–174
18. Zanetti M, Welshaupt D, Jost B et al (1999) MR imaging for traumatic tears of rotator cuff: high prevalence of greater tuberosity fractures and subscapularis tendon tears. AJR Am J Roentgenol 172:463–467
19. Zuckerman JD, Sahajpal DT (2009) Proximal humeral fractures: classification, diagnosis and conservative treatment. In: Iannotti JP, Williams Jr GR Shoulder diseases: diagnosis and treatment .Verduci Publisher. 2: 833–836
20. Green A, Izzi J Jr (2003) Isolated fractures of the greater tuberosity of the proximal humerus. J Shoulder Elbow Surg 12(6):641–649
21. Mora Guix JM, Gonzalez AS, Brugalla JV et al (2006) Proposed protocol for reading images of humeral head fractures. Clin Orthop Relat Res 448:225–233
22. Sjoden GO, Movin T, Guntner P et al (1999) Poor reproducibility of classification of the proximal humerus fractures. Additional CT of minor value. Acta Orthop Scand 68:239–242
23. Mattyasovszky SG, Burkhart KJ, Ahlers C et al (2011) Isolated fractures of the greater tuberosity of the proximal humerus: a long term retrospective study of 30 patients. Acta Orthop 82(6):714–720
24. Bigliani LU, Flatow EL (1998) Fractures of the proximal humerus. In: Rockwood CA, Matsen FA (eds) The shoulder, 3rd edn. WB Saunders, Philadelphia, pp 337–389
25. Resch H, Kathrein A, Golser K et al (1992) Arthroscopic and percutaneous bone screw techniques with a new screw system. Unfallchirurg 95(2):91–98
26. Braunstein V, Wiedemann E, Plitz W et al (2007) Operative treatment of greater tuberosity fractures of the humerus: a biomechanical analysis. Clin Biomech (Bristol, Avon) 22(6):652–657
27. Bhatia DN, van Rooyen KS, du Toit DF et al (2006) Surgical treatment of comminuted displaced fractures of the greater tuberosity of proximal humerus: a new technique of double row suture anchor fixation and long terms results. Injury 37:946–952
28. Baudi P, Rasia Dani E, Campochiaro G et al (2013) The rotator cuff tear repair with a new arthroscopic transosseous system: the Sharc-FT®. Musculoskelet Surg 97(Suppl 1):57–61
29. Gartsman GM, Taverna E (1996) Arthroscopic treatment of rotator cuff and greater tuberosity fracture nonunion. Arthroscopy 12:242–244

30. Taverna E, Sansone V, Battistella F (2004) Arthroscopic treatment for greater tuberosity fractures: rationale and surgical technique. Arthroscopy 20(6):53–57
31. Ji JH, Kim WY, Ra KH (2007) Arthroscopic double-row suture anchor fixation of minimally displaced greater tuberosity fractures. Arthroscopy 23(10):1133.e1-4
32. Ji JH, Shafi M, Song IS et al (2010) Arthroscopic fixation technique for comminuted, displaced greater tuberosity fracture. Arthroscopy 26(5):600–609
33. Song HS, Williams GR Jr (2008) Arthroscopic reduction and fixation with suture-bridge technique for displaced or comminuted greater tuberosity fractures. Arthroscopy 24(8):956–960
34. Lin CL, Hong CK, Jou IM et al (2012) Suture anchor versus screw fixation for greater tuberosity fractures of the humerus – a biomechanical study. J Orthop Res 30(3):423–428
35. Greiner S, Scheibel M (2011) Bony avulsion of the rotator cuff: arthroscopic concepts. Orthopade 40(1): 21–24, 26–30
36. Rose SH, Melton LJ, Morrey BF et al (1982) Epidemiologic features of humeral fractures. Clin Orthop Relat Res 168:24–30
37. Goeminne S, Debeer P (2012) The natural evolution of neglected lesser tuberosity fractures in skeletally immature patients. J Shoulder Elbow Surg 21(8):e6–e11
38. Neogi DS, Bejjanki N, Ahrens PM (2013) The consequences of delayed presentation of lesser tuberosity avulsion fractures in adolescents after repetitive injury. J Shoulder Elbow Surg 22(4):e1-5
39. Vezeridis PS, Bae DS, Kocher MS et al (2011) Surgical treatment for avulsion injuries of the humeral lesser tuberosity apophysis in adolescents. J Bone Joint Surg Am 93(20):1882–1888
40. Levine B, Pereira D, Rosen J (2005) Avulsion fractures of the lesser tuberosity of the humerus in adolescents: review of the literature and case report. J Orthop Trauma 19(5):349–352
41. Ogawa K, Takahashi M (1997) Long-term outcome of isolated lesser tuberosity fractures of the humerus. J Trauma 42(5):955–959
42. Robinson CM, Teoh KH, Baker A et al (2009) Fractures of the lesser tuberosity of the humerus. J Bone Joint Surg Am 91(3):512–520

13 Malunion of Humeral Tuberosity Fractures

Marco Saporito, Giovanni Merolla, Fabrizio Campi, Paolo Paladini, and Giuseppe Porcellini

13.1 Introduction

Proximal humeral head fractures account for 5 % of all fractures, and 20 % require surgical management [1].

Whereas the treatment and complications of humeral fractures have exhaustively been described, the management of malunited fractures of the proximal humeral end is not as well explored.

A malunited proximal humeral end fracture is one where healing has not restored the anatomic relationships between tuberosities, humeral head, and humeral diaphysis.

The increased incidence of fractures of the proximal humeral end seen over the past 50 years, favored by population aging and a reduction of the bone mass in younger patients, has been accompanied by a higher rate of malunited fractures [2]. In particular, these fractures can be classified into three types (avulsion, depression, split). Previous studies have demonstrated that even 2 mm of superior displacement of isolated greater tuberosity fractures leads to subacromial impingement [3].

A large number of patients with proximal humeral fractures can be managed conservatively, using an immobilizer, with a high rate of success.

However, a small proportion of these fractures and some of those managed by surgery may heal with malunion.

These patients typically present with pain, impaired mobility, loss of strength, and stiffness and usually require further treatment [4].

Whereas in the past fracture malunion was largely treated nonsurgically or by arthrotomy when surgery was required, today surgeons opt where feasible for arthroscopic approaches, because they enable treating associated conditions.

13.2 Etiology

Malunion of proximal humeral fractures may result from incorrect conservative treatment, inadequate surgical reduction of the fracture fragments, or postoperative loss of reduction after successful surgical management of the fragments.

The majority of cases of malunion are secondary to conservative treatment.

Malunion in surgery patients is often related to misdiagnosis or failure to identify displaced fractures.

Other factors that may contribute to malunion include soft tissue interposition, inadequate immobilization, and inappropriate rehabilitation.

M. Saporito, MD (✉) • G. Merolla • F. Campi
P. Paladini • G. Porcellini
Unità di Chirurgia Della spalla e gomito,
"D. Cervesi" Hospital, Via L. van Beethoven, 46,
Cattolica 47841, Italy
e-mail: saporitomarco@alice.it;
giovannimerolla@hotmail.com; fcampi@me.com;
palpaolo@tin.it; gporcellini@tin.it

F. Castoldi et al. (eds.), *Simple and Complex Fractures of the Humerus*,
DOI 10.1007/978-88-470-5307-6_13, © Springer-Verlag Italia 2015

13.3 Clinical Examination

Pain and functional impairment are the main symptoms of proximal humeral fracture malunion.

Physical examination should explore length differences between the affected and the contralateral limb and any signs of infection.

Pain, an abnormal orientation of the articular surface and the tuberosities, and retraction of capsular, ligamentous, and musculotendinous structures may considerably reduce active and passive range of motion (ROM).

ROM should be assessed especially in external rotation, with the arm adducted and in 90° of abduction, internal rotation, abduction, and anterior elevation.

A classic albeit non-conclusive sign of greater tuberosity malunion is loss of external rotation with the arm in maximum abduction.

Rotator cuff integrity should be assessed with routine tests. If one or both tuberosities have healed in abnormal anatomic position, the rotator cuff, albeit intact, may however be weakened. For instance, loss of strength in external rotation may result from greater tuberosity malunion [5].

Positive anterior instability tests may be related to healing of the greater tuberosity in a more posterior position than the anatomic position, which entails a greater anterior translation of the humeral head with respect to the glenoid, mimicking anterior instability.

Clinical examination should include a neurological assessment of the shoulder and of major brachial plexus nerves.

The trauma may have affected the brachial plexus or individual nerves such as the circumflex, suprascapular, or long thoracic nerve [6].

Electromyographic findings of upper limb neurological lesions are found in more than 50 % of patients over 50 years of age.

13.4 Diagnostic Imaging

The first-line instrumental examination that can provide confirmation of a diagnosis of proximal humeral head fracture malunion is radiography.

X-rays should be taken in the classic three views of the trauma series, i.e., true anteroposterior in internal and external rotation, axillary, and Y view.

The suspected length defect of the affected limb should be investigated with views of the whole humerus and of the contralateral humerus.

3D CT is the gold standard in the work-up of fracture malunion. A 3D CT scan demonstrates the extent of malunion and the relationships between tuberosities, humeral head, and surgical neck and between humeral head and glenoid surface [7].

MRI enables assessment of rotator cuff and glenoid rim integrity and early diagnosis of avascular necrosis of the humeral head, a frequent complication of displaced fractures of the proximal humeral epiphysis. However, fixation means increase the rate of imaging artifacts, often hampering scan interpretation.

13.5 Treatment

The management of malunited proximal humeral fractures depends on a variety of factors that include patient age, general condition, functional impairment, pain level, job, and sports practiced.

The main indications for surgical management are pain and ROM limitation.

Although age is not an absolute contraindication for surgery, the older the patient, the likelier the presence of comorbidities that have to be entered into the risk-benefit evaluation.

Management decisions must consider the type and mechanism of the initial trauma, any associated neurovascular conditions, the earlier treatment, and any fixation means used.

Further important factors are a history of shoulder trauma, the dominant limb, osteoporosis, and any associated metabolic conditions (e.g., diabetes).

Infection, such as erythema and secreting fistulas, must be excluded.

A conservative approach is preferred in the absence of severe functional impairment or pain and in patients where significant clinical improvement is reasonably expected; these are typically elderly individuals with varus healing of the surgical neck and a congruent articular surface without signs of arthrosis.

In symptomatic patients, conservative treatment does not relieve pain or improve the ROM.

The surgical approach entails either preservation or replacement of the humeral head [8].

Preservation is indicated when the articular surfaces are still intact, and there are no vascular problems [9].

Such findings are more common in malunion of two- and three-part fractures [10].

These patients undergo osteotomy and fixation of the tuberosities to the surgical neck, capsulotomy, and release and reconstruction of periarticular soft tissue [11].

Arthroscopic capsulotomy and smoothing of the tuberosities are associated with significantly better outcomes and prompter functional recovery [12, 13].

The rare cases of malunion associated with severe neurological impairment or previous infection should be managed with glenohumeral arthrodesis [14].

Malunion secondary to a two-part surgical neck fracture can be treated by varus, valgus, or derotating osteotomy; soft tissue release; and fixation with plate and screws [15–17].

Malunion of the greater or lesser tuberosity is managed in relation to fragment size and the extent of displacement.

Malunion involves most commonly the greater tuberosity, which may be displaced superiorly or posteriorly due to traction by the rotator cuff muscles; in such cases, the articular surface is intact with preserved anatomic relationship with the diaphysis.

Patients with superior displacement of the greater tuberosity will show loss of abduction and pain in extreme elevation; those with posterior displacement will show impaired external rotation.

Medial displacement of the lesser tuberosity impairs internal rotation due to impingement on the anterior edge of the glenoid or the coracoid [18].

A small fragment showing <5 mm displacement (Fig. 13.1) can be managed arthroscopically by fragment removal (tuberoplasty), circumferential capsulotomy, subacromial debridement, and rotator cuff reconstruction (Fig. 13.2).

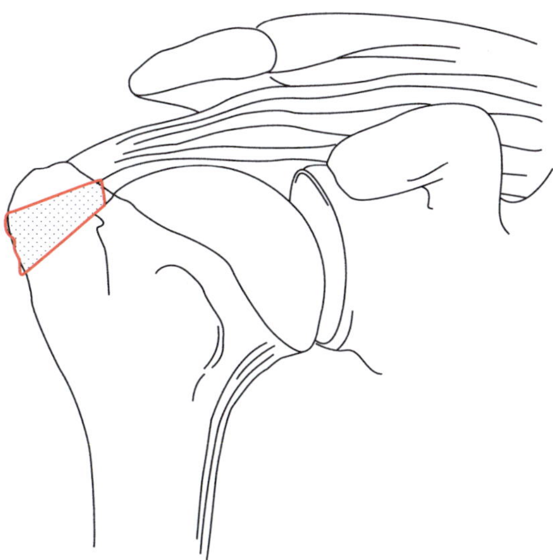

Fig. 13.1 Schematic drawing: displacement of the greater tuberosity >5

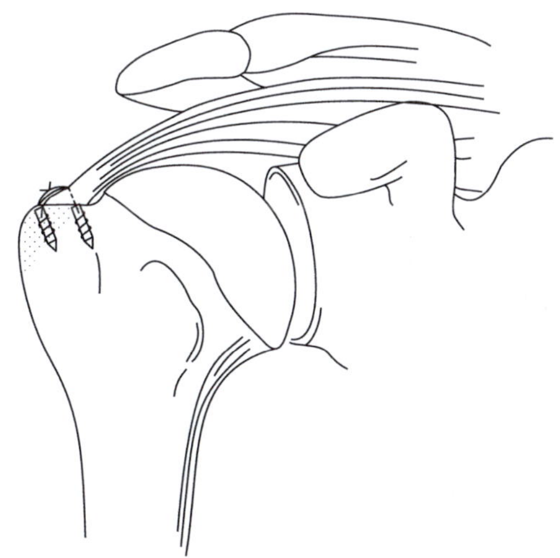

Fig. 13.2 Schematic drawing: arthroscopic fragment removal and rotator cuff reconstruction

Displacement >5 mm of a larger fragment is managed by fragment osteotomy, soft tissue release, capsulotomy through the rotator cuff interval, or a subscapularis split and fixation with plate, cannulated screws, and bone suture [19, 20].

If the fragment is still retracted and not sufficiently mobile after capsular and subacromial release, the rotator cuff interval must be opened completely.

Fragment reduction and fixation must be preceded by accurate decortication of bone surfaces, since bleeding is indispensable for the healing process; in some cases, autologous or synthetic bone grafts may be used [21].

If the fragment cannot be mobilized completely, it should be fixed in a more appropriate position with the arm in internal or external rotation and restored to its anatomic location as closely as possible [22].

In malunion secondary to three- or four-part fractures with congruent articular surfaces and no avascular necrosis or pain, surgery should be considered in relation to the residual ROM and to functional impairment.

Anterior elevation >120° and external rotation >30° rule out osteotomy and should entail arthroscopic capsulotomy and subacromial debridement, whereas elevation <120° and external rotation <30° require corrective osteotomy and fragment fixation [23].

Prosthetic replacement is indicated when malunion has severely damaged the head joint surface resulting in incongruent articular surfaces or head necrosis [24] (Figs. 13.3 and 13.4).

This situation is found more commonly in three- and four-part fractures, humeral head-splitting fractures, posttraumatic arthrosis, and head bone defects due to impact trauma involving >40 % of the articular surface [25, 26].

Implant selection is a function of the anatomopathological findings. Young patients with head necrosis are usually treated with hemiarthroplasty or resurfacing, whereas an anatomic prosthesis is preferred in patients with concentric posttraumatic arthrosis and a damaged glenoid articular surface [27].

In patients older than 65 years with a poor or absent rotator cuff, reverse shoulder arthroplasty is preferred [28].

Prosthesis implantation in a shoulder with a malunited fracture is a complex procedure, due to the abnormal position of the tuberosities and humeral head and to the retraction of capsular, ligamentous, and musculotendinous structures.

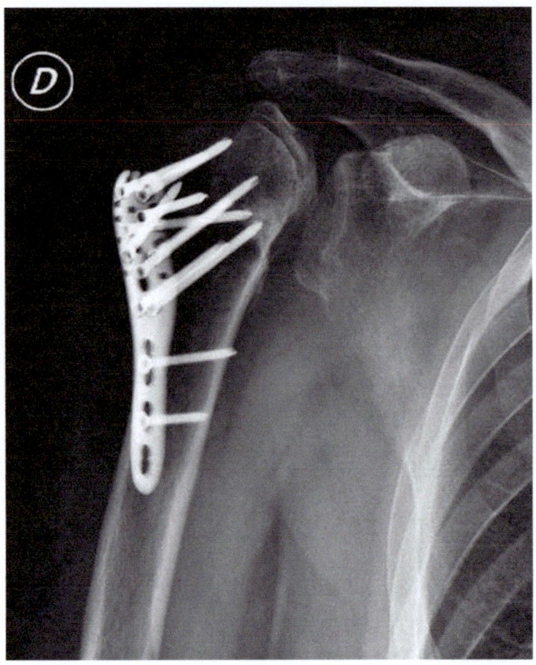

Fig. 13.3 Preoperative X-ray: malunion and necrosis of the humeral head in proximal humerus fracture sequelae

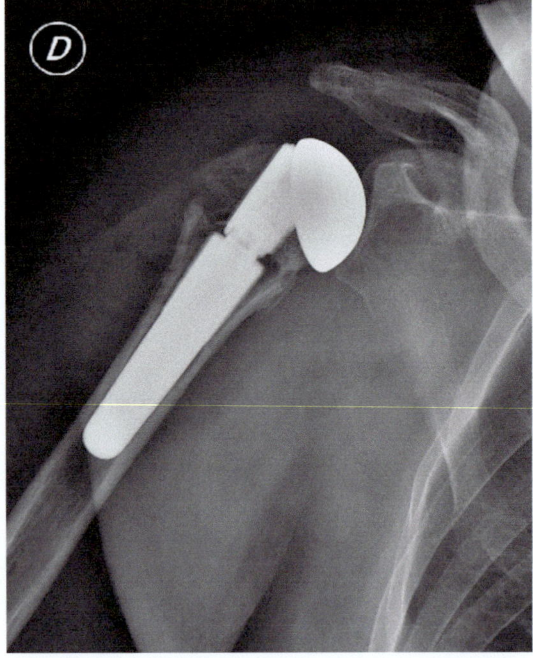

Fig. 13.4 X-ray view at 2 years of follow-up of the same patient: hemiarthroplasty with tuberosity osteotomy and reconstruction. The greater tuberosity appears healed and in the right position

All precautions should be enacted to achieve optimum capsular and subacromial release.

The risk of postoperative complications is high due to the complex nature of malunited proximal humeral fractures.

Besides the general risks related to surgery, procedure-specific complications may also arise, such as resorption of the tuberosities, fragment pseudarthrosis, and loosening of fixation [29].

Most patients are elderly with poor bone stock due to osteoporosis, a condition that greatly increases failure rates [30].

Humeral head vascularization is often damaged by the initial trauma, increasing the risk of necrosis after osteotomy [31].

Neurological lesions and infections are further potential complications whose incidence is related to the quality of surgery and antibiotic prophylaxis.

13.6 Results

Moineau and co-workers reported a gain of ca. 60° in elevation and external rotation after osteotomy and repositioning and fixation of the malunited greater tuberosity [32].

Beredjiklian and colleagues described significant pain reduction after osteotomy and soft tissue release in 8 of 11 patients with greater tuberosity malunion [33].

There are few published data regarding the treatment outcomes of malunited three- or four-part fractures of the proximal humerus.

In general, management by arthroplasty provides better outcomes in patients with acute fractures than in those with malunited three- or four-part fractures.

Pain reduction is often accompanied by residual functional and strength reduction [34].

In a study of 39 consecutive patients with malunion of three- or four-part fractures treated by hemiarthroplasty, Bosch and co-workers described outcomes that were inversely related to the duration of the interval from trauma to prosthesis implantation.

Conclusions

Malunion of proximal humeral fractures is a challenging condition to treat. Pain relief and improvement of mobility are the main objectives of surgical management.

The treatment of malunited two-part fractures envisages osteotomy and fragment fixation or arthroscopic tuberoplasty and capsulotomy.

When treating malunion of three- or four-part fractures, it is crucial to establish whether the head can be preserved or a prosthesis is required.

The outcomes of surgical management are a function of the correction of the bone problems and of soft tissue release.

References

1. Lind T, Kroner K, Jensen J (1989) The epidemiology of the proximal humerus. Arch Orthop Trauma Surg 108:285–287
2. Bengner U, Johnell O, Redlund-Johnell I (1988) Changes in the incidence of fracture of the upper end of the humerus during a 30-year period. Clin Orthop 231:179–182
3. Mutch J, Wang L, Yves Laflamme G, hagemeister N, Rouleau D (2013) Fractures of the greater tuberosity of the humerus: a study of function, muscular atrophy and fracture morphology. AAOS 2013 annual meeting, Chicago; Poster no. P339
4. Conner P, Flatow E (1997) Complications of internal fixation of proximal humeral fractures. Instr Course Lect 46:25–37
5. Craig EV (1995) Open reduction and internal fixation of greater tuberosity fractures, malunions, and nonunions. In: Craig EV (ed) Master techniques in orthopaedic surgery, the shoulder. Raven Press, New York, pp 289–307
6. Boileau P, Chuinard C, Le Huec JC et al (2006) Proximal humerus fracture sequelae: impact of a new radiographic classification on arthroplasty. Clin Orthop Relat 442:121–130
7. Morris ME, Kilcoyne RF, Shuman W et al (1987) Humeral tuberosity fractures: evaluation by CT scan and management of malunion. Orthop Trans 11:242
8. Iannotti J, Sidor M (1997) Malunions of the proximal humerus. In: Warner J, Iannotti J, Gerber C (eds) Complex and revision problems in shoulder surgery. Lippincott-Raven, Philadelphia, pp 245–264
9. Galatz LM, Iannotti JP (2000) Management of surgical neck nonunions. Orthop Clin North Am 31: 51–61
10. Beredjiklian PK, Iannotti JP, Norris TR et al (1998) Operative treatment of malunion of a fracture of the proximal aspect of the humerus. J Bone Joint Surg Am 80:1484–1497

11. Siegel JA, Dines DM (2000) Proximal humerus malunions. Orthop Clin North Am 31:35–50
12. Porcellini G, Campi F, Paladini P (2002) Articular impingement in malunited fracture of the humeral head. Arthroscopy 18:E39
13. Duparc F (2013) Malunion of the proximal humerus. Orthop Traumatol Surg Res 99:S1–S11
14. Calvo E, Merino-Gutierrez I, Lagunes I (2010) Arthroscopic tuberoplasty for subacromial impingement secondary to proximal humeral malunion. Knee Surg Sports Traumatol Arthrosc 18:988–991
15. Jupiter JB, Mullaji AB (1994) Blade plate fixation of proximal humerus non-unions. Injury 25:301–303
16. Solonen KA, Vastamaki M (1985) Osteotomy of the neck of the humerus for traumatic varus deformity. Acta Orthop Scand 56:79–80
17. Benegas E, Zoppi Filho A, Ferreira Filho AA et al (2007) Surgical treatment of varus malunion of the proximal humerus with valgus osteotomy. J Shoulder Elbow Surg 16:55–59
18. Kowalsky MS, Bell JE, Ahmad CS (2007) Arthroscopic treatment of subcoracoid impingement caused by lesser tuberosity malunion: a case report and review of the literature. J Shoulder Elbow Surg 16:e10–e14
19. Lädermann A, Denard PJ, Burkhart SS (2012) Arthroscopic management of proximal humerus malunion with tuberoplasty and rotator cuff retensioning. Arthroscopy 28:1220–1229
20. Burkhart SS (1996) Arthroscopic subscapularis tenolysis: a technique for treating refractory glenohumeral stiffness following open reduction and internal fixation of a displaced three-part proximal humerus fracture. Arthroscopy 12:87–91
21. Cheung EV, Sperling JW (2008) Management of proximal humeral nonunions and malunions. Orthop Clin North Am 39:475–482
22. Gerber C (1990) Reconstructive surgery following malunion of fractures of the proximal humerus in adults. Orthopade 19:316–323
23. Siegel JA, Dines DM (2003) Techniques in managing proximal humeral malunions. J Shoulder Elbow Surg 12:69–78
24. Mansat P, Guity MR, Bellumore Y et al (2004) Shoulder arthroplasty for late sequelae of proximal humeral fractures. J Shoulder Elbow Surg 13: 305–312
25. Dines DM, Warren RF, Altchek DW et al (1993) Posttraumatic changes of the proximal humerus: malunion, nonunion, and osteonecrosis. Treatment with modular hemiarthroplasty or total shoulder arthroplasty. J Shoulder Elbow Surg 2:11–21
26. Norris TR, Green A, McGuigan FX (1995) Late prosthetic shoulder arthroplasty for displaced proximal humerus fractures. J Shoulder Elbow Surg 4: 271–280
27. Boileau P, Trojani C, Walch G et al (2001) Shoulder arthroplasty for the treatment of the sequelae of fractures of the proximal humerus. J Shoulder Elbow Surg 10:299–308
28. Willis M, Min W, Brooks JP et al (2012) Proximal humeral malunion treated with reverse shoulder arthroplasty. J Shoulder Elbow Surg 21: 507–513
29. Wiesel BB, Nagda S, Williams GR (2013) Technical pitfalls of shoulder hemiarthroplasty for fracture management. Orthop Clin North Am 44:317–329
30. Maier D, Jäger M, Strohm PC et al (2012) Treatment of proximal humeral fractures – a review of current concepts enlightened by basic principles. Acta Chir Orthop Traumatol Cech 79:307–316
31. Dilisio MF, Noble JS, Bell RH et al (2013) Postarthroscopic humeral head osteonecrosis treated with reverse total shoulder arthroplasty. Orthopedics 36:e377–e380
32. Moineau G, McClelland WB Jr, Trojani C et al (2012) Prognostic factors and limitations of anatomic shoulder arthroplasty for the treatment of posttraumatic cephalic collapse or necrosis (type-1 proximal humeral fracture sequelae). J Bone Joint Surg Am 94:2186–2194
33. Beredjiklian PK, Iannotti JP (1998) Treatment of proximal humerus fracture malunion with prosthetic arthroplasty. Instr Course Lect 47:135–140
34. Antuña SA, Sperling JW, Sánchez-Sotelo J et al (2002) Shoulder arthroplasty for proximal humeral malunions: long-term results. J Shoulder Elbow Surg 11:122–129

14 Nerve Injuries in Proximal Humeral Fractures

Pierluigi Tos, Stefano Artiaco, Alessandro Crosio, and Bruno Battiston

14.1 Introduction

Nerve lesions are not frequently considered a problem in proximal humeral fractures and only a few studies exist concerning this matter. Nerve lesions in fractures of the proximal humerus are produced by the same mechanism occurring in an anterior dislocation of the shoulder and they are even more frequent than in glenohumeral dislocations. They are caused by extreme movements of the arm beyond physiological limits leading to traction injury. Less commonly they occur for a direct compression exerted by dislocated fracture fragments. Exposed fractures combined with nerve and/or vascular lesions have been rarely reported. Moreover, nerve injuries can also occur as a complication during surgical procedures on the shoulder performed to treat proximal humeral fractures.

The axillary nerve is the most frequently injured nerve in proximal humerus fractures, followed by the suprascapular nerve. Instead, musculocutaneous and median nerves are rarely involved in such kind of fractures. Nerve lesions can be isolated or combined usually in high-energy trauma when terminal branches of brachial plexus are stretched.

P. Tos (✉) • S. Artiaco • A. Crosio • B. Battiston
Reconstructive Microsurgery Unit, Department of Orthopaedics, Trauma Center CTO Città della Salute e della Scienza, Turin, Italy
e-mail: pierluigi.tos@unito.it

When the nerve lesion is due to neurapraxia or minor grade of axonotmesis according to the Sunderland classification, spontaneous recovery is frequent within 3–6 months after injury. If after 3 months there are no signs of reinnervation, a surgical revision of the nerve trunk could be a good indication depending on the characteristics of patient and the residual function of the involved nerves.

14.2 Anatomy

Knowledge of the anatomic course of nerves in the shoulder area is very important in order to understand the origin and the mechanisms that may lead to nerve lesions. Nerves may lie near to bone and joint surfaces which may produce a direct compression on nerve trunks. Furthermore, nerves may pass through narrow spaces in which they are exposed to traction injuries due to the reduced mobility. These mechanisms of injury are relatively common in proximal humeral fractures and/or dislocations of the glenohumeral joint when forced movements of the arm beyond physiological limits can occur [1].

The most commonly injured nerves around the shoulder are the axillary, the suprascapular, and the musculocutaneous nerves. Isolated median and radial nerve lesions are rare. Combined nerve injuries are often observed and should make one suspect brachial plexus injuries. The shoulder joint and the surrounding structures are supplied by the brachial plexus. The posterior

F. Castoldi et al. (eds.), *Simple and Complex Fractures of the Humerus*,
DOI 10.1007/978-88-470-5307-6_14, © Springer-Verlag Italia 2015

cord gives off the axillary nerve at the lower border of the subscapularis muscle and continues along the inferior and posterior surface of axillary artery as the radial nerve.

The axillary nerve surrounds the surgical neck of the humerus and supplies the shoulder joint, the deltoid, and the teres minor before ending as the superior lateral brachial cutaneous nerve. Inside the axillary hiatus, the nerve is limited proximally by the lower margin of the teres minor muscle, distally by the upper margin of the teres major muscle, laterally by the humerus, and medially by the long head of the triceps muscle. The axillary nerve enters this space from its position over the subscapular with the posterior circumflex artery and then passes deep to the deltoid muscle. This is the major site of risk for traction injuries of the axillary nerve. It has been estimated that axonotmesis may occur when the elastic limit of the nerve is exceeded of about 10–20 % of its initial length [2].

The suprascapular nerve originates from the superior trunk of brachial plexus. It passes in a superoposterior fashion through the supraclavicular fossa and the scapular notch (incisura scapulae) before reaching the supraspinatus fossa. The transverse scapular ligament forms a strong bridge over the notch and nerve which can occasionally be replaced by a foramen called foramen scapulae. At the incisura scapulae, the suprascapular nerve gives branches to the supraspinatus muscle, the acromioclavicular joint and bursa, and the subacromial bursa. In this limited space, the suprascapular nerve may be stretched by excessive scapular movements. Another critical point is the supraclavicular notch in which the nerve may be stretched in case of strain such as fractures or shoulder dislocation [3].

The musculocutaneous nerve originates from the anterolateral cord of the brachial plexus. It reaches the arm piercing the coracobrachialis muscle 3–8 cm distal to the coracoids and passes in the arm between biceps brachii and brachialis anterior muscles. The musculocutaneous muscle gives branches for coracobrachialis, biceps brachii, and brachialis muscles. The nerve could be at risk during surgical procedure with deltopectoral approach during dissection or medial retraction of conjoined tendon [3].

Median, radial, and ulnar nerve injuries following proximal humeral fractures are unusual. Throughout its course in the arm, the median nerve is protected from direct contact with the humerus by several muscles including the brachialis and coracobrachialis. Rare cases of isolated median nerve lesion have been reported in literature. Veilleux and Richardson [4] described a case of median nerve injury after a severe comminuted fracture of the proximal humerus in which the lesion was due to traction and direct compression of bony fragments on the median nerve. The radial nerve originates from posterior branch of the brachial plexus. It courses posterior to the axillary artery lying on the subscapular muscle, the tendons of the latissimus dorsi, and the teres major muscles before reaching the posterior surface of the humerus. In shoulder dislocation, the radial nerve is injured in about 7 % of cases usually in combination with other nerve injuries [5]. Injuries of the radial nerve in shoulder fractures are very rare. Liveson [6] reported a case of radial nerve injury after fractures of the proximal humeral head probably due to hematoma formation at the site of injury. Ulnar nerve originates from the medial cord of the brachial plexus and lies posteromedial to the brachial artery in the upper part of the arm. The nerve does not have a critical point of compression at shoulder girdle, but it can be injured following a traction force due to dislocation or fracture dislocation of the shoulder.

At infraclavicular level, the brachial plexus is made up of cords and terminal branches for the upper arm and shoulder girdle. Injuries of this part of the brachial plexus are possible in shoulder trauma with several mechanisms and different forms of clinical presentation. According to Hems, who reviewed 101 patients with this kind of injuries, four patterns of lesion can be identified: (1) anterior humeral dislocation, (2) isolated axillary nerve injury without dislocation, (3) displaced proximal humeral fractures, and (4) hyperextension of the arm. Both traction and compression observed in fractures and fractures/dislocations of the proximal humerus may lead to nerve injuries [7].

14.3 Epidemiology and Etiology of Nerve Injuries in Proximal Humeral Fractures

Nerve injuries may present after fractures or fractures/dislocations of the proximal humerus due to direct effect of trauma. Furthermore, they may be related to primary surgical procedures for reduction and fixation of fracture and to secondary treatment of fracture sequelae. A special consideration should be also given to nerve injuries associated with humeral fractures in children.

14.3.1 Fractures and Dislocations

Proximal humeral fractures are the second most common upper extremity fracture, after distal radius fractures. In patients older than 65 years of age, they are the third most common fracture, after hip fractures and distal radius fractures [8]. In most cases, they are osteoporosis-related fractures and occur in women more frequently than in men [9]. In the 1970s, nerve lesions were not frequently considered a major problem in proximal humeral fractures, but during that decade some studies focused their attention on this issue [10, 11].

The authors observed that incidence of nerve injuries after dislocation and humeral neck fractures was, respectively, in 36 [10] and 30 [11] percent of the cases reported.

In 1994, deLaat [12] in a prospective study including 101 patients with dislocation or fracture of the proximal humerus observed an incidence of nerve lesions slightly higher than previously reported with 45 % of all the patients presenting nerve involvement. Furthermore, the author observed that such lesions were more common in elderly patients and in those with posttraumatic hematoma formation.

Subsequently, Visser analyzed nerve injuries in shoulder dislocations and proximal humeral fractures with the EMG in two prospective studies [13, 14]. In glenohumeral dislocations, axonal loss was reported in 48 % of cases with the axillary nerve most frequently involved in 45 % of patients [13]. He hypothesized that the axillary nerve was probably damaged so frequently due to its anatomic position close to the anterior aspect of glenohumeral joint and its course around the surgical neck of the humerus. Nerve course makes it liable to be stretched or compressed due to the humeral head when the arm is forced in abduction and external rotation. In inferior dislocation (luxatio erecta), the incidence rises up to 60 %, while it is rare after posterior dislocation when less than 5 % of all the patients suffered from nerve injuries [15].

In proximal humeral neck fractures, nerve injuries with axonal loss detected by means of EMG were recorded in 67 % of cases. Solitary nerve injuries were seen in 21 out of 143 cases and multiple nerve injuries in 75 out of 143 cases. Furthermore, an association was observed between grade of fracture according to the Neer classification of proximal humeral fractures and incidence of nerve injuries. Such lesions were seen more commonly in displaced fractures (82 %) than in nondisplaced fractures (59 %). In displaced fractures, the risk of additional nerve injury was 4 times as high as that in nondisplaced fractures, and the severity of lesion was superior. As for nerve involvement, the most common injured nerve in Visser's clinical series was the axillary (58 %) followed by the suprascapular (48 %), radial (32 %), musculocutaneous (29 %), median (17 %), and ulnar (6 %). According to the author, the relevance of nerve lesions could be explained by the greater force of trauma and the position of arm at the moment of fracture. A fall on the arm positioned with internal rotation may stretch the neurovascular bundle over the humeral head causing major tension on the brachial plexus and all the nerves [5].

In complex four-part fractures of the proximal humerus, Stableforth reported an incidence of 6.1 % of brachial plexus injuries (5 out of 49 patients) with complete recovery in 2 and partial recovery in 3 cases [16].

14.3.2 Iatrogenic

Nerve injuries can occur also after surgical procedures for proximal humeral fractures and can be the reason for delayed or incomplete postsurgical clinical recovery. Neurological monitoring during fracture reduction and fixation showed that these kinds of injuries are seldom common [13–17], showing that nerve lesions can occur during surgical procedures. The most frequent iatrogenic nerve lesion is observed during positioning of the interlocking screw of humeral shaft nails and during positioning of locking plates through an anterolateral deltoid splitting approach [18, 19]. Nerves may also be injured during open surgery, especially in plate fixation of the proximal humerus, which requires significant retraction of the deltoid muscle [20]. Furthermore, intraoperative nerve lesions may occur during elective surgery for the treatment of traumatic sequelae with implantation of shoulder prostheses.

14.3.3 Fixation of Proximal Humeral Fractures

Open reduction and internal fixation procedures are not free of risk. Traditionally, the transdeltoid lateral and the deltopectoral approaches are used in reduction and internal fixation of proximal humeral fractures, depending on fracture type and surgeon experience. Preservation of the anterior humeral circumflex artery and the axillary nerve, which can be potentially injured during this type of operation, should always be considered because this may prevent AVN and early collapse of the humeral head. Minimally invasive lateral deltoid splitting approach has been described in order to treat two- and three-part valgus impacted humeral fractures. Although external fixation is not common in proximal humeral fractures, it can be useful in particular situations and selected patients as those affected by exposed fractures. The anatomic study by Kuang on axillary nerve in the Chinese population showed that the nerve may be at risk in either humeral fixation of intramedullary nail or external skeletal fixation also in the so-called safe zone [21]. In order to prevent nerve lesion, the surgeon must use drill protective guidance on bone surface, sleeve instrument to split deltoid muscle, and small incision.

14.3.4 Shoulder Arthroplasty

Shoulder arthroplasty is a common procedure for early or secondary treatment of complex proximal humeral fractures. Many authors reported series in which nerve injuries occurred during total arthroplasty implantation. Associated nerve injuries are more frequent than single nerve damage in this kind of surgery. In his clinical series, Nagada [22] reported that intraoperative electromyography (EMG) and transcranial motor evoked potential (MEP) showed sufferance of cord or trunk in 46 % of cases, especially for upper trunk (43 %) and for posterior cord (20 %). The most dangerous operative step was the preparation of glenoid, and the worst position for the patient was that with the arm in external rotation, abduction, and extension in which neurovascular bundles are potentially stretched. During surgical procedure, to reduce the sufferance of nerve, it is necessary to limit traction on retractors and leave the arm in neutral position when possible. Moreover, Nagada [22] reported that 57 % of patients that at the end of procedure presented an abnormal PEM showed also EMG and clinical signs positive for nerve injuries. Nevertheless, all patients recovered complete function of the nerve in 6 months confirming that the injuries were due to reversible axonal damage.

14.3.5 Nerve Injuries in Children

Fractures of the proximal humerus are relatively uncommon injuries in the pediatric population, representing approximately 0.5 % of all pediatric fractures and 4–7 % of all epiphyseal fractures in children [23, 24]. Approximately one third of these fractures involve the physis, and two thirds involve the metaphysis. Although displaced fractures theoretically expose neurological structures at risk, there is a paucity of information regarding the incidence and prognosis for these injuries [25, 26]. In literature, this kind of lesion has rarely been described having an estimated rate of 0.7 % of nerve involvement in proximal humeral fractures. Hwang et al. in 2008 reported four cases of nerve lesion in children. All patients presented high displaced fracture (Salter-Harris I–II with 50–100 % displacement) with combined nerve lesion of median-radial-ulnar nerve [26].

We reported a schematic view (Fig. 14.1) of relations between upper limb peripheral nerves and bones of the arm and frequency of axonal lesions according to Visser [5].

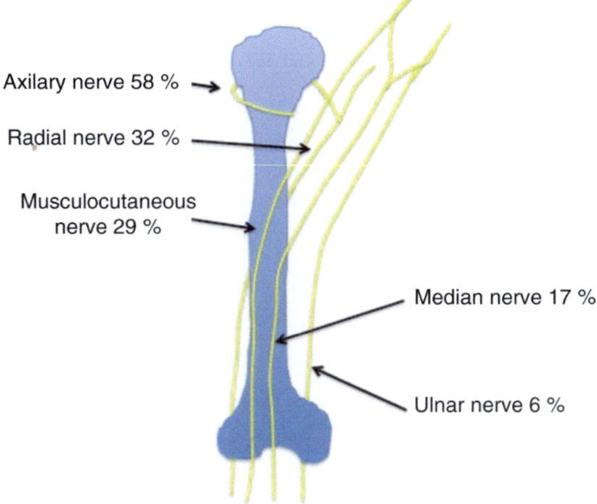

Fig. 14.1 Epidemiology of damaged nerves after proximal humeral fractures according to Visser's description

14.4 Clinical and Instrumental Diagnosis

Every dislocation or fracture of the proximal humerus with or without concomitant dislocation should be carefully examined in order to detect clinical signs of nerve injuries. Clinical exam should be performed at admittance and after conservative and/or surgical treatment in order to recognize and document every kind of lesion. This aspect is fundamental also for forensic implications [27]. In Table 14.1, upper limb muscles and their innervations are reported; it is mandatory to examine every muscle to identify the real level of nerve lesion.

Table 14.1 Innervations and main action of shoulder muscles

Muscle name	Innervation	Action
Trapezius	Spinal accessory nerve	Stabilize the scapula to allow normal shoulder motion especially shoulder abduction beyond 90°
Serratus anterior	Long thoracic nerve	Abduction and stabilization on the thorax of the scapula
Rhomboid major and minor	Dorsal scapular nerve	Scapular adduction or retraction, elevation, and downward rotation
Pectoralis major	Lateral and medial pectoral nerve	Adducts and medially rotates the humerus
Pectoralis minor	Medial pectoral nerve	Thrusts shoulder forward; tilts scapula anteriorly; aids respiration
Levator scapulae	Cervical (C3, C4) nerve, dorsal scapular nerve	Elevates the scapula
Coracobrachialis	Musculocutaneous nerve	Flexes and adducts the shoulder joint
Latissimus dorsi	Thoracodorsal nerve	Abducts, extends, and internally rotates the shoulder
Deltoid (anterior, middle, posterior)	Axillary nerve	Shoulder joint abduction, flexion (anterior), extension (posterior)
Teres major	Subscapular nerve	Internally rotates, adducts, and extends the shoulder joint
Rotator cuff muscles		
Supraspinatus	Suprascapular nerve	Abduction of the shoulder
Infraspinatus	Suprascapular nerve	Externally rotates the shoulder
Teres minor	Axillary nerve	Externally rotates the shoulder
Subscapularis	Upper subscapular nerve, lower subscapular nerve	Internally rotates the shoulder joint; stabilizes the head of the humerus

Nonetheless, in early phase after trauma, clinical testing could be difficult to interpret and of low value in detecting axonal nerve lesions in these fractures just after trauma. This happens because nearly all patients show muscle weakness at testing in the first weeks after the trauma due to pain making it difficult to distinguish between this condition and paresis due to a nerve lesion [14].

Clinical exam requires competence and knowledge of motor and sensory innervations of brachial plexus primary and secondary trunks and terminal nerves for the upper limb. Clinical signs of axillary nerve lesions may depend on the nerve branches that have been compromised. They may range from paresthesia and hyperesthesia around the shoulder and upper arm to deltoid atrophy manifested by contour changes around the shoulder (this becomes evident at least 3 weeks after the palsy). Active deltoid muscle contraction should be evaluated. Compensatory activity of the supraspinatus muscle in conjunction with the long head of the biceps should be checked. The sensibility has a minor role in initial diagnosis because clinical sensory loss in deltoid area was present only in 7 % of all the patients with lesion of the axillary nerve detected by means of EMG. A similar pattern of clinical presentation is observed also for the musculocutaneous nerve. Clinical exam includes examination of active elbow flexion in order to test biceps brachii and brachialis muscle. Sensory exam of the lateral cutaneous antebrachial nerve shows loss of sensory in only 4 % of all the patients in which a lesion of musculocutaneous nerve was detected by means of EMG [14].

The suprascapular and radial nerves have common root origins, so painful stimulation may overlap. Pain is more commonly appreciated over the posterior portion of the shoulder along the border of the trapezius muscle, with pain worsening at night. Loss of abduction and external rotation of the arm may be observed in such cases depending on to the extent of nerve impairment. Radial, median, and ulnar nerve injuries are rarely isolated and usually observed in case of stretching of infraclavicular terminal branches of brachial plexus. Diagnosis of nerve lesions can be suspected by examining antebrachial motor activity and activity and sensitivity of the hand.

In the presence of clinical suspicion of nerve injury, the first instrumental evaluation is electrophysiologic study by EMG. EMG is the initial investigation of choice, and it is recommended about 3–4 weeks after the nerve injuries (and not earlier) in order to detect site and entity of the lesions [6]. The exam can be subsequently repeated in order to follow the progression of nerve regeneration/healing or to plan an eventual surgical treatment when the absence of nerve recovery is documented after an adequate waiting time. Improved results of EMG without voluntary muscle activity warrant further conservative treatment. In most cases, the clinical evidence of a recovery is detected earlier than the electrophysiologic detection. Operative treatment of shoulder girdle neuropathy can be considered if no clinical and electrophysiologic recovery is present within 3–6 months after injury (9–18 cm of axonal regeneration proceeding 1 mm/day). This approach is indicated also after axillary isolated lesions and also after dislocations, fractures, or iatrogenic injuries without evidence of neurotmesis [28].

In every "closed" nerve lesion, the Tinel sign [29] ("tingling" feeling or "pins and needles" felt at the lesion site or more distally along the course of a nerve when it is tapped) should be tested. This test is one of the most important physical exam maneuvers in peripheral nerve injury evaluation to assess regeneration progress in the site of lesion and along the nerve distally to the lesion. If the Tinel sign progresses distally along the nerve over time, it means that something is recovering (1 mm/day) and the regeneration is possible and occurs; if the Tinel sign is stationary (stays in one place over time), a fourth, fifth, or sixth degree of injury is to be suspected. Unfortunately at the shoulder region, a Tinel sign is very difficult to arouse because of the anatomic depth of nerves around the shoulder (median and ulnar nerves at the axilla and distally are easy to test and radial nerve posteriorly and at the arm level, but suprascapular and axillary nerves at the shoulder are very difficult to test).

A magnetic resonance imaging (MRI) and/or an ultrasound (US) examination of the rotator cuff is always a fundamental and complementary diagnostic step studying a paralytic shoulder to verify the integrity of the rotator cuff [30].

14.5 Prognosis

Prognosis of nerve lesions in proximal humeral fractures depends on the grade of axonal and nerve damage. According to Seddon's [31] classification, we can describe neurapraxia when there is an alteration in nerve conduction, axonotmesis when axons have been cut, and neurotmesis when the nerve continuity is lost. In case of axonotmesis and neurotmesis, a Wallerian degeneration occurs losing the connection among proximal axons and the distal part of the nerve. Subsequently, Sunderland subclassified [32] these injuries into five types in order to better define the entity of injury and the optimal therapeutic approach. Besides neurapraxia (I degree), the axonotmesis was divided into axonal injuries with or without an intact basil lamina (II and III degree) or with complete scar block (IV degree). Neurotmesis is the complete transection (V degree) of the nerve trunk. A combination of conduction block and transection (VI degree) was added later by Mackinnon. From a therapeutic and practical point of view, according to the Sunderland classification, (1) I and II degree injuries will recover spontaneously and should be treated conservatively, (2) V and VI degree injuries should be surgically repaired, and (3) III and IV degree injuries have partial recovery and will likely need surgery.

Posttraumatic nerve injuries following shoulder fractures and dislocations commonly have a good prognosis, and recovery of function may be expected in a period of 3–6 months [6]. In the clinical series reported by Visser including 96 cases of nerve lesions, 73 % of patients reported no or only slight limitations in general function and activities of daily life, 19 % had limitations in such situations, and 6 % presented severe disabilities in daily life activities [14]. Regarding axillary nerve lesions, that is, the most common kind of nerve injury occurring in proximal humeral fractures, recovery is observed in the vast majority of cases [33]. According to Steinmann baseline, EMG should be obtained within 4 weeks after injury with a follow-up evaluation at 12 weeks. When no clinical or EMG improvement is noted, then operative treatment should be performed within 3–6 months from injury [33]. Recently, Hems reported a large study in which he defined four patterns of injuries of the terminal branches of the infraclavicular brachial plexus. In case of anterior glenohumeral dislocation, axillary and ulnar nerves are commonly injured, but rupture is rare. Instead, axillary nerve lesions without dislocation have the highest probability of rupture. In displaced humeral fractures, nerve injury may be due to direct compression of the proximal aspect of the humeral shaft. Last but not least in hyperextension injuries, the musculocutaneous nerve is commonly injured and disrupted. Therefore, the author suggested conservative treatment in most cases of infraclavicular injuries of the terminal branches of brachial plexus with some exceptions. Early exploration was indicated for axillary and musculocutaneous nerve injury without dislocation, and urgent operation was indicated for dislocated proximal humeral fractures in order to relieve pressure on suffering nerves [7].

Regarding iatrogenic injuries, some important prognostic data are given by intraoperative electrodiagnostic analysis [17]. Warrenders et al. [17] reported that the majority of alerts (65 % of the nerve events) occurred during fracture reduction, whereas 31 % occurred during plate application. During that phase of surgical procedure, the humeral shaft and tuberosities were subjected to traction in order to aid fracture reduction. Therefore, removing traction and positioning the arm in neutral position could be useful when an intraoperative delay or a prolonged procedure occurred [17]. Alert signal started when the arm is positioned in flexion abduction and external rotation in 58 % of cases, and positioning of the arm in neutral position and removing of retractors turned off alert signal. In 64 % of cases, there was a return at baseline at the end of surgery, but in 36 % there was no return of MEP at the baseline, and these patients corresponded clinical weakness of muscles especially in radial and axillary nerve territories. All of these patients recovered muscle function by 3 weeks postoperatively [17].

The quality of recovery after a nerve repair depends on many local and general factors. Regarding the age of the patient, nerve function recovery begins to decline after the second decade (75 % good results in children vs 50 % good results in adults) and may be poor after the fifth/sixth decade. Other factors considered are the mechanism of injury, elapsed time from injury, level of injury, type of nerve, specific nerve injured, associated injuries, and tension across the repair.

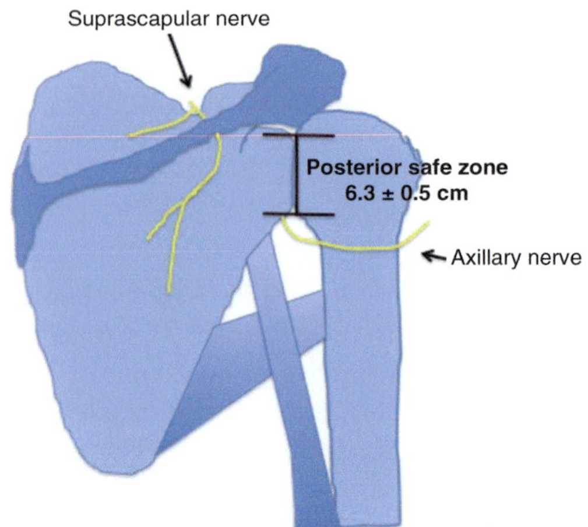

Fig. 14.2 Posterior anatomy of suprascapular and axillary nerve. Distance from the posterior acromion to the axillary nerve—safe zone

14.6 Prevention of Iatrogenic Lesion

Some anatomic considerations are useful to prevent iatrogenic nerve injuries especially concerning the axillary nerve. Landmarks of the location of the axillary nerve are taken from the acromion or from the greater tuberosity. When the acromion is considered as landmark, the mean distance from the superior border of the axillary nerve to the anteroinferior border of the acromion is about 6.3±0.5 cm [34]. When the greater tuberosity is considered as reference, the distance between this landmark and the axillary nerve is relatively constant from 3.5±0.2 to 4.6 cm [35]. The surgeon must take into account that the greater tuberosity may be displaced after a fracture. In this case, the course of the axillary nerve can be estimated from the acromion [36].

Another important consideration is the position of the arm during surgical procedures. When the arm is moved, both nerves and arteries may modify their position. In fact in neutral position (0° rotation, 20° abduction, 0° forward flexion), the axillary nerve is located about 6 cm from the acromion; when the arm is placed in 60° of abduction, the distance from the nerve to the acromion decreases to 5.4 cm. The safe zone for hardware placement in neutral shoulder position is up to 5 cm distal from the mid-acromion. The danger area has been reported with slight differences among authors from 5 to 9 cm according to Cheung, Ruedi, and Yung-Fen [36–38]. Distal to 9 cm, the deltoid may be safely split again with minimal risk of injuring the axillary nerve [38], but in any case, rough handling and strenuous retraction of the deltoid muscle should be avoided to minimize risk of axillary nerve damage [36].

These anatomic considerations are valid not only for open reduction and internal fixation by means of plates but also for synthesis with anterograde nails and for percutaneous fixation when screws and pins are used around the shoulder region. In particular, during humeral nailing, screw positioning should be as close as possible to the acromion in order to reduce the risk of nerve injuries. Moreover, the arm should be left in neutral position avoiding internal rotation that comes near the nerve to the entry site of screw [18].

In Fig. 14.2, we reported a schematic view of the anatomy of suprascapular and axillary nerve in the posterior aspect.

14.7 Treatment

Treatment options for nerve palsy in association with proximal humeral fractures include expectant observation, early exploration, late exploration, or tendon transfers.

As abovementioned, the most common mechanism of nerve lesion of the terminal branches of the plexus at the shoulder level is the stretching of the nerve trunk (for both traumatic and iatrogenic causes); this produces a lesion in continuity, without the section of the nerve, determining a Sunderland neurapraxia or minor grade of axonotmesis [32]. If after 3–6 months there are no signs of spontaneous recovery, a surgical revision of the nerve trunk could be a good indication depending on the characteristics of the patient (age, general condition) and the residual function and involved nerve(s).

Clear immediate indication for early exploration include, as in other district, combined vascular injury, severe soft tissue injury, sharp or penetrating injury, or high suspicion of nerve laceration. Hems [7] reported that axillary nerve lesions without dislocation and musculocutaneous nerve injuries due to hyperextension forces are likely to be severe. Thus, he suggests a conservative treatment in most cases of infraclavicular injuries of terminal branches of the brachial plexus and an early exploration in the abovementioned axillary and musculocutaneous nerve injury without dislocation [7].

Late exploration of injured nerves is performed in young patient if no electric or clinical activity can be identified by 3–6 months postinjury (depending of the site of the nerve lesion) [28–40].

During surgical exploration, nerves may present macroscopically various degrees of lesion.

A neurolysis should be performed if the nerve is in continuity and does not present, when inspected and palpated, signs of neuroma (scar inside the nerve); this situation corresponds to grades I and II of nerve injuries according to the Sunderland classification.

When a neuroma in continuity with a residual function is observed (grade III of the Sunderland classification), a neurolysis with eventually a cable graft according to Millesi is performed [41].

When a nonfunctional neuroma in continuity is observed or a complete lesion is found (grades III, IV, and V of the Sunderland classification), nerve reconstruction should be immediately performed by means of direct suture if nerve stumps are not under tension. When a nerve gap is present after neuroma or stump resection, the nerve should be reconstructed by means of autograft using microsurgical techniques. In particular circumstances (i.e., revision for open fractures and/or infections) if local conditions are not favorable for nerve reconstruction or when a microsurgeon is not present in the surgical staff, it is advisable to approximate nerve stumps with two stitches waiting for a secondary reexploration and grafting.

Some authors described that nerve repairing could be performed also at 15 months after trauma and stated also that patients under the age of 40 have better results [42]. Nevertheless, in case of very late reconstructions after 12–18 months from the time of injury, a reinnervation of a denervated muscle is not possible, and a fatty degenerative evolution occurs to the muscle belly.

Thus, an attempt at reconstruction can be performed at this time only in selected cases (i.e., very young patients) but with unpredictable results.

Neurotization (nerve transfer of a functioning nerve to the distal stump of the severed nerve) is indicated if a double-level lesion is suspected or if the proximal stump is not adequate for reconstruction. The most frequent neurotizations are for the suprascapular nerve (with a branch of the spinal accessory nerve) [43] and for the axillary nerve (with a branch of the radial nerve for a part of triceps) [44].

As abovementioned, before performing axillary nerve repair, it is fundamental to verify cuff integrity with clinical evaluation and MRI study [30] and eventually combine the repair of the nerve with the cuff lesion [42]. Supraspinatus integrity is fundamental because this muscle is the main motor of arm abduction.

Tendon transfers are indicated in patients not experiencing neurological recovery 1 year after nerve repair or if the nerve repair was not possible for clinical conditions, comorbidities, or age [45].

In Fig. 14.3, a flow chart for diagnosis, follow-up, and timing of treatment of nerve lesions is reported.

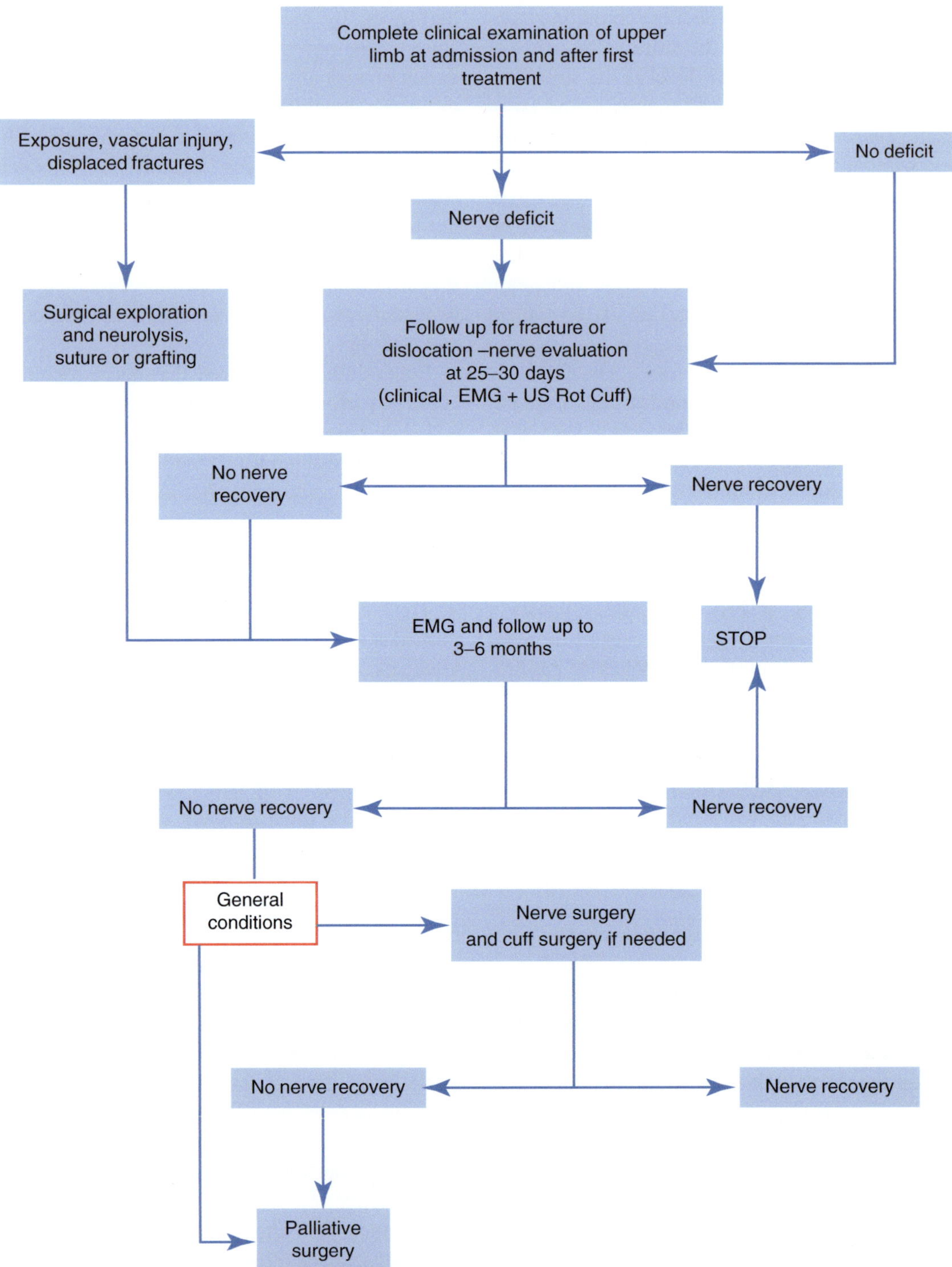

Fig. 14.3 Flow chart for diagnosis and timing of treatment of nerve injuries in proximal humeral fractures. Sunderland I = neurapraxia, Sunderland II = axonotmesis, Sunderland III = neuroma in continuity with or without nerve function, Sunderland IV = neuroma in continuity without nerve function, and Sunderland V = neurotmesis

References

1. Coene LNJEM (1993) Mechanisms of brachial plexus lesions. Clin Neurol Neurosurg 95(Suppl):S24–S29
2. Adams JH, Duchen LW (1992) Greenfield's neuropathology, 5th edn. Oxford University Press, New York
3. Snell RS (1973) The upper limb. In: Snell RS (ed) Clinical anatomy for medical students. Little, Brown and Co, Boston, pp 359–488
4. Veilleux M, Richardson P (2000) Proximal median neuropathy secondary to humeral neck fracture. Muscle Nerve 23:426–429
5. Visser C, Coene L, Brand R, Tavy D (2001) Nerve lesions in proximal humeral fractures. J Shoulder Elbow Surg 10:421–427
6. Liveson JA (1984) Nerve lesions associated with shoulder dislocation; an electromyographic study of 11 cases. J Neurol Neurosurg Psychiatry 47:742–744
7. Hems TE, Mahamood F (2012) Injuries of the terminal branches of the infraclavicular brachial plexus: patterns of injury, management and outcome. J Bone Joint Surg Br 94:799–804
8. Baron JA, Barrett JA, Karagas MR (1996) The epidemiology of peripheral fractures. Bone 18(3 Suppl): 209S–213S
9. Lind T, Krøner K, Jensen J (1989) The epidemiology of fractures of the proximal humerus. Arch Orthop Trauma Surg 108:285–287
10. Blom S, Dahlbäck LO (1970) Nerve injuries in dislocations of the shoulder joint and fractures of the neck of the humerus. Acta Chir Scand 136:461–466
11. Ebel R (1973) Uber die ursachen der axillaris paresen bei schulter luxationen. Monatsschr Hunfallheilck D 76:445–449
12. de Laat EA, Visser CP, Coene LN, Pahlplatz PV, Tavy DL (1994) Nerve lesions in primary shoulder dislocations and humeral neck fractures. J Bone Joint Surg Br 76:381–383
13. Visser CP, Coene LN, Brand R, Tavy DL (1999) The incidence of nerve injury in anterior dislocation of the shoulder and its influence on functional recovery. A prospective clinical and EMG study. J Bone Joint Surg Br 81:679–685
14. Visser CPJ, Tavy DLJ, Coene LNJEM, Brand R (1999) Electromyographic findings in shoulder dislocations and fractures of the proximal humerus: comparison with clinical neurological examination. Clin Neurol Neurosurg 101:86–91
15. Mallon WJ, Bassett FH, Goldner RD (1990) Luxatio erect: the inferior glenohumeral dislocation. J Orthop Trauma 4:19–24
16. Stableforth PG (1984) Four-part fractures of the neck of the humerus. J Bone Joint Surg Br 66:104–108
17. Warrenders WJ, Oppenheimer S, Abboud JA (2011) Nerve monitoring during proximal humeral fracture fixation: what have we learned? Clin Orthop Relat Res 469:2631–2637
18. Logters TT, Wild M, Windolf J, Linhart W (2008) Axillary nerve palsy after retrograde humeral nailing: clinical confirmation of an anatomical fear. Arch Orthop Trauma Surg 128:1431–1435
19. Nicandri GT, Trumble TE, Warme WJ (2009) Lessons learned from a case of proximal humeral locked plating gone awry. J Orthop Trauma 23:607–611
20. Tubbs RS, Oakes WJ, Blount JP, Elton S, Salter G, Grabb PA (2001) Surgical landmarks for the proximal portion of the axillary nerve. J Neurosurg 95: 998–1000
21. Kuang-Yi K, Tien-Hua C, Jia-Fwu S, Shih-Tien W, Jenn-Yuan L, Po-Hsin C (2011) Anatomic study of the axillary nerve in a Chinese cadaveric population: correlation of the course of the nerve with proximal humeral fixation with intramedullary nail or external skeletal fixation. Arch Orthop Trauma Surg 131:669–674
22. Nagada SH, Roger KJ, Sestokas AK, Getz LC, Ramsey ML, Glaser DL, Williams GR (2007) Neer award 2005: peripheral nerve function during shoulder arthroplasty using intraoperative nerve monitoring. J Shoulder Elbow Surg 16:3S–7S
23. Di Gennaro GL, Spina M, Lampasi M, Libri R, Donzelli O (2008) Fractures of the proximal humerus in children. Chir Organi Mov 92:89–95
24. Kohler R, Trillaud JM (1983) Fracture and fracture separation of the proximal humerus in children: report of 136 cases. J Pediatr Orthop 3:326–332
25. Drew SJ, Giddin GEB, Birch R (1995) A slowly evolving brachial plexus injury following a proximal humeral fracture in a child. J Hand Surg Br 20B(I):24–25
26. Hwang RW, Bae DS, Waters PM (2008) Brachial plexus palsy following proximal humeral fractures in patients who are skeletally immature. J Orthop Trauma 22:286–290
27. Ameh V, Crane S (2006) Nerve injury following shoulder dislocation: the emergency physician's perspective. Eur J Emerg Med 4:233–235
28. Grant GA, Goodkin R, Kliot M (1999) Evaluation and surgical management of peripheral nerve problems. Neurosurgery 44:825–839
29. Tinel J (1917) Nerve wounds. Baillère, Tindall and Cox, London
30. Degeorges R, Lebellec Y, Alnot JY (2004) Prognostic factors of axillary nerve surgery. Rev Chir Orthop Reparatrice Appar Mot 90(2):103–110
31. Seddon H (1943) Three types of nerve injury. Brain 66:247–288
32. Sunderland SS (1978) Nerves and nerve injuries, 2nd edn. Churchill Livingstone, Edinburgh
33. Steinmann SP, Moran EA (2001) Axillary nerve injury: diagnosis and treatment. J Am Acad Orthop Surg 9:328–335
34. Vathana P, Chiarapattanakom P, Ratanalaka R, Vorasatit P (1998) The relationship of the axillary nerve and the acromion. J Med Assoc Thai 81(12): 953–957

35. Lin J, Hou SM, Inoue N, Chao EY, Hang YS (1999) Anatomic considerations of locked humeral nailing. Clin Orthop 368:247–254
36. Yun-Feng C, Nai-Feng Z, Chang-Qing Z, Lei W, Hai-Feng W, Ye L (2012) The relevance of the anatomic basis of fracture for the subsequent treatment of the anterior humeral circumflex artery and the axillary nerve. Int Orthop (SICOT) 36:783–787
37. Ruedi TP, Murphy WM (2000) AO principles of fractures management. Thieme Stuttgart, New York
38. Cheung S, Fitzpatrick M, Lee QT (2009) Effects of shoulder position on axillary nerve positions during the split lateral deltoid approach. J Shoulder Elbow Surg 18:748–755
39. Saran N, Bergeron S, Bnoit B, Reindl R, Harvey EJ, Berry GK (2010) Risk of axillary nerve injury during percutaneous proximal humerus locking plate insertion using an external aiming guide. Injury 41: 1037–1040
40. Alnot JY, Livernaux P, Silberman O (1996) Lesions of the axillary nerve. Rev Chir Orthop Reparatrice Appar Mot 82(7):579–589
41. Millesi H (1980) Microsurgical nerve grafting. Int Surg 65(6):503–508
42. Prudnikov OE (1994) Simultaneous lesions of the rotator cuff and the brachial plexus. Rev Chir Orthop Reparatrice Appar Mot 80(7):602–609
43. Terzis JK, Kostas I (2006) Suprascapular nerve reconstruction in 118 cases of adult posttraumatic brachial plexus. Plast Reconstr Surg 117(2):613–629
44. Bertelli JA, Kechele PR, Santos MA, Duarte H, Ghizoni MF (2007) Axillary nerve repair by triceps motor branch transfer through an axillary access: anatomical basis and clinical results. J Neurosurg 107(2):370–377
45. Wolfe SW, Hotchkiss RN, Pederson WC, Kozin SH (2011) Green's operative hand surgery, 6th edn. Elsevier – Churchill Livingstone, Philadelphia

15 Fracture-Dislocations

Raffaele Russo, Fabio Cautiero, Alberto Fontanarosa, and Giuseppe Della Rotonda

15.1 Introduction

Fracture-dislocations of the shoulder are very rare, their prevalence being 1/100,000/year in the UK population [1, 2]. These are complex joint injuries characterized by the association of two or more fragments in the proximal humeral epiphysis with static dislocation of the articular component anteriorly, inferiorly, or posteriorly [3–5]. They are often associated with soft issue lesions and osteochondral glenoid fractures mostly in the anteroinferior corner of the glenoid. The involvement of soft tissue (tendon, capsule, and ligaments) explains the frequent scar contractures and heterotopic ossifications in patients after treatment [3, 6, 7]. These lesions must be recognized, and reduction maneuvers must be avoided. In fact, inappropriate maneuvers may transform two-part fracture-dislocations into four-part dislocations. They can also aggravate the injury of soft tissues, especially the rotator cuff, the axillary artery, or the plexus [2, 8]. Neer [3] classified these fractures based on the number of fragments involved and the direction of the displacement (anterior, posterior, or inferior). Head splitting and head impression after the shoulder dislocation have also been described [9–11].

15.2 Clinical and Radiological Evaluation

Fracture-dislocations of the shoulder are generally due to high-energy trauma but may also be due to banal domestic incidents, particularly in women. The most common running deck cause is a fall on the shoulder or trauma transmitted from the hand with the elbow extended [2, 4, 8]. In rare cases, these lesions may be due to an electric shock or to epileptic convulsions [2, 8]. Patients present to the emergency room with the affected limb supported by the contralateral hand in the throes of violent pain, and there is swelling of the shoulder. The patient is unable to make active movements and feels pain at the slightest movement, which is accompanied by a rattling noise in some cases. Ecchymosis is rarely seen at this time. Ecchymosis is more common in older people and in patients undergoing anticoagulation therapy. In young people, ecchymosis appears 24–48 h later in the arm and chest.

In case of a two-part anterior dislocation of the shoulder, the acromion prominence is more evident, whereas the deltoid pectoral groove appears edematous and prevents palpation of the coracoid. It is more difficult to observe the acromion prominence in three- and four-part anterior fracture-dislocations. The clinical aspect of the

R. Russo, MD, PhD (✉) • F. Cautiero, MD
A. Fontanarosa, MD • G.D. Rotonda, MD
Department of Orthopaedics and Traumatology, Ospedale dei Pellegrini, Via Portamedina 41, Napoli 80134, Italy
e-mail: raffrusso@tin.it; fabiocau@inwind.it; fontanarosa.alberto@libero.it; peppedellarotonda@libero.it

F. Castoldi et al. (eds.), *Simple and Complex Fractures of the Humerus*, DOI 10.1007/978-88-470-5307-6_15, © Springer-Verlag Italia 2015

shoulder is completely different in posterior fracture-dislocations. In fact, in the latter, the morphology of the back of the shoulder changes because the posterior aspect of the deltoid seems more prominent and round, whereas in the contrary the coracoid process is more evident on the front part of the shoulder, particularly in thin subjects.

Another aspect to consider in these patients is the position of the upper limb. In the case of a two-part fracture-dislocation, passive mobility of the limb is locked in a position of relative abduction and external rotation; attempts by the examiner to rotate the arm internally cause fierce pain. Instead, in case of a two-part posterior dislocation, the limb is intrarotated and external rotation is impossible. When the fracture rime affects the surgical neck, the axis of the humerus is in a neutral position [4].

15.3 Radiology

In fracture-dislocations, the X-ray study performed in the emergency department is crucial for a correct diagnosis and treatment. The fact that the glenoid is anteverted by 30–40° with respect to the frontal plane can confound the diagnosis. Indeed, in the frontal projection X-ray, the glenoid overlaps the humeral head so that the joint seems intact. This situation occurs because the patient cannot place the forearm in extrarotation. To overcome this problem, it was suggested the contralateral shoulder be rotated by 40° from the AP projection with the affected shoulder turned toward the film. But a better technique is to use the axillary view. This view must be performed with the patient in the supine decubitus position with the shoulder abducted 30°. The cassette is placed above the patient's shoulder, and the X-ray tube is angled into the axilla. If this abduction is not possible, it is advisable to use the Velpeau technique that can be performed with the patient's arm in a sling.

In case of doubts, a computerized tomography scan should be performed. This shows the fracture rimes, the direction of humeral head dislocation, the plurifragmentary aspect of the tuberosities, and the damage of the glenoid component [12–14]. In patients older than 40 years, it is advisable to carry out a magnetic resonance imaging (MRI) study to evaluate the condition of rotator cuff and capsule [7].

15.4 Associated Injuries

15.4.1 Rotator Cuff Injuries

The rotator cuff is frequently lesioned in two-part fracture-dislocations of the greater tuberosity. Robertson et al. [2] reported an incidence of rotator cuff lesions in 33.4 % of 3,633 fracture-dislocations. This lesion can affect the rotator interval and/or the junction between the supraspinatus and subscapularis muscles. Cuff tears can be particularly severe in three- and four-part complex fracture-dislocations. These lesions are often identified and treated during osteosynthesis. However, they can be identified presurgery with MRI. This technique will also show whether the biceps stabilization system is damaged and is consequently subluxed. Such cases should be treated with a tenotomy and tenodesis. In elderly patients, such lesions are often beyond repair.

15.4.2 Neurological Injuries

Neurological damage of the brachial plexus or of selected peripheral nerves consequent to fracture-dislocations or during reduction occurs in 2–30 % of cases. Robinson et al. [2] reported nerve injury in 13.5 % of a consecutive series of 3,633 anterior dislocation fractures (2,250 men and 1,383 women; average age, 47.6 years). The entity of damage depends on age, energy of trauma, type of lesion, and time between lesion and reduction. Electromyography is more accurate than clinical observation in identifying the severity of nerve lesion. The axillary nerve is the most frequently injured nerve in fracture-dislocations of the shoulder, and they resolve within 4–5 months. In the rare cases that axillary nerve damage requires surgery, this can be done with either direct suturing or graft reconstruction.

In 2012, Frank et al. 15] reported a rare case of irreducible head dislocation in which the axillary nerve was entrapped inferiorly.

15.4.3 Vascular Injuries

Fracture-dislocations are rarely associated with vascular injury. In such cases, the axillary artery or vein can be damaged. These injuries are more frequent in the elderly due to atherosclerosis of the vessel. These lesions are associated with 50 % mortality during surgery. The anatomopathological lesions are thrombosis or avulsion of arterial branches [2].

15.4.4 Impression Fractures and Glenoid Fractures

Impacted fractures of the humeral head in dislocations were first described by Hill Sachs and McLaughlin [16, 17]. It was widely reported in the nineteenth century and was subsequently classified by Neer [3]. In fact, in all dislocations, the head impacted against the glenoid margin undergoes an impacted fracture. The severity of this lesion depends on the age of the patient, the violence of the trauma, and the time elapsed between the event and the reduction. Impression fractures can occur anteriorly near the subscapularis attachment in case of a posterior dislocation or posterosuperiorly in case of an anterior or inferior dislocation. Thanks to recent CT and MRI advances, these lesions can now be assessed accurately, and treatment can be targeted. This is important because an anterior or posterior impression fracture is often unrecognized.

An impression fracture secondary to a dislocation is a transitory or static lesion that can be acute or chronic. The transitory form is an anterior or posterior dislocation followed by spontaneous relocation of the head into glenoid fossa. The subdivision of the static form, which is more easily unrecognized, into acute or chronic is debated. It has been defined as chronic for periods that range from 24 h to 6 months post-trauma. Schulz et al. [18] defined "chronic" static impression fractures 24 h after trauma, whereas Rowe and Zarins [19] defined such cases chronic 3 weeks after trauma.

Detailed knowledge of the pathological anatomy and of the time between the trauma and treatment is essential to decide treatment. Deep large impacted lesions should be treated with tendon remplissage or graft, particularly in young people and in case of a defect less than 45 % [20]. In cases of fracture impacted secondary to dislocation above 50 %, prosthetic replacement is needed. Less frequent are glenoid bone fractures in anteroinferior dislocations, which can change the entity of the lesion from a few millimeters to 20–25 % of the osteocartilaginous surface. Such acute injuries should be treated with synthesis of the fragments. Implantation of a prosthesis in the rare forms of anterior locked dislocations with impacted or nonimpacted glenoid must be associated with a glenoid bone graft.

15.5 Treatment

15.5.1 Two-Part Fracture-Dislocations

The shape of two-part fracture-dislocations depends on the pathological involvement of the tuberosities and the surgical neck of the humerus. Two-part anterior fracture-dislocations of the surgical neck are very rare. First, the surgeon must try to relocate the head in the glenoid fossa. If the first attempt is not successful, the patient should be given an analgesic. After reduction, the surgeon should check the morphology of the surgical neck fracture, and in case of displacement, surgery is required. A two-part fracture involving the greater tuberosity is the most frequent shoulder dislocation (10–33 %).

Bahrs et al. [21] in a review of over 100 patients with greater tuberosity fractures found that over 50 % of them were associated with a traumatic anterior glenohumeral dislocation. In these forms, attempts to reduce the humeral head in the glenoid fossa must be gentle and atraumatic and should be carried out after completing the radiographic protocol with a trauma series

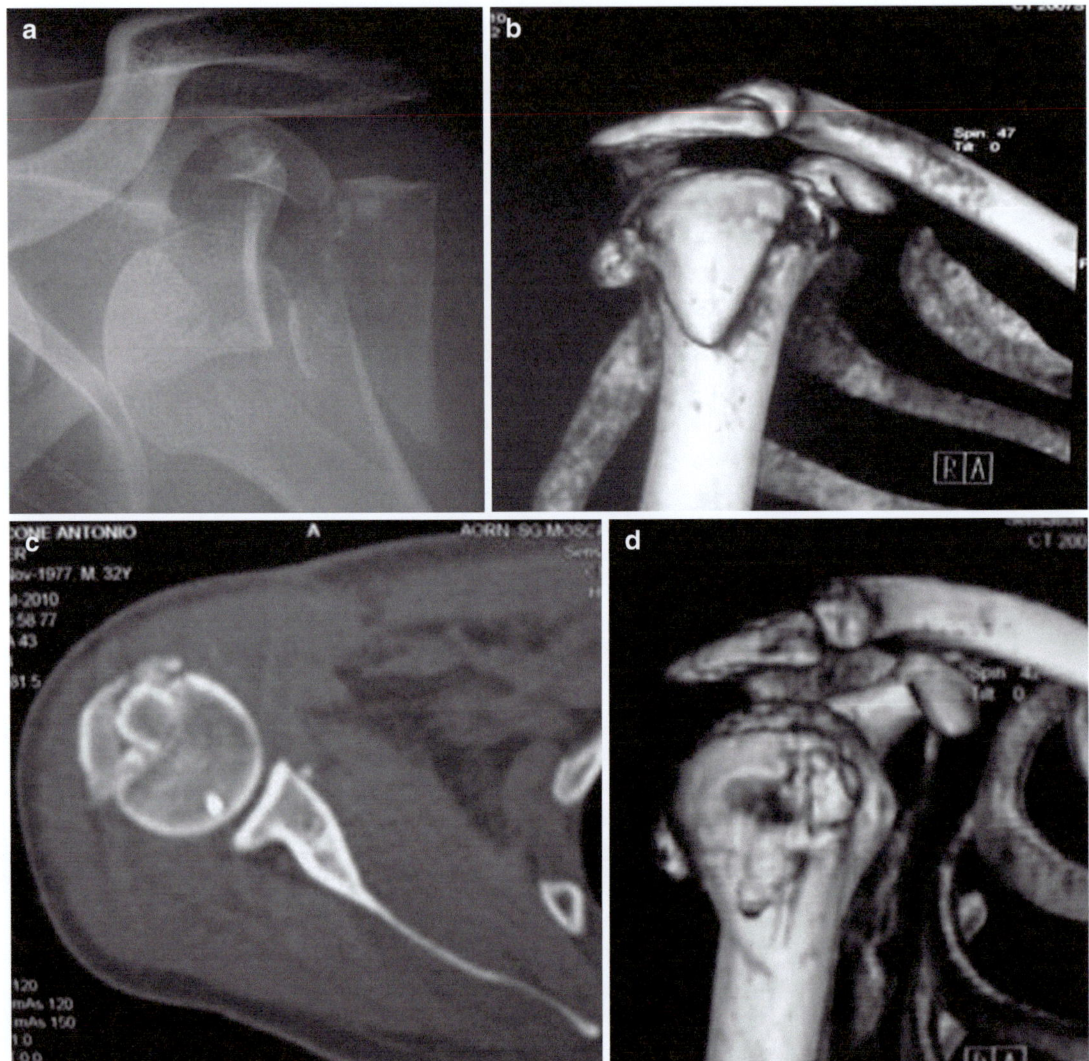

Fig. 15.1 Complex three-part fracture-dislocation with bone loss between the lesser and greater tuberosities. (**a**) Anteroposterior X-ray showing the anterior dislocation of the head and the fracture of the lesser and greater tuberosities. (**b**) 3D CT scan reconstruction showing displacement of fragments after reduction. (**c**) Axial projection CT scan showing postoperative reconstruction with minimal osteosynthesis (screws) and bone block, which is an important mechanical and biologic element that fills the secondary bone loss between the head and the greater tuberosity. (**d**) 3D CT scan reconstruction of the humeral head 2 years postsurgery

and/or CT. After reduction of the head, the greater tuberosity is often spontaneously reduced on the fractured rime. Surgery is indicated only when the displacement exceeds 5 mm (Fig. 15.1).

Two-part fractures involving the lesser tuberosity are rare. A posteriorly displaced humeral head must be evaluated with a trauma series and CT scan. The main cause of this fracture is the posterior dislocation with avulsion of the lesser tuberosity. The management protocol is the same as other two-part fracture-dislocations and consists in applying force, with the arm in extension, to promote longitudinal traction so that the head is relocated in the glenoid fossa. Surgical reduction and fixation of a lesser tuberosity fracture is indicated when the displacement exceeds 1 cm. A deltopectoralis approach is the best surgical access for the treatment of anterior and posterior fracture-dislocations. After the cephalic vein is exposed by blunting the groove and saved, the deep fascia is opened. The space below the deltoid is opened to expose the hemorrhagic subacromial bursa which is then resected. Using a brown retractor, the deltoid muscle is displaced laterally, and the coracobrachialis muscle is displaced medially. Thus, the surgeon can check for any damage of the superficial part of the rotator cuff and can see the biceps brachii interposed between fracture rimes. In cases in which the dislocation cannot be reduced, even when maneuvering with the patient under anesthesia, the biceps tendon is generally imprisoned between the two main fragments. In such cases, the rotator interval must be opened, and a tenotomy performed at the level of the glenoid tubercle. Thus, the head is well exposed, and the surgeon can see if an intra-articular humeral impact fracture hinders reduction. The head can be reduced using open reduction and internal fixation (ORIF). The patient is kept at rest with the shoulder in a sling for 4–6 weeks. This is followed by passive and active elbow and wrist motion.

15.5.2 Three-Part Anterior Fracture-Dislocations

The most frequent three-part anterior fracture-dislocation is an anterior dislocation of the humeral head with two rimes affecting the greater tuberosity and the surgical neck. In such cases, the lesser tuberosity remains attached to the head. This is a positive sign in terms of clinical outcome because vascularization is intact. The Laing artery should be respected during the surgical approach because it carries the blood supply to the humeral head. In three-part fracture-dislocations, the humeral neck is usually broken, and the two tuberosities are fractured and displaced. We use a deltopectoralis approach and identify the biceps as a landmark to reduce the head into the glenoid fossa. Sometimes we performed a bicep tenotomy and tenodesis and use ORIF to stabilize the fragments. In the more difficult case of a glenoid fracture that requires synthesis, we split the subscapularis muscle and perform a vertical capsulotomy, after which we reduce the glenoid fragment and stabilize it with cannulated screws.

15.5.3 Three-Part Posterior Fracture-Dislocations

Three-part posterior fracture-dislocations are characterized by rimes involving the surgical neck and the lesser tuberosity. Fragments are identified with CT scanning, and surgery is planned. A deltopectoralis approach is generally used. The rime between the lesser tuberosity and the intertubercular groove is opened to locate the posteriorly dislocated humeral head and reduce it into the glenoid fossa. The decision to reconstruct the fracture or replace it with a prosthesis depends on the patient's age, bone quality, comminution of fragments, and soft tissue lesions.

15.5.4 Four-Part Anterior and Posterior Fracture-Dislocations

Four-part fracture-dislocations are very complex lesions whose treatment is still debated [4, 5, 7, 8, 18, 22, 23]. The common denominator of this type of lesion is humeral head ischemia because of disruption of the blood supply [24, 25]. Various studies report a high percent of humeral head osteonecrosis [2, 3, 5, 8, 11, 13, 26]. Based on this observation, we replace the head with a humeral prosthesis, particularly in middle-aged and in elderly subjects, and use ORIF only in very young patients.

Recently, Hertel et al. [23] reported that the length of the dorsomedial extension and the integrity of the medial hinge can predict fracture-induced humeral head ischemia. However, although their study was an advance in the field of classification-surgical indications, it does not address the issue of whether osteosynthesis or prosthesis should be performed.

The implant of a prosthesis for a four-part anterior or posterior fracture-dislocation differs slightly from the implant of a standard four-part fracture. The level of difficulty depends on the expulsion zone of the humeral head. In some cases, it is positioned anteriorly near the glenoid rime; in others, the head is ejected outside the subscapularis muscle and must be sought below the plexus and vascular fascia. In rare cases, it lies on the chest wall, and even more rarely, it is displaced intrathoracically [27]. One should always assess for glenoid damage, which can consist in labrum and capsule injury, subscapularis muscle lesion, and even a bony Bankart fracture. In the latter case, osteosynthesis is necessary. In case of a posterior head dislocation, we have to consider the possibility of capsule avulsion from the posterior edge of glenoid and secondary posterior instability also after surgery.

Internal fixation of the humeral head in a four-part fracture-dislocation is difficult mainly because the fragments are unstable and the points of contact of fracture lines are difficult to identify; the same applies in case of humeral replacement.

15.5.5 Treatment-Related Classification of Four-Part Fracture-Dislocations

The gold standard treatment for four-part fractures and fracture-dislocations is the implant of a humeral prosthesis. However, there is now a trend toward humeral reconstruction in patients between 50 and 65 years old [4, 22, 28], whereas in patients older than 65 years the question is whether to implant an anatomic or a reverse prosthesis. We recently proposed a classification to guide this treatment decision [26]. This revisited Neer classification of four-part fractures [3] was prompted by the observation that previous classifications, from Codman [33] to Neer [3] and more recently Hertel et al. [23], do not correlate the traumatic lesion with surgical indications, namely, osteosynthesis versus prosthesis implant. Our classification is based on the study of "missing" fifth fragment, namely, the humeral calcar (Fig. 15.2a, b), which was not considered in previous classifications. To study the calcar,

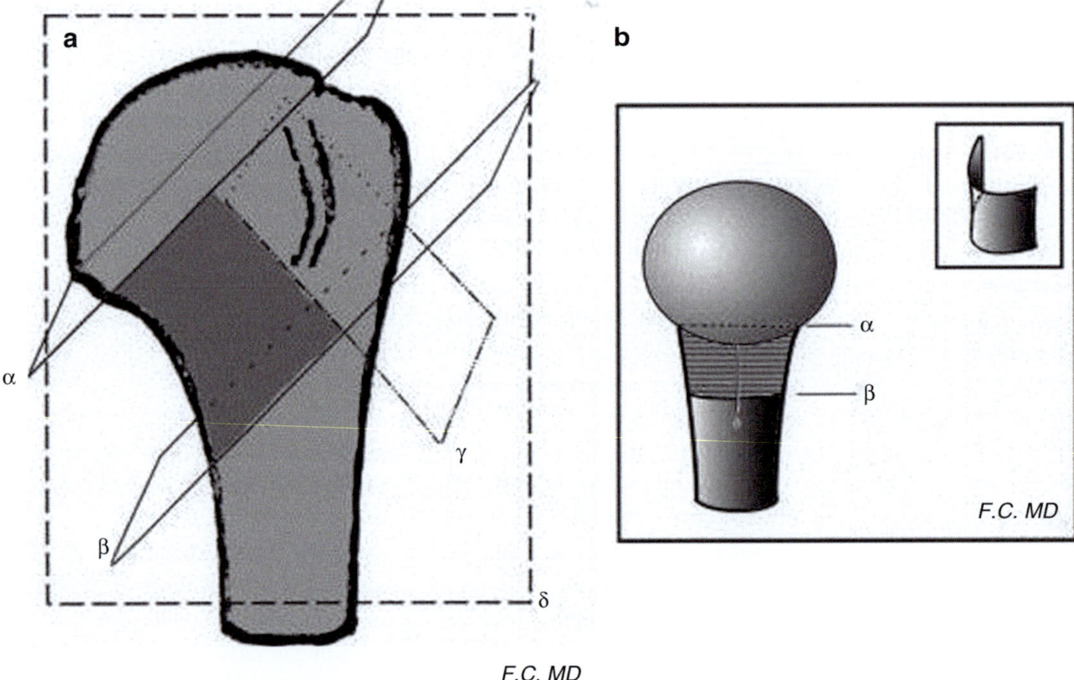

Fig. 15.2 Drawing showing the four planes delimitating the area of calcar. Studio in frontal plane (**a**) and in coronal plane (**b**)

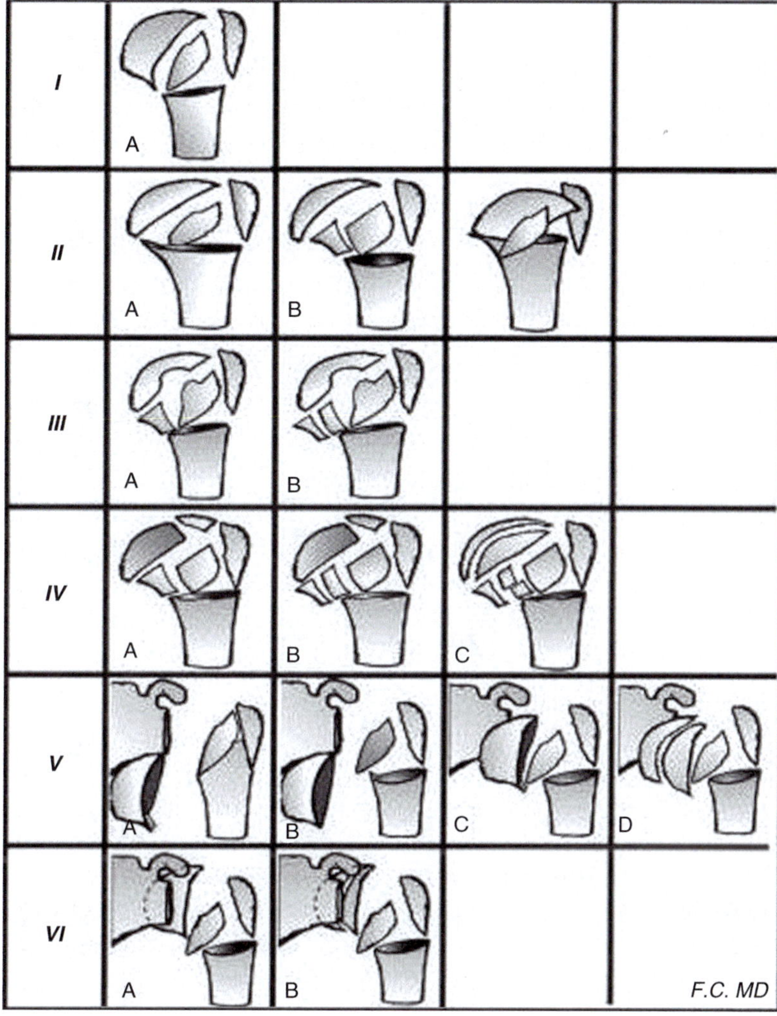

Fig. 15.3 The revisited Neer classification of four-part fracture-dislocations, which is based on the complexity of the *V* fragment. Groups *V* and *VI* are divided into subgroups of anterior and posterior fracture-dislocations according to the severity of the fracture of the *V* fragment

we delimit the calcar area on the medial column using four planes. These planes intersection at well-defined points. The calcar lies between two axial parallel planes denoted as "alpha" and "beta" (see Fig. 15.2a) that cross the anatomic and surgical neck, respectively. A third plane denoted as "gamma" intersects these planes orthogonally on the medial border of the lesser tuberosity. The fourth and last plane denoted as "delta" is coronal oblique and passes central to the humeral calcar, thereby dividing it into two parts: anterior and posterior. Thus, we can define the involvement of the calcar in the fracture, particularly on the CT scan, and determine the relationship between its fracture and cephalic cup with the other three fragments (i.e., the lesser and greater tuberosities and the surgical neck). This enables us to forecast the difficulties in case of reconstruction and the most appropriate technique to use.

This process resulted in six main fracture types divided into 16 subgroups (see Fig. 15.3). Fracture-dislocations are types V and VI. Type V is characterized by anterior displacement of the humeral head, which may be outside the articulation due to a tear in the capsule and outside the subscapularis muscle or outside the capsule but retained on the subscapularis muscle. Type V is divided into four subtypes. Subtype VA is extra-subscapular; the calcar is fractured on the beta plane, the entire tuberosity complex is fractured, and the greater tuberosity is displaced, whereas the lesser tuberosity can remain linked to the

Table 15.1 Surgical treatment according to the proposed revisited classification

Fracture type	Treatment group
I, II, IIIA, **VA, VC, VIA**	Reconstruction and osteosynthesis
IVC, **VD, VB, VIB**	Prosthesis: anatomic or reverse
IIIB, IVA, IVB, **VB**	Borderline group

Bold indicates the decision-making for four-part fracture-dislocations. We systematically apply this treatment-related classification

periosteum. Subtype VB is extracapsular with a fracture of the calcar on the alpha plane and with tuberosities displaced and often multifragmented. Subtype VC is intrasubscapular with a fracture in the beta plane. Type VD is intrasubscapular with a fracture on the alpha and beta planes and head splitting. Type VI fractures are characterized by posterior displacement of the head and are divided into VIA, which is an avulsion fracture of the lesser and greater tuberosities, and VIB, which is characterized by head splitting with the upper part of the head linked or not to the greater tuberosity.

To test our classification, we examined all the data (emergency room radiographs, CT scans, Neer classification, surgical technique used, type and results of surgery) related to 173 cases of complex fractures of the proximal third of the humerus. On the X-rays, we evaluated bone parameters in relation to the position of the calcar, humeral head inclination, and the position of the tuberosities. We focused on the morphology of the calcar fracture that serves as a landmark for implantation of the prosthesis at the correct height and retroposition (Table 15.1). If the humeral head is expelled anteriorly, outside the glenoid cavity after a shoulder dislocation, we carry out the bone block technique [29] that enables an anatomic reconstruction and stable fixation.

15.5.6 Technical Note Regarding the Bone Block and Titanium Block Techniques

If, in an anterior four-part fracture-dislocation, the CT evaluation of calcar shows that the hinge is linked on the alpha plane and if it is intact on the delta plane, osteosynthesis is indicated in young and middle-aged patients (Fig. 15.4a). As a technical note, below we report some steps of this operation:

- Recover the humeral head from the extra-articular side (usually the subscapularis fossa in anterior fracture-dislocations and the retroglenoid space in posterior fracture-dislocations) (Fig. 15.4b). Check for osteo-cartilaginous lesions, and if necessary reduce them and stabilize them with bone sutures using n. 1 nonabsorbable wires.
- After the recovery of the humeral head from the anterior subscapularis fossa, we identify the inferior fracture line between the calcar and cephalic cup, and then we identify the position of the superior aspect of the head. These two points enable us to determine the correct inclination. We then identify the junction with anterior and posterior rimes.
- Once ascertained the anatomic junction points of the humeral head, we position the metaphyseal part of the humerus ensuring the perfect correspondence between these two medial rimes (cup and calcar) that reconfigure the correct humeral retrotorsion and inclination (Fig. 15.4c).
- With the arm of the patient in complete external rotation to allow correct visualization of the proximal third of the humerus in its medial and posterior area, positioning the cephalic bone cup on the metaphyseal bone, we ensure the correct retroversion and inclination of the head on the calcar and fill the space between the cup and diaphysis with a modeled tricortical trapezoidal iliac crest bone graft or with a pyramidal titanium cage (especially in cases of osteoporosis). Having obtained a partial stabilization of this reconstructed proximal part with the bone block or titanium technique [30], we use three wires (or three screws at the end of the treatment) (Fig. 15.4d) crossing them through the humeral head and through the block (bone or titanium cage) to the diaphysis starting from the upper part of the cephalic cup and then drawing them down 4–5 mm under the cartilage.
- We replace the reconstructed humeral head stabled with the proximal humeral diaphysis in the glenoid fossa. With C-arm X-ray, we

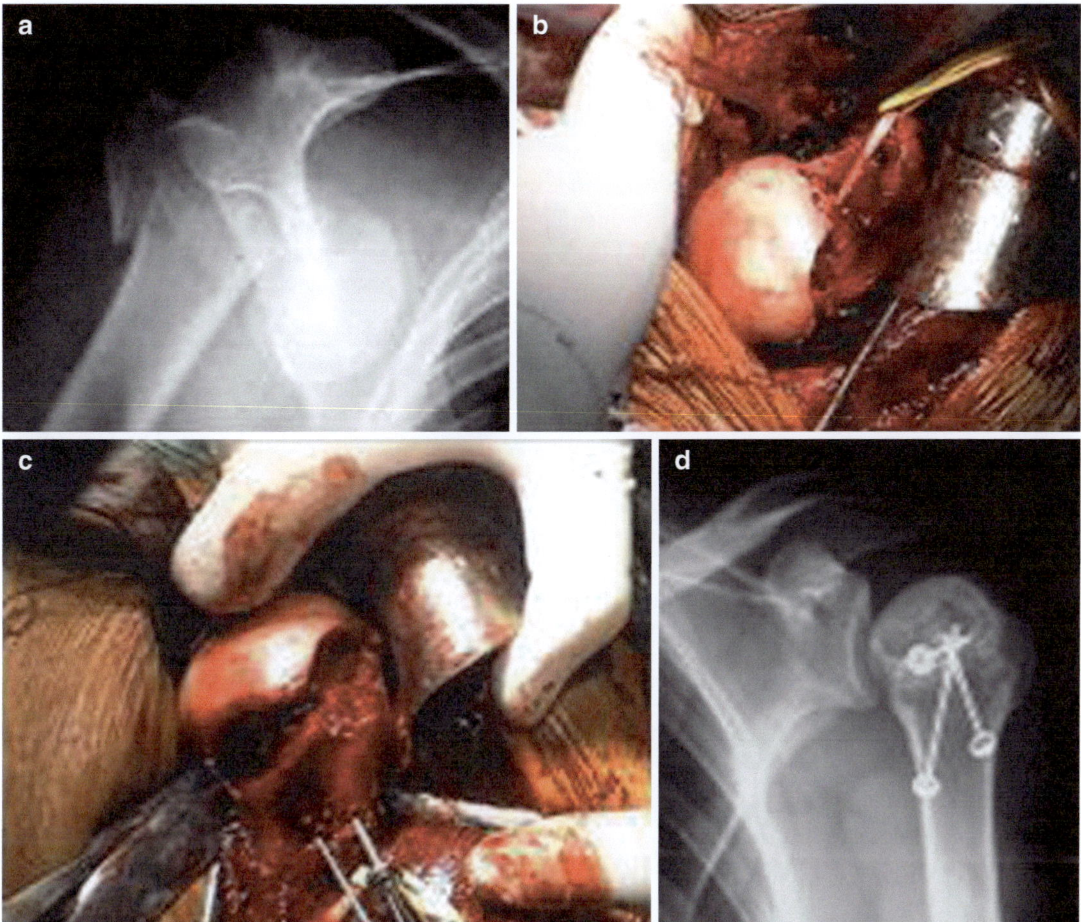

Fig. 15.4 Complex four-part anterior fracture-dislocation (type VC of the revisited Neer classification). (**a**) Anteroposterior X-ray showing a four-part anterior dislocation fracture (type VC of the revisited Neer classification). (**b**) Image of the humeral head after being recovered from the subscapularis fossa; four-part pathological position of the long head of the biceps on the fracture rimes. (**c**) Image of a perfect reconstruction of the medial calcar after we had filled the bone loss and replaced the wires with cannulated free screws. (**d**) Anteroposterior X-ray 5 years postsurgery

control the reduction of fracture and the orientation of the humeral head in different shoulder rotations.

- If the orientation of the head is good, we fill the remaining space with bone chips and very easily reconstruct the greater and lesser tuberosities on the original site. We fix everything with transosseous sutures using n. 2 or n. 5 nonabsorbable wires and/or screws or a small plate and screws.

If the alpha plane is not intact, we decide for prosthesis implant. We prefer an anatomic noncemented humeral prosthesis in patients between the age of 50 and 70 years if the rotator cuff is intact. Patients with a non-plurifragmented greater tuberosity are candidates for an anatomic implant. In cases of a plurifragmented greater tuberosity, we systematically use a reverse prosthesis in patients from 70 to 85 years old.

The revisited Neer classification, which reveals the pathomechanics of fractures between the humeral head and calcar, provides landmarks that enable reconstruction of the correct retrotorsion and height of the prosthesis. Moreover, starting from this medial reconstruction, with landmark points, it is possible to use the Brems puzzle piece technique [31] to implant anatomic humeral prostheses.

15.6 Postoperative Management

Patients with fracture-dislocations treated with osteosynthesis or prosthesis implants remain with their arm in a sling for 4 weeks and are allowed only active movements of the wrist and elbow. After 4 weeks of rest, we recommend rehabilitation with the Lyon technique [32] for 6 weeks, after which patients can resume active movement.

Acknowledgments We thank Jean Ann Gilder (Scientific Communication srl., Naples, Italy) for revising and editing the text.

References

1. Court-Brown CM, Garg A, McQueen MM (2001) The epidemiology of proximal humeral fractures. Acta Orthop Scand 72:365–371
2. Robinson CM, Akhtar A, Mitchell M, Beavis C (2007) Complex posterior fracture-dislocation of the shoulder. Epidemiology, injury patterns, and results of operative treatment. J Bone Joint Surg Am 89:1454–1466
3. Neer CS 2nd (1970) Displaced proximal humeral fractures: I. Classification and evaluation. J Bone Joint Surg Am 52:1077–1089
4. Bigliani LU (1998) Fractures of the proximal humerus. In: Rockwood CA, Matsen FA (eds) The shoulder, 2nd edn. WB Saunders, Philadelphia, pp 278–334
5. Ackermann C, Lam Q, Linder P, Kull C, Regazzoni P (1986) [Problems in classification of fractures of the proximal humerus]. Z Unfallchir Versicherungsmed Berufskr 79:209–215
6. Rouleau DM, Hebert-Davies J (2012) Incidence of associated injury in posterior shoulder dislocation: systematic review of the literature. J Orthop Trauma 26:246–251
7. Shrader MW, Sanchez-Sotelo J, Sperling JW, Rowland CM, Cofield RH (2005) Understanding proximal humerus fractures: image analysis, classification, and treatment. J Shoulder Elbow Surg 14:497–505
8. Duparc J, Largier A (1976) Fracture-dislocations of the upper end of the humerus. Rev Chir Orthop Reparatrice Appar Mot 62:91–110
9. Kristiansen B, Andersen UL, Olsen CA, Varmarken JE (1988) The Neer classification of fractures of the proximal humerus. An assessment of interobserver variation. Skeletal Radiol 17:420–422
10. Sidor ML, Zuckerman JD, Lyon T, Koval K, Cuomo F, Schoenberg N (1993) The Neer classification system for proximal humerus fractures. An assessment of interobserver reliability and intraobserver reproducibility. J Bone Joint Surg Am 75:1745–1750
11. Brien H, Noftall F, MacMaster S, Cummings T, Landells C, Rockwood P (1995) Neer's classification system: a critical appraisal. J Trauma 38:257–260
12. Bernstein J, Adler LM, Blank JE, Dalsey RM, Williams GR, Iannotti JP (1996) Evaluation of the Neer system of classification of proximal humeral fractures with computerized tomographic scans and plain radiographs. J Bone Joint Surg Am 78:1371–1375
13. Auffarth A, Mayer M, Kofler B et al (2013) The interobserver reliability in diagnosing osseous lesions after first-time anterior shoulder dislocation comparing plain radiographs with computed tomography scans. J Shoulder Elbow Surg 22(11):1507–1513. S1058-2746(13)00210-3
14. Bono CM, Renard R, Levine RG, Levy AS (2001) Effect of displacement of fractures of the greater tuberosity on the mechanics of the shoulder. J Bone Joint Surg Br 83:1056–1062
15. Frank MA, Laratta JL, Tan V (2012) Irreducible luxatio erecta humeri caused by an aberrant position of the axillary nerve. J Shoulder Elbow Surg 21:e6–e9
16. McLaughlin HL (1952) Posterior dislocation of the shoulder. J Bone Joint Surg Am 24-A-3:584–590
17. Hill SA, Sachs MD (1940) The grooved defect of the humeral head. A frequent unrecognized complication of dislocation of the shoulder Joint. Radiology 35:690
18. Shultz TJ, Jacobs B, Patterson LR (1969) Unrecognized dislocation of the shoulder. J Trauma 9:1009–1023
19. Rowe CR Zarins B (1982) Chronic unreduced dislocations of the shoulder. J Bone Joint Surg Am 64:494–505
20. Assom M, Castoldi F, Rossi R, Blonna D, Rossi P (2006) Humeral head impression fracture in acute posterior shoulder dislocation: new surgical technique. Knee Surg Sports Traumatol Arthrosc 14:668–672
21. Bahrs C, Lingenfelter E, Fischer F, Walters EM, Schnabel M (2006) Mechanism of injury and morphology of the greater tuberosity fracture. J Shoulder Elbow Surg 15:140–147
22. Duparc F, Huten D (1998) Conservative treatment of fractures of the upper end of the humerus. Rev Chir Orthop Reparatrice Appar Mot 84(Suppl 1):121–189
23. Hertel R, Hempfing A, Stiehler M, Leunig M (2004) Predictors of humeral head ischemia after intracapsular fracture of the proximal humerus. J Shoulder Elbow Surg 13:427–433
24. Gerber C, Schneeberger AG, Vinh TS (1990) The arterial vascularization of the humeral head. An anatomical study. J Bone Joint Surg Am 72:1486–1494
25. Meyer C, Alt V, Hassanin H et al (2005) The arteries of the humeral head and their relevance in fracture treatment. Surg Radiol Anat 27:232–237
26. Russo R, Cautiero F, Della Rotonda G (2012) The classification of complex 4-part fracture revisited: the missing fifth fragment and indication for surgery. Musculoskelet Surg 96(Suppl 1):S13-9
27. Salhiyyah K, Potter D, Sarkar PK (2012) Fracture-dislocation of humeral head with intrathoracic displacement. Asian Cardiovasc Thorac Ann 20: 196–198

28. Boileau P, Walch G (1997) The three-dimensional geometry of the proximal humerus. Implications for surgical technique and prosthetic design. J Bone Joint Surg Br 79:857–865
29. Russo R, Visconti V, Lombardi LV, Ciccarelli M, Giudice G (2008) The block–bridge system: a new concept and surgical technique to reconstruct articular surfaces and tuberosities in complex proximal fractures. J Shoulder Elbow Surg 17:29–36
30. Russo R, Cautiero F, Ciccarelli M, Vernaglia Lombardi L (2013) Reconstruction of unstable, complex proximal humeral fractures with the da Vinci cage: surgical technique and outcome at 2 to 6 years. J Shoulder Elbow Surg 22:422–431
31. Brems JJ (2002) Shoulder arthroplasty in the face of acute fracture: puzzle pieces. J Arthroplasty 17:32–35
32. Liotard JP, Edwards TB, Padey A, Walch G, Boulahia A (2003) Hydrotherapy rehabilitation after shoulder surgery. Tech Shoulder Elbow 4:44–49
33. Codman EA (1934) The shoulder. TT Todd, Boston. Reprinted Robert E Krieger Publishing, Malabar, Florida 1984

16 Treatment of the Sequelae

Mark Tauber

16.1 Introduction

Since proximal humerus fractures are increasing [46], posttraumatic conditions have to be faced in a growing number by orthopedic surgeons, as well. For the patients' satisfaction, two factors are relevant: pain and shoulder function. Usually, with increasing age, the functional expectations of the patients decrease. Thus, for elderly patients, priority in posttraumatic case management should focus on a low pain level, and shoulder function should at least allow for performance of daily activities.

Generally, fractures can result in various sequelae. It is important to distinguish between mechanical and biologic complications. Mechanical problems result from a changed anatomy due to fragment displacement, which can be primary after nonoperative treatment or poor fracture reduction or secondary after loss of reduction. Displacement of the tuberosities is associated with changed lever arms of the rotator cuff resulting in decreased shoulder function. Additionally, superior displacement of the greater tuberosity leads to a mechanical conflict with the acromion in terms of an impingement syndrome. Posterior displacement of the greater tuberosity with step formation toward the articular segment may limit external rotation in terms of a mechanical conflict between displaced tuberosity and posterior glenoid rim. The same problem is possible at the anterior aspect of the humeral head regarding the lesser tuberosity. In a biomechanical fracture model of the proximal humerus, Bono et al. [10] evaluated different amounts and directions of greater tuberosity malposition. They found that the deltoid abduction force was significantly increased by 16 and 27 % by superior displacements of 0.5 and 1 cm, respectively, while combined superior and posterior displacement of 1 cm gave an increase in force of 29 %. These data suggest that small amounts of residual displacement may alter the balance of forces required to elevate the arm at the glenohumeral joint.

In addition, tuberosity malunion limits the clinical outcome in posttraumatic shoulder arthroplasty. In an own study [58], the relevance of preoperative tuberosity malunion in 38 patients undergoing secondary shoulder arthroplasty for posttraumatic avascular humeral head necrosis was evaluated. Two novel radiological parameters were introduced, the greater tuberosity offset (GTO) in the AP view for lateralization of the greater tuberosity and the posterior offset (PO) in the axillary view to determine the widening at the intertubercular groove. Although general substantial improvement according to the Constant score (CS) was achieved (27 points preoperatively to 57 points postoperatively), patients with a near anatomic tuberosity alignment had a significantly better functional benefit.

M. Tauber, MD
Shoulder and Elbow Service, ATOS Clinic Munich,
Effnerstrasse 38, Munich, Bavaria 81925, Germany
e-mail: tauber@atos-muenchen.de

F. Castoldi et al. (eds.), *Simple and Complex Fractures of the Humerus*,
DOI 10.1007/978-88-470-5307-6_16, © Springer-Verlag Italia 2015

Greiner et al. [29] confirmed these findings and found out that tuberosity position correlates with fatty infiltration of the rotator cuff after hemiarthroplasty for proximal humeral fractures. The CS of patients with greater tuberosity displacement of 0.5–1 cm was significantly higher than that in patients with nonunited greater tuberosities. For the lesser tuberosity, patients with displacement of <0.5 cm showed significantly higher outcome scores than patients with displacement of >1 cm and nonunited lesser tuberosities. There was a significant correlation between fatty infiltration of the supraspinatus and infraspinatus muscles and greater tuberosity malposition and between fatty infiltration of the subscapularis and lesser tuberosity malposition.

All these data underline the importance of the anatomic configuration of the humeral head for a satisfying posttraumatic outcome. Another mechanical problem refers to the inclination angle according to varus and valgus malalignment of the humeral head. The current literature is scant regarding critical values for fragment displacement or angulation in the frontal plane. Solberg et al. reported that varus deformities exceeding 20° are associated with a significantly impaired outcome [54, 55]. Valgus deformities seem to be better tolerated.

Biologic complications refer to the vascularity of the humeral head. Depending on the fracture pattern, the vascular supply of the articular head segment can be interrupted and lead to a mid- or long-term evolution of partial or complete head necrosis. The incidence after surgical treatment has been reported to range between 4 and 33 % after open reduction and internal fixation [13] and between 8 and 11 % after percutaneous treatment [7, 49]. Nevertheless, the natural potential of revascularization, especially in young patients, has to be considered. After intraoperative documentation of avascularity of the articular segment, Bastian and Hertel [5] reported radiological signs of posttraumatic head necrosis after 5 years in 20 % and structural radiological alterations in 80 %. Thus, it was proven that a high number of initially avascular articular segments could be preserved in terms of revascularization after stable osteosynthetic treatment with associated satisfying clinical results.

A combination of mechanical and biologic complications leads to fracture nonunions. Usually, mechanical instability is the main reason for fragment nonunion at the surgical neck. In addition, extended displacement with disruption of blood vessels and the periosteum represents a biologic factor favoring delayed fracture union or even nonunion. For tuberosity nonunion, the mechanical aspect of insufficient fragment stability alone has to be considered due to a preserved fragment blood supply along the attached rotator cuff tendons.

In addition to fracture-related factors associated with posttraumatic complications such as comminution, fragment displacement, open injuries, involvement of the articular surface, fracture-dislocation, and delayed operative treatment, if indicated, general unfavorable factors have to be considered. These are advanced age of the patient, reduced general health status, metabolic diseases as diabetes, and nicotine or alcohol abuse. In many cases, the destiny of the fracture is designated by its personality already at the time of injury.

16.2 Classification

Posttraumatic deformities and pathologies show a complex heterogeneity with often coexisting and overlapping entities. Thus, it is not always easy to clearly define and classify these alterations. In order to obtain the correct diagnosis, a detailed imaging diagnostic should be performed in every case. In addition to biplane radiographs (AP and axillary views), a computed tomography (CT) scan is of utmost importance to acquire precise anatomic information about fragment position, grade of bony consolidation, bone quality, and joint alignment. 3D reconstruction allows for better visualization and preoperative planning for both, either reconstructive procedures or shoulder arthroplasty.

In 2001, Boileau et al. [9] presented a new classification system for proximal humerus fracture sequelae based on 71 cases undergoing prosthetic replacement with an anatomic design. This classification system has been established in the meantime and is still valid (Fig. 16.1).

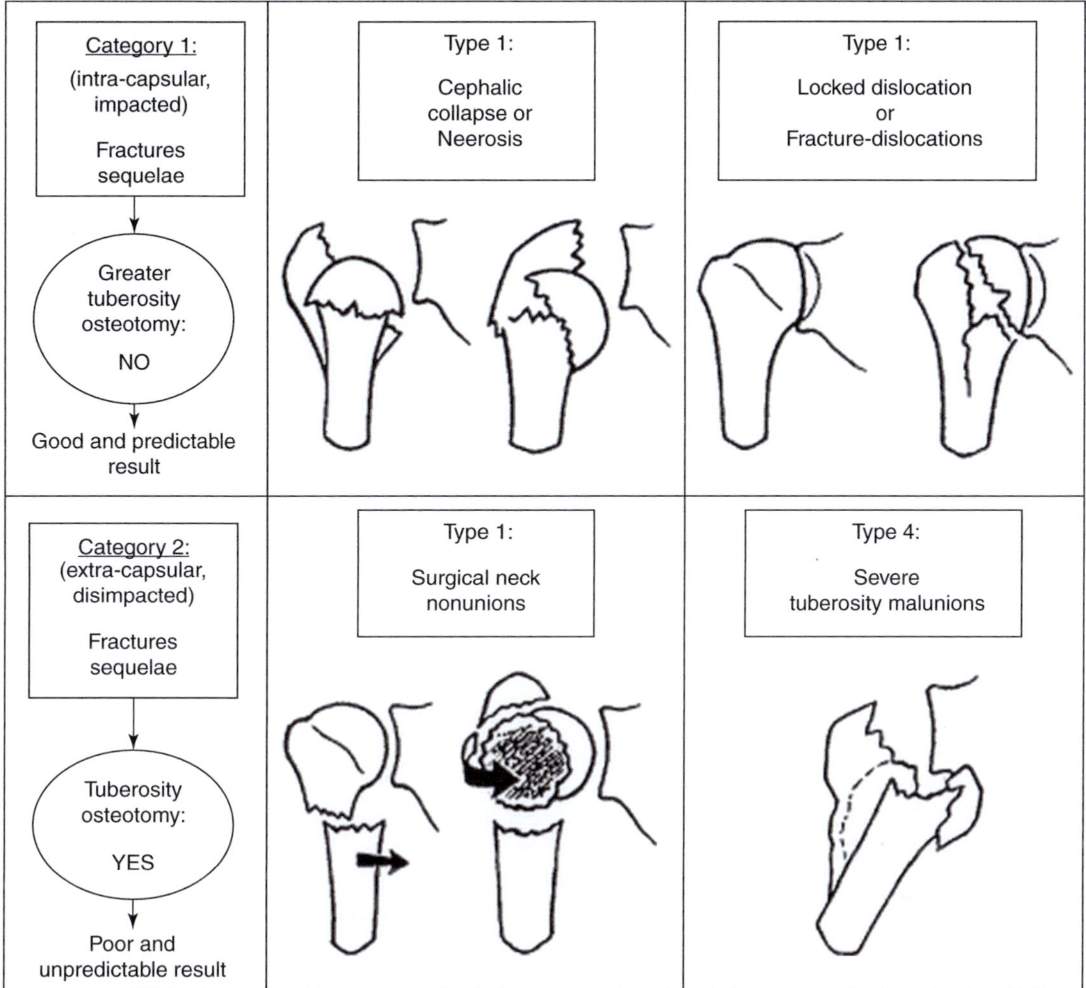

Fig. 16.1 Surgical classification of proximal humerus fracture sequelae according to Boileau et al. [9]: four types of sequelae including posttraumatic avascular humeral head necrosis as type 1, locked dislocation or fracture-dislocation as type 2, surgical neck nonunion as type 3, and severe tuberosity malunion as type 4

Two categories of fracture sequelae were implemented: Category 1 includes the intracapsular, impacted fracture sequelae, where no greater tuberosity osteotomy was necessary performing humeral head replacement. These were type 1 represented by the cephalic collapse or necrosis and type 2 represented by chronic locked dislocations or fracture-dislocations. Forty patients had cephalic collapse or necrosis, 35 of them with primary nonoperative treatment. Nine patients had a type 2 fracture sequelae including seven patients with posterior locked dislocation and each one patient with a posterior and anterior fracture-dislocation.

Category 2 included the extracapsular, disimpacted fracture sequelae with the need for tuberosity osteotomy when performing shoulder arthroplasty. Type 3 was surgical neck nonunion including each two 2-part surgical neck displaced fractures, 3-part greater tuberosity fractures, and 4-part fractures. One of them had already previous surgery. Type 4 fracture sequelae referred to severe tuberosity malunion including 16 4-part displaced or dislocated fractures, two undergoing revision surgery.

The main purpose was to correlate the clinical outcome after shoulder arthroplasty with an unconstrained stemmed design with the type of fracture sequelae. All patients in types 3 and 4, who underwent a greater tuberosity osteotomy, had either a fair or poor result and did not regain active elevation above 90°. Out of their findings, the authors recommended avoidance of greater tuberosity osteotomy whenever possible in secondary shoulder replacement using an unconstrained design with the use of a modular and adaptable prosthesis with both adjustable offsets and inclination.

16.3 Fracture Sequelae Type 1: Posttraumatic Avascular Necrosis

Vascular supply of the humeral head is provided by the anterior and posterior circumflex arteries, both originating from the axillary artery. Whereas at the beginning the role of the anterior circumflex artery was overestimated [12, 27], the importance of the posterior circumflex artery's contribution was highlighted later by several authors [20, 34, 39]. Decisive for the development of posttraumatic avascular head necrosis (PAVN) is the vascularity of the articular segment. In vivo measurement of this parameter is technically difficult and allows only assessment of the situation directly after the trauma. Posttraumatic processes of revascularization cannot be determined or quantified in a sufficient manner despite modern imaging tools. In 2004, Hertel et al. [33] published a pioneering work regarding this topic and identified 3 primary predictors of humeral head ischemia in 100 acute fractures after an average time period of 4 days after the trauma. These predictors were a calcar segment <8 mm, a disrupted hinge (>2 mm), and a fracture line at the anatomic neck (fracture types 2, 9, 10, 11, and 12 according to the classification of Hertel [33]). The combination of all 3 predictors was associated with a risk for humeral head ischemia of 0.97.

Thus, the risk for development of PAVN is mostly determined by the type of fracture. An incidence between 3 and 14 % has been reported for three-part fractures and 13–34 % for four-part fractures [18, 43, 56].

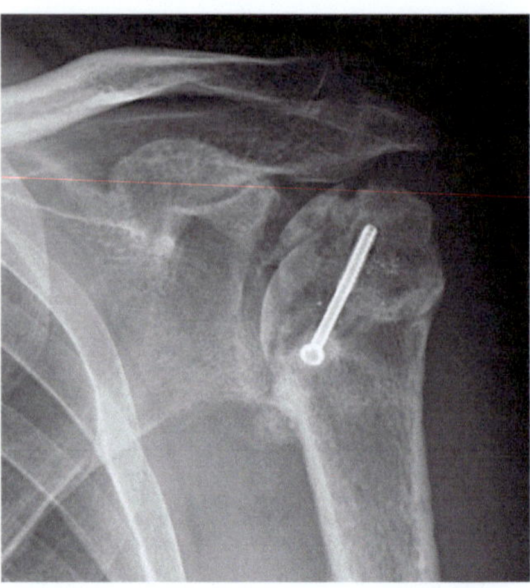

Fig. 16.2 Posttraumatic avascular necrosis of the humeral head after locking plate osteosynthesis of a four-part fracture. The anteroposterior screw for fixation of the lesser tuberosity is still in place. Note the medialization of the center of rotation following loss of sphericity of the articular segment with beginning glenoid erosion in terms of stage V according to the classification of Cruess [17]

Avascular necrosis has been classified by Ficat and Arlet [24] and was modified by Cruess [17] for the humeral head:

- Stage I: no radiographic evidence of necrosis
- Stage II: presence of mottled sclerosis
- Stage III: subchondral fracturing, crescent sign, occasional with flattening of articular surface
- Stage IV: collapse of subchondral bone, loss of humeral head sphericity
- Stage V: stage IV plus glenoid arthrosis (Fig. 16.2)

Stages I to III affect only the subchondral bone and cartilage, whereas the soft tissue envelope including capsule and rotator cuff is not involved. Due to the collapse of the head in advanced cases (stages IV and V), the center of rotation (COR) of the humeral head is shifted medially (medialization of COR) associated with capsular restriction and shortening of rotator cuff muscles adapted to the changed position of COR. This has to be taken into consideration when inserting a humeral head component of normal size and even more when total shoulder arthroplasty is planned with insertion of a glenoid component. Extended soft tissue management with bifocal capsular release on the humeral as well as on the glenoid side is of utmost importance in these cases to avoid overstuffing followed by pain and postoperative stiffness. Furthermore, release of the subscapularis tendon represents a key step of the procedure. A 270° tenolysis according to Matsen is performed mobilizing the tendon from the conjoint tendon, beneath the coracoid, and from the glenoid and scapular neck. Hereby, care must be taken not to harm the axillary nerve. In cases with malunion of the lesser tuberosity, correction osteotomy should be performed with lateralization of the lesser tuberosity.

Gerber et al. [26] stated that in cases with humeral head necrosis, the deformity rather than the necrosis itself creates disability underlining the importance of anatomic configuration of the proximal humerus with acceptable tuberosity alignment.

Treatment strategies are first of all stage dependent. Quite often a discrepancy is seen between advanced radiological changes with collapse of the head and low pain and moderate functional restriction and vice versa. Thus, the indication for surgical treatment has to be set individually depending on patients' complaints. However, range of shoulder motion should not be limited too much and for too long time in order to avoid soft tissue shortening and degenerative alterations as atrophy and fatty infiltration of the rotator cuff muscles. A functional and compensated soft tissue envelope represents a prerequisite for a good clinical outcome after posttraumatic shoulder arthroplasty.

If radiological signs of PAVN are present and the full spectrum of nonoperative treatment is exhausted, humeral head replacement represents the only sensible treatment solution. As standard implant stemmed humeral prosthesis has been established. A key aspect for adequate shoulder function is a correct COR. In order to restore anatomic glenohumeral joint kinematics, it is necessary to restore the COR, which in PAVN with loss of sphericity and possible additional tuberosity malunion has changed. Out of this rationale, it is important to use a shoulder prosthetic design of the fourth generation with 3D adaptability (inclination, retroversion, and eccentricity). In order to choose the right head size, preoperative radiographs of the uninjured shoulder are recommended to be made. If the surgeon is in doubt regarding the head size, a smaller one should be chosen in order to avoid joint overstuffing, especially if total shoulder arthroplasty is carried out. A major problem of stem designs in PAVN is that implantation of the humeral component refers always to the humeral shaft limiting the possibility of COR restoration in severely distorted anatomy. One option is to choose a smaller stem size and to implant it cemented. Nevertheless, some varus or valgus malalignment (Fig. 16.3) has to be tolerated, and sometimes it is even impossible to restore the COR due to severe malunion. In a recent retrospective study, Moineau et al. [40] followed up (mean follow-up time of 52 months) 55 patients undergoing anatomic shoulder arthroplasty (80 % TSA) without greater tuberosity osteotomy for type 1 fracture sequelae. The Constant score improved from 32 to 69 points, the Simple Shoulder Value was 81 %, and the revision rate was 7 %. As negative prognostic factors, proximal humeral deformity, specifically varus more than valgus malunion of the greater tuberosity, and fatty infiltration of the rotator cuff muscles have been identified. The authors concluded that anatomic shoulder arthroplasty for PAVN with acceptable deformation of the proximal humerus provides good and predictable outcomes. When negative predictive factors are present, reverse shoulder arthroplasty may be more appropriate, especially in elderly patients. The findings of Moineau et al. are consistent with those reported in the literature [8, 11, 19, 29, 36], including the author's own experience [58].

Out of the complex posttraumatic situations requiring independency from the humeral shaft, stemless designs were developed. Usually, the metaphyseal bone at the resection plane corresponding to the anatomic neck is of good, sclerotic bone quality allowing for stable fixation of various stemless designs. In the author's practice, the Eclipse prosthesis is used (Arthrex, Naples, Florida). This stemless implant offers a dual primary fixation mechanism. First, the so-called trunnion, a certain kind of baseplate, has cortical support on the resection plane, and a

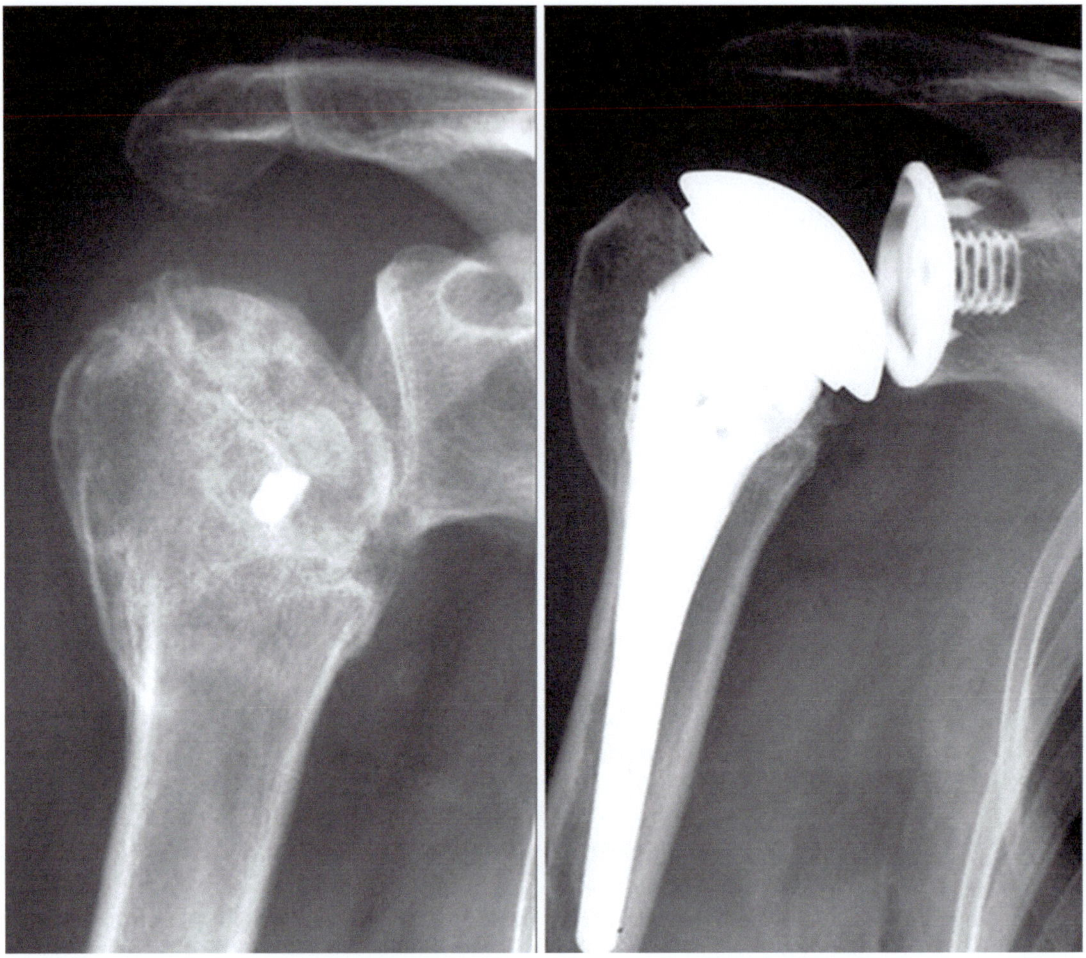

Fig. 16.3 Posttraumatic avascular head necrosis stage III according to Cruess [17] with valgus malalignment between shaft and head. Using a stem design introduction in valgus malalignment is unavoidable in order to restore COR. Note the relative overstuffing performing total shoulder arthroplasty with an increased acromiohumeral index

second stabilizing mechanism is provided by the cage screw, which is inserted through a central hole in the baseplate. Both, the trunnion and the cage screw, are coated with hydroxyapatite allowing for a reliable bony ingrowth. Finally, the head component is set on the top of the baseplate, which completes the three-component implant (Fig. 16.4). The plane of resection is defined using a 135° inclination resection guide. The amount of retrotorsion should be decided individually and ranges between 20° and 40°. During the resection using an oscillating saw, care must be taken not to harm the rotator cuff insertion which in some cases overlaps the resection plane due to tuberosity malunion and collapse of the articular segment. Small bone cysts, if encountered, can be filled with autologous or

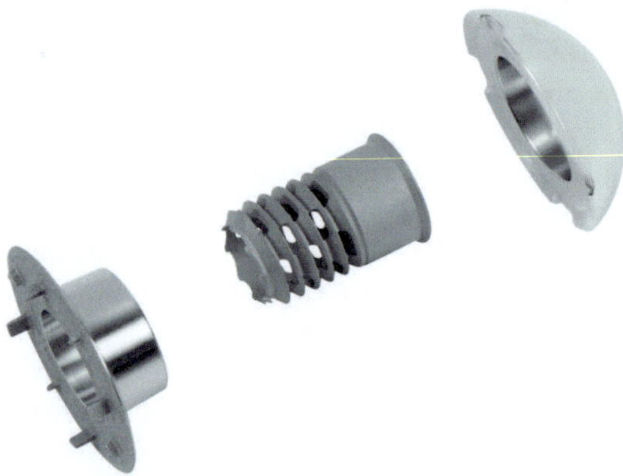

Fig. 16.4 The Eclipse prosthesis (Arthrex, Naples, FL), a stemless humeral head prosthetic design consisting of three components: trunnion (coated baseplate with antirotation fins at its undersurface), cage screw available in four length sizes, and the head

allogeneic bone material and usually do not set primary fixation stability of the cage screw at risk. However, if the metaphyseal bone is weak and/or soft with insufficient primary fixation of the cage screw, a stemmed prosthesis should be implanted. Thus, both arthroplasty systems should be at disposal in the surgical unit, when posttraumatic arthroplasty is performed. In a retrospective multicenter study, the outcome of the stemless Eclipse prosthesis has been evaluated [14]. From a total of 233 patients, 70 were posttraumatic cases type 1 with an average age of 59 years and a follow-up period of 27 months; 71 % of the patients had previous surgery. The age- and sex-related Constant score increased from 48 % preoperatively to 72 % postoperatively. Regarding the subgroups, the pain score improved from 7 to 12 points, activities of daily living from 8 to 13, range of motion from 16 to 21, and strength remained unvaried at 8 points. Range of motion increased in all planes significantly with flexion from 91° to 109°, abduction from 67° to 106°, and external rotation from 11° to 32°. Previous surgery seemed to negatively influence the final outcome (79 % according to the age- and sex-related Constant score for primary surgery and 69 % for revision surgery, respectively) without achieving statistical significance ($P = .18$). In comparison to the 100 cases operated on for primary osteoarthritis (53 % Constant score preoperatively to 84 % postoperatively), the posttraumatic results were moderately inferior (Fig. 16.5).

If PAVN is in an early stage with preserved sphericity of the articular segment (stages I to III, which is rarely the case), humeral head resurfacing can be performed. Initially designed for primary osteoarthritis, these cup prostheses replace only the cartilage and the subchondral bone. Therefore, it should be warranted that the necrotic process has ended without any further progression and loss of epiphyseal bone stock. Implants of the first generation were nonanatomic due to a geometric mismatch creating a glenohumeral overstuffing. With introduction of the new cup generation, this problem can be avoided. As main disadvantages, the risk for secondary glenoid erosion and the difficulty of glenoid component implantation have to be mentioned, which in PAVN is not always necessary.

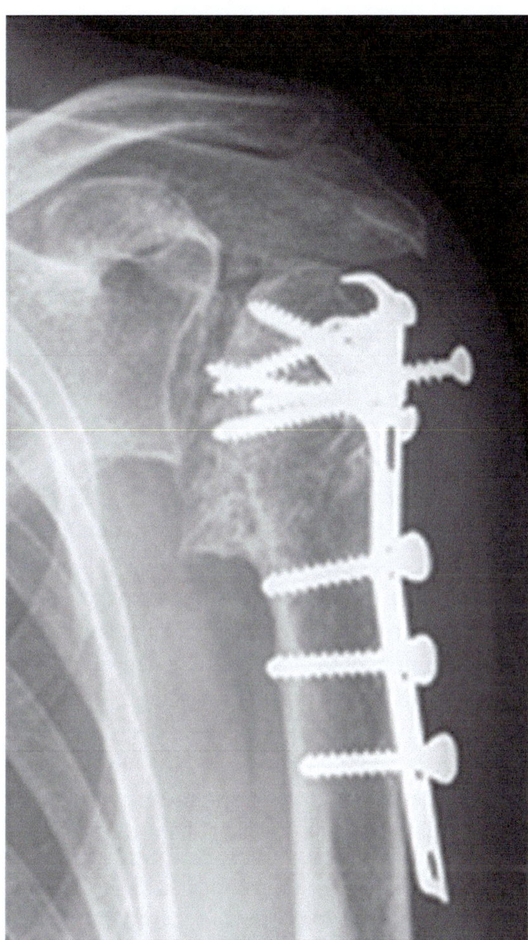

Fig. 16.5 AP radiogram showing PAVN stage IV after plate osteosynthesis of a four-part fracture in a 79-year-old female patient. One screw is loosened. Note the massive osteophyte at the calcar area

In a retrospective study, Raiss et al. [48] compared the functional results after cementless humeral replacement between posttraumatic ($n = 8$) and nontraumatic ($n = 9$) osteonecrosis of the humeral head. They included even stage 4 osteonecrosis with the presence of bone loss of as much as 31 % of the humeral head. After an average follow-up period of 3 years, significant improvement was observed for both groups (average age 48 years) with superior benefit in favor to the nontraumatic group (34 preoperatively to 70 points postoperatively in the Constant score for the nontraumatic group and 28–52 points for the PAVN, respectively). Signs of implant loosening were not observed in this short-term follow-up period. In 2010, comparable results were published by Pape et al. [47] reporting on 28 shoulders undergoing humeral head resurfacing after PAVN. The average age of the patients was 60 years with an average follow-up of 31 months. Three types of PAVN were distinguished according to the inclination of the impacted head: type 1, an impacted fracture with the head in an anatomic position; type 2, a valgus impacted fracture; and type 3, a varus impacted fracture. The overall Constant score improved from 23 to 55 points, with the best results for valgus impacted fractures. No loosening was reported with one patient suffering from mild secondary glenoid erosion. One patient required revision arthroplasty using a reverse design due to anterosuperior instability and persistent pain.

If PAVN is combined with severe tuberosity malunion or nonunion, shoulder arthroplasty using a reverse design should be considered. It is well documented in the literature that combined humeral head replacement and greater tuberosity osteotomy is associated with poor and unpredictable functional outcomes [9, 36, 45]. Thus, a constrained prosthetic design should be preferred in cases with PAVN and severely distorted anatomy of the tuberosities with secondary functional cuff deficiency.

16.3.1 Hemi- Versus Total Shoulder Arthroplasty

The decision to perform hemi- (HAS) or total shoulder arthroplasty (TSA) is dependent primarily from the integrity and shape of the glenoid but from the integrity of the cuff and capsular tension, as well. Small rotator cuff tears can be reconstructed. It is crucial to achieve centering of the head into the glenoid component with adequate tension and translation. If this is not possible, eccentric component positioning consequently is associated with increased loading and risk for glenoid component loosening in terms of the so-called rocking horse phenomenon [38]. Regarding the clinical outcome, LeHuec et al. [35] did not find a correlation between posttraumatic HSA or TSA and the clinical result, with the exception of PAVN. In this group, TSA showed significant better outcomes than HSA. This advantage was maintained even after complications and revisions [21]. These results were confirmed also in a later retrospective multicenter study [8]. In theory, implantation of a glenoid component provides superior support and containing in cases of glenoid erosion. However, survivorship of the glenoid component is more likely at risk than that of the humeral component. Thus, in younger patients with sufficient glenoid bone stock, implantation of the glenoid is dispensible [42], or reaming of the glenoid alone ("ream and run") can be performed. The results of glenoid replacement and "ream and run" have been reported to be comparable for glenohumeral arthritis [15].

16.4 Fracture Sequelae Type 2: Chronic Locked Dislocations or Fracture-Dislocations

These severe shoulder injuries are rare but still occur due to the fact that mainly posterior shoulder dislocations or fracture-dislocations represent the most commonly misdiagnosed dislocations of the body with devastating consequences. Main reasons are high-energy trauma or seizures [53]. The purpose is to primarily recognize such dislocations, to reduce them, and to reconstruct bony impression defects such as Hill-Sachs or Malgaigne lesions and bony glenoid rim lesions in order to prevent recurrence. Patients with type 2 fracture sequelae are younger [4, 31], and the main objective of shoulder arthroplasty is pain relief [4]. Anatomic shoulder arthroplasty (HSA or TSA) is recommended in type 2 fracture sequelae [8, 9]. Besides management of bony lesions, soft tissue balancing represents a challenging but key step procedure regarding the functional outcome. Capsule and rotator cuff muscles have been adapted to the chronic dislocated position of the joint and have to be addressed adequately and accurately during arthroplasty. In chronic posterior shoulder dislocation with fixed glenohumeral internal rotation and static decentration, the anterior soft tissue structures are shortened, which means to perform an extended anterior capsular and subscapularis tendon release together with tendon lengthening. In addition, a posterior capsular plication sometimes might be necessary in order to re-center the humeral head. However, the risk for recurrent instability of the shoulder arthroplasty might be given, so that a constrained prosthetic design becomes necessary in some cases.

Boileau et al. [9] reported on shoulder replacement in 9 patients with type 2 fracture sequelae, 7 had locked posterior dislocation, 1 locked posterior fracture-dislocation, and 1 locked anterior fracture-dislocation. After a mean delay of 19 months, 8 had HSA and 1 TSA with partial greater tuberosity in only one patient. The Constant score improved from 22 to 71 points, which was the highest improvement compared to other types of fracture sequelae. Although the overall clinical results are good, an increased complication rate up to 32 % has to be considered. Most frequent complications are infection, restriction of range of motion, persistent posterior instability, and heterotopic ossifications [4]. Similar good results have been reported for the outcome after reverse shoulder arthroplasty in type 2 fracture sequelae. Gwinner et al. [30] published their results of reverse shoulder arthroplasty for fracture sequelae treatment including 4 type 2 sequelae with combined rotator cuff pathology. The Constant score improved from 19 to 75 points (27–101 % age- and sex-adjusted) which was again the best result of all types of fracture sequelae treated with a reverse design. Neyton et al. [44] observed comparable results (16–57 points according to the Constant score), which are equivalent to anatomic shoulder arthroplasty. Thus, reverse shoulder arthroplasty is recommended by those authors in chronic locked anterior and posterior dislocations or fracture-dislocations with associated rotator cuff deficiency.

16.5 Fracture Sequelae Type III: Surgical Neck Nonunion

Humeral surgical neck nonunions are rare, but they cause considerable disability for the patient in terms of pain and functional impairment. Epidemiological data indicate a prevalence of proximal humeral nonunions of 1.1 % (11 out of 1.027 fractures) or up to 8 % if metaphyseal comminution is present and 10 % if there is between 33 and 100 % translation of the surgical neck [16]. In that study, the high percentage of fractures (89 %) treated nonoperatively with a nonunion rate of 0.8 %, in contrast to a 3.4 % nonunion rate in the operatively treated group, should be noted. However, other authors have reported a 20 % rate of proximal humerus nonunions with nonoperative fracture treatment identified as the principal cause [61]. Surgical treatment of fracture sequelae may be challenging due to patient-associated factors, such as advanced age, osteoporosis, medical illness, reduced compliance, alcoholism, and nicotine abuse. In addition, fracture and fracture care-associated factors, such as comminution, severe bone loss, cavitation of the humeral head resulting in a small articulating fragment, insufficient reduction and stabilization, and contracture of the glenohumeral joint following long-term disuse, are of major relevance. Several surgical techniques have been described for the treatment of humeral surgical neck nonunions, including reconstructive procedures using intramedullary nails [63], blade plates [25, 50, 57], locking plates [1], Rush rods with tension-band wiring [23, 41], and intramedullary bone pegging with internal plate fixation [60]. On the other hand, shoulder arthroplasty has been described using anatomic humeral head replacement [2, 8, 23, 32], as well as reverse shoulder arthroplasty [37, 44, 62].

Out from the current literature, shoulder arthroplasty seems not to provide reliable and satisfying results for type 3 fracture sequelae. Implantation of an anatomic design showed the poorest outcomes of all types of sequelae [8, 9] and a high tuberosity-related complication rate in terms of nonunion, resorption, and need for revision [22] influencing negatively the outcome. Even shoulder arthroplasty using a reverse design is associated with only moderate results and a surprisingly high complication and revision rate ranging from 27 % [37] up to 71 % (5 out of 7) [44] including infection, instability, and stiffness.

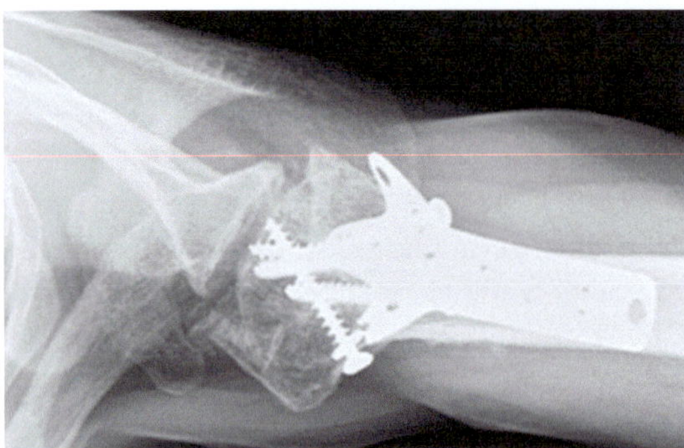

Fig. 16.6 Axillary view: complete collapse of the articular segment with medialization of the center of rotation. The joint is still centered with near anatomic alignment of the tuberosities

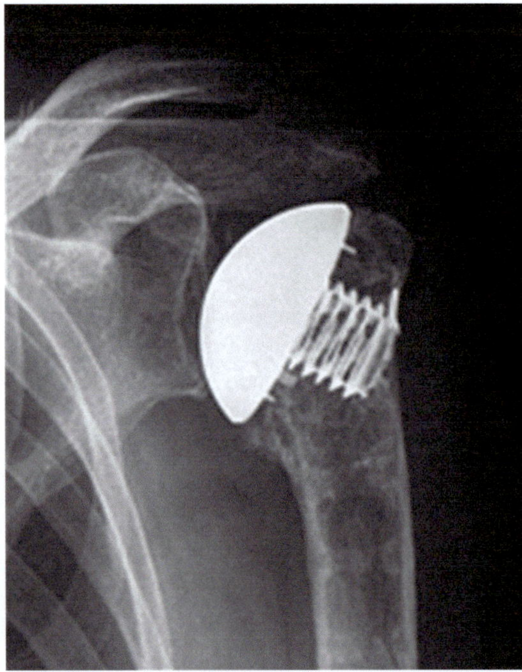

Fig. 16.7 Postoperative AP view 1 year after plate removal and HSA using a stemless design (Eclipse, Arthrex, Naples, FL). The center of rotation is restored

Thus, surgical reconstruction of surgical neck nonunion represents the first choice of treatment (Figs. 16.6, 16.7, and 16.8).

The rate of success in reconstructive surgical procedures in terms of bone healing varies from 50 % [23] to 100 % [1, 63]. In contrast to the mainstream trend to perform autologous bone grafting using either iliac crest or fibular/tibial

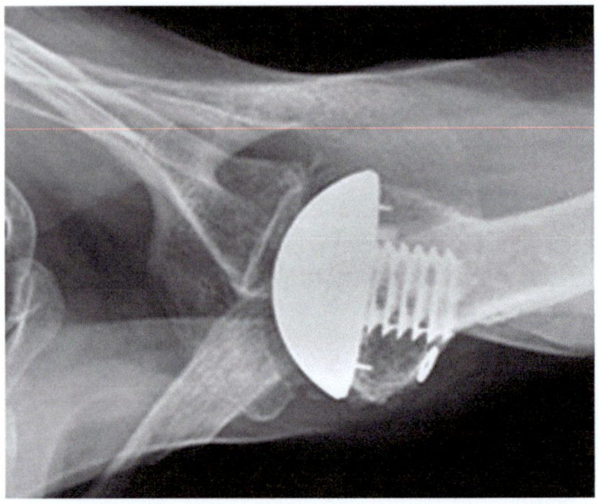

Fig. 16.8 Postoperative axillary view: well-centered glenohumeral joint without signs of implant loosening. The joint space is still preserved

bone grafts, in the author's experience, bone grafting seems not to be necessary to achieve bone union [57]. Magnetic resonance imaging demonstrates vitality of the humeral head, which indicates preserved vascularity of the head fragment. Thus, we are confronted with the challenge of treating loss of stability with intact vascularity. For this reason, only aggressive and accurate debridement of the nonunion gap without bone grafting is recommended to focus on achieving sufficient compression for osteosynthesis. This is achieved using a blade plate with an angle of 100° which exerts compression at the calcar side when fixed to the shaft by screws. According to the principle of tension banding, compression results from the tension forces of the rotator cuff. In patients with a small and cavitated head fragment, difficulties can be encountered when it is fixed by a blade plate. In these cases, the Humerusblock device (Synthes, Bettlach, Switzerland) is used, which was developed for percutaneous acute fracture management [7, 49]. In a series of 55 patients (mean age 66 years), the results using a blade plate (45 patients—group 1) or the Humerusblock device (10 patients—group 2) without bone grafting have been evaluated [57]. After a mean follow-up time of 74 months, the overall mean age- and sex-adjusted Constant score improved from 30.4 % preoperatively to 83.2 % postoperatively. The improvement was from 30.5 to 85.3 % in group 1 and from 32.2 to

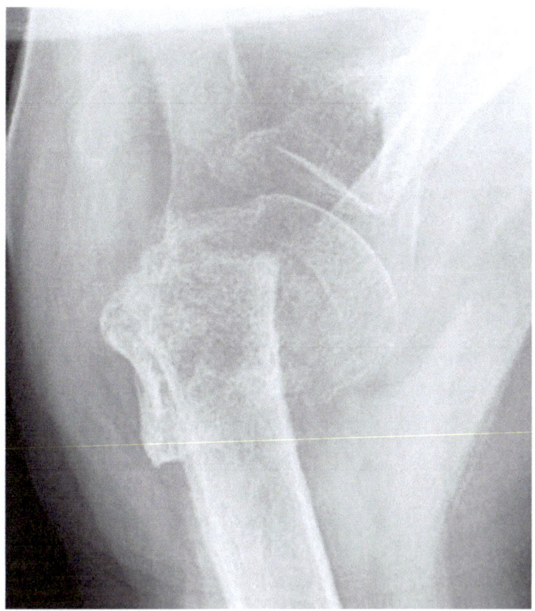

Fig. 16.9 Axillary view of a surgical neck nonunion after nonoperative treatment in an 80-year-old female patient. The head fragment is vital but unstable with malposition in hyperextension

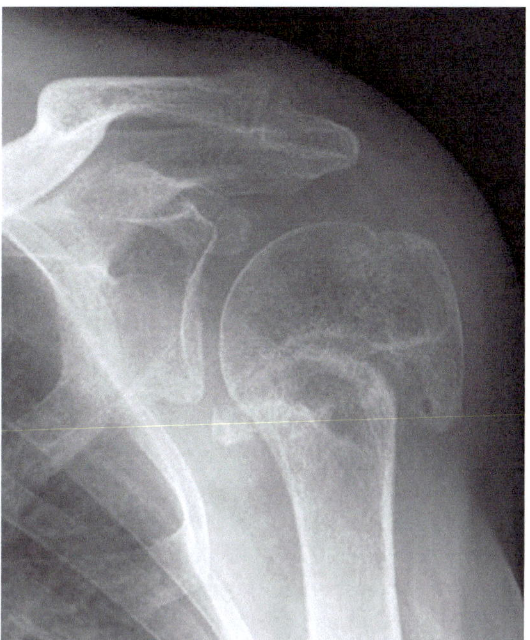

Fig. 16.10 The AP view shows bone deficiency at the surgical neck without bony contact at the lateral side. The head configuration is quite anatomic with minimal varus inclination

75.4 % in group 2, which represented statistically significant improvements for both groups ($P<.01$). Radiological bone healing was achieved in 51 patients (93 %). The overall complication rate was high (15 %) including plate loosening, avascular head necrosis, persistent nonunion, and infection. However, nonunion of humeral surgical neck fractures can be successfully treated by surgical reconstruction without bone grafting using either a blade plate (Figs. 16.9, 16.10, and 16.11) or the Humerusblock for small head fragments. The surgeon must be aware of the increased complication rate associated with this challenging posttraumatic pathology and has to inform the patient in the preoperative setting in a detailed manner.

16.6 Fracture Sequelae Type IV: Severe Malunion of the Tuberosities

Type 4 fracture sequelae are dealt with in the Chap. 13, p. 157 contributed by Giuseppe Porcellini.

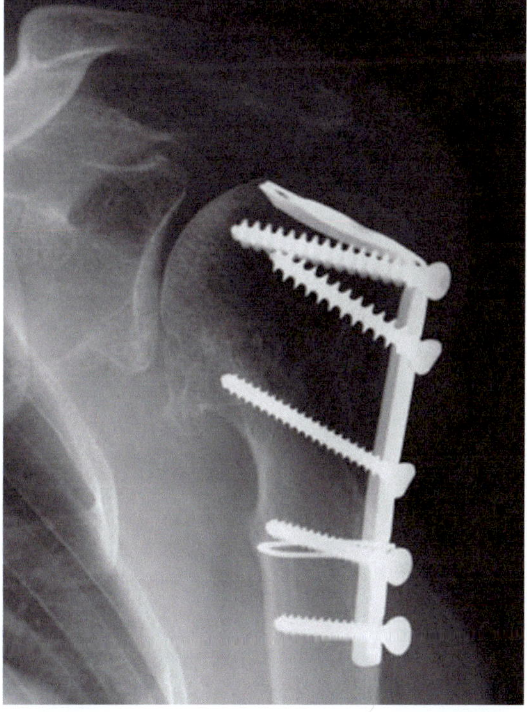

Fig. 16.11 AP view 2 years after angular blade plate stabilization without bone grafting shows complete bone union at the surgical neck with anatomic alignment. Note the broken drill tip at the second inferior plate hole

16.7 Severe Varus or Valgus Malunion of the Humeral Head

This type of fracture sequelae is not included in the classification system of Boileau. However, posttraumatic deformity relating only to the level of the surgical neck with malalignment in the frontal plane in terms of varus or valgus position does occur after both surgical and nonoperative treatments. Thereby, varus malalignment is more disabling than valgus deformity [54, 55]. From a biomechanical aspect, acromiohumeral impingement appears due to a relatively higher position of the greater tuberosity creating a subacromial conflict during abduction and flexion. In addition, the insertion point of the rotator cuff is medialized which is associated with shortened lever arms and reduced force vectors resulting in inability to gain full range of motion. If the anatomic shape of the humeral head is preserved without osteoarthritic changes, corrective metaphyseal valgus osteotomy at the surgical neck can be performed. The aim is to correct the inclination angle in order to restore normal joint kinematics. It is crucial to assess the amount of malunion using adequate imaging diagnostics. In addition to conventional radiographs with the forearm in neutral rotation, a CT scan is recommended. Accurate preoperative planning is necessary in order to exactly calculate the width of the valgus wedge. A deltopectoral approach is performed, and the surgical neck is presented. Two horizontally parallel pins are inserted through shaft and proximal humerus as references for the resection planes. In order to achieve healing of the osteotomy, the varus forces of the rotator cuff have to be neutralized during the healing period. For osteosynthesis purposes, either plate fixation or tension banding can be used [3, 6, 28, 51, 52]. The results reported in the literature are consistently good with bone union in all cases and significant functional improvement. Patients' subjective satisfaction is high and the complication rate low. Even complex two-plane and three-plane osteotomies are possible and provide functional improvement [52]. Nevertheless, the high technical demands of this procedure have to be considered.

In contrast to adults, varus deformity of the proximal humerus in children or adolescents usually is due to disturbs at the epiphyseal plate. Reasons for humerus varus caused by growth arrest in skeletally immature patients can be traumatic injuries of the epiphysis, infection, or acquired secondary to benign bone cysts. Ugwonali et al. [59] reported on the results after valgus osteotomy with tension-band fixation in six cases. Shoulder function improved significantly with flexion from 76° to 148° and abduction from 63° to 116°. The mean inclination angle increased from 95° preoperatively to 130° postoperatively. Two patients required tension-band removal due to local soft tissue irritation.

References

1. Allende C, Allende BT (2009) The use of a new locking 90 degree blade plate in the treatment of atrophic proximal humerus nonunions. Int Orthop 33(6):1649–1654
2. Antuna SA, Sperling JW, Sanchez-Sotelo J, Cofield RH (2002) Shoulder arthroplasty for proximal humeral nonunions. J Shoulder Elbow Surg 11(2):114–121
3. Aoki SK, Anderson LA, Marchese JW (2011) Recession wedge osteotomy of the greater tuberosity for proximal humeral varus. Orthopedics 34(5):398
4. Armengol-Barallat J, Trojani C, LeHuec JC (2000) Results of shoulder arthroplasty in locked dislocation and fracture dislocation (Type 2 sequelae). In: Boileau P, Walch G, Mole D (eds) Protheses d'Epaule recul de 2 a 10 ans. Sauramps Medical, Montpellier, pp 307–315
5. Bastian JD, Hertel R (2008) Initial post-fracture humeral head ischemia does not predict development of necrosis. J Shoulder Elbow Surg 17(1):2–8
6. Benegas E, Zoppi Filho A, Ferreira Filho AA et al (2007) Surgical treatment of varus malunion of the proximal humerus with valgus osteotomy. J Shoulder Elbow Surg 16(1):55–59
7. Bogner R, Hubner C, Matis N, Auffarth A, Lederer S, Resch H (2008) Minimally-invasive treatment of three- and four-part fractures of the proximal humerus in elderly patients. J Bone Joint Surg Br 90(12): 1602–1607
8. Boileau P, Chuinard C, Le Huec JC, Walch G, Trojani C (2006) Proximal humerus fracture sequelae: impact of a new radiographic classification on arthroplasty. Clin Orthop Relat Res 442:121–130
9. Boileau P, Trojani C, Walch G, Krishnan SG, Romeo A, Sinnerton R (2001) Shoulder arthroplasty for the treatment of the sequelae of fractures of the proximal humerus. J Shoulder Elbow Surg 10(4):299–308
10. Bono CM, Renard R, Levine RG, Levy AS (2001) Effect of displacement of fractures of the greater

tuberosity on the mechanics of the shoulder. J Bone Joint Surg Br 83(7):1056–1062
11. Bosch U, Skutek M, Fremerey RW, Tscherne H (1998) Outcome after primary and secondary hemiarthroplasty in elderly patients with fractures of the proximal humerus. J Shoulder Elbow Surg 7(5):479–484
12. Brooks CH, Revell WJ, Heatley FW (1993) Vascularity of the humeral head after proximal humeral fractures. An anatomical cadaver study. J Bone Joint Surg Br 75(1):132–136
13. Brorson S, Rasmussen JV, Frich LH, Olsen BS, Hrobjartsson A (2012) Benefits and harms of locking plate osteosynthesis in intraarticular (OTA Type C) fractures of the proximal humerus: a systematic review. Injury 43(7):999–1005
14. Brunner H, Fruth M, Rueckl K, Magosch P, Tauber M, Resch H, Habermeyer P (2012) Die schaftfreie Eclipse-Prothese – Indikation und mittelfristige Ergebnisse. Obere Extremität 7(1):22–28
15. Clinton J, Franta AK, Lenters TR, Mounce D, Matsen FA 3rd (2007) Nonprosthetic glenoid arthroplasty with humeral hemiarthroplasty and total shoulder arthroplasty yield similar self-assessed outcomes in the management of comparable patients with glenohumeral arthritis. J Shoulder Elbow Surg 16(5):534–538
16. Court-Brown CM, McQueen MM (2008) Nonunions of the proximal humerus: their prevalence and functional outcome. J Trauma 64(6):1517–1521
17. Cruess RL (1985) Corticosteroid-induced osteonecrosis of the humeral head. Orthop Clin North Am 16(4): 789–796
18. Darder A, Darder A Jr, Sanchis V, Gastaldi E, Gomar F (1993) Four-part displaced proximal humeral fractures: operative treatment using Kirschner wires and a tension band. J Orthop Trauma 7(6):497–505
19. Dines DM, Warren RF, Altchek DW, Moeckel B (1993) Posttraumatic changes of the proximal humerus: malunion, nonunion, and osteonecrosis. Treatment with modular hemiarthroplasty or total shoulder arthroplasty. J Shoulder Elbow Surg 2(1):11–21
20. Duparc F (2008) Proximal humerus arterial blood revisited. In: Boileau P (ed) Proximal humerus fractures and fractures sequelae. Sauramps Medical, Montpellier, pp 31–37
21. Duparc F, Trojani C, Boileau P (2000) Results of shoulder arthroplasty in cephalic collapse or necrosis following proximal humerus fractures. In: Boileau P, Walch G, Mole D (eds) Protheses d'Epaule recul de 2 a 10 ans. Sauramps Medical, Montpellier, pp 279–289
22. Duquin TR, Jacobson JA, Sanchez-Sotelo J, Sperling JW, Cofield RH (2012) Unconstrained shoulder arthroplasty for treatment of proximal humeral nonunions. J Bone Joint Surg Am 94(17):1610–1617
23. Duralde XA, Flatow EL, Pollock RG, Nicholson GP, Self EB, Bigliani LU (1996) Operative treatment of nonunions of the surgical neck of the humerus. J Shoulder Elbow Surg 5(3):169–180
24. Ficat RP (1985) Idiopathic bone necrosis of the femoral head. Early diagnosis and treatment. J Bone Joint Surg Br 67(1):3–9
25. Galatz LM, Williams GR Jr, Fenlin JM Jr, Ramsey ML, Iannotti JP (2004) Outcome of open reduction and internal fixation of surgical neck nonunions of the humerus. J Orthop Trauma 18(2):63–67
26. Gerber C, Hersche O, Berberat C (1998) The clinical relevance of posttraumatic avascular necrosis of the humeral head. J Shoulder Elbow Surg 7(6):586–590
27. Gerber C, Schneeberger AG, Vinh TS (1990) The arterial vascularization of the humeral head. An anatomical study. J Bone Joint Surg Am 72(10): 1486–1494
28. Gill TJ, Waters P (1997) Valgus osteotomy of the humeral neck: a technique for the treatment of humerus varus. J Shoulder Elbow Surg 6(3):306–310
29. Greiner SH, Diederichs G, Kroning I, Scheibel M, Perka C (2009) Tuberosity position correlates with fatty infiltration of the rotator cuff after hemiarthroplasty for proximal humeral fractures. J Shoulder Elbow Surg 18(3):431–436
30. Gwinner C, Greiner S, Gerhardt C, Scheibel M (2013) Reverse shoulder arthroplasty for fracture sequelae. Orthopade 42:531–541
31. Hawkins RJ, Neer CS 2nd, Pianta RM, Mendoza FX (1987) Locked posterior dislocation of the shoulder. J Bone Joint Surg Am 69(1):9–18
32. Healy WL, Jupiter JB, Kristiansen TK, White RR (1990) Nonunion of the proximal humerus. A review of 25 cases. J Orthop Trauma 4(4):424–431
33. Hertel R, Hempfing A, Stiehler M, Leunig M (2004) Predictors of humeral head ischemia after intracapsular fracture of the proximal humerus. J Shoulder Elbow Surg 13(4):427–433
34. Hettrich CM, Boraiah S, Dyke JP, Neviaser A, Helfet DL, Lorich DG (2010) Quantitative assessment of the vascularity of the proximal part of the humerus. J Bone Joint Surg Am 92(4):943–948
35. LeHuec JC, Trojani C, Boileau P (2000) Sequelae of proximal humeral fractures: validation of the surgical classification. In: Boileau P, Walch G, Mole D (eds) Protheses d'Epaule recul de 2 a 10 ans. Sauramps Medical, Montpellier, pp 317–324
36. Mansat P, Guity MR, Bellumore Y, Mansat M (2004) Shoulder arthroplasty for late sequelae of proximal humeral fractures. J Shoulder Elbow Surg 13(3): 305–312
37. Martinez AA, Bejarano C, Carbonel I, Iglesias D, Gil-Albarova J, Herrera A (2012) The treatment of proximal humerus nonunions in older patients with reverse shoulder arthroplasty. Injury 43(Suppl 2):S3–S6
38. Matsen F (1994) Smothness. In: Matsen FA, Lippitt SB, Sidles JA, Harryman DT (eds) Practical evaluation and management of the shoulder. Saunders, Philadelphia, p 190
39. Meyer C, Alt V, Hassanin H et al (2005) The arteries of the humeral head and their relevance in fracture treatment. Surg Radiol Anat 27(3):232–237
40. Moineau G, McClelland WB Jr, Trojani C, Rumian A, Walch G, Boileau P (2012) Prognostic factors and limitations of anatomic shoulder arthroplasty for the treatment of posttraumatic cephalic collapse or

necrosis (type-1 proximal humeral fracture sequelae). J Bone Joint Surg Am 94(23):2186–2194
41. Nayak NK, Schickendantz MS, Regan WD, Hawkins RJ (1995) Operative treatment of nonunion of surgical neck fractures of the humerus. Clin Orthop Relat Res 313(4):200–205
42. Neer C (1990) Old trauma in glenohumeral shoulder arthroplasty. In: Neer CS (ed) Shoulder reconstruction. Saunders, Philadelphia, pp 222–234
43. Neer CS 2nd (1970) Displaced proximal humeral fractures. II. Treatment of three-part and four-part displacement. J Bone Joint Surg Am 52(6):1090–1103
44. Neyton LG, Garaud P, Boileau P (2006) Results of reverse shoulder arthroplasty in proximal humerus fracture sequelae. In: Boileau P, Walch G, Mole D (eds) Reverse shoulder arthroplasty. Sauramps Medical, Montpellier, pp 81–101
45. Norris TR, Green A, McGuigan FX (1995) Late prosthetic shoulder arthroplasty for displaced proximal humerus fractures. J Shoulder Elbow Surg 4(4): 271–280
46. Palvanen M, Kannus P, Niemi S, Parkkari J (2006) Update in the epidemiology of proximal humeral fractures. Clin Orthop Relat Res 442:87–92
47. Pape G, Zeifang F, Bruckner T, Raiss P, Rickert M, Loew M (2010) Humeral surface replacement for the sequelae of fractures of the proximal humerus. J Bone Joint Surg Br 92(10):1403–1409
48. Raiss P, Kasten P, Baumann F, Moser M, Rickert M, Loew M (2009) Treatment of osteonecrosis of the humeral head with cementless surface replacement arthroplasty. J Bone Joint Surg Am 91(2):340–349
49. Resch H, Hubner C, Schwaiger R (2001) Minimally invasive reduction and osteosynthesis of articular fractures of the humeral head. Injury 32(Suppl 1): SA25–SA32
50. Ring D, McKee MD, Perey BH, Jupiter JB (2001) The use of a blade plate and autogenous cancellous bone graft in the treatment of ununited fractures of the proximal humerus. J Shoulder Elbow Surg 10(6): 501–507
51. Robinson CM, Inman D, Phillips SA (2011) The Plate-Joystick technique to reduce proximal humeral fractures and nonunions with a varus deformity through the extended deltoid-splitting approach. J Orthop Trauma 25(10):634–640
52. Russo R, Vernaglia Lombardi L, Giudice G, Ciccarelli M, Cautiero F (2005) Surgical treatment of sequelae of fractures of the proximal third of the humerus. The role of osteotomies. Chir Organi Mov 90(2):159–169
53. Schliemann BS, Schildhauer TA, Seybold D (2010) Die dorsal verhakte Schulterluxation. Obere Ex tremität 5(4):9
54. Solberg BD, Moon CN, Franco DP, Paiement GD (2009) Locked plating of 3- and 4-part proximal humerus fractures in older patients: the effect of initial fracture pattern on outcome. J Orthop Trauma 23(2): 113–119
55. Solberg BD, Moon CN, Franco DP, Paiement GD (2009) Surgical treatment of three and four-part proximal humeral fractures. J Bone Joint Surg Am 91(7): 1689–1697
56. Sturzenegger M, Fornaro E, Jakob RP (1982) Results of surgical treatment of multifragmented fractures of the humeral head. Arch Orthop Trauma Surg 100(4): 249–259
57. Tauber M, Brugger A, Povacz P, Resch H (2011) Reconstructive surgical treatment without bone grafting in nonunions of humeral surgical neck fractures. J Orthop Trauma 25(7):392–398
58. Tauber M, Karpik S, Matis N, Schwartz M, Resch H (2007) Shoulder arthroplasty for traumatic avascular necrosis: predictors of outcome. Clin Orthop Relat Res 465:208–214
59. Ugwonali OF, Bae DS, Waters PM (2007) Corrective osteotomy for humerus varus. J Pediatr Orthop 27(5): 529–532
60. Walch G, Badet R, Nove-Josserand L, Levigne C (1996) Nonunions of the surgical neck of the humerus: surgical treatment with an intramedullary bone peg, internal fixation, and cancellous bone grafting. J Shoulder Elbow Surg 5(3):161–168
61. Warner JJP, Costouros JG, Gerber C (2006) Fractures of the proximal humerus. In: Heckman JD, Bucholz RW, Court-Brown CM (eds) Rockwood and Green's fractures in adults. Lippincott, Williams & Wilkins, Philadelphia, pp 1161–1210
62. Wellmann M, Struck M, Pastor MF, Gettmann A, Windhagen H, Smith T (2013) Short and midterm results of reverse shoulder arthroplasty according to the preoperative etiology. Arch Orthop Trauma Surg 133(4):463–471
63. Yamane S, Suenaga N, Oizumi N, Minami A (2008) Interlocking intramedullary nailing for nonunion of the proximal humerus with the Straight Nail System. J Shoulder Elbow Surg 17(5):755–759

17 Conservative Treatment of Proximal Humeral Fractures: Prognostic Factors and Outcome

Antonio M. Foruria and Virginia Ruiz-Almarza

17.1 Introduction

Proximal humerus fracture treatment decision-making continues to be controversial. The majority of trauma and shoulder surgeons use the Neer classification to decide if a patient should be treated surgically or not. Neer-promulgated fractures were produced in reproducible planes, individualizing four main fragments: the articular segment, the greater tuberosity, the lesser tuberosity, and the diaphysis. A fragment was displaced when it was separated more than 1 cm from its origin or rotated more than 45°, independent of which was the involved fragment or the direction of the displacement [1]. Nondisplaced fractures would be treated conservatively with good results, whereas displaced ones would be treated surgically because of the poor results that could be obtained with nonsurgical treatment [2]. Although these guidelines have been very useful, the majority of authors recognize now the important limitations of this system: Neer classification was developed in the 1970s, when CT scans were not readily available, and was based on simple X-rays with their well-known limitations [3]; some fracture patterns were not included [4]; the description of the fragments were not accurate [5]; it has a low interobserver and intraobserver reproducibility [6, 7]; and the most important point is that it was based on a personal experience of a great shoulder surgeon, but not on the analysis of comparative data from patients with different injuries treated with different methods, and the criteria selected by Neer, 1 cm or 45° of displacement, were arbitrarily set [8]. As a consequence, we can affirm that the main classification system used currently is just an expert opinion.

After Neer's, other authors have tried to develop classifications, but all failed in giving a clear guideline for treatment. Some examples are the AO system [9], which has too many fracture types and did not improve Neer's system reproducibility; Edelson [10] tridimensional system, which included only displaced fractures assuming Neer's criteria; and others such as Duparc's [11] and Tamai's [12].

Trying to select the patients that would benefit from surgery, there has been also a great interest in trying to establish the factors that could predict the development of avascular necrosis. On this regard, several studies have described the vascular supply of the humeral head [13, 14] and the interruption of the vascularization in different fracture patterns [12]. Hertel established two important criteria that determined the isolation and ischemia of the humeral cephalic segment: the lack of integrity of the posteromedial periosteal hinge and a posteromedial metaphyseal segment extension in continuity with the articular segment lesser than 8 mm [15]. However, despite the initial enthusiasm with which this article was received, the same authors recognized in a

A. M. Foruria, MD, PhD (✉) • V. Ruiz-Almarza, MD
Shoulder and Elbow Reconstructive Surgery Unit, Department of Orthopedic Surgery, Fundación Jiménez Díaz, Avda. Reyes Católicos, 2, Madrid 28040, Spain
e-mail: antonio.foruria@gmail.com; ruiz.almarza.v@gmail.com

F. Castoldi et al. (eds.), *Simple and Complex Fractures of the Humerus*,
DOI 10.1007/978-88-470-5307-6_17, © Springer-Verlag Italia 2015

subsequent paper that the incidence of avascular necrosis in the same patients used for the first study was not related to the initial ischemia encountered, leading to the interpretation that there must be revascularization phenomena and other factors that preclude the possibility of predicting avascular necrosis [16]. After reviewing the literature, we should recognize we still are unable to reliably predict which patients will develop this complication.

When we finally analyze the evidence available, there is still a lack of evidence supporting surgical options over conservative treatment [17]. At this point, the need of further research to establish how we should treat our patients is clear. Until this new evidence is available, we believe we should fully understand the results of conservative treatment in the entire spectrum of injuries when establishing the treatment for a given patient; in our opinion, conservative treatment continues to be the best treatment option for the majority of patients, including some with "displaced" fractures. We will offer in this chapter a review of the results of conservative treatment and describe the prognostic factors determining the results of proximal humeral fractures treated conservatively.

17.2 Outcome of Conservative Treatment

Conservative treatment of proximal humeral fractures is the treatment of choice for the majority of patients. Early mobilization (1 week postinjury) offers a sooner and better outcome, with less pain and without compromising the final result [18, 19]. In minimally displaced [19] and impacted fractures [20], immediate mobilization allows a faster recovery. Patients receiving instructions to perform the physical therapy at home without supervision obtain satisfactory results [21].

Patients sustaining minimally displaced fractures according to Neer's criteria obtain good results in a high percentage of cases, but not in all of them. Good or excellent results can be expected in 80–90 % of patients [22, 23]. Sixty percent of cases can be expected to be pain-free and 10 % to have moderate to severe pain. Mobility can be 90 % of the contralateral shoulder in 80 % of the shoulders; however, complete recovery is only seen in 46 % [24].

Patients with displaced fractures obtain worse results compared to those with undisplaced ones when treated conservatively. Mobility is usually reduced, with values between 90° and 120° of elevation, and Constant scores were lower [25]. However, 30–60 % of patients can obtain reasonably good results [26], and patients' satisfaction can be also good in 60 % of cases [27].

When recommending a specific treatment, it should be taken into account that contrary to what is generally thought, displaced fractures can be successfully treated with nonoperative methods. Furthermore, there is no evidence supporting that surgical treatment would obtain a better outcome; in addition, more surgical patients have a reoperation—one reoperation every nine surgical cases—compared to the need of secondary surgery in conservatively treated cases (relative risk 3.3) [17]. As a consequence, we can say that "displaced fractures have a worse outcome when treated without surgery," but not "displaced proximal humeral fractures have a better outcome when treated surgically" as this last assumption is not supported by the literature.

17.3 Prognostic Value of Facture Pattern and Fragment Displacement

With the evidence available, we could easily reach a point of agreement saying that minimally displaced fractures should be treated conservatively and extremely displaced ones—i.e., a surgical neck fracture without fragment contact or a four-part fracture-dislocation—probably would be better treated surgically to avoid disabling and painful complications. However, after knowing the displacement thresholds published by Neer were arbitrarily set, it could be very difficult to make an unequivocal choice based on the literature for injuries in which an evident deformity exists, but fragments are near each other to allow an easy consolidation; on this regard, how do we

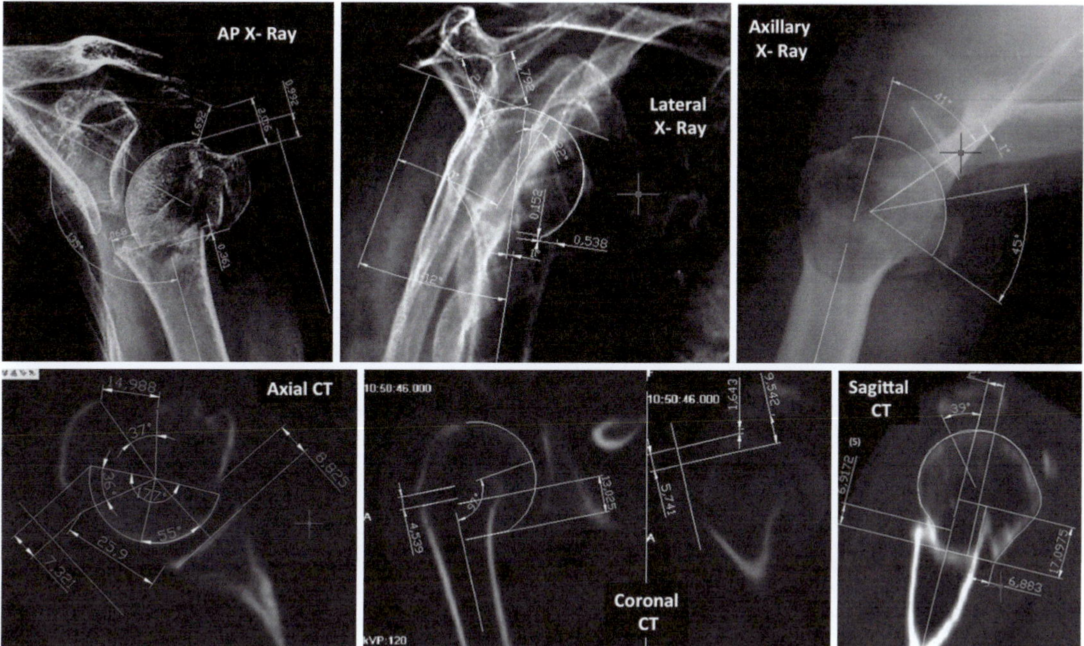

Fig. 17.1 Examples of computed tomography-assisted measurements performed after correction for magnification (Modified with permission and copyright © of the *British Editorial Society of Bone and Joint Surgery* [5])

know an initial deformity is severe enough to produce pain or a significant functional impairment? What is exactly the displacement limit from which the patient will develop a symptomatic malunion?

Some case series dealing with specific fracture patterns are available. It has been published that varus surgical neck impacted fractures have up to 80 % of good results independent of varus angulation [28] and that valgus impacted fractures have a similar outcome, but in these, the displacement appears to have a role in final results [29]. Surgical neck two-part proximal humeral fractures have worse outcome as they are more displaced, but surgery apparently did not improve their result [30]. Greater tuberosity displacement lesser than 5 mm can reach up to 97 % of good results [31].

With the hypothesis that fracture pattern and fragment displacement determine the outcome of conservatively treated proximal humeral fractures, we performed a prospective study including a consecutive series of 93 patients treated conservatively with a year of follow-up, in which standardized X-rays and tridimensional CT scans were performed [5]. We obtained a representative spectrum of injuries, as 40 % of the shoulders had a displaced fracture according to Neer's criteria. Patients were asked the day they had the fracture about their functional status and pain before the injury, and this information was compared to that recovered after 1 year of follow-up. Injured shoulder motion and strength was compared to that of the contralateral healthy shoulder. The same physician with the same home-based exercise program treated all patients nonsurgically. A set of standardized measurements was performed with dedicated software in both X-rays and CT scans (Fig. 17.1), and these values were related with clinical data, represented as the variation of function, motion, pain, and strength obtained by comparing the status "previous" to the injury to that at 1 year of follow-up.

Our study identified four main fracture types including 90 % of fractures (Fig. 17.2):

1. Posteromedial varus impaction with or without tuberosities involvement—54 %
2. Valgus impaction—14 %

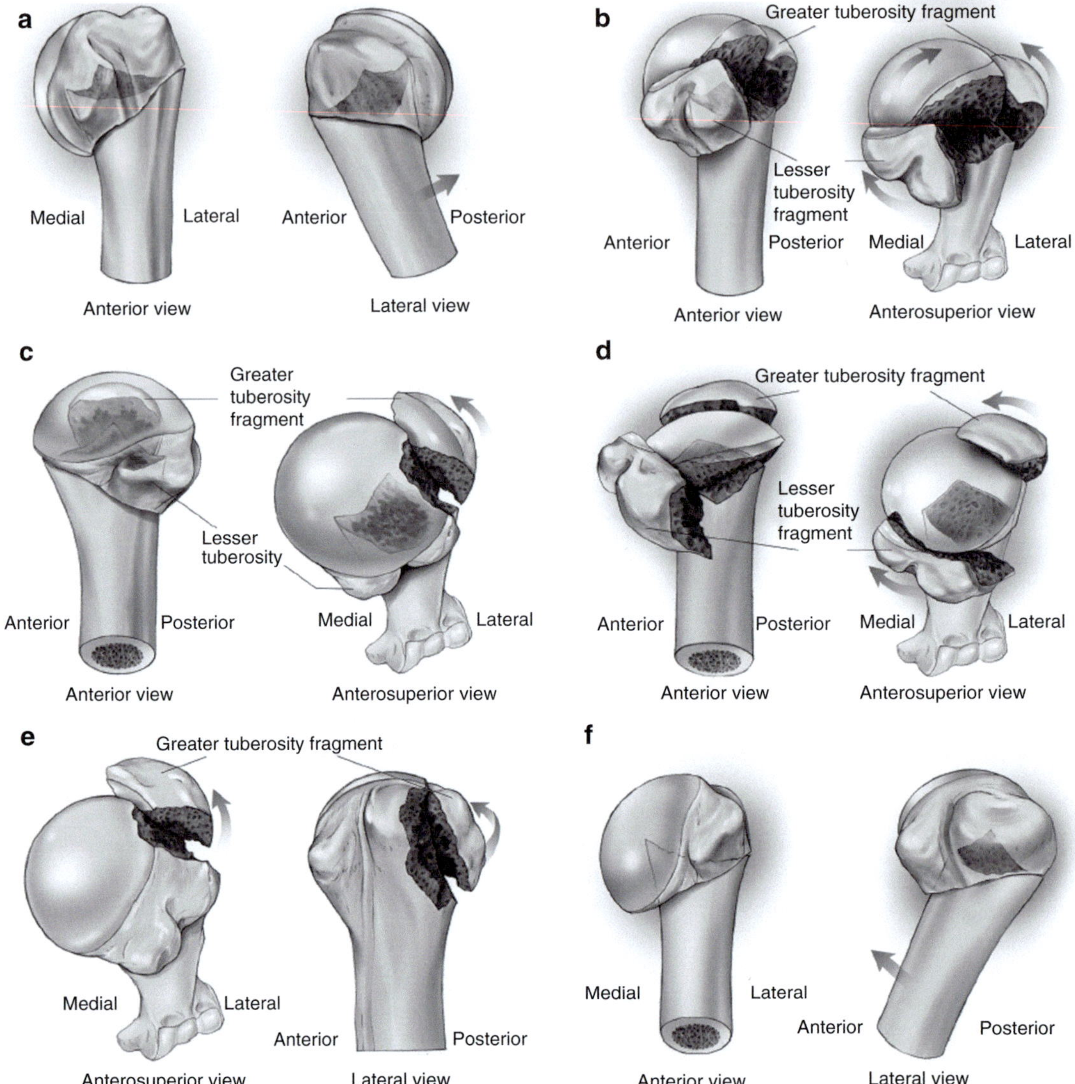

Fig. 17.2 Diagrams of some fracture patterns identified. (**a**) Posteromedial impaction fracture. (**b**) Posteromedial impaction fracture with fracture of both tuberosities. (**c**) Lateral neck valgus impaction fracture with involvement of the greater tuberosity. (**d**) Lateral neck impaction fracture with involvement of both tuberosities. (**e**) Fracture of the greater tuberosity. (**f**) Anteromedial impaction fracture (Reproduced with permission and copyright © of the *British Editorial Society of Bone and Joint Surgery* [5])

3. Isolated fractures of the greater tuberosity—16 %
4. Anteromedial impaction—9 %

A miscellanea group included the rest of the fractures. We found that different fracture patterns had different outcome (Fig. 17.3). Fifty-four percent of valgus impacted fractures had an unsatisfactory result, as well as 25 % of posteromedial varus impacted fractures. The great majority of isolated greater tuberosity and anteromedial impacted fractures had excellent results.

When analyzing fragment displacement in the posteromedial varus impacted fractures with or without tuberosity displacement, we were able to verify that specific fragment displacements correlated with loss of specific outcome parameters (Table 17.1). Motion loss was related to the change of orientation of the cephalic segment and the

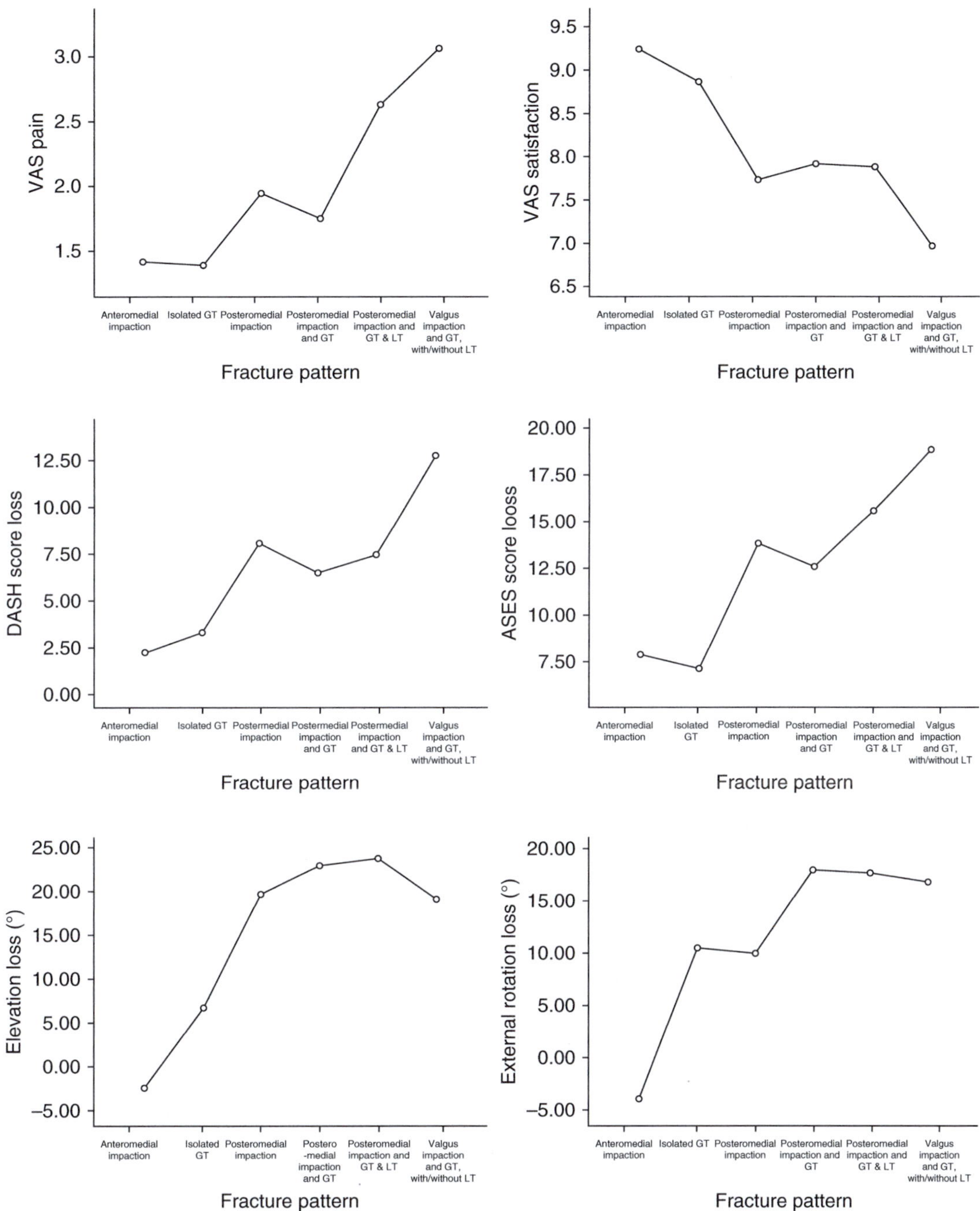

Fig. 17.3 Graphs showing the correlation with the patterns of fracture. (**a**) The visual analog scale for pain. (**b**) The visual analog scale for satisfaction. (**c**) The Disabilities of the Arm, Shoulder, and Hand (DASH) score loss. (**d**) The American Shoulder and Elbow Society (ASES) score loss. (**e**) The elevation loss. (**f**) The external rotation loss. *GT* greater tuberosity, *LT* lesser tuberosity (Reproduced with permission and copyright © of the *British Editorial Society of Bone and Joint Surgery* [5])

interference between fragments surrounding structures: the greater the varus impaction, the greater the elevation loss; the greater the posterior greater tuberosity displacement, the greater the loss of external rotation because of impingement with the posterior glenoid rim; the greater the retroversion,

Table 17.1 Clinical value and statistical signification of correlations between measurements performed in CT triplane reconstructions and outcome variables in all patients ($N=93$)

		Univariate linear regression parameter*/*P* value				
Measurement variable	Measured displacement	ASES change (points)	DASH change (points)	Elevation change (degrees)	External rotation change (degrees)	Internal rotation change (spinal levels)
Axial CT						
AS to Gle angle[a]	>45° retroversion	−15.2 $p=0.008$	+8.7 $p=0.05$	−14.6 $p=0.009$	−14.9 $p=0.02$	−2.1 $p=0.05$
% GT to AS superposition	20 %	−11.0 $p<0.001$	+8.4 $p<0.001$	−9.4 $p=0.002$	−12.8 $p<0.001$	$p=0.06$
Intertuberosity distance	10 mm	−4.3 $p=0.007$	+4 $p=0.001$	−3.3 $p=0.03$	−4.3 $p=0.01$	−0.8 $p=0.009$
GT medial displacement	10 mm	−8.8 $p<0.001$	+5.6 $p=0.005$	−6.6 $p=0.008$	−11.0 $p<0.001$	$p=0.09$
%LT-AS superposition	20 %	$p=0.65$	$p=0.22$	$p=0.47$	$p=0.39$	−6.2 $p<0.001$
Coronal CT						
Increase AS-AC distance	10 mm	−29.7 $p<0.001$	+20.9 $p<0.001$	−26.2 $p<0.001$	−21.7 $p<0.001$	−3.1 $p=0.002$
GT-AS distance (GT above AS)	10 mm	−10.9 $p<0.001$	+7.8 $p=0.002$	−15.5 $p<0.001$	−8.8 $p=0.02$	−1.5 $p=0.02$
Medial impaction	10 mm	−4.0 $p=0.04$	$p=0.09$	−7.5 $p<0.001$	$p=0.11$	$p=0.94$
AS-shaft (varus) angulation	20°	$p=0.32$	$p=0.81$	−4.6 $p=0.003$	$p=0.50$	$p=0.84$
Sagittal CT						
Extension surgical neck	20°	$p=0.11$	+3.6 $p=0.02$	−5.6 $p=0.003$	$p=0.13$	$p=0.44$
Posterior neck impaction	10 mm	$p=0.07$	$p=0.07$	−8.6 $p<0.001$	−5.9 $p=0.02$	$p=0.50$

*Model parameters represent change in outcome from baseline to follow-up for the given displacement (independent variable). Model parameters are not reported for nonsignificant associations
AS articular surface, *Gle* glenoid, *GT* greater tuberosity, *LT* lesser tuberosity, *AC* acromion, *Post* posterior
[a]Angle between the articular surface axis and the perpendicular line to the glenoid face, greater than 45°

the lesser the loss of external rotation. Finally, multivariate analysis defined prognostic models for the loss of motion and function based on combinations of measurements of displacement (Table 17.2).

In a subsequent analysis of image test—X-ray and CT scan—performed at 1 year of follow-up, we observed that initial humeral neck deformity increased during fracture healing in a significant number of patients. However, tuberosity progression of displacement seldom occurred. This fracture settling was significantly greater in older patients and in those fractures that were initially more displaced. This finding represents another source of outcome variability that had not been well studied yet—study pending of publication.

Using the most modern imaging techniques available and dedicated software, up to 57 % of outcome variability could be explained by the initial morphology of the fracture. Other patient, treatment, fracture healing process, or environmental factors could be influencing the final outcome after a proximal humeral fracture.

17.4 Patient-Related Prognostic Factors

Patient characteristics influence fracture pattern, displacement, and outcome after conservative treatment.

Table 17.2 Outcome multivariable models

Outcome variable	Measurement variables to use	Increase in measurement variable displacement	Resultant change in outcome	*P*	R^2
Posteromedial impaction fracture pattern ($N=50$)					
Change ASES (points)	AS-AC distance (mm). Coronal CT	10 mm	−32.4	$p<0.001$	0.40
Change DASH (points)	AS-AC distance (mm). Coronal CT	10 mm	25.6	$p<0.001$	0.34
Change elevation (degrees)	AS-AC distance (mm). Coronal CT	10 mm	−22.1	$p<0.001$	0.48
	AS-diaphysis angle. Lat X-ray	50°	−9.9	$P=0.004$	
Change external rotation (degrees)	GT medial displacement (mm). Axial CT	10 mm	−15	$p<0.001$	0.46
	LT-Glen distance (mm). Axial CT	10 mm	−20	$p<0.001$	
Change internal rotation (spinal levels)	LT-AS % overlapping. Axial CT	10 %	−4.3	$P=0.009$	0.22
	AS-AC distance (mm). Coronal CT	10 mm	−2.5	$P=0.044$	
Change pain (points)	AS-AC distance (mm). Coronal CT	10 mm	2.9	$p<0.001$	0.23
Posteromedial impaction and greater tuberosity fracture ($N=32$)					
Change ASES (points)	Cephalic axis-diaphyseal axis angle[a]. Axillary X-ray	20°	−4.6	$P=0.037$	0.39
	AS-AC distance (mm). Coronal CT	10 mm	−20.4	$P=0.003$	
Change DASH (points)	AS-AC distance (mm). Coronal CT	10 mm	15	$p<0.01$	0.57
	LT-Glen distance (mm). Axial CT	10 mm	8	$p=0.01$	
	Neck extension angle. Sagittal CT	20°	6	$p=0.007$	
Change elevation (degrees)	AS-diaphysis angle. Lat X-ray	20°	−6.6	$P=0.001$	0.45
	Intertuberosity Angle. Axial CT	20°	−4.2	$P=0.004$	
Change external rotation (degrees)	GT medial displacement. Axial CT	10 mm	−16.8	$P<0.001$	0.45
	Cephalic axis-glenoid axis angle[a]. Axial CT	20°	9.6	$P=0.013$	
Change internal rotation (spinal levels)	LT-AS overlapping angle. Axial CT	20°	−4	$P=0.044$	0.44
	Anterior head translation. Sagittal CT	10 mm	−10.5	$P<0.001$	

Each multivariable linear regression model provides the predicted change in the outcome variable for the given displacement (independent variables) defined on the model. The predicted model-based decrease in DASH after a posteromedial impaction and greater tuberosity fracture with an increase of 5 mm of the AS-AC distance, a decrease of 5 mm of the LT-Glen distance, and an extension of the neck of 40° will be 7.5 − 4 + 12 = 15.5 points

AS articular surface, *AC* acromion, *GT* greater tuberosity, *LT* lesser tuberosity, *Glen* glenoid, *Lat* lateral

[a]Measured as increased retroversion

Age is related to displacement; in our sample, displaced fractures according to Neer's criteria occurred in individuals 7 years older compared to those with undisplaced fractures, and this has been found also by other authors [32]. Furthermore, older patients had more often fracture patterns with worse results, as valgus impacted fractures. When only final results are evaluated and they are not related to the previous status, older patients seem to have a worse outcome [22, 33], but this apparent conclusion finding is a consequence of their initial status.

We found in our study that comorbidity did not correlate with age, but it was associated with sustaining a displaced fracture according to Neer's criteria—odds ratio of 4. Those comorbidities were diabetes, cardiac, lung, kidney or digestive diseases, and neoplasm. Furthermore, patients with severe diseases had a worse recovery along the follow-up, with more strength, motion, and functional loss.

Other authors found that patients without underlying diseases had fewer complications and lower consumption of drugs; mortality in patients with associated severe illness was also greater. However, they found no significant differences in final function, Constant-Murley scores, pain, or range of motion [34].

Finally, rotator cuff integrity at the moment of sustaining a proximal humeral fracture is not a predictor of shoulder function; therefore there is no clinical indication for routine imaging of the rotator cuff in patients for whom conservative management is the preferred treatment option [35].

Conclusion

Conservative treatment continues to be the best treatment option for the majority of patients sustaining a proximal humeral fracture. However, specific fracture patterns, such as valgus impaction, and cases with important displacement are associated with pain, motion loss, and functional impairment. Such injury consequences can be anticipated based on the fracture configuration and specific displacement measurements. Patients with advanced age and/or comorbidities have displaced injuries more frequently, but such conditions are not independently associated with greater functional loss. These findings are very useful in counseling our patients; however until information regarding the theoretical superiority of surgery over conservative treatment in the more severe injuries is available, cautious and informed decisions should be made and treatment established in an individual basis.

References

1. Neer CS 2nd (1970) Displaced proximal humeral fractures. I. Classification and evaluation. J Bone Joint Surg Am 52(6):1077–1089
2. Neer CS 2nd (1970) Displaced proximal humeral fractures. II. Treatment of three-part and four-part displacement. J Bone Joint Surg Am 52(6):1090–1103
3. Brorson S, Bagger J, Sylvest A, Hrobjartsson A (2002) Low agreement among 24 doctors using the Neer-classification; only moderate agreement on displacement, even between specialists. Int Orthop 26(5):271–273
4. Jakob RP, Miniaci A, Anson PS, Jaberg H, Osterwalder A, Ganz R (1991) Four-part valgus impacted fractures of the proximal humerus. J Bone Joint Surg Br 73(2):295–298
5. Foruria AM, de Gracia MM, Larson DR, Munuera L, Sanchez-Sotelo J (2011) The pattern of the fracture and displacement of the fragments predict the outcome in proximal humeral fractures. J Bone Joint Surg Br 93(3):378–386, Epub 2011/03/02
6. Kristiansen B, Andersen UL, Olsen CA, Varmarken JE (1988) The Neer classification of fractures of the proximal humerus. An assessment of interobserver variation. Skeletal Radiol 17(6):420–422
7. Sidor ML, Zuckerman JD, Lyon T, Koval K, Cuomo F, Schoenberg N (1993) The Neer classification system for proximal humeral fractures. An assessment of interobserver reliability and intraobserver reproducibility. J Bone Joint Surg Am 75(12):1745–1750
8. Neer CS 2nd (2002) Four-segment classification of proximal humeral fractures: purpose and reliable use. J Shoulder Elbow Surg 11(4):389–400
9. Müller ME, Nazarian S, Koch P (1987) Classification AO des fractures. Springer, Berlin/Heidelberg
10. Edelson G, Safuri H, Salami J, Vigder F, Militianu D (2008) Natural history of complex fractures of the proximal humerus using a three-dimensional classification system. J Shoulder Elbow Surg 17(3):399–409
11. Duparc J (1995) [Classification of articular fractures of the upper extremity of the humerus]. Acta Orthop Belg 61(Suppl 1):65–70
12. Tamai K, Hamada J, Ohno W, Saotome K (2002) Surgical anatomy of multipart fractures of the proximal humerus. J Shoulder Elbow Surg 11(5):421–427
13. Duparc F, Muller JM, Freger P (2001) Arterial blood supply of the proximal humeral epiphysis. Surg Radiol Anat 23(3):185–190
14. Gerber C, Schneeberger AG, Vinh TS (1990) The arterial vascularization of the humeral head. An anatomical study. J Bone Joint Surg Am 72(10): 1486–1494
15. Hertel R, Hempfing A, Stiehler M, Leunig M (2004) Predictors of humeral head ischemia after intracapsular fracture of the proximal humerus. J Shoulder Elbow Surg 13(4):427–433
16. Bastian JD, Hertel R (2008) Initial post-fracture humeral head ischemia does not predict development of necrosis. J Shoulder Elbow Surg 17(1):2–8
17. Handoll HH, Ollivere BJ, Rollins KE (2012) Interventions for treating proximal humeral fractures in adults. Cochrane Database Syst Rev 12:CD000434. Epub 2012/12/14
18. Kristiansen B, Angermann P, Larsen TK (1989) Functional results following fractures of the proximal humerus. A controlled clinical study comparing two periods of immobilization. Arch Orthop Trauma Surg 108(6):339–341
19. Hodgson SA, Mawson SJ, Saxton JM, Stanley D (2007) Rehabilitation of two-part fractures of the neck of the humerus (two-year follow-up). J Shoulder Elbow Surg 16(2):143–145

20. Lefevre-Colau MM, Babinet A, Fayad F, Fermanian J, Anract P, Roren A et al (2007) Immediate mobilization compared with conventional immobilization for the impacted nonoperatively treated proximal humeral fracture. A randomized controlled trial. J Bone Joint Surg Am 89(12):2582–2590
21. Lungberg BJ, Svenungson-Hartwig E, Wikmark R (1979) Independent exercises versus physiotherapy in nondisplaced proximal humeral fractures. Scand J Rehabil Med 11(3):133–136
22. Gaebler C, McQueen MM, Court-Brown CM (2003) Minimally displaced proximal humeral fractures: epidemiology and outcome in 507 cases. Acta Orthop Scand 74(5):580–585
23. Tejwani NC, Liporace F, Walsh M, France MA, Zuckerman JD, Egol KA (2008) Functional outcome following one-part proximal humeral fractures: a prospective study. J Shoulder Elbow Surg 17(2): 216–219
24. Koval KJ, Gallagher MA, Marsicano JG, Cuomo F, McShinawy A, Zuckerman JD (1997) Functional outcome after minimally displaced fractures of the proximal part of the humerus. J Bone Joint Surg Am 79(2):203–207
25. Zyto K (1998) Non-operative treatment of comminuted fractures of the proximal humerus in elderly patients. Injury 29(5):349–352
26. Kristiansen B, Christensen SW (1987) Proximal humeral fractures. Late results in relation to classification and treatment. Acta Orthop Scand 58(2):124–127
27. Rasmussen S, Hvass I, Dalsgaard J, Christensen BS, Holstad E (1992) Displaced proximal humeral fractures: results of conservative treatment. Injury 23(1):41–43
28. Court-Brown CM, McQueen MM (2004) The impacted varus (A2.2) proximal humeral fracture: prediction of outcome and results of nonoperative treatment in 99 patients. Acta Orthop Scand 75(6):736–740
29. Court-Brown CM, Cattermole H, McQueen MM (2002) Impacted valgus fractures (B1.1) of the proximal humerus. The results of non-operative treatment. J Bone Joint Surg Br 84(4):504–508
30. Court-Brown CM, Garg A, McQueen MM (2001) The translated two-part fracture of the proximal humerus. Epidemiology and outcome in the older patient. J Bone Joint Surg Br 83(6):799–804
31. Platzer P, Kutscha-Lissberg F, Lehr S, Vecsei V, Gaebler C (2005) The influence of displacement on shoulder function in patients with minimally displaced fractures of the greater tuberosity. Injury 36(10):1185–1189
32. Court-Brown CM, Garg A, McQueen MM (2001) The epidemiology of proximal humeral fractures. Acta Orthop Scand 72(4):365–371
33. Keser S, Bolukbasi S, Bayar A, Kanatli U, Meray J, Ozdemir H (2004) Proximal humeral fractures with minimal displacement treated conservatively. Int Orthop 28(4):231–234
34. Olsson C, Petersson CJ (2006) Clinical importance of comorbidity in patients with a proximal humerus fracture. Clin Orthop Relat Res 442:93–99
35. Nanda R, Goodchild L, Gamble A, Campbell RS, Rangan A (2007) Does the presence of a full-thickness rotator cuff tear influence outcome after proximal humeral fractures? J Trauma 62(6): 1436–1439

Part II

The Diaphysis

18 The Diaphysis: Nonsurgical Treatment

Konrad Mader, Simone Mader, and Per-Olof Berntsson

18.1 Introduction

Fractures of the humeral shaft are common, account for approximately 3 % of all orthopedic injuries, and result in a significant burden to society from lost productivity and wages [1]. Treatment modalities have greatly evolved since their first description in ancient Egypt (circa 1600 BC); however, fundamental management principles have remained consistent throughout time [2]. Nonoperative management continues as the mainstay for treatment of the majority of these injuries, with acceptable healing in more than 90 % of patients. The treatment of humeral shaft fractures may be the only fracture treatment concept left in the human body, in which nonoperative measures will survive. There is no evidence to this, and we want to cite one of the great orthopedic trauma surgeons on the topic, Ernest Amory Codman: "there is one very striking thing about fractures of the humerus, and that is that most cases eventually recover to pretty good use of the shoulders in spite of any kind of treatment" [3]. This chapter will shed some light on the concept and the actual treatment and evaluate the results we can expect from this treatment.

K. Mader (✉)
Department of Trauma, Hand Surgery and Upper Extremity Reconstruction, Ortopedisk Avdeling, Sentralsykehuset Førde, Førde 6807, Norway

Department of Surgical Sciences, Medical Faculty, University of Bergen, Bergen, Norway

Medical Faculty, University of Cologne, Cologne, Germany
e-mail: konrad.mader@helse-forde.no

S. Mader
Section Trauma, Hand and Upper Extremity Reconstruction, Ortopedisk Avdeling, Sentralsykehuset Førde, Førde 6807, Norway

P.-O. Berntsson
Section Trauma, Hand and Upper Extremity Reconstruction, Ortopedisk Avdeling, Sentralsykehuset Førde, Førde 6807, Norway

Orthopaedisk Avdeling, Danderyds Sykehuset, Stockholm, Sweden

18.2 Relevant Anatomy

The humeral shaft is defined as the expanse between the proximal insertion of the pectoralis major and the distal metaphyseal flare of the humerus. Cylindrical in shape, the shaft inherently provides strength and resistance to both torsional and bending forces. Distally the bone transitions into a triangular geometry with the base posterior; the supracondylar region maintains a narrow anteroposterior dimension. Important osseous landmarks of the humeral shaft include the deltoid tuberosity at the midanterolateral aspect, which serves as the insertion for the deltoid muscle, and the spiral groove posteriorly, which houses the profunda brachii

F. Castoldi et al. (eds.), *Simple and Complex Fractures of the Humerus*,
DOI 10.1007/978-88-470-5307-6_18, © Springer-Verlag Italia 2015

artery and radial nerve as they traverse proximally to distally in a posterolateral direction. The humeral shaft serves as the insertion and origin site for several major muscles of the upper extremity. These play an important role in the biomechanical consequences of different fracture patterns. Muscles inserting on the shaft include the deltoid, pectoralis major, teres major, latissimus dorsi, and coracobrachialis; those originating on the shaft include the brachialis, brachioradialis, and the medial and lateral heads of the triceps brachii. In fractures occurring between the more proximal pectoralis insertion and the more distal deltoid insertion, the proximal fragment is adducted by the pull of the pectoralis and the force of the deltoid pulls the distal fragment upward and laterally. In comparison, fractures occurring distal to both insertions cause abduction of the proximal fragment due to the deltoid, whereas the distal fragment is drawn proximally due to the pull of the biceps brachii, coracobrachialis, and triceps muscles [1].

18.3 The History of Conservative Treatment of Humeral Shaft Fractures

Methods and materials used for immobilization of humeral shaft fractures have remained unchanged over the past several thousand years. In the Edwin Smith Papyrus, circa 1600 BC, Egyptians first described treatment of three humeral shaft fractures with splints made of cloth, alum, and honey [2]. Thirteen hundred years later, the Greeks, in De Fracturis (415 BC), described the use of weights for traction during closed reductions and elaborated on specific methods of splinting with bandages soaked in cerate (an ointment composed of lard mixed with wax) after reduction was performed. The Roman author Celsus (25 BC to AD 50) described in the medical text "De Medicina" different humeral shaft fracture patterns, as well as benefits of fracture reduction including length restoration and reduction of pain. Since the first narrative description, other various splinting techniques have come into vogue, including hanging arm casts, Thomas arm splints, modified Velpeau dressings, coaptation splints, shoulder spica casts, and abduction-type splints, and have been advocated and used, then it will make sense. Despite the various modifications in theme, the basic principle of fracture stabilization has remained unchanged throughout time. The main limitation of many of these earlier splinting techniques was the impairment imparted to the patient with regard to activities of daily living. These apparatuses extended from the shoulder to past the elbow, and the prolonged use required for healing of humeral shaft fractures often resulted in stiffness in both the shoulder and elbow. It was not until 1977, when Sarmiento et al. first described functional bracing, that a major advancement was made and the modern era of splinting was introduced [4]. Since its first inception, functional bracing has become the gold standard for definitive management of the majority of midshaft humeral fractures. A functional brace is an orthosis with an anterior and posterior prefabricated shell that is contoured to accommodate the arm musculature (Fig. 18.1).

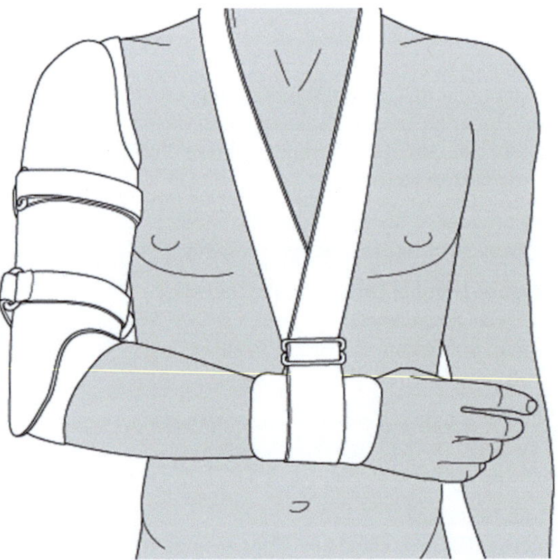

Fig. 18.1 Schematic image of a Sarmiento (functional) brace. The material is a Thermoplastic moldable splint with Velcro straps that can be tightened as swelling subsides to allow continued compression on the fracture. The brace is applied in a manner that allows shoulder and elbow motion

Fracture stabilization is accomplished via the hydrostatic compressive forces of the surrounding soft tissues and is not dependent on the rigidity of the splinting material [5]. As demonstrated by Sarmiento et al. through laboratory analysis, the fracture callous created through functional activity during the reparative process is more robust and is mechanically stronger than that gained through rigid immobilization [4]. The advantage of this type of bracing is that it avoids unnecessary immobilization of other joints and allows for earlier restoration of motion and function to the injured extremity.

18.4 Four Different Types of Conservative Measures Can Be Used

Although good to excellent results have been reported using each of these different treatment modalities, functional fracture bracing has become the most common treatment for closed humeral shaft fractures [6].

18.4.1 The Hanging Arm Cast

The hanging arm cast uses gravity traction provided by the weight of the cast to maintain fracture reduction. Therefore, for this technique to be effective, the patient ideally should remain semierect at all times. The hanging arm cast may be the definitive fracture treatment or can be exchanged for a functional fracture brace. Treatment with the hanging arm cast requires meticulous attention to detail. The cast should be lightweight and applied with the elbow at 90° and the forearm in neutral rotation. The cast should extend at least 2 cm proximal to the fracture. Three plaster or wire loops are applied at the distal forearm in dorsal, neutral, and volar positions; a stockinette is passed through one of these loops and around the patient's neck. Apex anterior angulation is corrected by shortening the sling; apex posterior angulation is corrected by lengthening the sling; apex medial angulation is corrected by using the volar loop; and apex lateral angulation is corrected by using the dorsal loop (Fig. 18.2).

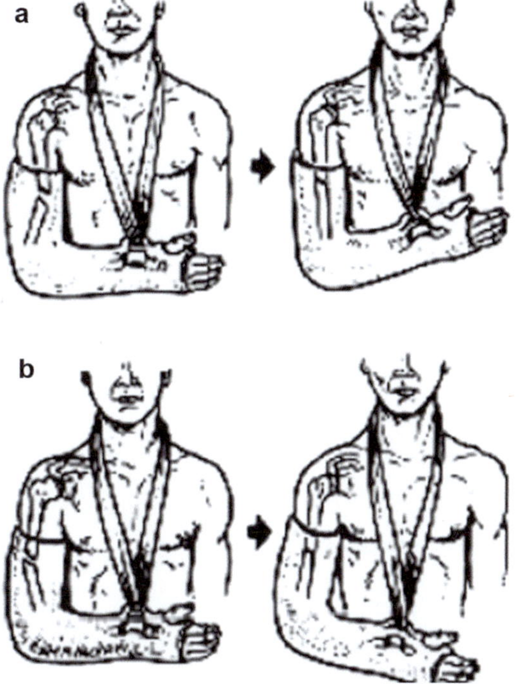

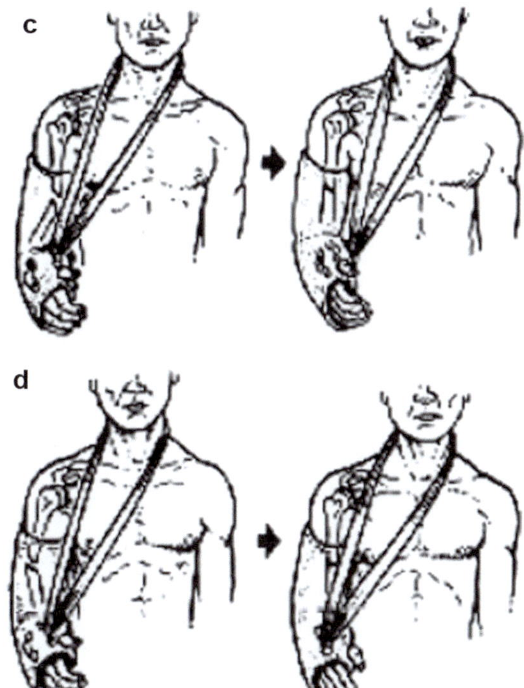

Fig. 18.2 (**a**) With a hanging cast, apex anterior angulation can be corrected by shortening the sling; (**b**) apex posterior angulation is corrected by lengthening the sling; (**c**) apex medial angulation is corrected by using the volar loop; (**d**) apex lateral angulation is corrected by using the dorsal loop (Modified after Taha [6])

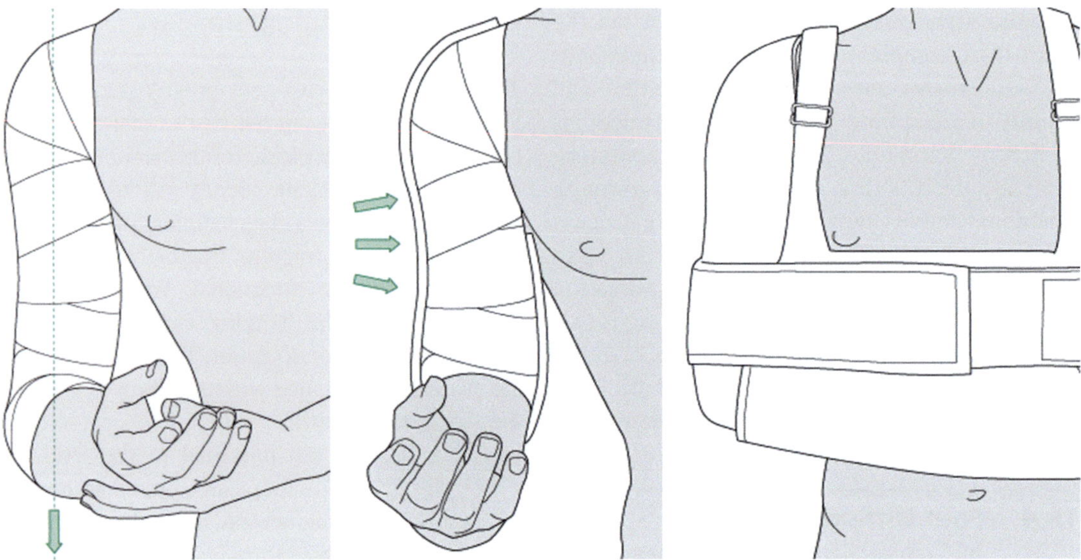

Fig. 18.3 Schematic image of the fabrication of a U-shaped coaptation splint

18.4.2 Coaptation Splint

The U-shaped coaptation splint with collar and cuff is indicated for the acute treatment of humeral shaft fractures with minimal shortening. A carefully molded plaster slab is placed around the medial and lateral aspects of the arm, extending around the elbow and over the deltoid and acromion (Fig. 18.3). The forearm is suspended by a collar and cuff. The splint should hang free of the body. The patient is instructed in range of motion exercises of the shoulder, elbow, wrist, and hand. Similar to the hanging arm cast, the coaptation splint is frequently exchanged for a functional cast brace 1–2 weeks after injury as the patient's pain permits.

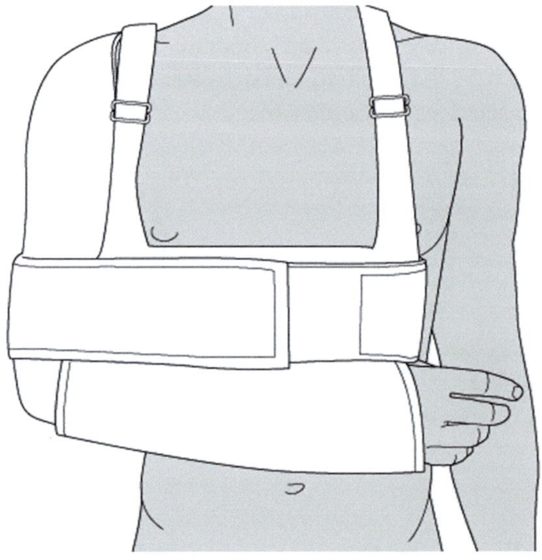

Fig. 18.4 Schematic image of a Velpeau shoulder dressing, which can be fabricated from a single piece of stockinette

18.4.3 Thoracobrachial Immobilization

A stockinette Velpeau shoulder dressing is used for immobilization of the shoulder girdle. This over-the-shoulder device is inexpensive, comfortable, and easily applied (Fig. 18.4). This device is most useful in nondisplaced or minimally displaced fractures in children or the elderly who are unable to tolerate other methods of management.

18.4.4 Functional Bracing

The humeral functional brace was first described by Sarmiento et al. [4]. A functional brace is an orthosis that affects fracture reduction through soft tissue compression. The use of this device allows for shoulder and elbow motion. This brace initially was custom-made and designed as a

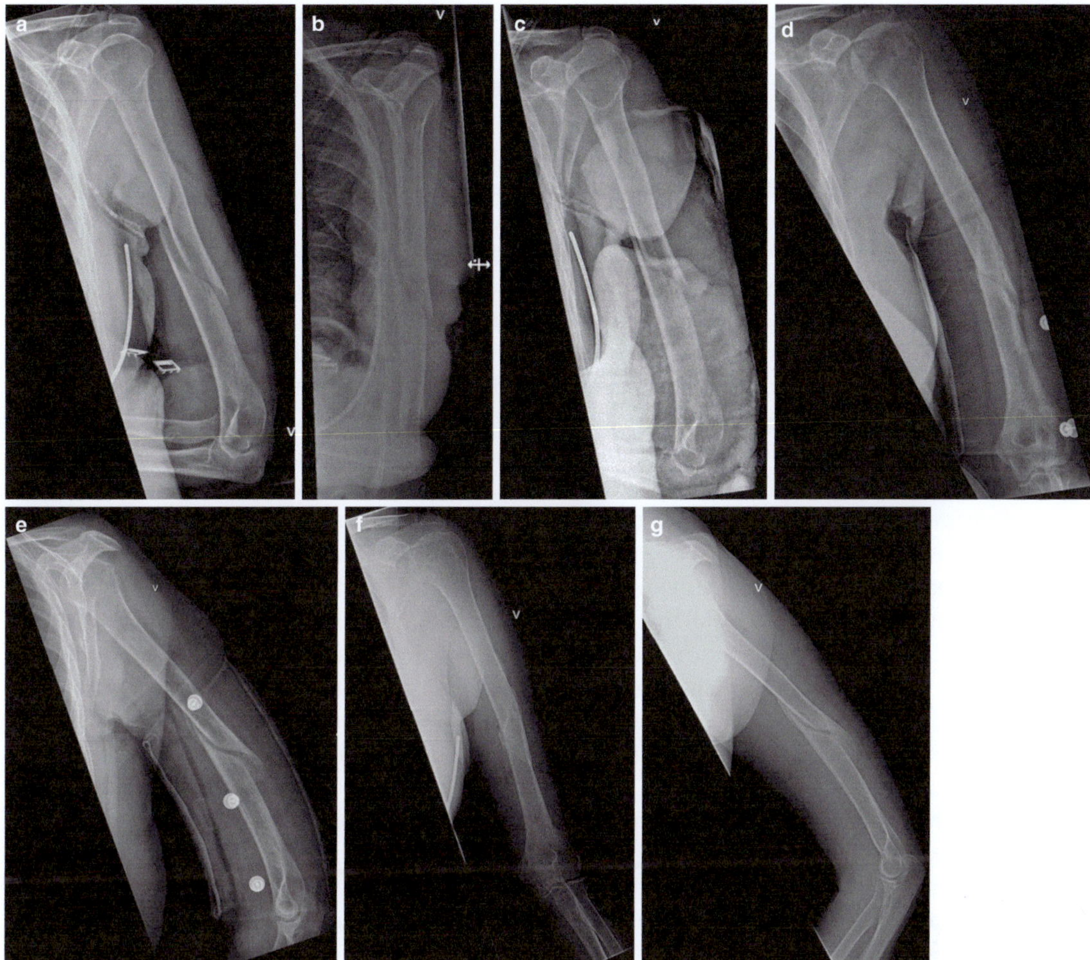

Fig. 18.5 X-ray series of the left humerus in a 66-year-old female patient: (**a**, **b**) trauma X-rays, (**c**) after application of a coaptation cast, (**d**, **e**) after application of a custom-made Sarmiento brace, and (**f**, **g**) after healing of the fracture 10 weeks after trauma

wraparound sleeve. However, current braces are prefabricated and consist of an anterior shell (contoured for the biceps tendon distally) and a posterior shell (Fig. 18.1). These shells are circularized with Velcro straps, which can be tightened as swelling decreases. Sometimes a custom-made Sarmiento brace is necessary (Fig. 18.5).

18.5 Discussion of Current Nonoperative Management

It is important to stress here that virtually nearly all transverse to short oblique humeral shaft fractures are amenable to nonoperative management and recommendations by some authors for immediate surgical intervention are not at all supported by orthopedic evidence (there is only level II study evidence and one randomized controlled trial underway); the Cochrane analysis from 2012 is even more characteristic [7–9]: six completed studies that appeared to meet the Cochrane inclusion criteria. After scrutiny, all six studies were excluded: five were retrospective studies and one was a prospective study without randomization. There is no evidence available from randomized controlled trials to ascertain whether surgical intervention of humeral shaft fractures gives a better or worse outcome than no surgery. One sufficiently powered good quality randomized controlled trial comparing surgical (MIPO plating) versus non-surgical intervention (bracing) for treating humeral shaft fractures in adults is actually ongoing, and it is likely that the results from this and two other ongoing randomized trials will help inform practice in due course [9]. In addition a level III comparative study of extra-articular distal-third diaphyseal humeral fractures brings into play complications: the authors concluded that although operative treatment resulted in more predictable alignment and a potentially quicker functional return, the operative risks were not insignificant and included loss of fixation; infection, which is concerning; and postoperative radial nerve palsy, which is of serious concern [10]. Among the 19 patients treated surgically, a 26 % complication rate was reported. Comparatively, in the group that underwent brace treatment, the end result in each case was a healed fracture with excellent functional outcome, with only minor skin complications due to local brace irritation. Advocates for surgical treatment should acknowledge that even in cases in which brace treatment is a challenge, the literature does not support the superiority of operative treatment [10]. Our current strategy for conservative management of humeral shaft fractures begins with immediate immobilization of the injured extremity via a coaptation splint and/a cuff and collar shoulder sling to provide initial fracture stability, pain control, and resolution of the swelling. Once the soft tissue envelope is adequate, typically after 7–10 days, the initial splint is exchanged for a functional brace that provides circumferential soft tissue compression. When fitted properly, the brace extends medially from 2.5 cm beneath the axilla to 1 cm proximal to the medial epicondyle. On the lateral aspect of the arm, the brace should be placed so that it spans from just below the lateral acromion to a point just above the lateral epicondyle [11]. Velcro straps that are fashioned around the brace are tightened periodically as the swelling subsides to maintain the constant compressive environment during fracture healing. Adequate placement of the orthosis will provide nearly unhindered range of motion of the shoulder and elbow. Active motion of these joints should begin as soon as tolerated. The use of the brace is typically continued for a period of approximately 8 weeks, at which time it is discontinued after clinical and radiological confirmation of fracture healing. In the largest clinical analysis to date, Sarmiento et al. reported on 922 patients treated with a functional brace for both closed and open humeral shaft fractures [11]. In total, 67 % of patients were available for follow-up, and among these patients, 98 % of all closed injuries and 94 % of all open fractures healed. Frequently debated concerns regarding closed management of humeral shaft fractures pertain to the amount of angulation that is acceptable for a good outcome and the proper management of an associated radial nerve injury [1]. Fjalestad et al. added a further concern in treating humeral shaft fractures conservatively, a substantial deficit in external rotation in the shoulder using standardized CT scan [12]. With regard to angular deformities, given the mobility afforded by the shoulder and elbow, malunions of the humeral shaft are well tolerated with minimal functional impairment [1, 10, 11, 13]. Parameters in the acceptable range therefore have included up to 30° of varus angulation, 20° of anterior bowing, and up to 15° of internal rotation; beyond these limits, cosmetic deformity and functional impairment may show clinically [11, 14]. In terms of neurological sequelae, injury to the radial nerve with neurapraxia is the most frequently encountered nerve deficit associated with humeral fractures and is found in up to a fifth of all patients [15]. Spontaneous recovery over a period of 4 months occurs in 70–92 % of patients managed expectantly; therefore, its presence is not an indication for open management and nerve exploration [14–16]. Conversely, nerve loss after application of a brace or closed reduction of the fracture is sometimes considered a relative indication for nerve exploration; however, no studies document improvement with such management, and most authors continue to recommend against operative intervention [17].

18.6 Limitations to Functional Bracing Do Exist (Relative Contraindications)

Open fractures, specifically Gustilo type III injuries with extensive soft tissue stripping, are not amenable to bracing because of the wound contamination, soft tissue deficits, and inherent difficulties with dressing care. These fractures are best managed with immediate stabilization through internal or external fixators. Conversely, in situations where the patient is not hemodynamically stable because of severe head or chest trauma and has several long-bone fractures in a *polytrauma scenario*, external fixation in a "damage control orthopedics"—strategy of the humeral fracture—can aid in nursing care when access to the chest or positioning of the arm is vital to proper ventilation and oxygenation of the patient. *Fracture patterns with a high propensity for nonunion* are also believed to be best managed by immediate fixation to potentially improve the healing rate [18]. Fractures at particular risk include humeral fractures associated with ipsilateral brachial plexus involvement and long oblique fractures with proximal extension. A high risk of nonunion has also been observed in patients *with long oblique fractures* with proximal extension. Soft tissue interposition between the fracture fragments occurs due to buttonholing of the sharp distal fragment through the deltoid muscle belly. Relative indications for surgery also include the cases of "floating elbow" with *concomitant fractures of the humerus and both forearm bones*, *morbidly obese patients* whose bracing is uncomfortable or not feasible because of the impediments of the surrounding soft tissues, and *cases in which closed management has failed* [1]. An unreliable or uncooperative patient will be a challenge for both conservative and operative treatment (Table 18.1). In modern orthopedic times, DRG revenue plays unfortunately a more active role (Table 18.2), the modern DRG-driven reimbursement policy shifts the pendulum more and more toward operative therapy, and it is nearly a shame that financial implications will influence the treatment concept substantially.

Table 18.1 Indications of ORIF in fractures of the humeral shaft

Open fracture
Associated vascular injury
Floating elbow
Bilateral humerus fractures
Humerus fracture in polytrauma patients
Failure of conservative treatment
Radial nerve dysfunction after fracture manipulation
Pathological fracture
Nonunion
Unacceptable malunion
No compliance, uncooperative patient

Table 18.2 Payment for conservative treatment and operative treatment of a humeral fracture

Treatment	DRG	CM	Revenue
Conservative	I17B	0.539	1,569.92€
Nail or plate	I13C	1.528	4,450.53€

Mean costs in the German DRG refunding system, personal communication, Prof. Dr. med. Leonard Bastian, Klinikum Leverkusen, Germany

References

1. Walker M, Palumbo B, Badman B, Brooks J, Van Gelderen J, Mighell M (2011) Humeral shaft fractures: a review. J Shoulder Elbow Surg 2011:1–12
2. Brorson S (2009) Management of fractures of the humerus in Ancient Egypt, Greece, and Rome: an historical review. Clin Orthop Relat Res 467:1907–1914
3. Brorson S (2013) Fractures of the proximal humerus: history, classification, and management. Acta Orthop Suppl 351:1–30
4. Sarmiento A, Kinman PB, Galvin EG, Schmitt RH, Phillips JG (1977) Functional bracing of fractures of the shaft of the humerus. J Bone Joint Surg Am 59:596–601
5. Zagorski J, Latta L, Zych G, Finnieston A (1988) Diaphyseal fractures of the humerus. Treatment with prefabricated braces. J Bone Joint Surg Am 70:607–610
6. Taha MM (2011) The outcome of conservative treatment of closed fractures of the humeral shaft in adult patients. Am Med J 2:32–39
7. Denard A Jr, Richards JE, Obremskey WT, Tucker MC, Floyd M, Herzog GA (2000) Outcome of nonoperative vs operative treatment of humeral shaft fractures: a retrospective study of 213 patients. Orthopedics 11:33
8. Gosler MW, Testroote M, Morrenhof J, Janzing HMJ (2012) Surgical versus non-surgical interventions for treating humeral shaft fractures in adults. Cochrane Database Syst Rev 1:CD008832

9. Matsunaga FT, Tamaoki MJ, Matsumoto MH, dos Santos JB, Faloppa F, Belloti JC (2013) Treatment of the humeral shaft fractures–minimally invasive osteosynthesis with bridge plate versus conservative treatment with functional brace: study protocol for a randomised controlled trial. Trials 14:246
10. Jawa A, McCarty P, Doornberg J, Harris M, Ring D (2006) Extra-articular distal-third diaphyseal fractures of the humerus. A comparison of functional bracing and plate fixation. J Bone Joint Surg Am 88: 2343–2347
11. Sarmiento A, Zagorski JB, Zych GA et al (2000) Functional bracing for the treatment of fractures of the humeral diaphysis. J Bone Joint Surg Am 82: 478–486
12. Fjalestad T, Stromsoe K, Salvesen P et al (2000) Functional results of braced humeral diaphyseal fractures: why do 38 % lose external rotation of the shoulder? Arch Orthop Trauma Surg 120:281–285
13. Koch P, Gross D, Gerber C (2002) The results of functional (Sarmiento) bracing of humeral shaft fractures. J Shoulder Elbow Surg 11:143–150
14. Papasoulis E, Drosos GI, Ververidis AN, Verettas DA (2012) Functional bracing of humeral shaft fractures. A review of clinical studies. J Am Acad Orthop Surg 20(7):423–433
15. Ekholm R, Ponzer S, Tornkvist H, Adami J, Tidermark J (2008) Primary radial nerve palsy in patients with acute humeral shaft fractures. J Orthop Trauma 22:408–414
16. Shao Y, Harwood P, Grotz M, Limb D, Giannoudis P (2005) Radial nerve palsy associated with fractures of the shaft of the humerus: a systematic review. J Bone Joint Surg Br 87:1647–1652
17. Anglen J, Archdeacon M, Cannada L, Herscovici D Jr, Ostrum R (2009) Avoiding complications in the treatment of humeral fractures. Instr Course Lect 58:3–11
18. Spiguel AR, Steffner RJ (2012) Humeral shaft fractures. Curr Rev Musculoskelt Med 5:177–183

Radial Palsy and Humerus Fractures

19

Bruno Battiston, Teresa Benigno, and Pierluigi Tos

19.1 Introduction

Fractures of the humeral shaft are quite common and represent ~1 to 3 % of all fractures. The average age of incidence is older than 50 years [1–3]. Most fractures are simple and associated with low-energy injuries such as a simple fall. The incidence of humerus fractures and concomitant nerve injury can be significant. Noble et al. examined 444 patients with humerus fractures for incidence of concomitant nerve injury and reported a 9.5 % incidence of radial nerve injury, 3 % incidence of median nerve trauma, and 1.5 % incidence of ulnar nerve problems [4]. The majority of these injuries (60 %) were associated with high-energy trauma such as motor vehicle accidents. From this and other reports, the radial nerve palsy seems to be the most common nerve lesion complicating fractures of the humeral shaft, with a frequence of 4–16 % according to the different series [5].

The radial nerve is in close contact with the humerus as it wraps around it into the spiral groove at the posterior aspect of the humeral shaft; it may be injured at the occasion of humeral fracture or entrapped into the fracture site or damaged during closed reduction maneuvers or open reduction and internal fixation procedure [6–8]. Ekholm et al. noted a radial nerve injury incidence of 8 % in their series of humerus fractures [2]. The authors further analyzed the data and found that radial nerve injury occurred in 2 % of proximal, 11.5 % of midshaft, and 20.7 % of distal third fractures. They concluded that fracture type, energy of injury, and patient age were not associated with a higher risk of concomitant radial nerve injury [2]. In 1963, Holstein and Lewis described a higher incidence of radial nerve injury associated with an oblique distal third of humerus fracture pattern [9]. They postulated that the obliquity of the fracture injured or lacerated the nerve as it courses alongside the humerus. Several subsequent investigators have supported their findings [2, 10, 11]. However, other studies demonstrated contradictory findings [12, 13]. Shao et al. performed a meta-analysis of the literature and concluded that there were not enough data to support Holstein and Lewis's original premise [14]. They noted that risk factors for concomitant radial nerve injuries included both middle and mid-distal fractures and both transverse and spiral fracture patterns [14]. Although causes of postoperative radial nerve paralysis are poorly documented in the literature, they have been attributed to several factors such as stretching and elongation of the nerve during fracture manipulation, extensive dissection of the nerve, and the direct compression of the nerve by bone clamps or plate or even because of direct accidental injury to the nerve by the surgical blade [7]. Additionally, the position

B. Battiston (✉) • T. Benigno • P. Tos
Unit of Musculoskeletal Traumatology,
Departmental Unit of Microsurgery,
Hospital Città della Salute e della Scienza, Turin, Italy
e-mail: bruno.battiston@virgilio.it;
teresabenigno@libero.it

F. Castoldi et al. (eds.), *Simple and Complex Fractures of the Humerus*,
DOI 10.1007/978-88-470-5307-6_19, © Springer-Verlag Italia 2015

of the nerve over the plate at the end of the operation may cause chronic friction and conflict between the nerve and the hardware with consequent secondary palsy.

As for nerve recovery possibilities, Ogawa and Ui reported 100 % recovery in one large series [15]. However, other authors as Shao found a statistically significant difference in the recovery between complete (77.6 %) and incomplete (98.2 %) radial nerve palsy and closed (97.1 %) versus open fractures (85.7 %) [14]. While reviewing 101 patients who experienced spontaneous nerve recovery in a meta-analysis of the literature, they also observed that the average time to recovery was 7.3 weeks [14]. One could consider this to be a minimum period of clinical observation.

All these observations may explain why several authors approach differently this type of lesion going from simple clinical control to early surgical exploration, and the debate on the subject is still open.

19.2 Anatomy

The radial nerve [1] is derived from the posterior cord of the brachial posterior cord of the brachial plexus, which receives contributions from all three trunks of the plexus and consequently from the cervical spine nerve roots 5 through 8, with inconsistent contribution from the first thoracic nerve root (T1). As the radial nerve leaves the axilla, it travels along the fibrotendinous junction of the latissimus dorsi and the long head of the triceps. It then continues distally between the long and the medial head of the triceps, sending off motor branches to supply these muscles, as well as the lateral head of the triceps. The motor branch to the medial head of the triceps continues on to innervate the anconeus. Sensory contributions include the posterior brachial cutaneous and posterior antebrachial cutaneous nerves, which supply the posterior aspect of the arm and forearm, respectively. As the radial nerve enters into the arm, it passes from medial to lateral and enters the spiral groove of the humerus. Approximately at the level of the deltoid, the radial nerve passes laterally around the humerus. Although the spiral groove of the radius is frequently described as containing the radial nerve, it is actually the origin of the brachialis muscle. During this path, the nerve has close relationship with the posterior aspect of the humerus as it lies directly on it without any interposed layer of soft tissue over a mean distance of 6.5 cm [16, 17]. The radial nerve continues on to pierce the intermuscular septum 10–12 cm proximal to the lateral epicondyle of the humerus and runs between brachialis and brachioradialis muscles; at this area of emergence, the nerve is relatively fixed to the diaphysis and is therefore more vulnerable [9, 18]. The nerve remains anterior to the humerus and passes along the lateral column, anterior to the capitellum at the elbow. The radial nerve divides into the superficial radial nerve and the posterior interosseus nerve at the level of the radial head.

Although the radial nerve is separated from the humerus by the fibers of the medial head of the triceps proximally and the brachialis laterally, it does travel directly on bone over the distal third of the humerus. Thus, the anatomic location of the Holstein-Lewis fracture is thought to predispose the radial nerve to injury via either laceration or entrapment.

19.3 Diagnosis and Prognosis

In the acute setting, diagnosis of radial nerve injury in patients with humerus fractures is based on clinical examination. Patients present with weakness or paralysis of wrist, finger, and thumb extension. Sensory examination frequently shows diminished or absent sensation of the dorsal and radial aspect of the hand in the distribution of the superficial branch of the radial nerve. The patient is observed clinically for any sign of recovery of the nerve, which is typically seen in the first muscles innervated distal to the injury: the brachioradialis and extensor carpi radialis brevis and longus. The patient should be given a cock-up wrist splint and instructed to perform daily passive wrist, finger, and thumb range of motion exercises to prevent the development of a flexion contracture [19]. Electromyography (EMG) can be a useful adjunct tool in the investigation of associated radial nerve palsy [20, 21]. A baseline EMG at 3–6 weeks after injury provides an index for following evaluations. Typical EMG findings at this initial evaluation include fibrillation potentials, positive sharp waves, and monophasic action potentials (MAPs) of short duration. Repeat examination at 12 weeks should show larger polyphasic action potentials in recovering nerves. Nerves that are not recovering generally show no change in the fibrillation potentials, sharp waves, or MAPs. EMG findings may precede clinical indications of reinnervation by up to 4 weeks.

Radiographic methods that directly verify the entrapment of the radial nerve at the fracture site are limited. Bodner et al. described a case of radial nerve palsy investigated by both magnetic resonance imaging (MRI) and ultrasound [22]. Ultrasound was then used to trace the radial nerve into the zone of injury, and an abrupt change was observed in its course over the site of the fracture, suggesting entrapment of the nerve that was later confirmed surgically. They then prospectively performed ultrasound on 11 patients with a high-energy humeral fracture and associated radial nerve palsy [23]. The examinations were performed between 1 and 8 weeks after the initial injury. In all cases, the radial nerve was easily identified and traced past the zone of injury. The uninjured side served as a control, as did the ultrasound examinations of 10 healthy patients. Surgical fixation and concomitant nerve exploration were performed in 5 of the 11 patients confirming the preoperative diagnosis, and the remaining 6 patients, who had benign findings on ultrasound, recovered fully.

Several characteristics of presentation of radial nerve palsy can be consistently correlated with rates of recovery. Fortunately, most of these lesions are neuropraxic injuries of the nerve: spontaneous recovery is the rule. Pollock et al. reported a recovery rate of 90 % in closed fractures [13], and Sarmiento et al. reported a 100 % recovery rate in 85 patients with distal humeral shaft fractures [24]. However, there is some evidence that the prognosis for recovery with high-energy or open fractures is not as good. Sanders et al. presented 12 cases of open humeral shaft fractures associated with radial nerve injury; only four recovered function [25]. Ring et al. described six radial nerve transections in 24 patients with high-energy humeral shaft fractures with an associated radial nerve palsy [26]. Connolly reported that 4 of 14 radial nerve injuries in patients with open fractures did not recover and required nerve grafting.

Shao agree with Green, Hotchkiss, and Pederson [14, 27], who stated that assuming a nerve regenerates at the rate of approximately 1 mm a day and adding 30 days (as suggested by Seddon [28]), the maximum length of time which may be required for motor recovery to first manifest itself could easily be calculated. This is achieved by measuring the distance on the radiograph from the fracture site to the point of innervation of the brachioradialis muscle, which is approximately 2 cm above the lateral epicondyle. The overall waiting time should not be longer than 6 months. The presence of an advancing Tinel sign can be helpful in suggesting recovery. In a series of patients with peripheral nerve palsies associated with closed fractures and dislocations, Birch noted that when a stronger Tinel sign was present at the level of injury, compared with the growing point, recovery was likely to be poor.

The significance of radial nerve palsy not present initially but that develops after iatrogenic treatment is another area of controversy. These cases are defined as secondary radial neuropathy. The incidence of these injuries ranges from 10 to 20 %. In 1967, Shaw and Sakellarides reported on 45 cases of radial nerve palsy, finding that only 40 % of primary nerve palsies recovered spontaneously, whereas all of the secondary nerve deficits recovered fully [29]. In Shao's meta-analysis of 1,045 cases of radial nerve palsy, 921 palsies resolved fully (88.1 %) [14]. Primary nerve palsy recovery was noted at a rate of 88.6 %; secondary nerve palsy recovery was 93.1 %. This difference between these two groups was not statistically significant. Other recent studies however contradict or at least fail to confirm this doctrine.

19.4 Treatment

Treatment options for radial nerve palsy with associated humeral fracture include expectant observation, early exploration, late exploration, or performing tendon transfers.

Whether or not early exploration of a radial nerve palsy associated with a humeral fracture is due or not is a continual subject of controversy. In some cases, such as an open fracture with radial nerve palsy, there is a clear need for early exploration.

There are differences in opinion regarding the treatment of choice. Early exploration of the radial nerve claims a variety of advantages. It is technically easier and safer than the delayed procedure. Direct examination of the nerve clarifies the diagnosis and the extent of the lesion. Open reduction of the fracture helps to lessen the risk of further neural damage from mobile bone ends. Shortening of the humerus to facilitate nerve repair is better done before healing of the fracture is complete [9, 30, 31]. Early stabilization of the fracture reduces the chance of the nerve being enveloped by scar tissue and callus. Besides, there are accepted indications for exploration of the radial nerve in the setting of a humeral shaft fracture. Clear indications for early exploration include vascular injury, high-velocity gunshot wounds, a high suspicion of nerve laceration, severe soft tissue injury, and sharp or penetrating injury [10, 13, 31–35].

However, opponents of early exploration have observed high rate of spontaneous recovery and have advised a policy of expectancy [10, 11, 13, 36–39], believing that this approach mitigates an unnecessary complications attendant on exploration. Late exploration may avoid unnecessary early surgery in patients who would otherwise obtain spontaneous recovery, may allow for nerve recovery in an environment more conducive to healing, and allows for nerve sheath to thicken providing for easier repair of the nerve if necessary. Finally, it may be easier to treat the nerve when the fracture is healed. Potential disadvantages include the possibility that nerve exploration can become more difficult due to scarring.

Late exploration of radial nerve injuries associated with humerus fractures is somewhat controversial. The findings at the time of surgery and outcomes following treatment are variable. Shao et al. noted that the incidence of nerve entrapment ranged from 6 to 25 %, and the incidence of nerve laceration noted was 20–42 %.

However, in the case of a closed humeral fracture with radial nerve palsy, consistent reports in the literature show that at least 70 % of patients experience spontaneous recovery [9, 11, 26, 28, 31, 33, 35–38, 40]. In a series of 59 patients with complete radial nerve palsy, half of which were treated with early exploration and the other half with expectant management, an overall recovery rate was found to be 78 %, 73 % in the early exploration group, and 83 % in the observation group. Eighty-five percent of the explored cases showed the nerve to be only contused.

In a review of 14 cases of radial nerve palsy associated with open humerus fracture, 64 % of patients were found to have a surgically correctable radial nerve injury [32]. Even after repair of the radial nerve, none of these patients recovered sensation, but only one patient failed to recover motor function and required tendon transfer.

Sonneveld et al. reviewed 17 humerus fractures with radial nerve injury, 16 of which were closed [39]. Fourteen underwent early exploration, and on inspection 13 appeared undamaged and 1 had a contusion with mild laceration. Twelve completely recovered, including the one case with gross injury; two partially recovered. All three patients that were observed recovered fully. The authors concluded that most concomitant radial nerve injuries recover and surgical exploration is unnecessary. Bostman et al. in two related studies, reported on 75 patients with humerus fractures and associated radial nerve injury [12, 41]. The authors concluded that routine early exploration could not be justified and the decision for exploration should be based on the nature of the fracture and not the function of the nerve.

Delay beyond 5 months is associated with poorer outcomes [10]. However, other reports suggest healing rates are comparable to early exploration and repair [42]. Although the optimal timing of late exploration has been debated, most investigators suggest it is best performed between 4 and 6 months postinjury [10, 43, 44]. Shaw and Sakellarides [29] reviewed a series of patients and concluded that the nerve should be explored at 7–8 weeks if there is no evidence of return of function. The reasons for this decision were that all patients in their series showed some signs of recovery of nerve function within the first 2 months and unnecessary operation would be avoided in most patients, in whom spontaneous nerve recovery would occur; furthermore, there is no interference with fracture healing, and the waiting period allows the neuroma to become well delineated and to be adequately resected but is short enough to minimize nerve retraction. Goldner and Kelley [45] advocated a similar position, but they considered the absence of an advancing Tinel sign to be an important added indication for exploration at 6–8 weeks. They go on to say, however, that "a longer waiting period could not be criticized, because some of the patients in this group recovered completely without sign of motor recovery for 20 weeks." Amillo and associates [10] recommended surgical exploration at 3 months if there are no clinical or electrophysiological signs of nerve recovery.

Some authorities recommend that baseline electromyography and nerve conduction studies be performed at 3 weeks postinjury so that later studies can be compared to them [46, 47]. The patient is observed clinically for any sign of recovery of the nerve, which is typically seen in the first muscles innervated distal to the injury: the brachioradialis and extensor carpi radialis brevis and longus. The electric equivalent is the development of action potentials where complete denervation or fibrillation was noted before. If no electric or clinical activity can be identified by 3–4 months postinjury (depending on the site of the fracture), then surgical exploration of the nerve is indicated [19]. This plan of management is based on the work of Seddon [48, 49] regarding nerve regeneration. Assuming that a nerve regenerates at the rate of approximately 1 mm/day and adding 30 days for an initial latent period as Seddon [48] suggested, the maximum length of time that may be required for motor recovery first to manifest itself can easily be calculated by measuring the distance on the X-ray from the fracture site to the point of innervation of the brachioradialis muscle (approximately 2 cm above the lateral epicondyle). In most midshaft humerus fractures, this distance is 90–120 mm. The major advantages of this plan of management are that unnecessary operative intervention is avoided in most patients, most of these patients achieve full recovery of the radial nerve without surgical treatment, and the humerus fracture usually is healed. A question that must be raised is whether the delay in nerve repair for the very few patients in whom neurorrhaphy becomes necessary is excessive and would lessen the chances for good functional recovery. According to Sunderland [50], a delay of 12 months or longer is not likely to jeopardize functional motor return after nerve repair. Seddon [51] reported that prognosis for good recovery worsens only after a 12-month delay, quoting Zachary's conclusions that the radial nerve can be repaired successfully 9–16 months after injury, depending on the level of injury.

In some cases of exploration of the radial nerve, a nerve graft may be indicated. Performing nerve repair free of any tension is essential for optimal nerve recovery [52]. Delayed exploration of a severed nerve can result in retraction of the nerve ends due to its elastic properties. Repair of a nerve in such a situation would necessitate grafting to ensure the repair is tension-free. Additionally, damaged areas of nerves, if present, should be resected back to healthy nerve tissue, requiring grafting. Functional recovery after nerve grafting is related to the length of the defect and the time interval from injury [53]. Nunley et al. reported that 85 % of patients grafted within 6 months of injury obtained M3 or better motor recovery, and no patient grafted after 12 months gained useful function [54]. The length of nerve graft does not appear to play a significant role in functional recovery until lengths exceed 10 cm. Shergill noted that no patient with a graft length >10 cm obtained good results.

Tendon transfers are most often advocated as secondary procedures for patients not experiencing neurological recovery 1 year after nerve

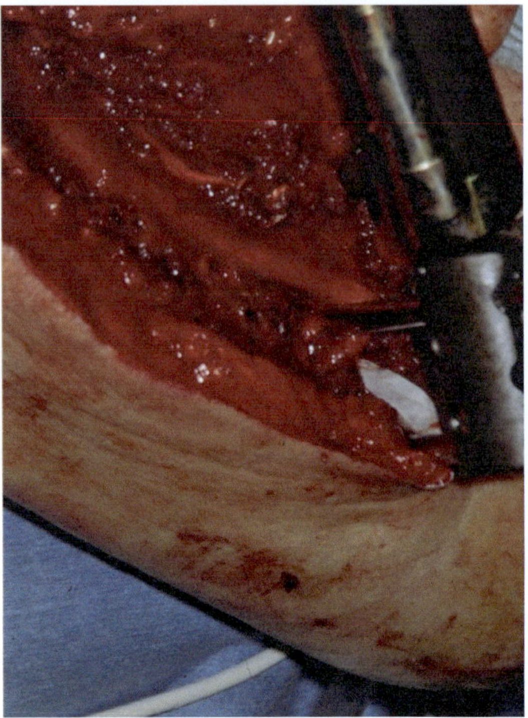

Fig. 19.1 Radial nerve entrapped by external fixation screw. The early exploration, following the secondary nerve palsy, allowed a simple decompression with screw reposition. The radial nerve recovered in 2 weeks

repair [55]. Some investigators have recommended simultaneous nerve repair along with tendon transfer [56]. Given the high rates of functional recovery after radial nerve repair, others find this combined approach unnecessary [57]. Tendon transfer is a reliable salvage for nerves that fail to recover, often resulting in excellent functional outcomes, and some authors advocate this even as a first choice in aged patients or even in noncompliant patients not wishing to wait for nerve repair and regeneration.

Another point regarding early exploration deals with patients who develop "secondary" radial nerve paralysis in conjunction with a fractured humerus, that is, the nerve is intact when the patient is first seen and subsequently goes out, usually after fracture reduction. In several articles [29, 33, 58], this situation was cited as an absolute indication for immediate nerve exploration (Fig. 19.1), although more than one study [12, 37] has offered convincing evidence that even secondary radial nerve paralysis can be treated nonoperatively with good expectation for full recovery in most cases.

19.5 Surgical Procedure

The majority of authors preferred a lateral approach of the humerus in semi-sitting position. This is also our standard approach. A lateral skin incision is made from the tip of the deltoid V to the lateral epicondyle; it can be extended proximally as for a deltopectoral approach if needed. The radial nerve is first identified at its emergence from the lateral intermuscular septum and dissected anteriorly and distally between brachialis and brachioradialis muscles. At this point, the nerve is isolated, and reduction and fixation of the fracture with plate and screws is finally achieved [6] (Fig. 19.2).

Many authors preferred the posterior approach [6–30, 40, 59–62], in lateral position to explore the radial nerve. A longitudinal incision is made in the midline of the posterior aspect of the arm, from 8 cm below the acromion to the olecranon fossa. The deep fascia of the arm is incised in line with skin incision. The gap is indentified between the lateral and long heads of the triceps muscle. The interval between the two heads is proximally developed by blunt dissection, retracting the lateral head laterally and the long head medially. Their common tendon is distally split along the line of the skin incision by sharp dissection. The radial nerve and the accompanying profunda brachii vessels are identified. The fracture is exposed and fixed with a plate that is put on the posterior surface of the humerus anterior to the radial nerve.

If the nerve is severed, there are no doubts on its reconstruction by means of suture or grafts. If the nerve is in continuity, its function of the nerve is tested by intraoperative electric nerve stimulation and also by detecting the nerve integrity by its normal glistening whitish color, soft in consistency with normal nerve sheath containing longitudinal blood vessels. The use of magnification facilitates the identification of healthy nerve tissue from the injured and edematous nerve

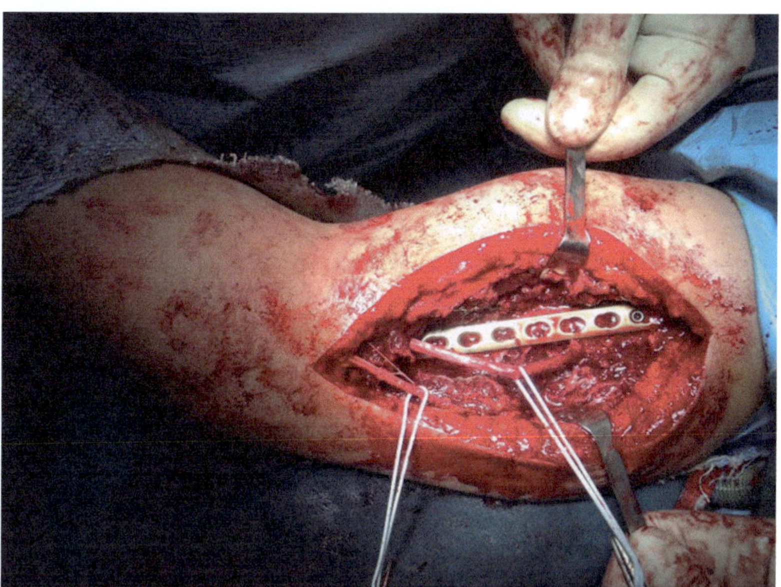

Fig. 19.2 Lateral approach to the humerus

tissues. Resection of the damaged portion of the nerve is followed by cable graft reconstruction using sural nerve. If nerve reconstruction is unsuccessful or not indicated, tendon transfers are an ideal procedure to restore function, since the major contribution of the radial nerve to the hand is the motor function.

Some authors reported trans-fracture transposition of the radial nerve through lateral approach [6, 7, 63, 64]. The authors believe that this procedure allows a better exposure of the fracture site, protects the radial nerve during manipulations and reduction, and facilitates the application of longer plates.

19.6 Proposed Algorithm Treatment

Humeral shaft fractures with radial nerve palsy has been the debate since this entity was originally described and continues to be a controversial subject among upper extremity surgery.

Generalized guidelines based on the literature can be stipulated as follows. Open fractures or any fracture with concomitant radial nerve palsy that warrants operative fixation should undergo exploration of the nerve at the time of fixation. Some types of injuries, i.e., high-energy trauma and/or oblique fractures of the lower third of the humerus, are highly suspicious for an important radial nerve lesion. In such cases, an open reduction and fixation of the fracture with early nerve exploration is more suggested than other fracture treatments. Then, the indication for early exploration of the radial nerve appears to be based best on the type of trauma and type of fracture and on the decision of how to treat the fracture than on the clinical suspect of severe nerve lesion.

Radial nerve status can be kept under clinical control in fractures that would otherwise be treated nonoperatively. Ultrasound shows promise as a useful adjunct for visualizing the radial nerve. If the nerve is intact, observation can be continued. If the nerve is clearly severed, exploration is warranted. Repairable nerves should be microsurgically reconstructed by means of suture or graft. When ultrasounds or MRI suggests the possibility of an entrapped nerve, it should be explored.

We agree with many authors that there is no need to be too aggressive and that, except the clear indications for an early exploration, we may wait for a spontaneous nerve recovery. In studies drawn from major trauma centers where consecutive series of patients with humeral shaft fractures complicated by radial nerve palsy were evaluated, virtually all the authors [12, 13, 37, 65,

66] agree that nonoperative management of the radial nerve palsy is the treatment of choice. However, the waiting time should not be too long: if no sign of recovery appears by 3–4 months from the injury, a radial nerve exploration is suggested. In fact, we think that an excessive delay would lessen the chances for good functional recovery (need of longer grafts, long denervation time of the muscles, etc.).

Tendon transfers are indicated for irreparable nerves or for patients with long persistent nerve palsy.

Finally, a different approach should be used for secondary nerve palsies: especially in cases where open procedures (plates) in which the nerve was not well visualized or even in closed reduction fixed by external devices with "dangerous positioned screws," we think that early nerve exploration could avoid to underestimate a severe nerve lesion, reducing the medicolegal sequelae.

References

1. Elton SG, Rizzo M (2008) Management of radial nerve injury associated with humeral shaft fractures: an evidence-based approach. J Reconstr Microsurg 24:569–574
2. Ekholm R, Adami J, Tidermark J, Hansson K, Tornkvist H, Ponzer S (2006) Fractures of the shaft of the humerus: an epidemiological study of 401 fractures. J Bone Joint Surg Br 88(11):1469–1473
3. Tytherleigh-Strong G, Walls N, McQueen MM (1998) The epidemiology of humeral shaft fractures. J Bone Joint Surg Br 80(2):249–253
4. Noble J, Munro CA, Prasad VS, Midha R (1998) Analysis of upper and lower extremity peripheral nerve injuries in a population of patients with multiple injuries. J Trauma 45(1):116–122
5. Venouziou AI, Dailiana ZH, Varitimidis SE, Hantes ME, Gougoulias NE, Malizos KN (2011) Radial nerve palsy associated with humeral shaft fracture. Is the energy of trauma a prognostic factor? Injury 42(11):1289–1293. doi:10.1016/j.injury.2011.01.020
6. Chamseddine AH, Zein HK, Alasiry AA, Mansour NA, Bazzal AM (2013) Trans-fracture transposition of the radial nerve during the open approach of humeral shaft fractures. Eur J Orthop Surg Traumatol 23(6):725–730. doi:10.1007/s00590-012-1065-1
7. El Ayoubi L, Karmouta A, Roussignol X, Auquil-Auckbur I, Milliez PY, Dupare F (2003) Transposition antérieure du nerf radiai dans les fractures du 1/3 moyen de l'humérus: bases anatomiques et applications cliniques. Rev Chir Orthop Reparatrice Appar Mot 89:537–543
8. Paris H, Tropiano P, Clouet D'Orval B, Chaudel H, Poitout DG (2000) Fracture diaphysaire de l'humérus: ostéosynlhèse systématique par plaque. Rev Chir Orthop 86:346–359
9. Holstein A, Lewis GM (1963) Fractures of the humerus with radial nerve paralysis. J Bone Joint Surg Am 45:1382–1388
10. Amillo S, Barrios RH, Martinez-Peric R, Losada JI (1993) Surgical treatment of the radial nerve lesions associated with fractures of the humerus. J Orthop Trauma 7(3):211–215
11. Samardzic M, Grujicic D, Milinkovic ZB (1990) Radial nerve lesions associated with fractures of the humeral shaft. Injury 21(4):220–222
12. Bostman O, Bakalim G, Vainionpaa S, Wilppula E, Patiala H, Rokkanen P (1986) Radial palsy in shaft fracture of the humerus. Acta Orthop Scand 57(4):316–319
13. Pollock FH, Drake D, Bovill EG, Day L, Trafton PG (1981) Treatment of radial neuropathy associated with fractures of the humerus. J Bone Joint Surg Am 63(2):239–243
14. Shao YC, Harwood P, Grotz MR, Limb D, Giannoudis PV (2005) Radial nerve palsy associated with fractures of the shaft of the humerus: a systematic review. J Bone Joint Surg Br 87(12):1647–1652
15. Ogawa K, Ui M (1997) Humeral shaft fracture sustained during arm wrestling: report on 30 cases and review of the literature. J Trauma 42(2):243–246
16. Yakkanti MR, Roberts CS, Murphy J, Acland RD (2008) Anterior transposition of the radial nerve: a cadaveric study. J Orthop Trauma 22:705–708
17. Guse TR, Ostrum RF (1995) The surgical anatomy of the radial nerve around the humerus. Clin Orthop Relat Res 320:149–153
18. Bonnevialle P (1996) Fraetures récentes el anciennes de la diaphyse humérale. Conférences d'enseignement de la SOFCOT 1996. Expansion Scientifique Paris 55:79–96
19. McKee MD (2006) Fractures of the shaft of the humerus. In: Rockwood CA, Green's DP (eds) Fractures in adults. Lippincott Williams & Wilkins, Philadelphia, pp 1119–1159
20. Lowe JB III, Sen SK, Mackinnon SE (2002) Current approach to radial nerve paralysis. Plast Reconstr Surg 110(4):1099–1113
21. Shah JJ, Bhatti NA (1983) Radial nerve paralysis associated with fractures of the humerus: a review of 62 cases. Clin Orthop Relat Res 172:171–176
22. Bodner G, Huber B, Schwabegger A, Lutz M, Waldenberger P (1999) Sonographic detection of radial nerve entrapment within a humerus fracture. J Ultrasound Med 18(10):703–706
23. Bodner G, Buchberger W, Schocke M et al (2001) Radial nerve palsy associated with humeral shaft fracture: evaluation with US: initial experience. Radiology 219(3):811–816
24. Sarmiento A, Horowitch A, Aboulafia A et al (1990) Functional bracing for comminuted extra-articular fractures of the distal third of the humerus. J Bone Joint Surg Br 72(2):283–287

25. Sanders R, Yach J, Dipasquale T et al (2000) Radial nerve palsy associated with humeral fractures. Presented at the 16th Annual Meeting of the Orthopaedic Trauma Association, San Antonio
26. Ring D, Chin K, Jupiter JB (2004) Radial nerve palsy associated with high-energy humeral shaft fractures. J Hand Surg Am 29:144–147
27. Green DP, Hotchkiss RN, Pederson WC (1999) Green's operative hand surgery, vol 2. Churchill Livingstone, New York, p 1492
28. Seddon HJ (1963) Nerve grafting. J Bone Joint Surg Br 45-B:447–461
29. Shaw JL, Sakellarides H (1967) Radial-nerve paralysis associated with fractures of the humerus: a review of forty-five cases. J Bone Joint Surg Am 49(5):899–902
30. Noaman H, Khalifa AR, El-Deen MA, Shiha A (2008) Early surgical exploration of radial nerve injury associated with fracture shaft humerus. Microsurgery 28(8):635–642. doi:10.1002/micr.20542
31. Dabezies EJ, Banta CJ II, Murphy CP, d'Ambrosia RD (1992) Plate fixation of the humeral shaft for acute fractures, with and without radial nerve injuries. J Orthop Trauma 6:10–13
32. Foster RJ, Swiontkowski MF, Bach AW, Sack JT (1993) Radial nerve palsy caused by open humeral shaft fractures. J Hand Surg Am 18(1):121–124
33. Garcia A Jr, Maeck BH (1960) Radial nerve injuries in fractures of the shaft of the humerus. Am J Surg 99:625–627
34. Modabber MR, Jupiter JB (1998) Operative management of diaphyseal fractures of the humerus: plate versus nail. Clin Orthop Relat Res 347:93–104
35. Packer JW, Foster RR, Garcia A, Grantham SA (1972) The humeral fracture with radial nerve palsy: is exploration warranted? Clin Orthop Relat Res 88:34–38
36. Larsen LB, Barfred T (2000) Radial nerve palsy after simple fracture of the humerus. Scand J Plast Reconstr Surg Hand Surg 34:363–366
37. Shah JJ, Bhatti NA (1983) Radial nerve paralysis associated with fractures of the humerus: a review of 62 cases. Clin Orthop 172:171–176
38. Kettelkamp DB, Alexander H (1967) Clinical review of radial nerve injury. J Trauma 7:424–432
39. Sonneveld GJ, Patka P, van Mourik JC, Broere G (1987) Treatment of fractures of the shaft of the humerus accompanied by paralysis of the radial nerve. Injury 18:404–406
40. Mast JW, Spiegel PG, Harvey JP Jr, Harrison C (1975) Fractures of the humeral shaft: a retrospective study of 240 adult fractures. Clin Orthop Relat Res 112:254–262
41. Bostman O, Bakalim G, Vainionpaa S, Wilppula E, Patiala H, Rokkanen P (1985) Immediate radial nerve palsy complicating fracture of the shaft of the humerus: when is early exploration justified? Injury 16(7):499–502
42. Omer GE Jr (1982) Results of untreated peripheral nerve injuries. Clin Orthop Relat Res 163:15–19
43. DeFranco MJ, Lawton JN (2006) Radial nerve injuries associated with humeral fractures. J Hand Surg Am 31(4):655–663
44. Mohler LR, Hanel DP (2006) Closed fractures complicated by peripheral nerve injury. J Am Acad Orthop Surg 14(1):32–37
45. Goldner J, Kelley JM (1958) Radial nerve injuries. South Med J 51:873–883
46. Swenson MR, Villasana DR (1991) Neurologic evaluation of the upper extremity. In: Kasdan ML (ed) Occupational hand and upper extremity injuries and diseases. Hanley and Belfus, Philadelphia, pp 115–130
47. Bodine SC, Lieber RL (1994) Peripheral nerve physiology, anatomy, and pathology. In: Simon SR (ed) Orthopaedic basic science. American Academy of Orthopaedic Surgeons, Rosemont, pp 325–396
48. Seddon H (1947) Nerve lesions complicating certain closed bone injuries. JAMA 135:691–694
49. Seddon H (1975) Surgical disorders of the peripheral nerves. Churchill Livingstone, Edinburgh
50. Sunderland S (1978) When are attempts at nerve repair no longer justified? In: Sunderland S (ed) Nerves and nerve injuries. Churchill Livingstone, Edinburgh, pp 507–509
51. Seddon H (1972) Factors influencing indications for operation. In: Seddon H (ed) Surgical disorders of the peripheral nerves. Williams & Wilkins, Baltimore, pp 240–245
52. Millesi H, Meissl G, Berger A (1972) The interfascicular nerve grafting of the median and ulnar nerves. J Bone Joint Surg Am 54(4):727–750
53. Shergill G, Bonney G, Munshi P, Birch R (2001) The radial and posterior interosseous nerves: results for 260 repairs. J Bone Joint Surg Br 83(5):646–649
54. Nunley JA, Saies AD, Sandow MJ, Urbaniak JR (1996) Results of interfascicular nerve grafting for radial nerve lesions. Microsurgery 17(8):431–437
55. Sunderland S (1991) Decision making in clinical management of nerve injury and repair. In: Sunderland S (ed) Nerve injuries and their repair. Edinburgh, Churchill Livingstone, pp 413–431
56. Burkhalter WE (1974) Early tendon transfer in upper extremity peripheral nerve injury. Clin Orthop Relat Res 104:68–79
57. Krishnan KG, Schackert G (2008) An analysis of results after selective tendon transfers through the interosseous membrane to provide selective finger and thumb extension in chronic irreparable radial nerve lesions. J Hand Surg Am 33(2):223–231
58. Duncan D, Johnson KA, Monkman GR (1974) Fracture of the humerus and radial nerve palsy. Minn Med 57:659–662
59. Friedlllan RJ, Smith RJ (1984) Radial nerve laceration, twenty six years after screw fixation or a humeral fracture. A case report. J Bone loint Surg Am 66-A:959–960
60. Postacchini F, Morace GB (1988) Fractures of the humerus associated with paralysis of the radial nerve. Ital J Orthop Traumatol 14(4):455–464
61. Connolly S, Nair R, Waddell JP et al (2000) Immediate plate osteosynthesis of open fractures of the humeral shaft. Proceedings of the 55th Canadian Orthopaedic Association annual meeting, Edmonton

62. Songcharoen P, Wongtrakul S, Mahaisavariya B, Spinner RJ (2001) Hemi-contralateral C7 transfer to median nerve in the treatment of root avulsion brachial plexus injury. J Hand Surg Am 26(6): 1058–1064
63. Olarte CM, Darowish M, Ziran BH (2003) Radial nerve transposition with humeral fracture fixation. Preliminary results. Clin Orthop Relat Res 413:170–174. doi:10.1097/01.blo.0000072470. 32680.60
64. Lee SU, Kim WY, Kang SH, Park YS, Rhee SK (2008) Medial transposition or radial nerve in distal humerus shaft fracture: a report of six cases. J Korean Fract Soc 21:240–243
65. Bleeker W, Nijsten MWN, ten Duis HJ (1991) Treatment of humeral shaft fractures related to associated injuries. Acta Orthop Scand 62:148–153
66. Szalay E, Rockwood CA Jr (1983) The Holstein-Lewis fracture revisited. Orthop Trans 7:516

Internal Fixation of Diaphyseal Humeral Fractures: Plate or Intramedullary Nail?

20

Michele James Ceglia, Stefano Bianco, Antonio Ciardullo, and Roberto Buzzi

20.1 Introduction

Humeral shaft fractures account for about 3 % of all fractures and 20 % of humeral fractures; therefore, they represent a common fracture in the adult [1, 2]. Most commonly they are represented by closed fractures: open fractures are 2–10 % of cases. Sixty percent involve middle third of the diaphysis.

Traditionally most humeral shaft fractures have been treated conservatively. The initial stabilization is usually achieved with a U-shaped splint. The splint is removed once swelling has subsided and a functional brace is applied [3]. Reduction occurs due to gravity and circumferential compression of the limb. The range of acceptable alignment of the fracture is quite wide [4] with up to 20–30° of angular and rotational deformities and up to 3 cm of shortening. With this treatment, encouraging results have been documented. Sarmiento et al. [3] reported an incidence of nonunion of less than 2 % in closed fractures and 6 % in open fractures. Time to union was 9 and 14 weeks in closed and open fractures, respectively. Varus deformity up to 10° was common and observed in 75–80 % of cases.

Also other authors have described positive outcomes of functional bracing. Koch et al. [5] retrospectively reviewed 67 humeral shaft fractures treated with a Sarmiento brace. Fifty-eight fractures (87 %) were clinically healed at a mean of 10 weeks after injury. Fifty-five cases treated conservatively (95 %) obtained an excellent or good clinical result. Three patients (5 %) had a slight limitation of active range of motion. All 58 patients returned to their job. Ekholm et al. [6] performed a retrospective study of 78 closed humeral shaft fractures. Ninety percent of the fractures healed with the brace. Almost 50 % of the patients reported full recovery. The short musculoskeletal functional assessment (SMFA) for arm/hand function was acceptable. The SF 36 score was slightly lower when compared to a Swedish reference population [6]. In conclusion, a high rate of union can be achieved with functional bracing, and these patients experience good functional outcome.

Not all diaphyseal humeral fractures can be treated conservatively, and absolute and relative indications to surgery have been defined [7, 8]. Intramedullary nailing (IMN) and plate fixation (PLT) techniques are the most common choices, and each one has advantages and disadvantages. Up to date there is an ongoing debate on whether treatment option is preferable. The purpose of this article is to describe the

M.J. Ceglia, MD (✉) • S. Bianco, MD
A. Ciardullo, MD • R. Buzzi, MD
Department of Traumatology and General Orthopaedics, AOU Careggi, Careggi Hospital, Largo Palagi 1, Florence 50139, Italy
e-mail: michaelceglia79@gmail.com

F. Castoldi et al. (eds.), *Simple and Complex Fractures of the Humerus*,
DOI 10.1007/978-88-470-5307-6_20, © Springer-Verlag Italia 2015

key points of such controversy as well as the data on which they are based.

20.2 Indications to Surgical Treatment

Surgical treatment is indicated in cases of failure to achieve and maintain acceptable reduction and alignment at fracture site. Bedridden patients and segmental fractures are examples. Open fractures require surgical treatment including debridement, lavage, and stabilization. Polytraumatized patients, fractures with articular extension either proximally or distally, associated fracture of the shoulder girdle or forearm benefit from surgical treatment to allow early motion and facilitate patient care. Humeral shaft fractures with a vascular injury require limb revascularization and stabilization. The presence of a nerve injury, more often regarding the radial nerve, may require nerve exploration and fracture stabilization. Pathological fractures are another good indication for surgery together with nonunions.

The growing importance of socioeconomic issues has expanded the indications for surgery. Some patients poorly tolerate the application of a brace. Others are concerned by the occasional occurrence of a malunion of the fracture. The possibility of active postoperative mobilization and of shorter sick leave also represents attractive advantages for some patients [9].

Operative techniques include plate fixation (PLT), intramedullary nailing (IMN), and external fixation. The choice depends on fracture characteristics, associated injuries, and surgeon's preference. Most surgeons use external fixators for acute fracture stabilization. Soft tissue injuries, burns, fractures in polytrauma patients, and associated vascular injuries are excellent indications for external fixation. The external fixator is usually converted to more stable constructs such as PLT or IMN.

Theoretically, both PLT and IMN have a rationale that justifies and favors their use. Topics of this debate include biologic insult, mechanical properties, as well as technical issues, results, and complications.

20.3 Plate and Screw Fixation

The theoretical advantages of plate and screw fixation include direct visualization, anatomic reduction, and compression of the fracture. Fracture gaps are poorly tolerated by the humerus and should be avoided. The radial nerve can be identified and explored. Neither the shoulder nor the elbow is harmed by the procedure therefore encouraging a full recovery of joint motion.

The disadvantages of PLT include a wide dissection, soft tissue stripping with biologic damage, and the potential for iatrogenic injury to neurovascular structures including the radial nerve.

The recommended surgical approach is influenced by the anatomic location of the fracture. The anterolateral approach is indicated in fractures of the proximal and middle third of the humeral shaft. It includes the deltopectoral approach which can be extended distally splitting the brachialis muscle in the middle [10]. The radial nerve is protected by the lateral third of the brachialis. The deltoid tendon requires to be elevated from the lateral surface of the humerus, but the consequences are limited if it is left continuous with the lateral half of the brachialis.

Fractures of the distal third are usually approached posteriorly; the advantage is a flat surface for the placement of the plate. There are different techniques to develop a posterior approach to the humerus. A triceps-splitting approach may be chosen: the lateral and long head of the triceps are separated proximally. The radial nerve may be visualized deep between the two heads. The deeper medial head is exposed and incised longitudinally. With the triceps-splitting approach and the mobilization of the radial nerve, 76 % of the humerus can be visualized [11]. Alternatively the triceps can be mobilized from lateral to medial, the so-called paratricipital approach. The lateral margin of the triceps is lifted off the lateral intermuscular septum. This approach avoids splitting the muscle and decreases scar formation and muscle denervation [12]. Using this approach over 90 % of humeral shaft can be exposed [11]. Regardless which approach is used, triceps splitting or paratricipital, the radial nerve must be identified and protected throughout the procedure.

Minimally invasive percutaneous osteosynthesis [13] technique has been recently developed for the treatment of humeral shaft fractures. The amount of soft tissue dissection is minimized compared to a traditional open approach. The approach is usually anterior with the arm maximally supinated to protect the posteriorly located radial nerve [14]. Excellent union rates without an iatrogenic injury to the radial nerve have been recently reported [13, 15].

The MIPO technique seems to enhance recovery of range of motion postoperatively [16]. Limited indications in terms of fracture type, increased technical difficulties, and prolonged use of fluoroscopy have so far limited this technique to spread among all surgeons.

As far as reduction techniques are concerned, indirect reduction is preferred to direct manipulation of bone fragments. Instruments with a small footprint like Weber clamps should be used whenever possible and preferred to more invasive instruments. The preliminary reduction is maintained with either K-wires or compression screws. A prominent screw head invariably interferes with the subsequent plate positioning. The use of smaller screws (2.4 or 2.7 mm in diameter) with low-profile heads adequately countersunk in the cortex is ideal to avoid interference with plate. Small plates applied with an antiglide function may be occasionally used to aid in preliminary reduction.

The type of fracture influences the plating technique: transverse and short oblique fractures should be plated with axial compression taking advantage of the oval shape of the holes. Prebending of the plate is mandatory to compress the opposite cortex. Alternatively the compressor device can be used but it requires a longer surgical approach. Oblique and spiral fractures can be treated with compression interfragmentary screws and a neutralization plate. Attention should be paid to minimize soft tissue dissection and interfragmentary screws should be placed through the plate if it all possible. Comminuted fractures are typically managed with bridge plating techniques to span the zone of comminution with minimal manipulation of the interposed bone fragments. A "wave plate" technique with autologous bone graft is advocated for the treatment of nonunions [17].

The most common implant employed is a narrow 4.5 mm straight plate. Smaller patients may require 3.5 mm plate. Fractures extended to the proximal metaphysis require plates with multiple locking screws to engage the humeral head. Fractures with extension to the distal metaphysis may require a preshaped plate with a "J" design to reach the lateral column of the distal humerus.

The ideal number of screws to be inserted on each fracture fragment is debated: two is the minimum, and three is wiser. This corresponds to six cortices to be engaged. More recent studies have emphasized that the working length of the plate may be more important than the number of screws [18, 19] and increased spacing between the screws may offer better mechanical properties. Nowadays the trend involves careful attention to optimal placement of the implants reducing at the same time the total amount of hardware.

The introduction of locking screws [20] has added a new dimension to the techniques, and this applies also to the treatment of humeral shaft fractures in the setting of osteoporosis. Plates are now available from many brands which accept both locking and non-locking screws, and locking screws may have a fixed or variable axis. Fixation with locking screws has been found to be mechanically superior to non-locking screws [21]. Hybrid fixation with a single non-locking screw and two locking screws has been found mechanically comparable to a fixation with three locking screws. Hybrid fixation offers some advantages in that the fracture can be preliminary reduced and compressed with the non-locking screws and then stabilized with locking screws [21]. The ideal number of locking screws has been investigated in the humeral shaft [22]. Other authors emphasized that two well-placed locking screws per fragment may offer sufficient mechanical stability which is not augmented by the placement of a third locking screw [22].

The advantage of the locking screws however seems to be less evident for fractures involving only the humeral shaft [23]. In conclusion until further data become available, locking screws may be advisable in osteopenic bone or nonunions or for a short proximal or distal fragment.

20.4 Intramedullary Nailing

Intramedullary nailing has theoretical advantages from a mechanical and biologic perspective.

Locked intramedullary humeral nails behave as load sharing devices [7] and promote the healing process without bone exposure at fracture site. IMN are positioned in line with the mechanical axis of the humeral shaft and therefore are subjected to lower bending loads.

Flexible nails including Kirschner wires or Ender nails have been used in the past, but they have been abandoned due to insufficient control of rotational and axial forces [24]. The main disadvantage of IMN is the production of an entry hole close to the proximal or distal epiphysis with possible pain and stiffness.

Currently the most common devices are represented by interlocking medullary nails which can be inserted in either an antegrade or a retrograde fashion.

To perform an antegrade nailing, the patient is positioned in either the beach-chair, supine, or lateral position. Antegrade nails are introduced through a deltoid-splitting incision followed by excision of the subdeltoid bursa and exposure of the supraspinatus tendon. The supraspinatus tendon is incised in line with its fibers in order to reach the correct entry point on bone surface. The insult to the rotator cuff may cause shoulder pain and stiffness [25].

The diameter of the medullary canal should be carefully evaluated preoperatively. The size of the nail should match the diameter of the medullary canal. The shape of the humerus is peculiar as it narrows along its course from proximal to distal and it ends 2 cm proximal to the olecranon fossa. The attempt to introduce a mismatched nail will invariably cause distraction at fracture site which predisposes to nonunion. Aggressive reaming to house an oversized nail has several potential drawbacks: cortical necrosis due to thermal injury [26], iatrogenic comminution at fracture site, and potential injuries to neurovascular structures.

Proximal locking should be performed before distal locking and it is preformed using the dedicated guide. Attention should be paid to the course of axillary nerve which runs about 5–6 cm distal to the acromion process. An oblique screw running proximal to distal is safer than a transverse screw. Before proximal locking, attention should be paid to avoid protrusion of the nail in the subacromial space in order to prevent postoperative shoulder impingement. After proximal locking, distraction at fracture site should be minimized. The fracture should be carefully reduced before proceeding to distal locking.

Distal locking is usually performed in the sagittal plane with "freehand" technique under fluoroscopic control. A 3 cm incision and two right angle retractors are useful to expose the bone and avoid accidental injuries to the soft tissues.

Retrograde nailing requires a prone position and triceps-splitting incision proximal to the olecranon. A substantial entry hole needs to be carefully produced proximal to the olecranon fossa and enlarged with high-speed burrs until it allows nail introduction. This procedure may significantly weaken the cortex of the distal humerus and predispose it to the feared complication of supracondylar fractures. Other possible complications include postoperative elbow pain and range of motion difficulties as well as the formation of periarticular ossifications. Distal locking is performed as previously described through the guide. Proximal locking is performed with "freehand" technique under fluoroscopic assistance usually in the frontal plane. Attention to avoid damage to neurovascular structures is essential also at this level.

20.5 Comparative Studies

A few comparative studies between PLT and IMN in diaphyseal humeral fractures have been published (Table 20.1).

Table 20.1 Randomized prospective studies of humeral shaft fracture fixation: intramedullary nails versus plates

Name, year	Patients	Time to healing	Nonunion	Infection	Postopeative radial nerve palsy	Shoulder problems	Elbow problems	Functional outcome	Complications	Second surgery
Chapman et al., 2000	84	Nonsignificant (ns)	ns	ns	ns	⇑ IMN	⇑ PLT	Not available (na)	ns	na
McCormack, 2000	44	(ns)	ns	ns	⇑ IMN	⇑ IMN	⇑ IMN	ns	⇑ IMN	⇑ IMN
Changulani, 2007	47	⇑ plate (PLT)	ns	⇑ PLT	⇑ PLT	ns	na	ns	⇑ PLT	na
Raghavendra, 2007	36	ns	ns	na	⇑ IMN	⇑ IMN	ns	⇓ IMN	⇑ IMN	⇑ IMN
Putti, 2009	34	ns	ns	ns	ns	ns	na	ns	⇑ IMN	ns
Khan, 2010	60	na	na	ns	ns	⇑ IMN	na	ns	na	na

Rodriguez-Merchan [27] prospectively studied 40 patients with closed transverse fractures of the diaphysis of the humerus without associated nerve palsies. All failed nonoperative treatment and were operated with either compression plating (PLT) or intramedullary fixation (IMN) with Hackethal nail. The patients were not randomized but the treatment was left to the surgeon's preference. The patients were reviewed with an average follow-up of 18 months. The patients in the IMN group required with one exception a second anesthesia to remove the symptomatic nails and had to be protected in the brace for 6 months. Patients in the PLT group performed the same rehabilitation protocol but did not use the postoperative brace. All fractures treated with IMN healed with a delayed union in one case. All the fractures treated by PLT healed with one exception who showed delayed union. The author concluded that there were no differences between the two groups and that either PLT or IMN can be used. Disadvantages of the IMN group included the need to use a postoperative brace and the need of a second procedure to remove the device.

Chapman et al. [28] performed a prospective randomized study including 84 patients which underwent IMN ($n=38$) or PLT ($n=46$). The devices implanted were either an antegrade humeral nail (Russell Taylor, Smith and Nephew) or a dynamic locking compression plate (DCP Synthes). The results were studied with a 13-month follow-up. Fracture healing by 16 weeks was present in 42 of 43 PLT, compared with 33 out of 38 in the IMN group (p=nonsignificant). Shoulder pain and decreased shoulder motion were significantly more frequent after IMN ($p=0.007$). A decreased range of motion of the elbow was significantly ($p=0.003$) more frequent after PLT of distal third fractures. The same patients did not experience increased elbow pain. The prevalence of other complications was not significantly different between the two groups. The authors concluded that both treatments can provide predictable methods for the treatment of these fractures.

McCormack et al. [29] prospectively randomized 44 patients with fractures of the shaft of the humerus to either intramedullary nail (IMN) or plating (DCP). After a minimum 6-month follow-up, there were no differences in shoulder and elbow function and pain and time to return to normal activity. Shoulder impingement was present in one case after plating and six after IMN. Complications were found in three DCP group patients compared with 13 in the IMN group. Secondary surgery was needed in 7 IMN nail patients but only one in the DCP group. The author concluded that DCP remained the best treatment for humeral shaft fractures, while IMN may have specific indications but is technically more demanding and shows a higher complication rate.

Changulani et al. [30] compared results of humerus IMN and DCP. Forty-seven patients with a diaphyseal fracture of the shaft were prospectively randomized. The IMN group included 23 patients, while in the DCP group there were 24 patients. Antegrade nailing was routinely employed and DCP plating was applied through an anterolateral or posterior approach. The outcome measurements included union time, union rate, functional outcome, and incidence of complications. Functional outcome assessed with the American Shoulder and Elbow Surgeons Score (ASES) showed no differences between the two groups. Union rate was similar, and time to union was significantly lower for IMN. Complications such as infection were higher with DCP. Shortening of the arm and restriction of shoulder movements due to impingement were more frequent with IMN compared with DCP. The authors concluded that IMN may be preferable because of shorter union time and lower incidence of infection. There were no differences between the two groups in terms of rate of union and functional results.

Raghavendra and Bhalodiya [31] prospectively studied 36 patients with fractures of the shaft of the humerus. The follow-up was from 1 to 2 years. There were two groups, each one of 18 patients. There were no differences in union time between the two groups but patients with an interlocking nail underwent more bone grafting procedures to achieve the union (six vs two). A good to excellent result was achieved by 12 patients in the DCP (66 %) compared to 4 patients

(25 %) in the nailing group. Locked nailing was associated with a significant reduction of shoulder function ($p=0.003$) and overall results ($p=0.02$). The authors concluded that there was no difference between the two groups in terms of time to union. However compression plating was preferable because of better preservation of joint function and lesser need for secondary bone grafting.

Putti et al. [32] randomized 34 patients with humeral shaft fractures to either antegrade IMN ($n=16$) or DCP ($n=18$). Fractures were classified according to the AO system (type A in 19 cases, type B in 15 cases). The outcome evaluation included functional results, union, and complications. The minimum follow-up was 24 months. The functional scores according to American Shoulder and Elbow Surgeons (ASES) were not significantly different. Complication rates were higher in IMN group versus DCP groups (50 % vs 17 %, $p=0.038$) and the nonunion rate was 0 % versus 6 % (ns). Two patients in the IMN group sustained an iatrogenic fracture at the time of insertion. Two had a radial nerve palsy and one patient needed nail removal for shoulder impingement. Three patients had adhesive capsulitis. The authors concluded that the complication rate was higher in the IMN group, while functional outcomes were similar in the two groups.

Khan et al. [33] compared two groups of 30 patients each treated with intramedullary interlocking nail and plating with DCP. In the IMN group 11 patients had moderate to severe shoulder dysfunctions and 8 of them were above 50 years of age. In the DCP group only one patient had severe shoulder dysfunction ($p=0.001$). There was no significant difference in infection rate and palsy between the two groups. The authors concluded that antegrade nailing may not be suitable in elderly patients as it can cause significant shoulder dysfunction.

20.6 Meta-Analysis

In an effort to enlarge the number of patients, several meta-analysis have been performed (Table 20.2).

Bhandari et al. [16] reviewed randomized trials from 1969 to 2000. Only three studies were included for a total of 155 patients. Plate fixation showed a lower risk of reoperation compared to the intramedullary nailing. The risk reduction was 74 %: one reoperation could be prevented every ten patients treated with plates. Plate fixation also reduced the risk of shoulder problems. The authors concluded that plate fixation may reduce the risk of reoperation and shoulder impingement.

Orthopedic Trauma Directions in 2007 performed a meta-analysis based on a MEDLINE search for randomized and quasi randomized studies published between 1995 and 2007. Three studies were identified. Common outcome measures included reoperation (any additional humeral surgery), nonunion, time to union, infection, and nerve injury. The authors identified an

Table 20.2 Meta-analysis of randomized prospective studies of humeral shaft fracture fixation: intramedullary nails versus plates

Author, year	Total complication rate	Reoperation	Time to union	Nonunion	Shoulder problems	Radial nerve palsy
Bhandari, 2006	Not available (na)	⇑ IMN	na	ns	⇑ IMN	ns
Orthop Tr Directions, 2007	na	⇑ IMN	ns	ns	na	ns
Orthop Tr Directions, 2010	na	⇑ IMN	ns	ns	na	⇑ IMN
Heineman, 2010	Nonsignificant (ns)	ns	ns	ns	na	ns
Heineman, 2010	⇑ nail (IMN)	ns	ns	ns	na	ns
Ouyang, 2013	na	⇑ IMN	na	ns	⇑ IMN	ns

increased risk of reoperation with IMN. Time to union ranged from 6.3 to 9.8 in the IMN group compared with 8.9–10.4 of the plating, and the difference was significant in only one study.

This study was updated by Orthopedic Trauma Direction in 2010 by adding the fourth study carried out by Putti et al. Outcome measures remained the same. There was a significantly increased incidence of reoperation and radial nerve palsy after IMN, while the time to union remained not significant.

Heineman et al. [34] performed a literature search between 1967 and 2007 in the main medical search engines. Four randomized trials were selected pooling a total of 203 patients. Primary outcome included the total complication rate. Secondary outcomes included nonunion, infection, nerve palsy, and reoperation rate. Results did not show significant differences between the IMN and PLT groups. These authors updated their conclusions adding Putti's study and found that total complication rates were higher after IMN nailing [35].

Ouyang et al. [36] conducted an updated meta-analysis on the optimal treatment of humeral shaft fractures and included ten randomized controlled trials comparing nailing and plating from 1969 to 2011. Primary outcomes were nonunion, delayed union, postoperative infection, reoperation, and radial nerve palsy. Secondary outcomes include shoulder motion, shoulder impingement, iatrogenic fracture comminution, and implant failure. Plating (PLT) reduced the risk of shoulder impingement and shoulder loss of motion in comparison to nailing (IMN). Reoperation risk was uncertain. No other significant difference was identified. The authors concluded that plating and nailing can achieve similar results, but plating may reduce the occurrence of shoulder problems.

Conclusion

The classic indications to surgical treatment of diaphyseal fractures of the humerus have broadened due to new considerations including cost-effectiveness, time of disability, functional outcome, and others [20]. Given this trend it would be helpful to define which surgical option, PLT or IMN, represents the gold standard technique.

Both plates and nails have relative advantages and disadvantages. IMN seems to be ideal from the biologic point of view since the technique may be employed without exposing the fracture site. The cosmetic advantage of IMN is also obvious. A disadvantage to be expected with IMN is the increased incidence of pain and stiffness at the site of introduction of the nail, namely, the shoulder or the elbow.

Plating techniques offer the opportunity to visualize fracture fragments and to manipulate these to achieve a more anatomic reduction of the fracture. If exploration of the radial nerve is needed, the use of a plate seems logical. The obvious disadvantage of plating is the wide dissection to be employed which can lead to a biologic insult and delayed healing.

Both techniques are demanding and require a careful operative execution. Technical difficulties are challenging to estimate and may be widely influenced by the surgeon's training and experience.

The type of fracture also has an influence on the choice of the procedure. When the fracture approach is to either the proximal or distal epiphysis, a plating technique is advisable. Segmental, comminuted, and pathological fractures are good indications for IMN; again the presence of a short proximal or distal fragment demands the use of a plate. The presence of a preoperative radial nerve palsy suggests avoidance of closed IMN for fear of further damage to the nerve.

The revision of comparative randomized trials between PLT and IMN suggest that significant differences occur (Table 20.1). We pooled six publications for a total 305 patients. We analyzed differences in 9 outcome measures for a total of 54 fields. We found that 25 (46 %) fields showed insignificant differences. A significant difference was identified in 18 (33 %) fields: in 14 (26 %) fields IMN performed less well, while in 6 (11 %) PLT was inferior. Differences in eight (15 %) fields could not be evaluated because data were not available. The results of meta-analysis (Table 20.2) further contribute to identification of significant differences. We pooled 6 meta-analysis and analyzed 6 outcome measures for a total of 36 fields. There were no differences in 18 (50 %) fields, while a significant difference was shown in eight (22 %), and IMN performed less well in all of them. Differences in ten (28 %) fields could not be evaluated because data were not available. Significant differences seem to suggest that IMN perform less well with increased incidence in reoperation rate, radial nerve palsy, and shoulder problems.

In conclusion published trials have been limited in size and have methodological limitations. Definitive larger trials should be conducted and should be prospective randomized with blinding of patients, care providers, and outcome assessors. The influence of new devices including locked plating and newly designed intramedullary nails along with the importance of new surgical techniques like MIPO should also be evaluated.

References

1. Tytherleigh–Strong G (1998) The epidemiology in humeral shaft fractures. J Bone Joint Surg Br 80(2):249–253
2. Igbigbi PS (2004) Epidemiology of humeral fractures in Malawi. Int Orthop 28:338–341
3. Sarmiento A, Zagorsky JB, Zych GA et al (2000) Functional bracing for the treatment of fractures of the humeral diaphysis. J Bone Joint Surg Am 82(4):476–488
4. Klenerman L (1966) Fractures of the shaft of the humerus. J Bone Joint Surg Br 48(1):105–111
5. Koch PP, Gross DF, Gerber C (2002) The results of functional bracing of humeral shaft fractures. J Shoulder Elbow Surg 11(2):143–150
6. Ekholm R, Tidermark J, Törnkvist H, Adami J, Ponzer S (2006) Outcome after closed functional treatment of humeral shaft fractures. J Orthop Trauma 20(9):591–596
7. Schemitsch EH, Bhandari M (1998) Fractures of the humeral shaft. In: Browner J, Levine T (eds) Skeletal trauma. Saunders, Philadelphia, pp 1481–1511
8. Rommens PM, McCormack R (2007) Humerus, shaft. In: Ruedi T, Buckley RE, Moran CG (eds) AO principles of fracture management. AO publishing, Davos Platz, pp 595–597
9. Bhandari M, Devereaux PJ, McKee MD, Schemitscch EH (2006) Compression plating versus intramedullary nailing of humeral shaft fractures – a meta-analysis. Acta Orthop 77(2):279–284
10. Hoppenfield S, deBoer P (2003) Surgical exposures in orthopaedics: the anatomic approach, 3rd edn. Lippincott Williams and Wilkins, Philadelphia
11. Gerwin M, Hotchkiss RN, Weiland AJ (1996) Alternative operative exposures of the posterior aspect of the humeral diaphysis with reference to the radial nerve. J Bone Joint Surg Am 78(11):1690–1695, Gerwin 1996
12. Zlotolow DA, Catalano LW III, Barron OA, Glickel SZ (2006) Surgical exposures of the humerus. J Am Acad Orthop Surg 14(13):754–765
13. Zhiquan A et al (2007) Minimally invasive plating osteosynthesis (MIPO) of middle and distal third humeral shaft fractures. J Orthop Trauma 21:628–633
14. Apivatthakakul T et al (2005) Minimally invasive plate osteosynthesis (MIPO) of the humeral shaft fracture. Is it possible? A cadaveric study and preliminary report. Injury 36:530–538
15. Jiang R, Luo CF, Zeng BF, Mei GH (2007) Minimally invasive plating for complex humeral shaft fractures. Arch Orthop Trauma Surg 127(7):531–535
16. Kobayashi M, Watanabe Y, Matsushita T (2010) Early full range of shoulder and elbow motion is possible after minimally invasive plate osteosynthesis for humeral shaft fractures. J Orthop Trauma 24(4): 212–216
17. Hsu TL, Chiu FY, Chen CM, Chen TH (2005) Treatment of nonunion of humeral shaft fracture with dynamic compression plate and cancellous bone graft. J Chin Med Assoc 68(2):73–76
18. Crow BD, Mundis G, Anglen JO (2007) Clinical results of minimal screw plate fixation of forearm fractures. Am J Orthop 36(9):477–480
19. Lindvall EM, Sagi HC (2006) Selective screw placement in forearm compression plating: results of 75 consecutive fractures stabilized with 4 cortices of screw fixation on either side of the fracture. J Orthop Trauma 20(3):157–162
20. Walker M et al (2011) Humeral shaft fractures: a review. J Shoulder Elbow Surg 20(5):833–844
21. Gardner MJ et al (2006) Hybrid locked plating of osteoporotic fractures of the humerus. J Bone Joint Surg Am 88(9):1962–1967
22. Hak DJ et al (2010) Locked plate fixation of osteoporotic humeral shaft fractures: are two locking screws per segment enough? J Orthop Trauma 24(4):207
23. O'Toole RV et al (2008) Are locking screws advantageous with plate fixation of humeral shaft fractures? A biomechanical analysis of synthetic and cadaveric bone. J Orthop Trauma 22(10):709–715
24. Zimmerman MC, Waite AM, Deehan M, Oppenheim W (1994) A biomechanical analysis of four humeral fracture fixation systems. J Orthop Trauma 8(3): 233–239
25. Cheng HR, Lin J (2008) Prospective randomized comparative study of antegrade and retrograde locked nailing for middle humeral shaft fracture. J Trauma 65(1):94–102

26. Leunig M, Hertel R (1996) Thermal necrosis after tibial reaming for intramedullary nail fixation. J Bone Joint Surg Br 78-B:584–587
27. Rodriguez-Merchan EC (1995) Compression plating versus Hackethal nailing in closed humeral shaft fractures failing nonoperative reduction. J Orthop Trauma 9(3):194–197
28. Chapman JR, Henley MB, Agel J, Benca PJ (2000) Randomized prospective study of humeral shaft fracture fixation: intramedullary nails vs plates. J Orthop Trauma 14(3):162–166
29. McCormack RG, Brien D, Bucley RE, McKee MD et al (2000) Fixation of fractures of the shaft of the humerus by dynamic compression plate or intramedullary nail. J Bone Joint Surg Br 82-B:336–339
30. Changulani M, Jain UK, Keswani T (2007) Comparison of the use of the humerus intramedullary nail and dynamic compression plate for the management of diaphyseal fractures of the humerus. A randomized controlled study. Int Orthop 31:391–395
31. Raghavendra S, Bhalodiya H (2007) Internal fixation of fractures of the shaft of the humerus by dynamic compression plate or intramedullary nail: a prospective study. Indian J Orthop 41(3):214–218
32. Putti AB, Uppin RB, Putti BB (2009) Locked intramedullary nailing versus dynamic compression plating for humeral shaft fractures. J Orthop Surg (Hong Kong) 17(2):139–141
33. Khan AS, Azfal W, Anwar A (2010) Comparison of shoulder function, radial nerve palsy and infection after nailing versus plating in humeral shaft fractures. J Coll Physicians Surg Pak 20(4):253–257
34. Heineman DJ, Poolman RW, Nork SF, Ponsen KJ, Bhandari M (2010) Plate fixation or intramedullary fixation of humeral shaft fractures. Acta Orthop 81(2):216–223
35. Heineman DJ, Bhandary MO et al (2010) Treatment of humeral shaft fractures – meta-analysis reupdated. Acta Orthop 81(4):517
36. Ouyang H, Xiong J, Xiang P, Cui Z, Chen L, Yu B (2013) Plate versus intramedullary nail fixation in the treatment of humeral shaft fractures: an updated meta-analysis. J Shoulder Elbow Surg 22: 387–395

21 Humeral Shaft Fractures and External Fixator

Domenico Aloj, Pietro Pellegrino, Eraclite Petruccelli, Giovanni Martino, and Daniele Santoro

21.1 External Fixation in Humeral Shaft Fractures

21.1.1 Introduction

Humeral shaft fractures account for about 1–3 % of all fractures [1]. The overall incidence rate is about 14.5/100,000 people/year, and open fractures amount to 2 %.

Two classes of patients are the most interested ones: young patients with a high-energy trauma or elderly patients with a low-energy injury. Nevertheless, the average age for both genders is 68 for females and 53 for males [2].

21.1.2 Diagnosis and Classification

The most common classification is the AO (Muller) classification, as shown in Fig. 21.1. The greatest part of all fractures could be classified with some standard AP and lateral X-rays. In less than 2 % of all cases, a vascular lesion involving the axillary or humeral artery can coexist; in selected cases with a doubtful clinic and a major trauma, a CT, a CTA, or an angiography could be performed to improve the diagnosis and to act immediately to repair the vascular damage. CT scan could also be useful, especially with 3D reconstructions.

Several mechanisms could be a cause of a humeral shaft fracture, and the mechanism normally correlates with the fracture type:

- A flexion trauma usually leads to a transverse fracture.
- A twisting trauma could lead to a spiral fracture.
- A mix of bending and twisting could lead to an oblique fracture.
- High loads, especially in axial direction, could lead to complex and epiphyseal fracture.

The most important biomechanical aspect in humeral shaft fractures is where the fracture occurs: if it is between the insertion of the deltoid and the pectoralis major, the proximal fragment will be displaced medially and adduced by the traction of the fibers of the pectoralis (Fig. 21.2); if it is under the insertion of the deltoid, the proximal fragment will be displaced laterally and abducted by the traction of the same deltoid (Fig. 21.3).

Although any randomized clinical trial does not exist confirming a safe, proven, and effective treatment, the first eligible treatment for these fractures is the conservative one [3]. Following recent meta-analyses, about 94–97 % of the humeral shaft fractures heal in cast or brace [4]; in low-energy fractures, this percentage could grow up to 99 % [5].

D. Aloj (✉) • P. Pellegrino • E. Petruccelli
D. Santoro
Department of Traumatology, Hospital Città della Salute e della Scienza, Presidio CTO, Via Zuretti, Turin, Italy
e-mail: aloj.domenico@katamail.com; pelle.pelle@gmail.com

G. Martino
AO Città della Salute e della Scienza di Torino, Presidio CTO, Via Zuretti, Turin, Italy

F. Castoldi et al. (eds.), *Simple and Complex Fractures of the Humerus*, DOI 10.1007/978-88-470-5307-6_21, © Springer-Verlag Italia 2015

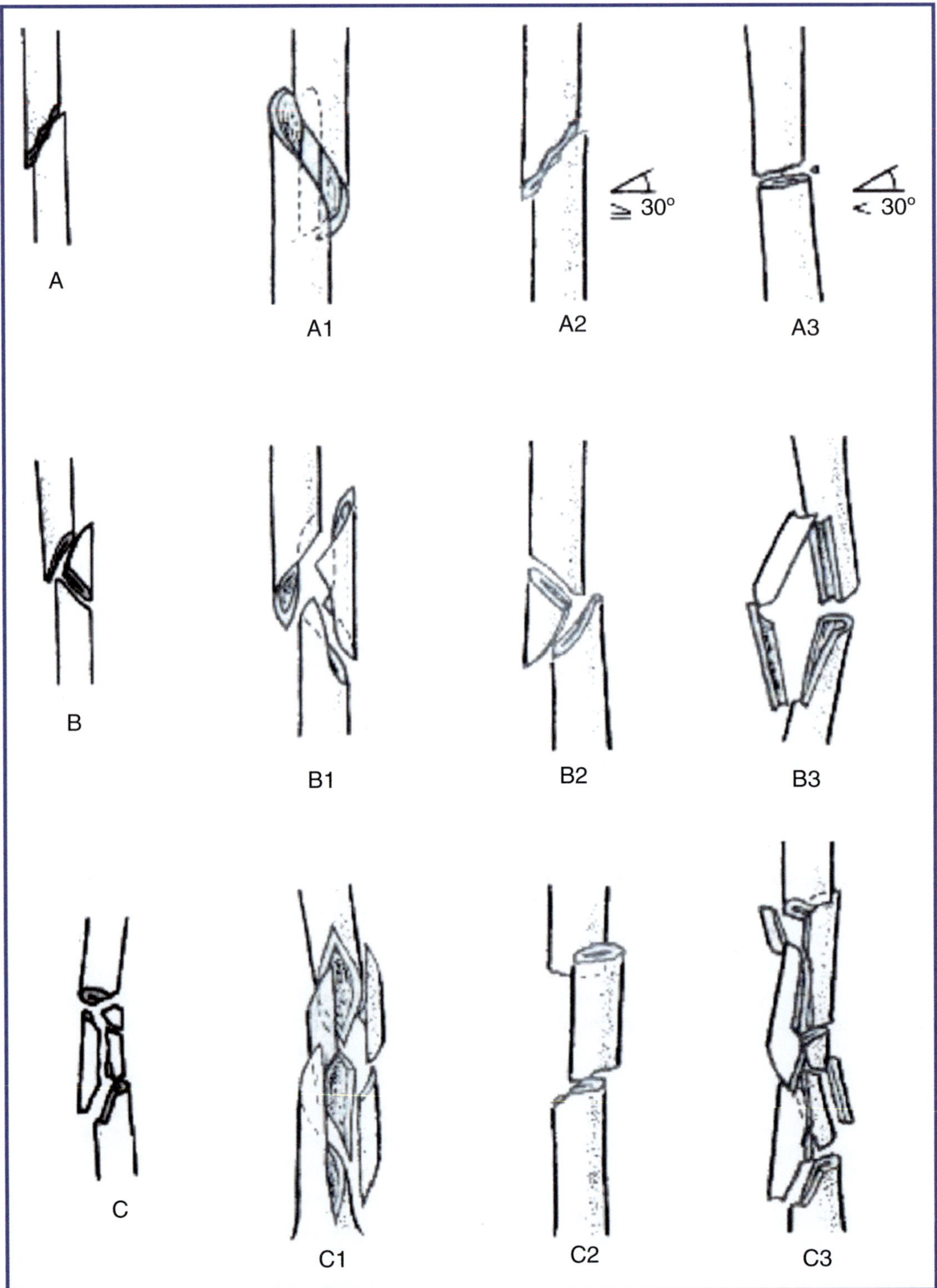

Fig. 21.1 AO classification of the humeral shaft fracture

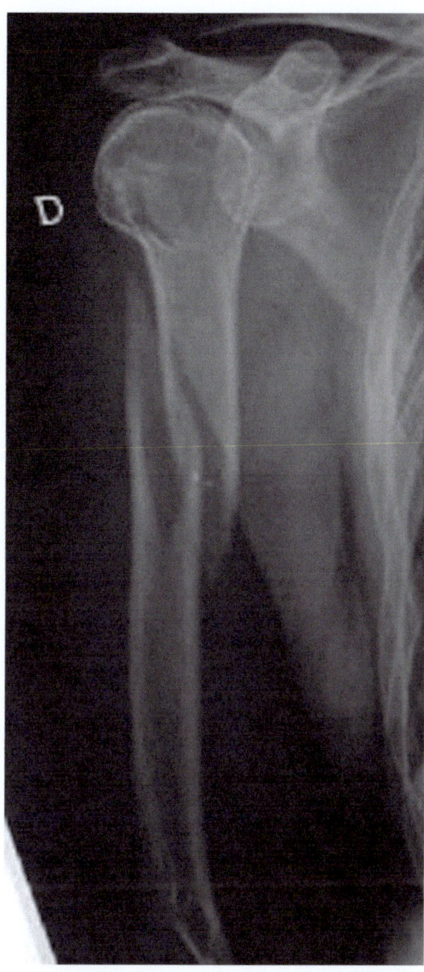

Fig. 21.2 Displacement mechanism #1: pectoralis major traction and adduction of the proximal fragment

In fact, the humerus can tolerate deformities of 20° in procurvatum and 30° in varus, shortening and translation up to 4 and 1 cm, respectively [6].

The remaining fractures are treated surgically, following AO indications with plating, with anterograde or retrograde nailing, and in some selected cases with external fixation.

21.1.3 Surgical Indications

Commonly accepted criteria for surgical treatment, with both open and closed reductions, are [7]:

- Exposed fractures
- Severe radial nerve injuries
- Multifragmentary fractures
- Bilateral fractures or polytrauma
- Stabilization in intensive trauma care unit
- Obese patients

Common indications for *external fixation* in humeral shaft fractures are:

- Bilateral fractures
- Poor cutaneous conditions
- Infections and infected nonunions
- Malunions
- Posttraumatic radial nerve palsy
- Severe displacement of the fracture
- Open fractures or comminuted fractures
- Failure of a previous treatment

Although these are commonly accepted indications, a standardized decision-making guideline does not exist for any surgical treatment: we suggest that external fixation, in the presence of an expert surgeon, could be a safe option for the greatest part of the humeral shaft fractures. External fixation is often a more safe, rapid, and low-complication-rate procedure; nevertheless, it needs a high patient compliance and an accurate surgical procedure.

21.1.3.1 External Fixation Technique

In our experience, external fixation has to be used more commonly, with the purpose of a simple management and a rapid mobilization. The advantage of this technique (which if performed by an experienced surgeon takes a little surgical time) is giving an excellent stability with minimizing soft tissue damage. Furthermore, the possibility of callus distraction and compression and alignment correction during the treatment could lead to excellent results [8, 9].

Considering these factors, our indication in acute trauma is given when the patient presents a severe nerve injury, exposed fractures, and bilateral or comminuted fractures but also in young patients with simple fractures.

Other indications could be given in chronic conditions like pseudarthrosis, both septic and non-septic.

Three steps are mandatory for a good reduction and positioning of a humeral external fixator: patient position, pin insertion, and subsequent reduction:

1. Patient position—the patient lies supine, with the head immobilized, under general or selective anesthesia: a support has to be

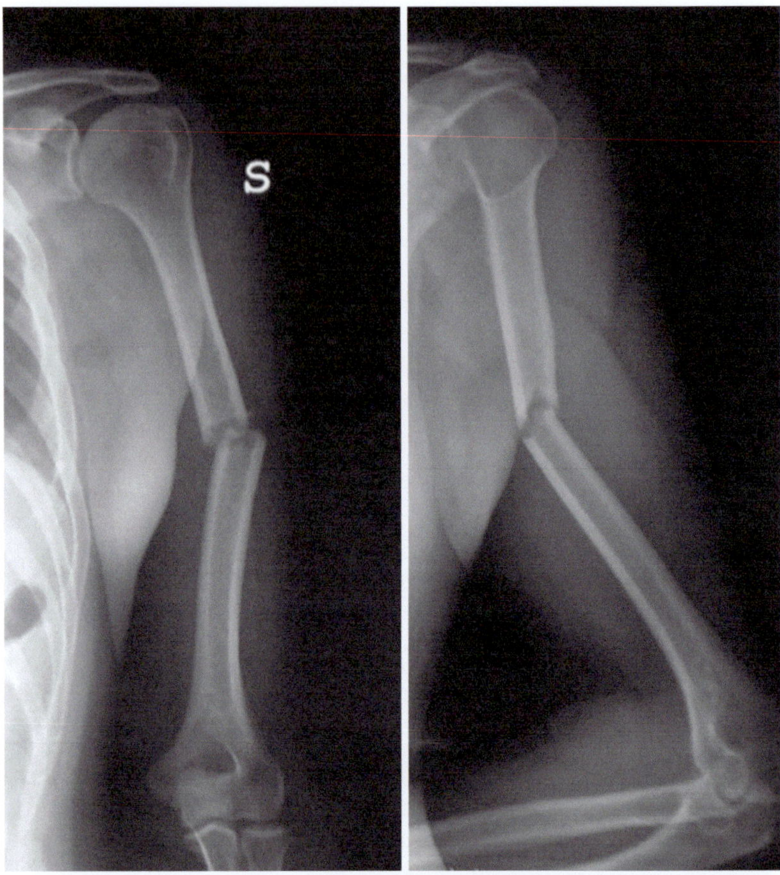

Fig. 21.3 Displacement mechanism #2: deltoid traction and abduction of the proximal fragment

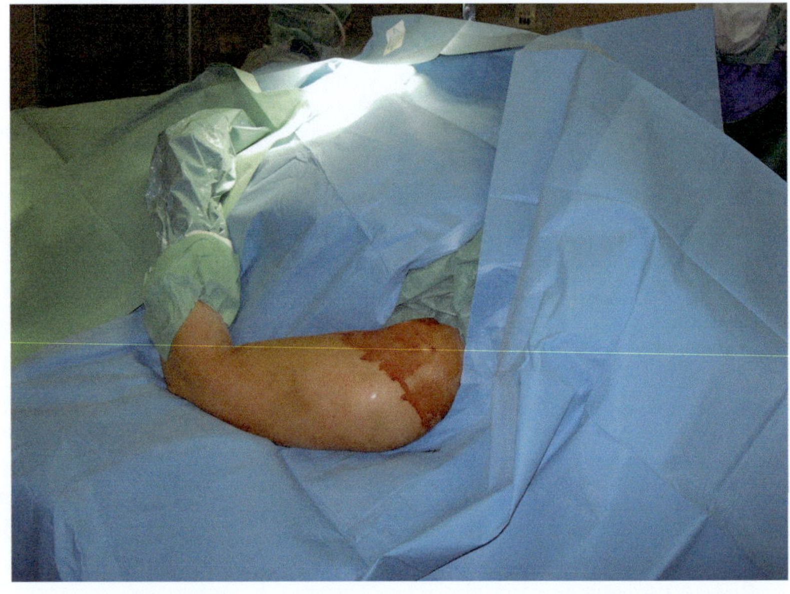

Fig. 21.4 Patient positioning

mounted under the humerus; surgical zone (in the absence of further lesions) goes from the axilla to the elbow included. Draping may leave free motion range to the entire arm. No fixed traction is needed (Figs. 21.4 and 21.5).

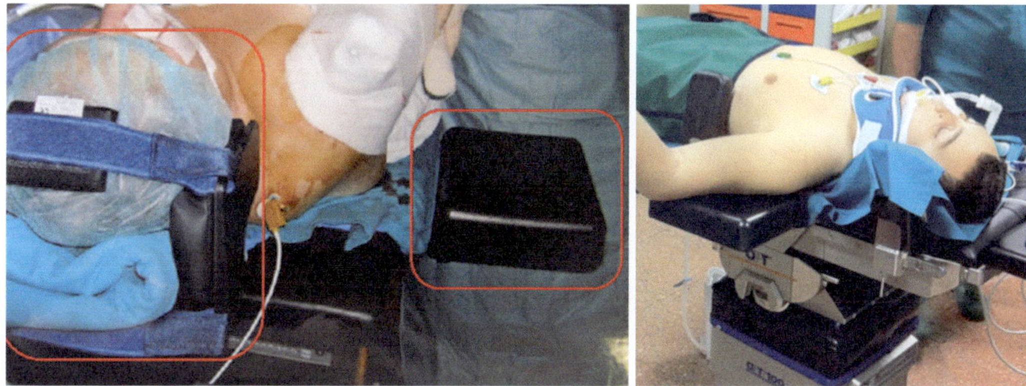

Fig. 21.5 Patient positioning

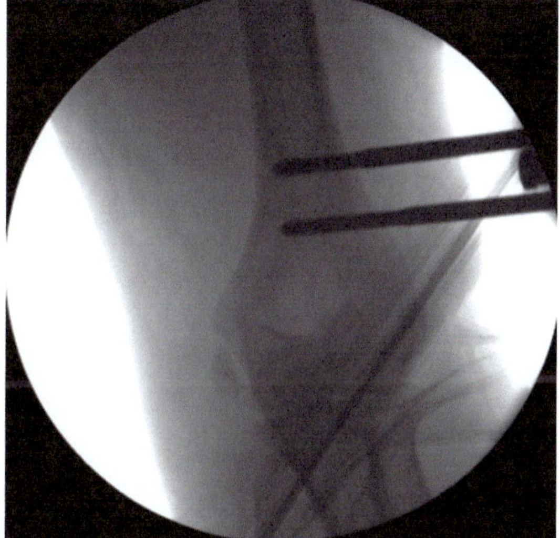

Fig. 21.6 Distal pins

2. Screw position and fracture reduction have to be done always under image intensifier control. Screws are placed on the lateral side of the humerus. The first screw is the most distal one, which has to be placed parallel to the articular line and in proximity to the epicondylar line (Fig. 21.6). The use of a K-wire to find a good zone for screw positioning is recommended. After finding a good point for the screw insertion, the bone has to be drilled and the screw positioned. The same procedure has to be repeated, without the use of the K-wire, for the second distal screw. Be careful of the radial nerve: we usually maintain a safe zone of 4 cm above the transepicondylar line.

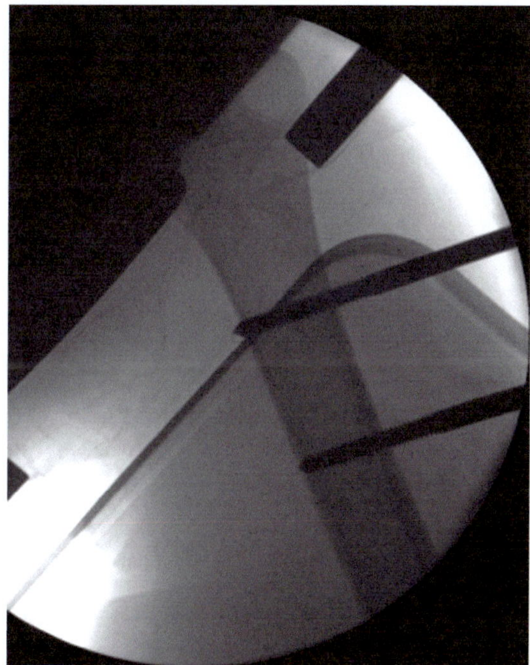

Fig. 21.7 Proximal pins

3. An analog procedure has to be performed for the two proximal screws, which have to be placed nearly perpendicular to the cortical bone; the main difference is the safe area (normally 5 cm under a line tangential to the most proximal part of the humeral head) to avoid an iatrogenic lesion of the axillary nerve (Fig. 21.7). Use the fixator without reducing the fracture to obtain a useful, simple, and correct guide for the insertion of the two proximal screws.

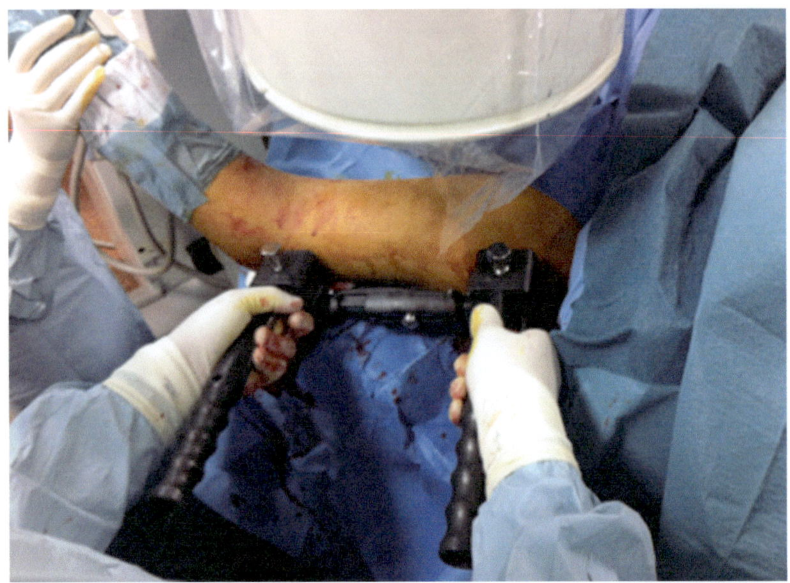

Fig. 21.8 Reduction of the fracture

4. Once placed the screws, lock the fixator to the screws leaving the same fixator free in movements and, using the designed devices, reduce the fracture (Fig. 21.8). Once a good reduction is achieved, lock the fixator (Fig. 21.9).

Do not mind of the alignment of the fixator till the fracture is reduced; if a good screw positioning and a good reduction have been performed, the fixator will appear aligned at the end of the procedure, and the screws will appear parallel in the AP X-rays. In case of an irreducible fracture, a mini approach in correspondence of the fracture line has to be considered.

If an exposition is present, always perform an irrigation and debridement of the wound before locking the fixator.

In case of a radial nerve palsy, vascular injury, or difficulty of reduction, a surgical approach is performed in correspondence of the site of injury.

The standard program includes an early mobilization without weight bearing for the first month; elbow and shoulder mobilization is conceded and is normally preserved, especially in young people, although pins through muscles could cause lesser stiffness problems. If other lesions do not coexist, monthly X-ray controls are performed, until the radiographic healing of the fracture (Fig. 21.10). The mean time of treatment with external fixator is about 12 weeks.

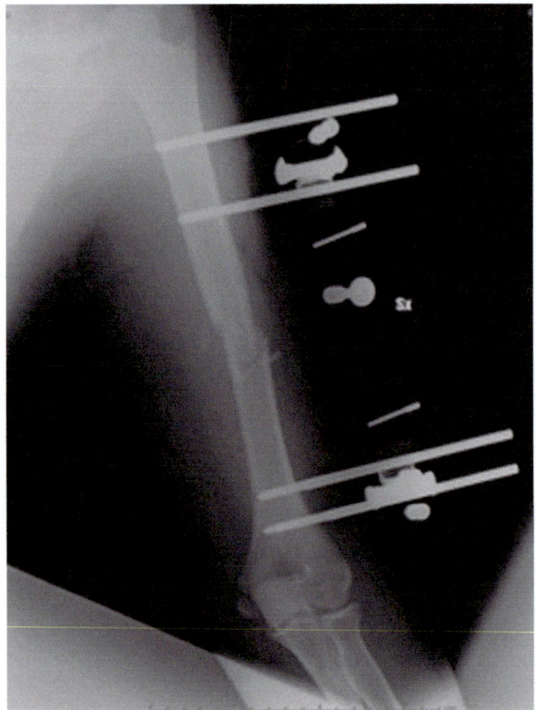

Fig. 21.9 Reduced fracture appearance at X-ray control

Complications are rare: except radial nerve palsy, which is a common complication of this kind of fractures, affecting up to 18 % of

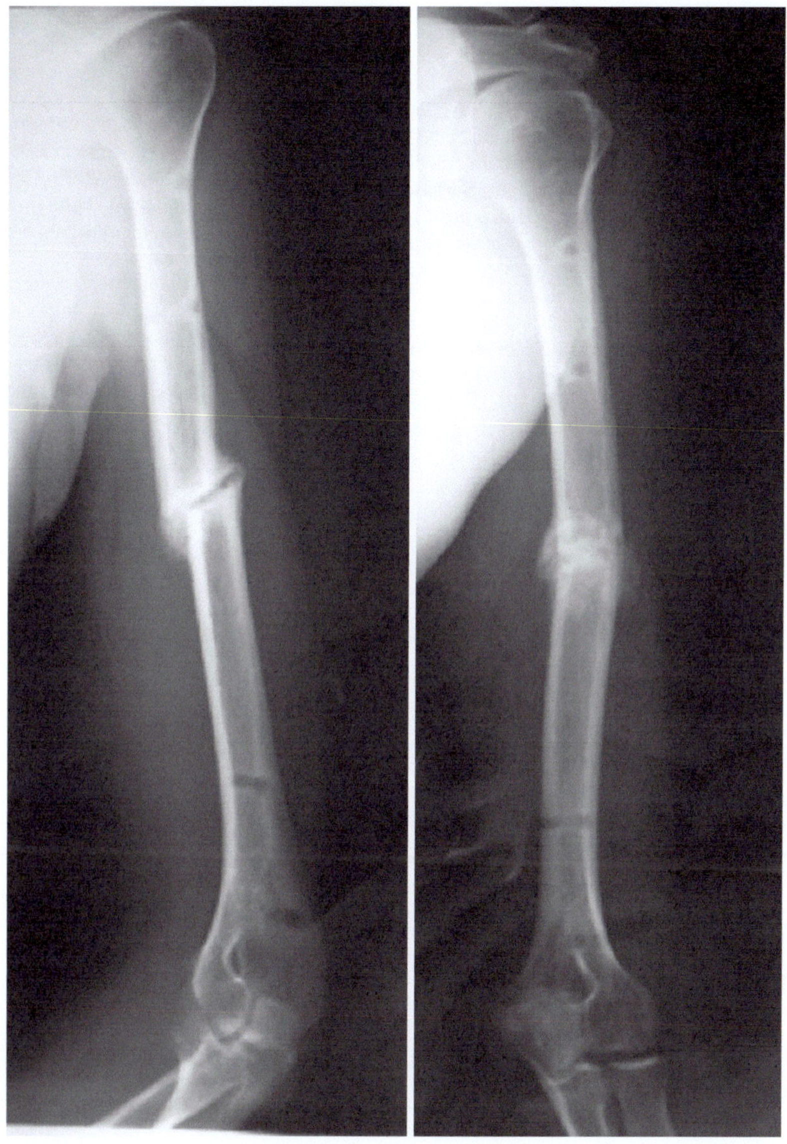

Fig. 21.10 Consolidated fracture

all fractures [10], infection and malunion rates are lower than in other surgical treatments.

Deep infection rate is consistently lower because of the smaller wounds and the little surgical exposition.

Superficial skin infections are quite common; about 10 % of all patients could experience a pin tract infection; normally, this kind of infections is auto-limiting or resolvable with light antibiotic and anti-inflammatory therapy. Infections are avoidable with a periodic careful cleaning and disinfection of pin tracts.

Malunions and malalignments could be avoided with callus compression or distraction and with axial correction and leaving the fixator in situ for a greater lapse of time, although a review over real pseudarthrosis rate does not exist yet. Probably pseudarthrosis accounts for about 1 % of all cases.

Wire breakage is another complication; this one could easily be avoided using adequate (normally 6 mm of diameter) HA screws.

References

1. Carrol EA et al (2012) Management of humeral shaft fractures. J Am Acad Orthop Surg 20(7):423–433
2. Ekholm R, Adami J, Tidemark J et al (2006) Fractures of the shaft of the humerus: an epidemiological study of 401 fractures. J Bone Joint Surg Br 88:1469–1473
3. Stannard JP, Schmidt AH, Kregor PJ (2007) Surgical treatment of orthopaedic trauma. Thieme, New York
4. Gosler MW, Testroote M, Morrenhof JW, Janzing HM (2012) Surgical versus non-surgical interventions for treating humeral shaft fractures in adults. Cochrane Database Syst Rev 1:CD008832. doi:10.1002/14651858.CD008832.pub2
5. Sarmiento A, Zagorski JB, Zych GA et al (2000) Functional bracing for the treatment of fractures of the humeral diaphysis. J Bone Joint Surg 82A(4): 478–486
6. Klenerman L (1966) Fractures of the shaft of the humerus. J Bone Joint Surg Br 48:105–111
7. Wallny T et al (1997) Functional treatments in humeral shaft fractures: indications and results. J Orthop Trauma 11(4):283–287
8. Ruland WO (2000) Is there a place for external fixation in humeral shaft fractures? Injury 31(Suppl 1):27–34
9. Catagni MA et al (2010) The external fixation in the treatment of humeral diaphyseal fractures: outcomes of 84 cases. Injury 41(11):1107–1111
10. Pollock FH, Drake D, Bovill EG, Day L, Trafton PG (1981) Treatment of radial neuropathy associated with fractures of the humerus. J Bone Joint Surg Am 63:239–243

22 Periprosthetic Fractures

Dario Petriccioli, Celeste Bertone, and Giacomo Marchi

22.1 Background

There are about 4,000 shoulder arthroplasty procedures in Italy annually. This number is expected to double over the next decade. In general, the incidence of periprosthetic humeral or scapular fracture associated with shoulder arthroplasty is approximately 0.6–4.5 % of all complications [1, 2]. The incidence of shoulder periprosthetic fractures is expected to increase not only for an increased number of primary and revision shoulder arthroplasties performed annually but also for the increased survivorship of the elderly with shoulder arthroplasties and the increased activity of patients after a shoulder arthroplasty [3–10].

Periprosthetic humeral or scapular fractures can occur intraoperatively or postoperatively after shoulder arthroplasty [8]. From the Swedish registry database, up to 76 % of humeral fractures have been reported to occur intraoperatively [1, 2]. Intraoperative fractures occur more commonly during revision surgery and with implantation of noncemented stems. The intraoperative humeral fractures in reverse shoulder arthroplasty (RSA) occur mainly during removal of the primary humeral stem or cement mantle in revision surgery in up to 24.1 % of all revisions [2]. Intraoperative glenoid fractures are rare in unconstrained and reverse shoulder arthroplasty and related to the reaming or fixation technique. Postoperative low-energy falls are the mechanism of injury in most patients; high-energy trauma accounts for only a small percentage of periprosthetic fractures, and these types are usually more comminuted fracture pattern than seen with low-energy fractures. General risk factors for periprosthetic shoulder fractures include osteopenia/osteoporosis, rheumatoid arthritis, neurological disorders, chronic steroid therapy, and revision surgery [1, 2, 5–10].

Most humeral and glenoid fractures can be treated conservatively with closed reduction and splinting or bracing. Early classification system focused on displacement as a guide to operative versus nonoperative treatment; however, current surgical techniques and the use of modular implants have made operative treatment the preferred choice for most of these fractures [3, 10]. The fracture management is dictated by type and location of the fracture in relation to the shoulder arthroplasty component and the stability of the prosthesis. Surgical methods of treatment include open reduction and internal fixation, revision arthroplasty, removal of prosthetic components, or arthrodesis. It is important to understand which options are most appropriate for each type of fracture pattern since no treatment option is optimal for all fracture types. The difficulty in management of periprosthetic fractures is evidenced by the array of treatment options described in the literature without a clear consensus emerging on the most appropriate method [11–17].

D. Petriccioli • C. Bertone (✉) • G. Marchi
Department of Orthopaedic Surgery,
"Città di Brescia" Clinical Institute,
Via Gualla, 15, Brescia 25128, Italy
e-mail: celeste.bertone@gmail.com

F. Castoldi et al. (eds.), *Simple and Complex Fractures of the Humerus*,
DOI 10.1007/978-88-470-5307-6_22, © Springer-Verlag Italia 2015

22.2 Clinical and Imaging Evaluation for Periprosthetic Fractures

The evaluation of a patient with an obvious or even suspected periprosthetic fracture should include a detailed history of the status of the arthroplasty. Any information about the date of implantation, the specific prosthesis used, and the index diagnosis for implantation (primary or revision surgery) should be recorded. Additional secondary procedures should be carefully cataloged as well as other complications, such as prior wound infection or recent change in symptoms related to the involved joint. In case of displaced fracture, a standard orthopedic clinical exam is sufficient to confirm the diagnosis. However, it is important to obtain a comprehensive history in order to identify potential etiologic factors to the acute fracture such as implant loosening, osteolysis, and infection that could influence the fracture treatment [4–8, 13].

Direct observation of periprosthetic fractures occurs when the fractures happen intraoperatively during reaming or impaction of a trial or final component. For example, a pitch change during malleting a component should alert the surgeon to the possibility of an intraoperative fracture; in this case, the surgeon should immediately proceed to a direct observation.

In case of a clinical suspicion of periprosthetic fracture, it is mandatory to obtain a standard radiographic evaluation. The standard radiographic evaluation should include two orthogonal plain radiographic views that include the joint in question and full length of the bone above and below the prosthetic components. On the fracture X-rays, the degree of angulation, amount of displacement, and fracture configuration should be evaluated. The radiographic evaluation should be made whether the humeral or glenoid component is tightly fixed or loose. In uncemented or cemented components, the presence of radiolucent lines at the implant-bone or cement-bone interface should be identified. If the lucent lines are 1.5–2 mm or greater in thickness and surround the implant, it should be seriously considered the presence of an implant loosening. A similar line extending entirely along one side of the implant or substantive osteolysis of the humeral shaft adjacent to the implant would also likely indicate prosthetic loosening [5–7, 9].

Previous radiographic images, when available, can provide insight to the time course of any existing or impending prosthetic failure, specifically osteolysis, progression of cortical erosions, and the presence of any cortical penetrations or notching.

The main risk factor for the occurrence of a periprosthetic fracture is osteopenia. On the fracture X-rays, the degree of osteopenia can be judged according to Campbell et al. [13]. Osteopenia is graded on the basis of the ratio of combined width of mid-diaphyseal cortices to the diameter of the diaphysis. It is graded as normal if the ratio is greater than 50 %, mildly osteopenic if the ratio is between 25 and 50 %, and severely osteopenic if ratio is less than 25 %.

A computed tomography scans could be required to evaluate small fractures or available bone stock for fracture treatment.

22.3 Classification System

There have been several fracture classifications described for periprosthetic humeral fractures.

Thomas W. Wright and Cofield have classified these fractures into three groups: type A (near the stem tip, extending proximally), type B (near the stem tip, extending distally), and type C (distal to the stem tip) [18].

Campbell et al. categorized fractures into four types related to the fracture site. Type 1 included the greater or lesser tuberosity, type 2 metaphyseal portion or surgical neck, type 3 proximal humeral diaphysis, and type 4 the mid- and distal diaphysis [13].

Groh et al., like Wright and Cofield classification, distinguished three types of humeral shaft fractures. Type I fractures occur proximal to the tip of the prosthesis; type 2 fractures originate proximal to the tip of the prosthesis and extend distal to it; type 3 fractures lie distal to the tip of the prosthesis [14].

Worland classified these fractures by fracture anatomic pattern and implant stability in order to provide a treatment algorithm. Type A (tuberosi-

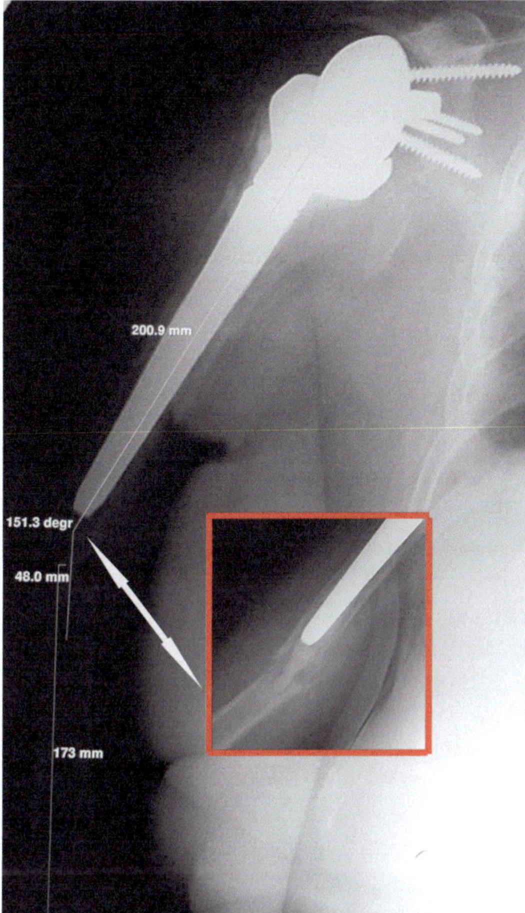

Fig. 22.1 Periprosthetic humeral shaft fracture distal to the tip of a cemented stem in an RSA, the Worland type C fracture

ties) and C (distal to the tip of the stem prosthesis; Fig. 22.1) fractures were considered to behave in the same manner as humeral fractures without a prosthesis. Fractures around the stem were designated type B, with type B1 being a spiral fracture with a stable stem, type B2 being a transverse or short oblique fracture with a stable stem, and type B3 being a fracture about the prosthesis with an unstable stem [19].

Periprosthetic scapular fractures most commonly occur intraoperatively to the glenoid. Due to the rarity of these fractures, no generally accepted fracture classification exists. Acromion and scapular spine fracture is a relatively common complication of reverse shoulder arthroplasty (RSA) and rates 2.2 % of all complications in RSAs [2]. In a series of seven patients (eight shoulders), Rittmeister et al. reported three cases of reoperations for nonunion of the acromion. These cases were all patients with rheumatoid arthritis, and the authors utilized a trans-acromial approach with a sagittal osteotomy [20]. Crosby and Hamilton proposed an anatomic classification system based on the relationship of the fracture to the acromioclavicular joint [21]. According to this system of classification, the scapular fractures after RSA are graded as:

- Type I: small avulsions of the anterior acromion that seemed to occur at the time of surgery
- Type II: fractures propagated from just posterior to the AC joint through the anterior acromion
- Type III: all displaced fractures of the posterior acromion or scapular spine

Recently, Otto et al. showed that the classification of Crosby and Hamilton has only moderate inter-rater reliability, which questions its validity and suggests that an alternative method of classifying these fractures is needed. The authors speculate that in many of type I fracture cases, the patients may have an os acromiale or preoperative acromial insufficiency or fragmentation; thus, the authors do not consider these to be fractures. The study also suggests that these fractures are not always detectable on plain radiographs and may require additional imaging studies to make a firm diagnosis [22].

Wahlquist et al. reported on five patients with "acromial base fracture" after RSA. The authors defined these fractures as a fracture occurring at the connection between the acromial process and the spine of the scapula at the level of the glenoid. This location is the foundation of the bony support for the entire deltoid, so a fracture of this region disables the deltoid function [23].

22.4 Surgical Techniques: Treatment Options and Outcomes/Results for Site

For shoulder arthroplasty, the preferred surgical approach is the deltopectoral exposure. When fracturing of the humeral shaft occurs during surgery or when periprosthetic humeral shaft fracture occurs after surgery and it requires to approach both the shoulder joint and the humeral shaft, this incision can be extended distally following the anterolateral aspect of the humerus. For displaced humeral shaft fractures associated with a stable implant, the preferred exposure is through a posterior approach. This exposure allows complete visualization of the humeral shaft and a clear identification of the radial nerve that can be protected during reduction, plating, and most importantly cable fixation in the zone of the prosthesis.

For primary RSA, some surgeons prefer the anterosuperior or transdeltoid approach. The main advantages of this approach during primary implant are simplicity, ease of axial preparation of the humerus, quality of the frontal exposure of the glenoid, and preservation of the subscapularis tendon. Its main drawback is the risk of neurological weakening of the anterior deltoid by damage to the distal branches of the axillary nerve in case of inferior extension incision to reach the humeral shaft for an intraoperative fracture [24, 25].

22.4.1 Periprosthetic Humeral Fractures

The majority of periprosthetic fractures of the greater tuberosity, type A according to the Worland classification, are stable [19]. They are usually non- or minimally displaced and, when occurring postoperatively, can be managed nonoperatively (immobilization in a sling or brace for about 4 weeks) with symptomatic treatment. Intraoperative stable fractures of the greater tuberosity can be managed similarly. Displaced, or otherwise unstable, intraoperative fractures are generally treated with a cerclage. Intraoperative fractures of the tuberosities have been considerably diminished by having the availability of trial humeral stems without associated heads that can be maintained in the humeral canal during posterior retraction of the proximal humerus during glenoid preparation. If there is an osteopenic bone condition that could weaken the greater and lesser tuberosity, it may be useful to perform a transdeltoid surgical exposure rather than a deltopectoral approach to avoid torsional stress on the tuberosities during performance of the procedure.

The Worland type C fractures are defined as being "distal" to the humeral stem. The literature demonstrates that these fractures with a well-fixed humeral component are similar to closed humerus fractures and may respond favorably to nonoperative treatment. Campbell et al. [13] reported on a multicenter series of periprosthetic humeral fractures. Each of the five postoperative fractures healed with nonoperative management. Four of these were distal to the tip of the humeral stem. When the humeral component of the prosthesis is loose, revision with a longer stemmed humeral component is the first choice. In case an acceptable closed reduction cannot be obtained with the use of a plastic orthosis, an open reduction and internal fixation (ORIF) could be considered. General principles are anatomic reduction and a stable fixation using a long plate to overlap the humeral stem. Fixation in the distal fragment is with multiple bicortical screws distal to the stem into the native bone and mono-cortical screws in the zone of the humeral prosthesis supplemented with multiple cables. Similar systems are generally used for periprosthetic fractures of the femur [5–8, 11–15, 26, 27].

Bone graft is also used in order to maximize the healing potential: allograft in acute cases and autograft (iliac crest) in cases with delayed healing or nonunion. In addition, one may consider supplementary fixation with a cortical strut onlay allograft in combination with a plate and screws/cables to obtain secure fixation. The specific revision strategy chosen depends on the quality of the remaining bone stock [28, 29].

In case of a periprosthetic humeral fracture with a loosening component, several strategies can be used, but all rely on obtaining secure distal fixation [30]. Only rarely a cemented long-stem component is used; the most effective strategies include noncemented distal fixation techniques. If the distal fragment maintains 5 cm of intact tubular diaphysis, then extensively coated uncemented long-stem prosthesis with or without plate augmentation could be used (Figs. 22.2, 22.3, and 22.4). The distal canal is reamed, and a trial stem is temporarily implanted. The proximal fragments can then be reduced using the trial component as a template. A lateral plate with cerclage cables is then applied in order to recover the normal length and obtain a stable fixation. Once length and stability are acceptable, the trial component is removed, and a definitive humeral stem is impacted; the cerclage cables are then retensioned and cut, and some screws are added to maximize the stability. The appropriate humeral length is selected combining different modular components (metaphysis and head), and a trial reduction is performed. After trialing, the definitive components are assembled and the shoulder reduction. These types of modular prosthesis have demonstrated excellent results in the revision setting and for periprosthetic fracture situations [30, 31]. This strategy is also effective for the Worland type B3 fractures (fractures about the prosthesis with an unstable stem).

Rarely, the proximal bone is so deficient that a modular proximal humeral replacement (so-called tumor prosthesis) could be used. In these situations, a cemented distal fixation is recommended. The proximal remaining bone and soft tissue can be cerclaged around the body of the proximal humeral replacing prosthesis with cable or heavy braided suture in order to maintain a stable shoulder.

For the Worland type B1 and B2 fractures with good alignment and a well-fixed humeral component, a nonoperative treatment could be considered. However, as reported in the literature, type B fractures treated nonoperatively have a high propensity to fail to heal and eventually require surgery. Wright and Cofield suggested that operative treatment should be considered for short oblique or transverse fractures that occur at the level of prosthesis tip. In addition, they recommended the use of autologous bone graft at the time of surgery. Type B fractures that have not progressed toward union by 3 months are also recommended for operative intervention.

For patients with a type B fracture and a well-fixed humeral component, the preferred current construct practice is a lateral plate with screw fixation in the distal portion and cerclage fixation in the proximal portion of the humerus. Distally, the plate should have a minimum of four to six holes covering the native humerus distal to the stem. If the diaphyseal bone is osteoporotic, as it is in many cases of periprosthetic fractures, locked screws are indicated. Locked screws should be placed after non-locked screws and appear to be most advantageous near the fracture site. Two or three equally spaced cables are used proximally between the surgical neck and the tip of the stem. The cables are sequentially tightened akin to the method of tightening a car wheel. This assures that tightening one cable does not result in loosening of an adjacent cable. Bone grafts are also used in order to maximize the healing potential, and strut allografts are reserved for situations with associated bone loss. The strut is secured with cables independent of an associated plate (cables over the strut and under the plate) and with cables around both.

The occurrence of humeral fractures after a shoulder prosthesis does not appear to significantly alter the final functional results.

22.4.2 Periprosthetic Scapular Fractures

Fractures of the glenoid usually occur intraoperatively when the glenoid is extremely osteopenic, such as in the patient with rheumatoid arthritis, and are related to the reaming or fixation technique. These complications concern only total shoulder replacements. Generally, the fracture fragments are small and comminuted and are not available to screw fixation. With inadequate bone support, the implant of a glenoid component should be abandoned and the defect bone grafted for a two-stage revision. After fracture healing, conversion of a hemiarthroplasty to a total unconstrained or RSA can be considered if symptoms require.

Postoperative acromial and spine fractures after RSA and their treatment have been described in the literature [32–35]. Because of the relatively brief history of the RSA, the management of these complications is poorly understood. The operative treatment is characterized

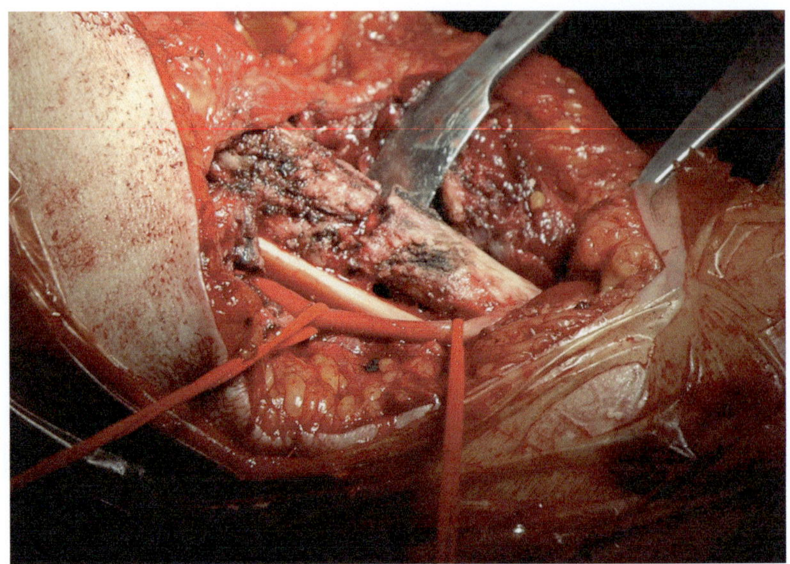

Fig. 22.2 Treatment of the fracture in Fig. 22.1. The glenoid component was well fixed at the time of surgery, and thus revision of the component was not necessary. The humeral component was removed and replaced with an uncemented long-stemmed component. The fracture was further secured with cortical strut allograft and plate with multiple cables. The radial nerve is precisely located and protected

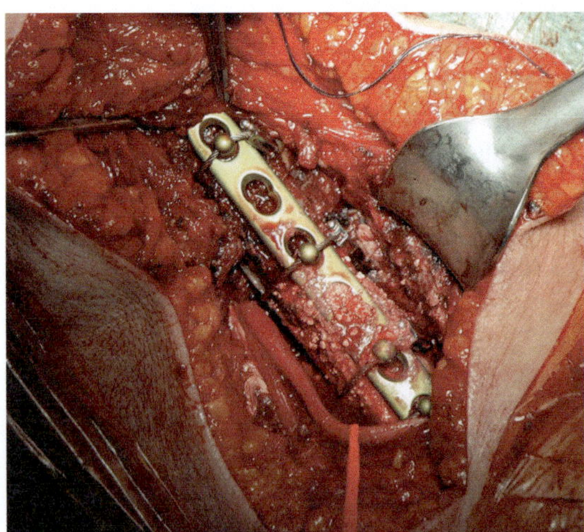

Fig. 22.3 Bone graft substitute was added at the fracture site in order to maximize the healing potential

by a high rate of nonunion due to the difficulty of stabilizing an osteoporotic bone under the increased tension of an elongated deltoid. The natural history of nonoperative management is characterized by reduced global shoulder function, but most of the patients who experienced this complication did not report chronic pain [36]. Given these patient outcomes, conservative treatment with an abduction splint for 6 weeks to limit pain and acromial tilt is a reasonable option for this complication.

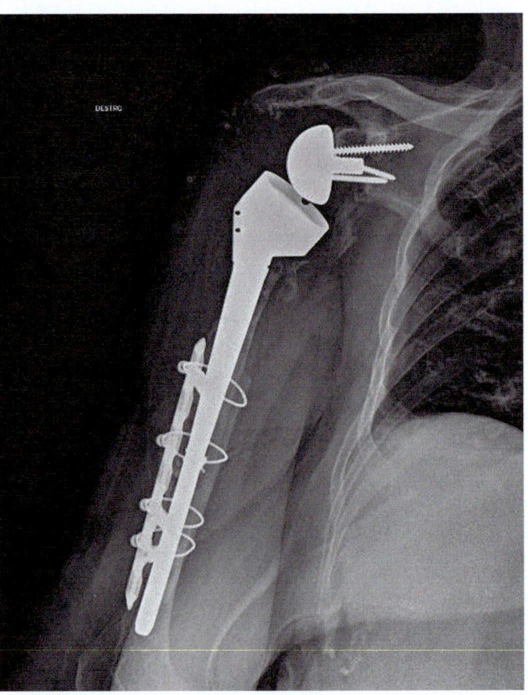

Fig. 22.4 Fracture healing 1 year after surgery

22.5 Postoperative Restrictions/ Rehabilitation

Patients with periprosthetic fractures often have numerous medical comorbid conditions that should be managed properly to mobilize the patients early and prevent life-threatening complications [1, 2, 5–8]. Physical therapy of the shoulder depends on type of fixation and bone quality; as in an acute fracture, early passive mobilization is recommended when adequate fixation has been achieved.

Few days after surgery, the hand, forearm, and elbow are gently exercised with active-assisted movement. Typically, passive external rotation outward to neutral position (0° degree with the arm at the side) and in elevation to 100–120° is also started early (2 weeks after surgery); however, it is important to avoid stress at the fracture site when doing this and also to continue with a passive program until healing has been ensured. When a long-stemmed implant has been implanted and the fracture is rotationally stable, we usually begin an active-assisted motion program at 4 weeks after the soft tissues have been allowed to heal.

In case of reverse shoulder replacement, due to the high incidence of instability, it is always recommended to delay the beginning of the therapy till the sixth week after surgery [2].

22.6 Complications

The complications of periprosthetic fracture can be related to the typical complications of an acute fracture in a native bone or the complications secondary to a joint replacement; sometimes the complications can occur in combination. These include nonunion, infection, axillary or radial nerve paresthesias or palsy, and stiffness as those with the major functional implications [5–8].

Nonunion is perhaps the most common complication, and the rate of nonunion in periprosthetic fracture is generally higher than the rate of a fracture in a native bone. The presence of an intramedullary stem implant could compromise the optimal fixation of the fracture, especially in osteopenic bone. Plate with cable fixation around the zone of prostheses has inferior strength compared with bicortical screw plating. Different operative strategies could be utilized in order to achieve fracture healing: long-stem prostheses in conjunction with extramedullary locked plates where mono-cortical locking screws augment cable fixation in the zone of the implant, the use of osteogenic and osteoinductive grafts or graft substitutes, and supplementation with osteogenic growth factors and cytokines [26–28].

Radial nerve injury may occur at the time of surgery because of the proximity of the nerve to the fracture site. Of course, appropriate choice of surgical approach is mandatory in order to avoid the nerve by careful dissection; the radial nerve should be precisely located and protected throughout the procedure. After a careful neurological clinical exam, the surgeon must be sure at the time of surgery that the radial nerve is not compromised [8].

Postoperative *infection* is a devastating complication in periprosthetic fracture that could compromise the fracture healing and the survivorship of the associated arthroplasty [5–7]. An acute infection could be managed by thorough debridement and irrigation, maintenance of the implanted internal fixation, and the use of antibiotics. In subacute or chronic infection, an implant revision could be considered in 1 or 2 stages using a temporary antibiotic-impregnated spacer. Failure to control the infection can lead sometimes to resection arthroplasty or even amputation.

Conclusions

Periprosthetic fractures continue to increase in frequency. In general, the goals of a periprosthetic fracture care include uncomplicated fracture union and return to preinjury level of pain and function. Treatment of periprosthetic fractures starts with prevention of intraoperative humeral or glenoid fracture. Meticulous surgical technique, good exposure, and gentle manipulation facilitate the procedure and reduce the risk of intraoperative fracture. In postoperative fractures, most authors favor nonoperative treatment and only consider open reduction and internal fixation when the fracture is unstable or in an unacceptable position. When the fracture leads to component loosening, revision of the component is indicated.

References

1. Gonzalez JF, Alami GB, Baque F, Walch G, Boileau P (2011) Complications of unconstrained shoulder prostheses. J Shoulder Elbow Surg 20(4):666–682. doi:10.1016/j.jse.2010.11.017
2. Zumstein MA, Pinedo M, Old J, Boileau P (2011) Problems, complications, reoperations, and revisions in reverse total shoulder arthroplasty: a systematic review. J Shoulder Elbow Surg 20(1):146–157. doi:10.1016/j.jse.2010.08.001
3. Boyd AD Jr, Thornhill TS, Barnes CL (1992) Fractures adjacent to humeral prostheses. J Bone Joint Surg Am 74(10):1498–1504
4. Kumar S, Sperling JW, Haidukewych GH, Cofield RH (2004) Periprosthetic humeral fractures after shoulder arthroplasty. J Bone Joint Surg Am 86-A(4):680–689
5. Singh JA, Sperling JW, Cofield RH (2011) Revision surgery following total shoulder arthroplasty: analysis of 2588 shoulders over three decades (1976 to 2008). J Bone Joint Surg Br 93(11):1513–1517. doi:10.1302/0301-620X.93B11.26938
6. Singh JA, Sperling JW, Cofield RH (2012) Risk factors for revision surgery after humeral head replacement: 1,431 shoulders over 3 decades. J Shoulder Elbow Surg 21(8):1039–1044. doi:10.1016/j.jse.2011.06.015, Epub 2011 Oct 5
7. Singh JA, Sperling J, Schleck C, Harmsen W, Cofield R (2012) Periprosthetic fractures associated with primary total shoulder arthroplasty and primary humeral head replacement: a thirty-three-year study. J Bone Joint Surg Am 94(19):1777–1785. doi:10.2106/JBJS.J.01945
8. Steinmann SP, Cheung EV (2008) Treatment of periprosthetic humerus fractures associated with shoulder arthroplasty. J Am Acad Orthop Surg 16(4):199–207
9. Athwal GS, Sperling JW, Rispoli DM, Cofield RH (2009) Periprosthetic humeral fractures during shoulder arthroplasty. J Bone Joint Surg Am 91(3): 594–603. doi:10.2106/JBJS.H.00439
10. Chin PY, Sperling JW, Cofield RH, Schleck C (2006) Complications of total shoulder arthroplasty: are they fewer or different? J Shoulder Elbow Surg 15(1): 19–22
11. Cameron B, Iannotti JP (1999) Periprosthetic fractures of the humerus and scapula: management and prevention. Orthop Clin North Am 30(2):305–318
12. Andersen JR, Williams CD, Cain R, Mighell M, Frankle M (2013) Surgically treated humeral shaft fractures following shoulder arthroplasty. J Bone Joint Surg Am 95(1):9–18. doi:10.2106/JBJS.K.00863
13. Campbell JT, Moore RS, Iannotti JP, Norris TR, Williams GR (1998) Periprosthetic humeral fractures: mechanisms of fracture and treatment options. J Shoulder Elbow Surg 7(4):406–413
14. Groh GI, Heckman MM, Wirth MA, Curtis RJ, Rockwood CA Jr (2008) Treatment of fractures adjacent to humeral prostheses. J Shoulder Elbow Surg 17(1):85–89
15. Bonutti PM, Hawkins RJ (1992) Fracture of the humeral shaft associated with total replacement arthroplasty of the shoulder. A case report. J Bone Joint Surg Am 74(4):617–618
16. Kligman M, Roffman M (1999) Humeral fracture following shoulder arthroplasty. Orthopedics 22(5): 511–513
17. Williams GR Jr, Iannotti JP (2002) Management of periprosthetic fractures: the shoulder. J Arthroplasty 17(4 Suppl 1):14–16
18. Wright TW, Cofield RH (1995) Humeral fractures after shoulder arthroplasty. J Bone Joint Surg Am 77(9):1340–1346
19. Worland RL, Kim DY, Arredondo J (1999) Periprosthetic humeral fractures: management and classification. J Shoulder Elbow Surg 8(6):590–594
20. Rittmeister M, Kersch-Baumer F (2001) Grammont reverse total shoulder arthroplasty in patients with rheumatoid arthritis and non reconstructible rotator cuff lesions. J Shoulder Elbow Surg 10(1):17–22
21. Crosby L, Hamilton A (2011) Scapula fractures after reverse shoulder arthroplasty: classification and treatment. Clin Orthop Relat Res 469:2544–2549. doi:10.1007/s11999-011-1881-3
22. Otto RJ, Virani NA, Levy JC, Nigro PT, Cuff DJ, Frankle MA (2013) Scapular fractures after reverse shoulder arthroplasty: evaluation of risk factors and the reliability of a proposed classification. J Shoulder Elbow Surg 22(11):1514–1521. doi:10.1016/j.jse.2013.02.007, pii: S1058-2746(13)00132-8
23. Wahlquist TC, Hunt AF, Braman JP (2011) Acromial base fractures after reverse total shoulder arthroplasty: report of five cases. J Shoulder Elbow Surg 20(7):1178–1183. doi:10.1016/j.jse.2011.01.029
24. Wall B, Nové-Josserand L, O'Connor DP, Edwards TB, Walch G (2007) Reverse total shoulder arthroplasty: a review of results according to etiology. J Bone Joint Surg Am 89(7):1476–1485
25. Molé D, Wein F, Dézaly C, Valenti P, Sirveaux F (2011) Surgical technique: the anterosuperior approach for reverse shoulder arthroplasty. Clin Orthop Relat Res 469(9):2461–2468. doi:10.1007/s11999-011-1861-7
26. Christofokaris J, Sadio S, Evans M (2003) Use of the Dall-Miles plate and cables for fixation of a periprosthetic humeral fracture. Acta Orthop Belg 69:562–565
27. De Smet L, Debeer I (2005) Fixation of a Periprosthetic Humeral Fracture with CCG-Cable System. Acta Chir Belg 105:543–544
28. Gerstenfeld LC, Edgar CM, Kakar S, Jacobsen KA, Einhorn TA (2007) Osteogenic growth factors and cytokines and their role in bone repair. In: Bronner F, Farach-Carson MC, Mikos AG (eds) Engineering of functional skeletal tissues topics in bone biology, 3rd edn. Springer, London, pp 17–45. doi:10.1007/978-1-84628-366-6_2
29. Trompeter AJ, Gupta RR (2013) The management of complex periprosthetic humeral fractures: a case

series of strut allograft augmentation, and a review of the literature. Strategies Trauma Limb Reconstr 8(1):43–51. doi:10.1007/s11751-013-0155-x
30. Owens CJ, Sperling JW, Cofield RH (2013) Utility and complications of long-stem humeral components in revision shoulder arthroplasty. J Shoulder Elbow Surg 22(7):e7–e12. doi:10.1016/j.jse.2012.10.034
31. Sommacal R, Bloch HR, Ghidelli A, Bettelli G, Dalla PP (2009) Comminuted periprosthetic humeral fracture after reverse shoulder prosthesis. Chir Organi Mov 93(Suppl 1):S83–S87. doi:10.1007/s12306-009-0013-7
32. Mottier F, Wall B, Nové-Josserand L, Galoisy Guibal L, Walch G (2007) Reverse prosthesis and os acromiale or acromion stress fracture. Rev Chir Orthop Reparatrice Appar Mot 93(2):133–141
33. Walch G, Mottier F, Wall B, Boileau P, Molé D, Favard L (2009) Acromial insufficiency in reverse shoulder arthroplasties. J Shoulder Elbow Surg 18(3):495–502. doi:10.1016/j.jse.2008.12.002
34. Hamid N, Connor PM, Fleischli JF, D'Alessandro DF (2011) Acromial fracture after reverse shoulder arthroplasty. Am J Orthop (Belle Mead NJ) 40(7):E125–E129
35. Cheung E, Willis M, Walker M, Clark R, Frankle MA (2011) Complications in reverse total shoulder arthroplasty. J Am Acad Orthop Surg 19(7):439–449
36. Hattrup SJ (2010) The influence of postoperative acromial and scapular spine fractures on the results of reverse shoulder arthroplasty. Orthopedics 12:33(5). doi:10.3928/01477447-20100329-04

Part III

Distal Humerus

23 Distal Humerus: Surgical Anatomy

Davide Blonna

23.1 Introduction

An overall prevalence of 12 % of acute radial nerve palsies after humeral shaft fractures has been reported [1]. An additional 10 % of the fractures treated surgically can develop an iatrogenic radial nerve palsy [2]. Forty percent of the patients that undergo open reduction and internal fixation for a distal humeral fracture can develop an acute or late ulnar neuropathy [3]. These data give a clear picture of the scope of the problem.

The surgical treatment of fractures of the elbow includes fractures of the distal humerus, coronoid and radial head fractures, and articular fractures of the trochlea and of the capitulum humeri. These fractures, whether they are treated with open or arthroscopic technique, can potentially injure the ulnar and radial nerves. The median nerve, on the contrary, is less frequently affected, as it is protected by the brachialis muscle. In this chapter, we will discuss the surgical anatomy of the ulnar and radial nerves with useful tips on how to avoid neurological injures. The median nerve, due to the rarity with which it is injured, will not be discussed here.

D. Blonna, MD, FACS
Department of Orthopaedics and Traumatology,
Mauriziano-Umberto I Hospital,
University of Turin Medical School,
Largo Turati 62, Turin 10128, Italy

23.2 Ulnar Nerve: Open Surgery

An understanding of the anatomic path of the ulnar nerve is critical to understand how to avoid ulnar nerve problems during fixation or replacement of distal humeral fractures. The first important concept regarding the anatomy of the ulnar nerve is the extreme variability of its course in the distal part of the humerus. Because of this variability, it is dangerous to blindly rely on precise anatomical landmarks when handling the ulnar nerve, without exploring its real position.

Key Points

The anatomy of the ulnar nerve is extremely variable in its course in the distal part of the humerus.

The ulnar nerve runs initially in the anterior compartment of the arm and goes posteriorly through the medial intermuscular septum at an average distance of about 6–8 cm proximal to the medial epicondyle with a range of between 5 and 11 cm [4, 5]. In approximately 40 % of cases, however, the ulnar nerve passes posteriorly without crossing the medial intermuscular septum and then transitions from anterior to posterior at a more distal point [6].

The online version of this chapter (doi:10.1007/978-88-470-5307-6_23) contains supplementary material, which is available to authorized users.

F. Castoldi et al. (eds.), *Simple and Complex Fractures of the Humerus*,
DOI 10.1007/978-88-470-5307-6_23, © Springer-Verlag Italia 2015

Further complicating the picture, the point of passage through the medial intermuscular septum can occur through a simple hole in the membrane or a fibrous channel formed by a splitting of the medial intermuscular septum. In some cases, the presence of a fibrous tissue in the vicinity of the medial intermuscular septum, particularly evident at the level of the passage of the nerve, led to the coining of the term *arcade of Struthers* whose existence and description, however, remain unclear. Several anatomical studies on cadavers have investigated the existence of the arcade of Struthers and have described its anatomical variants. The great variability reported in some articles is largely dependent on the terminology used to describe this structure. In articles in which the presence of any fibrous structure between the medial triceps and the medial intermuscular septum has been defined as the arcade of Struthers, the prevalence of this arcade exceeds 80 % in cadavers [4, 5].

In articles in which the description of the arcade is more adherent to the original description of the ligament of Struthers, the percentage drops to 0 % [7]. According to our clinical experience, the presence of a clear structure of a dense, fibrous, tendon-like membrane, stretched between the medial intermuscular septum and medial head of the triceps, is extremely rare. However, it is important to explore the nerve proximally, even in the absence of a clear ligament of Struthers, until it passes through the medial intermuscular septum, to avoid tardy neuropathies of the ulnar nerve.

At the level of the elbow, the ulnar nerve engages in the cubital tunnel, which is comprised proximally by the Osborne ligament (a fibrous structure stretched between the two heads of the FCU) and is formed distally by the deep flexor/pronator aponeurosis (approximately 5 cm distal to the medial epicondyle).

Considering the great variability of the ulnar nerve and its proximity to the medial epicondyle and the distal humerus, a cautious exploration of the ulnar nerve is usually recommended before proceeding with the treatment of the fracture. In elective surgery cases, the identification of the ulnar nerve is not particularly difficult. However, in fracture cases—especially those treated several days after the trauma—the identification of the ulnar nerve can be tricky because of the local edema and hematoma that usually infiltrates the triceps. To simplify the identification of the ulnar nerve, we recommend the application of a sterile tourniquet and to begin the identification of the ulnar nerve from proximal to distal (Fig. 23.1a, b).

Key Points

To simplify the identification of the ulnar nerve, we recommend the application of a sterile tourniquet and to begin the identification of the ulnar nerve from proximal to distal.

In extremely difficult cases, the identification of the nerve is made simpler by extending the exploration more proximally. Once isolated, the ulnar nerve must be released distally in order to allow a complete exposure of the medial epicondyle and to avoid a more distal compression. The exposure of the medial epicondyle is especially crucial for the synthesis of distal humeral fractures using parallel precontoured plates (Fig. 23.2). We recommend a neurolysis extending at least until the first motor branch followed by a transposition into a large subcutaneous pocket. During surgery, great care must be taken to avoid excessive traction on the nerve. For this reason, we prefer not to place heavy tools to clamp the vessel loop but instead use a simple knot (Fig. 23.3).

The postoperative management is extremely important to avoid tardy ulnar nerve complications. In this regard, we believe that it is important a drain be kept in place for 24 h to prevent the formation of large hematomas that may compress the ulnar nerve. The elbow must also be kept in extension for 24 h, hung above the head, to facilitate the resolution of local edema.

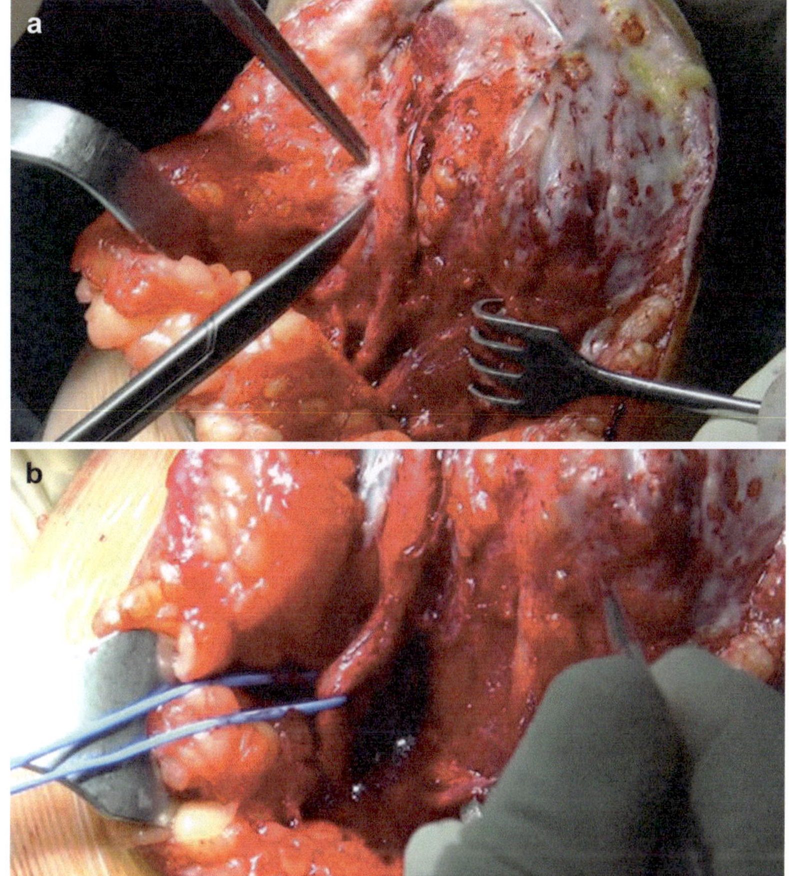

Fig. 23.1 (**a**) Posterior approach to the left elbow: the ulnar nerve is covered by abundant scar tissue. (**b**) The identification of the nerve is performed from proximal to distal

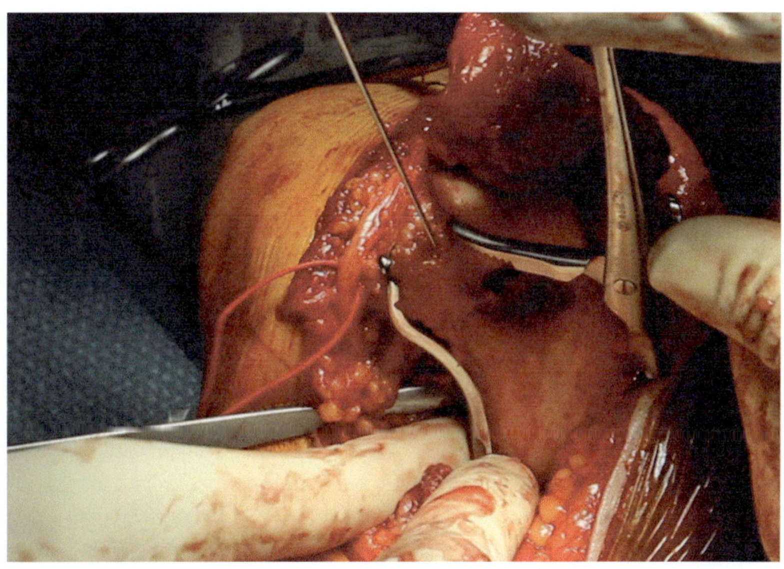

Fig. 23.2 The ulnar nerve is isolated before placing a medial precontoured plate for the distal humerus. In this case, a triceps-on technique has been used to fix the fracture

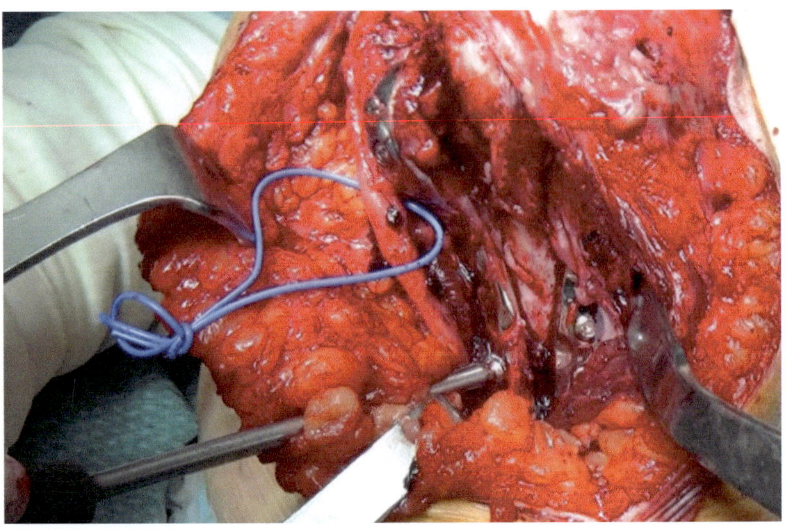

Fig. 23.3 A vessel loop without tension is placed around the ulnar nerve

23.3 Ulnar Nerve: Arthroscopic Surgery

The treatment of articular fractures of the elbow can be assisted by the use of arthroscopy in order to reduce the invasiveness of the surgical procedure and to obtain a better reduction. This can be done by following the principles that have led to the adoption of arthroscopic techniques for the repair of fractures in the shoulder such as in cases of bony Bankart fractures of the glenoid. Differently from the shoulder, however, the risk of injuring the three major nerves is greater in the elbow. The ulnar nerve is at risk especially during placement of the anteromedial portal. In the treatment of fractures, the risk is still higher than that in elective surgery due to the presence of edema and hematoma which reduces our ability to predict the position of the nerve. To reduce the risk of neurological injury, we advise to always perform an open exploration of the ulnar nerve without violating the joint capsule (so as not to lose the fluid pressure essential for proper arthroscopic visualization). The exploration of the ulnar nerve is also essential because a modest instability of the ulnar nerve at the level of the cubital tunnel is not uncommon—a factor that significantly increases the risk of iatrogenic nerve injury (Fig. 23.4a–c).

23.4 Radial Nerve: Open Surgery

The radial nerve has a course that puts it at high risk of iatrogenic damage in both fractures of the distal humerus and fractures of the radial head. The orthopedic surgeon's main difficulty is to correctly predict the position of the radial nerve with respect to the fracture line in order to ascertain during the preoperative planning stage if it will be necessary to isolate the radial nerve.

The importance of correct preoperative planning for the fixation of fractures of the proximal humerus is not to be underestimated. The knowledge, in advance, of the need to isolate the radial nerve has some advantages including (a) mental preparation of the surgeon, (b) a more accurate prediction of the length of the intervention and better management of the tourniquet, and (c) the ability to foresee the use of sterile tourniquet in cases of fractures with a more proximal extension.

The radial nerve arises, along with the axillary nerve, from the posterior cord of the brachial plexus. It runs posteromedially in the arm and descends into the arm moving laterally between the medial and lateral heads of the triceps closely to the radial nerve groove of the humerus. Here, the nerve is at high risk during the surgical treatment of diaphyseal fractures of the humerus (Fig. 23.5).

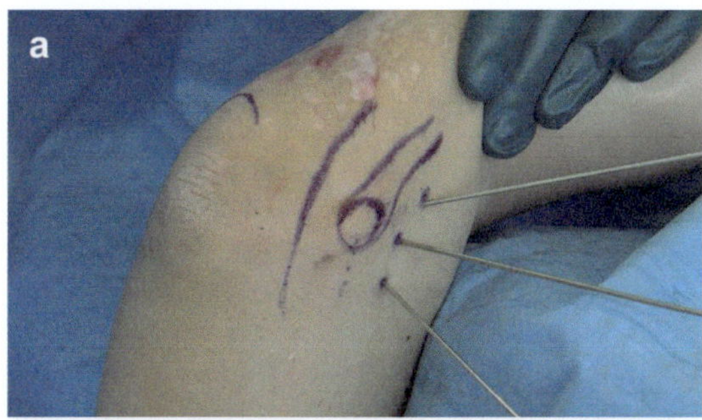

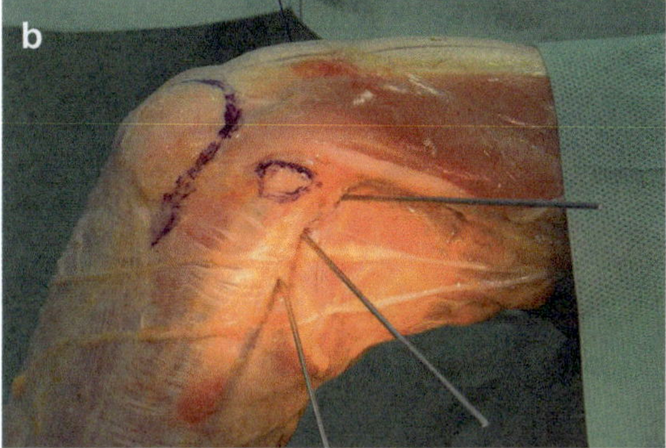

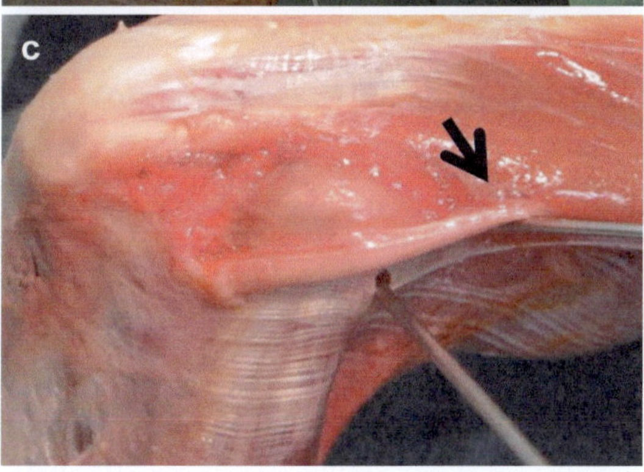

Fig. 23.4 (**a–c**) The more proximal anteromedial portals, during elbow arthroscopy, are at risk of damaging the ulnar nerve especially in cases of ulnar nerve instability (**c** *black arrow*). In this cadaver specimen, the proximal anteromedial portal is at the level of the ulnar nerve with a high potential risk of damaging the nerve

Moving laterally, the radial nerve pierces the intermuscular septum, and it runs in the anterior compartment of the arm between the biceps brachii muscle and the brachialis muscle. Approximately at the level of the elbow joint, it divides into its two terminal branches—the anterior and posterior interosseous nerve. The posterior interosseous nerve passes adjacent to the joint capsule at the level of the radial head. In this area, it is consistently located at the level of the middle aspect of the radial head. This site is of particular clinical importance because here the radial nerve is at risk in surgical procedures involving the removal of the joint capsule for stiff elbow. The posterior interosseous nerve passes from the anterior compartment to the posterior compartment of the forearm in the deep part of the supinator muscle adjacent to the proximal radius. The entrance of this channel is known as the arcade of Frohse. At this level, the posterior interosseous nerve is at risk of injury in surgery of the proximal radius (Fig. 23.6).

A prerequisite to the successful execution of preoperative planning is the knowledge of the path of the radial nerve in particular in relation to the lateral epicondyle (for fractures of the distal humerus) and radiohumeral joint (for fractures of the radial head).

The study of Kaminemi et al. [8] has demonstrated the importance of the intercondylar distance as a reliable measurement to predict the position of the radial nerve. This distance describes a secure area where we can manage the fracture of the distal humerus in relative safety. Increasing this measure by 40 %, we closely approach the radial nerve in its passage from the anterior to the posterior compartment of the arm. We commonly use this measure during preoperative planning to estimate the risk of damaging the radial nerve during repair of distal humeral fractures and thus know when it is necessary to explore the radial nerve posteriorly. This information is extremely important when an anatomical precontoured lateral plate is used for the fixation of the lateral column of a distal humeral fracture (Video 23.1).

Distal to the elbow, the radial nerve and its major branch, the posterior interosseous nerve, are at risk in different surgical procedures such as radial head replacement, fixation of radial head fractures, and reinsertion of the distal head of the biceps (Fig. 23.6).

The posterior interosseous nerve is in fact at risk both because of the close relationship between the nerve and the proximal radius and for the relative rarity with which orthopedic

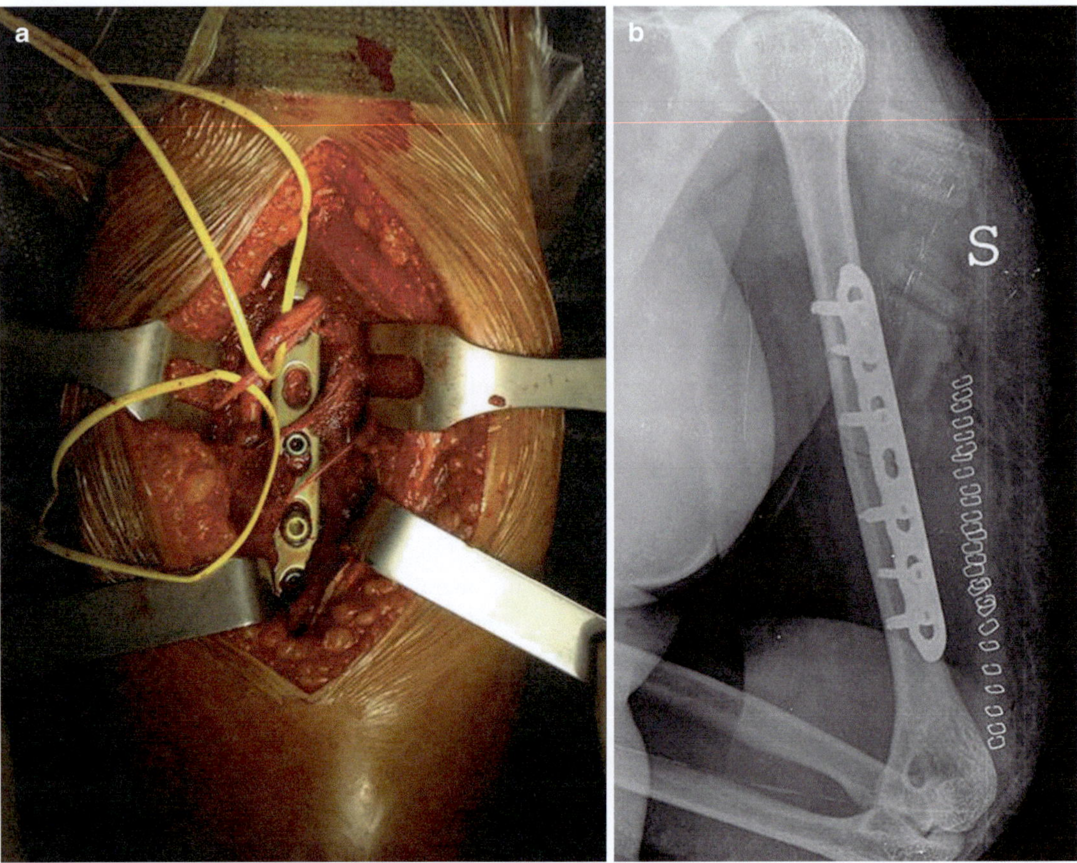

Fig. 23.5 Identification of the radial nerve through a posterior approach to the humerus to treat a fracture of the diaphysis

surgeons operate in this area. There are essentially two mechanisms of injury of the posterior interosseous nerve: (a) direct injury and (b) compression by retractors. In our experience, the second cause is far more frequent (Fig. 23.6). The placement of a retractor anterior to the radial diaphysis is very risky if it is not done with caution since the nerve passes close to the shaft and can be easily compressed by a retractor positioned incorrectly. The risk of a retractor damaging the posterior interosseous nerve is affected by the degree of pronation and supination of the forearm. The posterior interosseous nerve in fact changes position relative to the radial shaft during pronation-supination.

Forearm pronation tends to move the radial nerve more distally, while supination moves it more proximally. Based on the degree of pronation and supination, the radial nerve can therefore be, in theory, moved proximally or distally, making it more or less safe during the surgical procedure. However, this theory has been partially negated by recent studies of the anatomy of the posterior interosseous nerve where it appeared that pronation and supination change the orientation of the nerve without affecting its position relative to the articular surface [9].

As we have seen for fractures of the distal humerus, even in elbow surgery cases involving the proximal radius, preoperative planning is extremely important to prevent damage to the radial nerve.

What is important to know is the safety distance at which the nerve is located, with respect to the articular surface, in order to know whether it will be necessary to isolate and protect the posterior interosseous nerve during surgery. A study of Lawton et al. pointed out that the

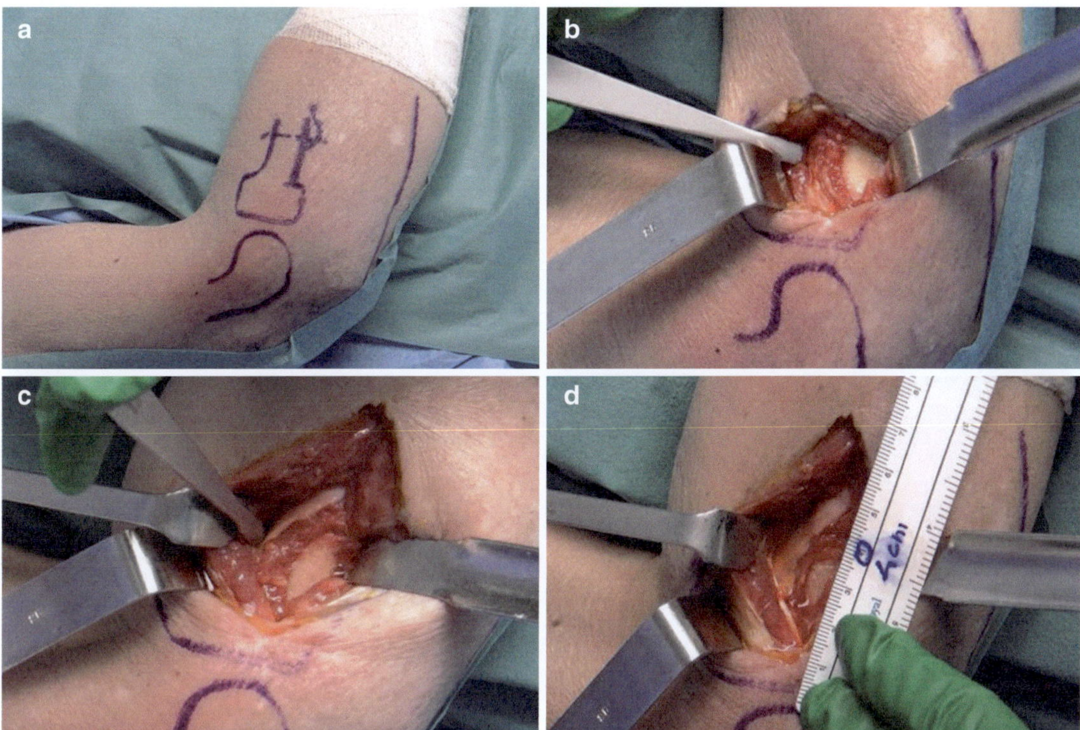

Fig. 23.6 The lateral approach to the proximal radius is at risk of damaging the posterior interosseous nerve (**a**). In this specimen, the Hohmann retractor is placed erroneously into the supinator muscle instead of in tight contact with the radius (**b**). By enlarging the approach (**c**), it is clear that the retractor is placed over the posterior interosseous nerve with an extremely high risk of neurological deficit after surgery. Four centimeters distally to the radiohumeral joint is generally considered a safe area in order to avoid damaging the posterior interosseous nerve (**d**)

average distance from the radiocapitellar joint to the posterior interosseous nerve was 4.6 cm with a minimum distance of 4 cm and limited nerve distal translation in pronation [9].

23.5 Radial Nerve: Arthroscopic Surgery

At the level of the elbow joint, the radial nerve is constantly in contact with the anterior joint capsule and crosses the joint at the level of the middle aspect of the radial head. This localization is very reproducible (Shawn O'Driscoll, personal communication) and exposes the radial nerve to iatrogenic injury during anterolateral access to the elbow. Three anterolateral arthroscopic portals have been described that can compromise the radial nerve in this area: the anterolateral portal, the proximal anterolateral portal, and the accessory proximal anterolateral portal. Although all three portals allow you to reach the joint cavity, the more proximal portals are likely to be safer because they are further from the path of the radial nerve (Fig. 23.7). For this reason, we recommend to those who favor the arthroscopic fixation technique to use a more proximal anterolateral portal.

Key Points

- Importance of preoperative planning.
- Intercondylar distance as a safe distance.
- Use proximal anterolateral portals for elbow arthroscopy.
- Do not rely on pronation and supination of the forearm to move the radial nerve away from iatrogenic injury.

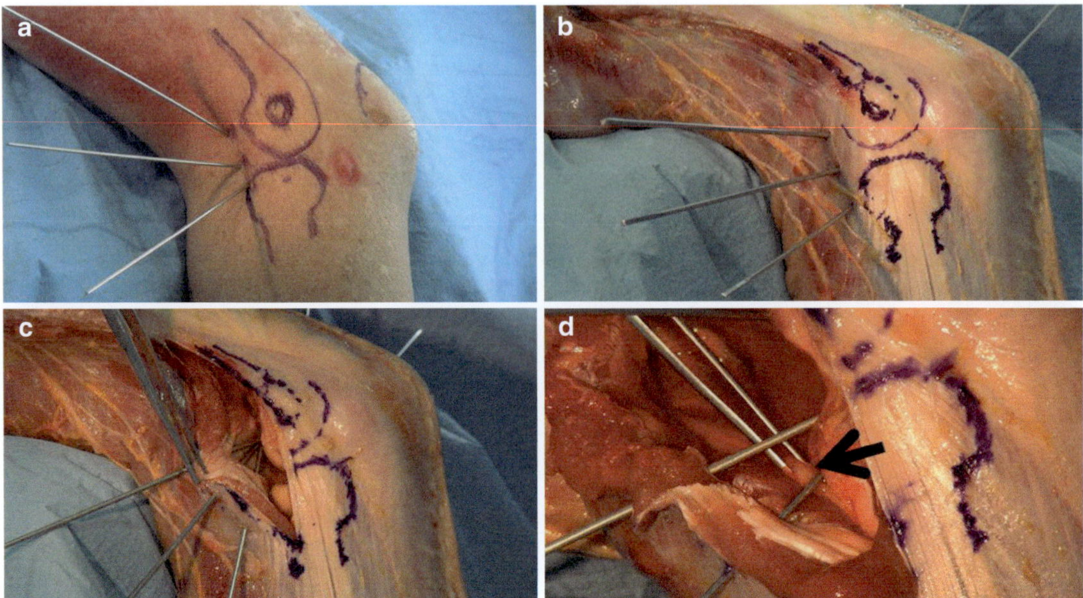

Fig. 23.7 Relationship between anterolateral portals and radial nerve from superficial (**a**) to deep anatomical layers (**b**). All the three portals can be used to reach the anterior joint (**c**). The more distal portal however is too close to the radial nerve (**d**, *black arrow*)

References

1. Shao YC, Harwood P, Grotz MR, Limb D, Giannoudis PV (2005) Radial nerve palsy associated with fractures of the shaft of the humerus: a systematic review. J Bone Joint Surg Br 87(12):1647–1652
2. Ouyang H, Xiong J, Xiang P, Cui Z, Chen L, Yu B (2013) Plate versus intramedullary nail fixation in the treatment of humeral shaft fractures: an updated meta-analysis. J Shoulder Elbow Surg 22(3):387–395
3. Worden A, Ilyas AM (2012) Ulnar neuropathy following distal humerus fracture fixation. Orthop Clin North Am 43(4):509–514
4. Amadio PC (1986) Anatomical basis for a technique of ulnar nerve transposition. Surg Radiol Anat 8:155–161
5. Tubbs SR, Deep A, Shoja MM, Mortazavi MM, Loukas M, Cohen-Gadol AA (2011) The arcade of Struthers: an anatomical study with potential neurosurgical significance. Surg Neurol Int 2:184
6. Won HS, Han SH, Oh CS, Chung IH, Kim SM, Lim SY (2011) Topographic relationship between the medial intermuscular septum and the ulnar nerve in the upper arm. J Neurosurg 114(6):1534–1537
7. Dellon A (1986) Musculotendinous variations about the medial humeral epicondyle. J Hand Surg Br 11:175–181
8. Kamineni S, Ankem H, Patten DK (2009) Anatomic relationship of the radial nerve to the elbow joint: clinical implications of safe pin placement. Clin Anat 22(6):684–688. doi:10.1002/ca.20831
9. Lawton JN, Cameron-Donaldson M, Blazar PE, Moore JR (2007) Anatomic considerations regarding the posterior interosseous nerve at the elbow. J Shoulder Elbow Surg 16(4):502–507

24 Surgical Approaches Based on Fracture Patterns

Alessandro Marinelli, Enrico Guerra, Graziano Bettelli, Michele Cavaciocchi, and Roberto Rotini

24.1 Introduction

Many surgical approaches have been described in the treatment of distal humerus fractures. Especially based on fracture patterns and surgeon's preference, the lateral, posterior, medial, and anterior approaches have been proposed. Of all the approaches described, only some are diffusely used in clinical practice: olecranon osteotomy, triceps-on (or triceps-preserving), triceps-splitting, triceps-reflecting anconeus pedicle (TRAP), Bryan-Morrey, and Kocher and Hotchkiss approaches and posterolateral extensile exposure. Each of these approaches presents inherent advantages in specific cases of trauma reconstruction, but no single approach can be considered optimal for the treatment of all the different patterns of distal humerus fractures. In fact, the complexity of different types of fractures along with the necessity to manage the extensor mechanism, to avoid neurovascular injuries, instability, and triceps weakness, requires to adapt the surgical exposure to the type of fracture.

The strategic choice of the surgical exposure is certainly the first basic step to obtain good functional results and minimize complications.

The choice of the surgical exposure requires an accurate comprehension of the lesion pattern, and it should be evaluated case by case; *general factors*, common to all the distal humerus fractures, along with *specific elements* of each case must be evaluated to choose the right approach. Also the possible intraoperative decision to have to convert surgery from ORIF to replacement can influence the choice of the approach.

The *general elements* that need to be considered in distal humerus exposure are:

- Obtaining an optimal visualization of all structures that require to be fixed (bone and soft tissues)
- Extending the exposure if required
- Minimizing the risk of injury of the neurovascular structures
- Preserving stability or allowing a strong repair if the ligaments are broken to allow early mobilization
- Handling the triceps in the best possible way in order to start an early rehabilitation

Specific patient's elements that need to be carefully considered for the choice of the exposure are:

- Osteopenia, age, and preexisting arthritis: In case of not fixable fracture in old and low-demand patients or in the presence of preexisting arthritis, a prosthesis has to be considered.

A. Marinelli (✉) • E. Guerra • G. Bettelli
M. Cavaciocchi • R. Rotini
Shoulder and Elbow Surgery Unit,
Rizzoli Orthopaedic Institute,
Via Pupilli 1, Bologna 40136, Italy
e-mail: alessandro.marinelli@ior.it;
enrico.guerra@ior.it; graziano.bettelli@ior.it;
michele.cavaciocchi@ior.it; roberto.rotini@ior.it

F. Castoldi et al. (eds.), *Simple and Complex Fractures of the Humerus*,
DOI 10.1007/978-88-470-5307-6_24, © Springer-Verlag Italia 2015

- Associated lesions: It is possible to take advantage of associated lesions (osseous, ligamentous, muscular) exploiting the broken structures as "windows" for the exposure and limiting the dissection of other healthy tissues.
- Previous surgical scars or skin lesions: The course of previous incisions should be followed whenever it is possible; conversely, skin lesions should be avoided modifying the line of the incision. In cases of severe skin lesions, the assistance of a plastic surgeon can be helpful to perform cutaneous or musculocutaneous flaps.

For practical purposes, to guide the best possible choice of the approach, it is possible to divide the distal humerus fractures in two main types: those requiring exposure of only one column, medial or lateral (A1, B1, B2, most of B3 types of the AO/OTA classification [1]) (Fig. 24.1), and those requiring both column exposures (A2, A3, C1, C2, C3) (Fig. 24.2).

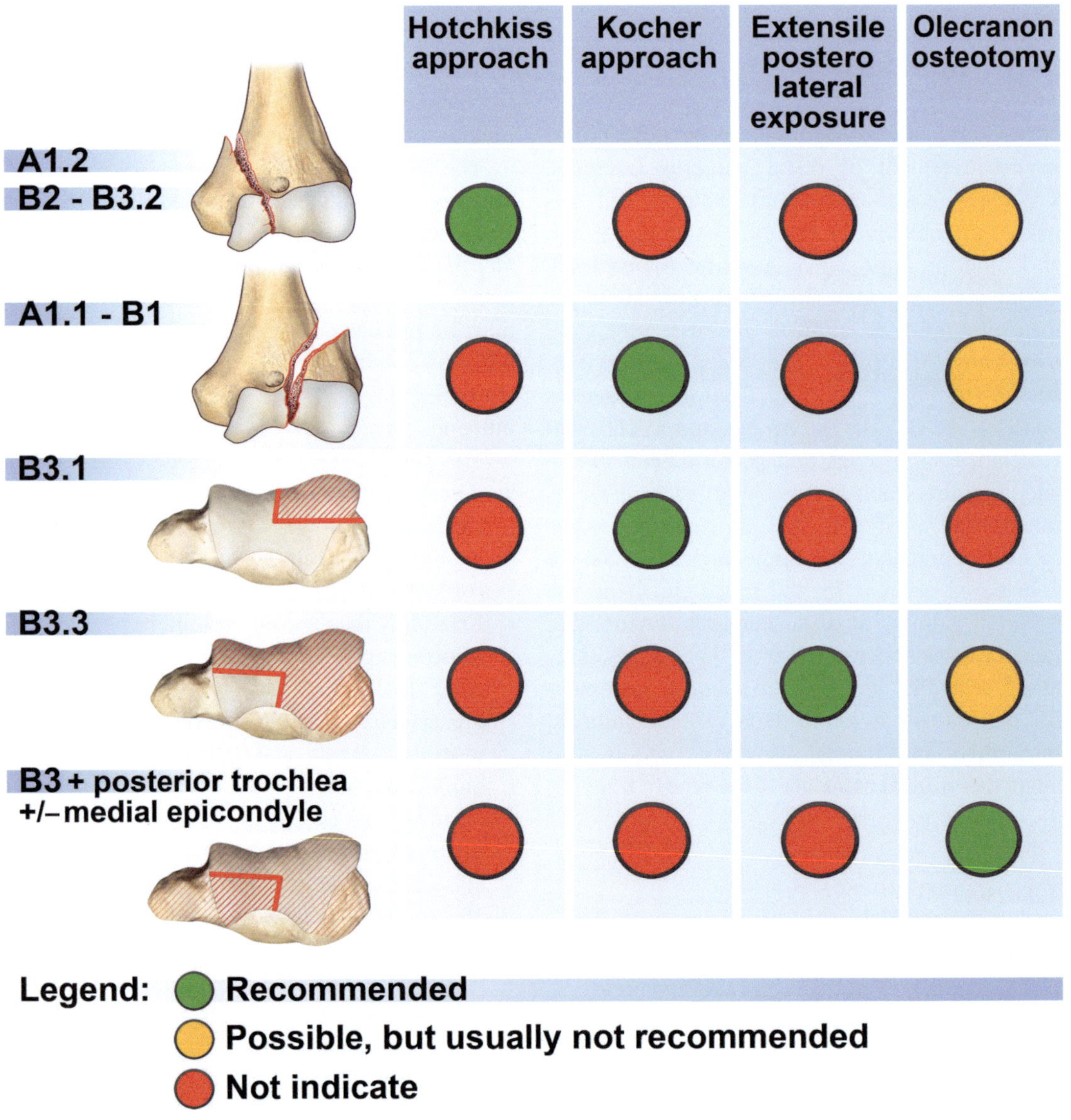

Fig. 24.1 Indications for surgical approaches based on fracture patterns

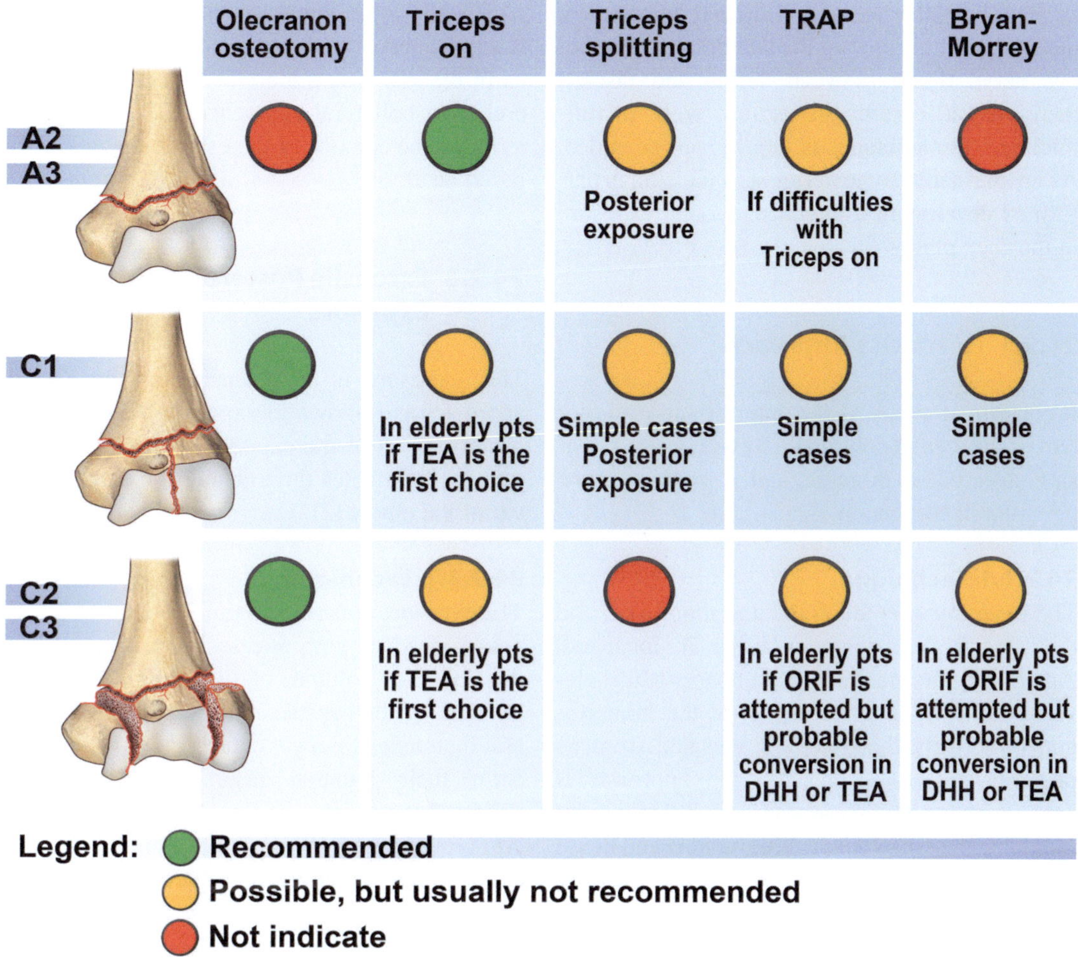

Fig. 24.2 Indications for posterior approaches based on fracture patterns

24.2 Lateral and Medial Approaches

In trauma reconstruction, a medial paratricipital approach, described by Hotchkiss [2], is indicated for the medial epicondyle fractures (A1.2) or the rare medial monocondylic fractures (B2) and the very rare isolated trochlear fractures (B3.2). Similarly, a Kocher approach with its variations (more or less extended proximally or distally) [2, 3] can be ideal to treat the lateral epicondylar fractures (A1.1), the lateral monocondylic fractures (B1), or the isolated capitellar fractures (B3.1, corresponding to the type I of the Dubberley classification [4]).

An extensile posterolateral exposure [2], feasible through a posterolateral skin incision, is indicated for capitellar and trochlear fractures (B3.3 type II of the Dubberley classification).

For the rare coronal plane fractures of the distal humerus involving not only the capitellum but also the posterior trochlea and the medial epicondyle (type of fracture not included in AO/OTA classification, corresponding to type 3B of the Dubberley classification [4] or to type 5 of the Ring classification [5]), the exposure of both columns is necessary, and therefore an olecranon osteotomy is the recommended approach. The indications for lateral and medial approaches are summarized in Fig. 24.1.

With both the lateral and medial approaches, there is a risk of injuring the antebrachial cutaneous nerve (lying between derma and fascia); therefore, a careful dissection with a full-thickness fasciocutaneous flap is recommended. As an alternative, a posterior skin incision is performed developing a lateral or medial exposure in the deep planes.

24.2.1 Hotchkiss Approach

It consists of exposing the anterior and posterior part of the medial column [2, 3] with distal extension toward the pronator and a portion of the common flexor tendon.

24.2.1.1 Technique

The ulnar nerve is identified and mobilized, and the medial supracondylar ridge is localized. Anteriorly, the brachialis is subperiosteally elevated from the anterior aspect of the humerus, and posteriorly the triceps is elevated from its posterior insertion. Distally, the approach is extended between pronator teres and flexor carpi radialis or between flexor carpi radialis and flexor carpi ulnaris (FCU). It is important to preserve the anterior band of the medial collateral ligament lying beneath the FCU.

24.2.2 Kocher Approach

In distal humerus fracture, the Kocher approach commonly used is the extensile variation [3] with exposure of the anterior and posterior part of lateral column (as described in lateral column procedure [6]), the lateral condyle, and the radial head as far as needed, preserving the LCL.

24.2.2.1 Technique

Anteriorly, the insertion of the brachioradialis, extensor carpi radialis longus, and brachialis is elevated from the lateral column; the triceps is elevated from its insertion on the posterior column. Proximally, the radial nerve is encountered approximately 8–10 cm above the lateral epicondyle as it crosses the lateral intermuscular septum.

Distally, the approach is extended in the Kocher interval between anconeus and extensor carpi ulnaris. It is important to preserve the lateral ulnar collateral ligament (LUCL) lying posterior to the equator of the capitellum and of the radial head.

24.2.3 Extensile Posterolateral Exposure

This exposure is an extension of the Kocher approach and allows to expose the anterior and posterior part of the capitellum and the anterior part of the trochlea through a dislocating maneuver of the elbow [2].

24.2.3.1 Technique

The exposure consists proximally of a lateral column procedure with release of the triceps from the posterior column, of the common extensor tendons, of the capsule, and of the lateral collateral ligament (if not yet detached by the fracture) from their humeral insertion. Distally, the approach consists of a Kocher approach. Applying a varus, flexion, and supination force, a subluxation maneuver is achieved, allowing a wide exposure of the anterior articular distal humerus surface.

24.3 Anterior Approach

The anterior approach is not usually required in the treatment of distal humerus fracture, even if it has been suggested to fix capitellar and trochlear fractures. This approach in our experience is not recommended in view of both the vicinity of neurovascular structures and the difficulties to obtain an accurate reduction of the fragments.

24.4 Posterior Approaches

In distal humerus fractures, the exposure is posterior in the great majority of cases because of its great versatility. This approach permits to reach not only the posterior but also the medial, lateral, and (albeit to a lesser extent) anterior part of the joint, and every type of distal humerus fracture can be treated with a posterior skin incision. "The front door to the elbow is at the back" is the famous sentence by Shawn O'Driscoll [7]. Precisely for its maximal versatility, the extensile posterior cutaneous incision has also been named the "universal approach."

Independently of the technique used to manage the triceps, the posterior approaches present some elements in common:

- *Patient's position*: Usually, a lateral decubitus with the arm supported over a bolster is preferred. Alternatively, a supine position with a bolster under the ipsilateral scapula and the arm crossing the chest with the humerus in a vertical position can be used. The choice between the two positions is essentially based on the surgeon's preference; however, the lateral decubitus allowing full elbow flexion can maximize the exposure of the articular surface.
- *A pneumatic tourniquet* during the ulnar nerve isolation and exposure/fixation of the fragments is helpful.
- *Skin incision:* A posterior midline straight incision just medial or lateral to the tip of the olecranon is performed. For most distal humeral fractures, a skin incision about 15 cm long is performed, but it can vary based on the proximal and distal extension of the fracture.
- The incision is carried down to the level of the deep fascia and triceps tendon, achieving two full-thickness fasciocutaneous flaps.
- *Ulnar nerve:* In the treatment of distal humerus fractures involving the medial column, the ulnar nerve requires to be always identified and dissected free throughout the cubital tunnel to its first motor branch, and—in our practice—it is always anteriorly transposed to protect it during the procedure and to prevent contact with the plate.
- *Radial nerve:* A proximal posterolateral extension over 10 cm requires to isolate the radial nerve.
- *Reconstruction surgery*: Independently of the triceps management, a careful reconstruction of the extensor mechanism is mandatory to avoid complications and to allow a rapid rehabilitation.

On the contrary, the posterior approaches differ in the way used to face the extensor mechanism. Based on the technique used to move the triceps off, the selective posterior approaches for distal humerus fixation can be classified in olecranon osteotomy, triceps splitting, Bryan-Morrey exposure, triceps on (or triceps preserving), and TRAP.

Olecranon osteotomy approach offers the maximum exposure, and therefore it is the exposure to be preferred in case of complex but fixable distal humerus fractures.

The triceps-on approach, allowing to maintain the triceps integrity, is recommended for fixation of extra-articular fractures (A2–A3 types of the AO/OTA classification [1]) to manage a not fixable fracture with a linked total elbow arthroplasty. In case of surgical difficulties, the triceps on can be converted in TRAP approach obtaining a greater articular exposure.

In case of open distal humerus fractures, it is possible to take advantage from the triceps muscle rupture to perform the triceps-splitting approach; however, because of the limited exposure of the joint, this approach is not indicated to treat the more complex distal humeral fractures.

TRAP and Bryan-Morrey approaches are especially indicated when the decision to proceed with internal fixation or arthroplasty needs to be taken intraoperatively.

We prefer to use the TRAP rather than the Bryan-Morrey approach for its better exposure of the lateral column permitting an easier placement of the plates with parallel configuration. The indications for each posterior approach are summarized in Fig. 24.2.

24.4.1 Olecranon Osteotomy

It is certainly the most frequently used approach, as it provides the widest exposure of the articular surface of the distal humerus.

This approach is however associated with possible complications as delayed union, nonunion, malunion, prominent hardware, intra-articular adhesions, and arthritis.

Moreover, if a total elbow arthroplasty (TEA) is considered in face of a fracture not certainly reconstructible, the olecranon osteotomy is contraindicated.

24.4.1.1 Technique

The ulnar nerve is identified along the medial border of the triceps, dissected at least 6 cm proximally and distally, and anteriorly transposed at the end of the procedure. Once the greater sigmoid notch is exposed medially and laterally to clearly visualize the bare area (the nonarticular portion between the olecranon articular facet and the coronoid articular facet), an apex-distal chevron-shaped osteotomy is performed at that level, initially using an oscillating saw and completing the procedure with an osteotome. The osteotomized proximal fragment is reflected proximally, exposing the medial and lateral columns and all the posterior articular part. With elbow hyperflexion, also a part of the anterior distal humerus can be exposed.

Athwal et al. [8] suggested a modification of the technique to preserve the anconeus muscle innervation, because the anconeus branch of the radial nerve comes from the lateral triceps muscle. This exposure, called "anconeus flap transolecranon approach," consists of combining the olecranon osteotomy with a proximally based anconeus flap, leaving the anconeus in continuity with the triceps muscle.

The anconeus is in fact a dynamic stabilizer of the elbow, and as it provides a vascular supply to the proximal fragment of the olecranon, it can play a role in reducing the risk of olecranon nonunion.

24.4.2 Triceps Splitting

The technique was originally described by Campbell [9]. This approach, consisting of a longitudinal splitting of triceps muscle and tendon to expose the distal humerus, is relatively easy to perform and allows a good exposure of the two columns and of the posterior part of the distal humerus articular surface. In patients with open intra-articular distal humeral fractures, the shaft of the humerus typically ruptures through the triceps muscle; this defect can be incorporated into a triceps-splitting approach [10]. The limited exposure of the joint makes this approach not indicated to treat the more complex distal humeral fractures.

24.4.2.1 Technique

A midline incision is performed through the triceps, fascia, and tendon and is continued distally across the insertion of the triceps tendon at the tip of the olecranon and down the subcutaneous crest of the ulna.

The ulnar nerve is identified and protected during the following time of triceps retraction.

The triceps muscle and its tendon are splitted, and two full-thickness flaps are created, leaving the extensor mechanism in continuity with the forearm fascia and muscle medially and laterally; the triceps insertion on the ulna is carefully subperiosteally reflected, laterally with the anconeus and medially with the flexor carpi ulnaris, exposing the olecranon.

It is possible to detach the triceps insertion by elevating osteoperiosteal flaps with a sharp osteotome from the olecranon as proposed by Gschwend [11].

In distal humerus fixation, attention must be paid not to detach the collateral ligaments; instead, they need to be released to allow the necessary elbow dislocation to implant a total elbow prosthesis.

Careful reconstructive surgery with transosseous suture on the olecranon of the triceps insertion is recommended because triceps detachment can occur, with olecranon buttonholing through the detached split triceps.

24.4.3 Triceps Reflecting or Bryan-Morrey

This approach permits to expose the posterior part of the distal humerus preserving the integrity of the extensor mechanism that is reflected from medial to lateral. Although this exposure has been described for total elbow arthroplasty [12], it can also be used for relatively not complex fractures of the distal humerus. Without detaching the collateral ligaments, it is possible with this approach to obtain an optimal exposure of the medial column; more difficulties can be encountered in fixing a fracture of the lateral column with proximal extension.

24.4.3.1 Technique

The ulnar nerve is identified, extensively isolated, and anteriorly transposed at the end of the procedure. The medial aspect of the triceps is proximally elevated from the humerus, and the posterior capsule is incised; more distally, Sharpey's fibers of the triceps attachment are sharply dissected from the proximal ulna. It is also possible to release the triceps with its osseous attachment as a thin wafer of bone [13]. With the elbow flexed 20–30° to relieve the tension on the extensor mechanism, it is entirely reflected over the lateral epicondyle.

In fracture fixation, careful attention must be paid not to detach the collateral ligaments from their humeral origins: in this way, mostly the medial column is exposed.

Instead, if a prosthesis is planned, the technique requires the surgical release of the collateral ligaments to allow elbow dislocation and to provide visualization of all the elbow joint.

A careful reinsertion of the extensor mechanism with heavy nonabsorbable sutures placed through crossed holes in the ulna is mandatory.

24.4.4 Triceps-On or Triceps-Preserving or Paratricipital Approach

This approach has been ideated in order to maintain the triceps integrity with visualization through medial and lateral windows, leaving the triceps insertion on the olecranon intact [14]. This provides an adequate exposure to treat extra-articular or simple intra-articular fractures; in case of difficulty due to an unexpectedly complex intra-articular fracture, this approach can be easily converted into a TRAP or a transolecranon approach.

This is the recommended approach to manage a not fixable fracture with a linked total elbow prosthesis [15]. Flexor and extensor tendons are released from the medial and lateral epicondylar regions, and the excision of the fractured condyles creates a distal working space to insert the components. The prosthesis is implanted by working on either side of the triceps mechanism. To have a better visualization of the ulna and to prepare the ulnar canal, about 20 % of the medial attachment of the triceps needs to be released.

24.4.4.1 Technique

The ulnar nerve is identified and isolated to the arcade of Struthers proximally and to the first motor branch in the flexor carpi ulnaris muscle belly distally. In case of medial column plating at the end of the procedure, our preference is to perform an anterior transposition of the ulnar nerve. The medial and lateral borders of the triceps muscle are elevated from their respective intermuscular septa. The lateral dissection is continued distally in the Kocher interval elevating the anconeus muscle along with the triceps and preserving its neurovascular supply.

The medial and lateral windows are connected with blunt dissection, elevating the triceps muscle from the posterior aspect of the humerus.

- Extreme flexion can be helpful to further visualize the posterior aspect of the distal part of the humerus.

Using the triceps-on approach, the reconstructive surgery at the end of the procedure is very limited, and a rehabilitation program can be started immediately.

24.4.5 Triceps-Reflecting Anconeus Pedicle (TRAP) Approach

This approach consists in detaching the triceps-anconeus unit from their ulnar and proximal humeral insertion with proximal reflection to expose the distal humerus. This exposure has been described by Shawn O'Driscoll [7], and although it does not allow an exposure as wide as that obtained with olecranon osteotomy, it is the approach suggested by O'Driscoll in many cases of distal intra-articular humeral fracture [7]. We can strongly support the author's opinion that this approach is easier to perform than it is imaginable by reading the description of the technique, and in our experience it is an effective elbow exposure in many situations both in trauma reconstruction and in replacement. This is our preferred approach when the decision to proceed with internal fixation or arthroplasty (distal humeral hemiarthroplasty, DHH, or total elbow arthroplasty, TEA) needs to be taken intraoperatively.

24.4.5.1 Technique

The ulnar nerve is identified, isolated, and usually anteriorly transposed at the end of the procedure. Laterally, a modified Kocher approach is performed. Opening the interval between the anconeus and the extensor carpi ulnaris, the anconeus is elevated subperiosteally off the ulna and the capsule. More proximally, the triceps is released from the lateral supracondylar ridge of the humerus. Medially, an exposure similar to the Bryan-Morrey approach is performed, with the triceps elevated from the medial supracondylar ridge and from the proximal ulna. More distally, the medial release of the anconeus from the ulna is connected with the previously performed lateral dissection. The triceps and anconeus are reflected proximally as a unique structure in an apex-distal V-shaped flap to expose the distal humerus. On both sides of the elbow, attention must be paid to preserve the lateral collateral ligaments.

In two studies performed on cadaver elbows, the distal articular surface exposure of different approaches has been calculated [16, 17]. It has been observed in both studies that the percentage of articular surface visible with a triceps splitting was about 35 % and with olecranon osteotomy about 55 %. The Bryan-Morrey approach allows to expose 46 % [16] and triceps on 26 % [17].

These studies indicate that all four tested approaches (olecranon osteotomy, Bryan-Morrey, triceps splitting, and triceps on) can provide good exposure to the medial and lateral columns; the olecranon osteotomy provides the greatest exposure of the distal humeral articular surface but leaves a substantial part of the anterior articular surface unvisualized (more than 40 %) [17], and the other three approaches (triceps on, splitting, Bryan-Morrey) provide even poorer exposure to the trochlear articular surface and almost no visualization of the capitellum [17].

24.5 Discussion and Conclusion

Controversy still exists regarding which is the best approach in optimizing fixation and minimizing complications for distal humerus fracture. However, even with limits and generalizations, it is possible to indicate that eight approaches can be effectively used to treat the different patterns of distal humerus fractures, each with specific indications and particular limits. In no other joint, so many exposures for trauma reconstruction have been described and should be known.

Certainly, the personal preference of the surgeon can be important in choosing the exposure, even if we think that the surgeon should adapt the exposure as much as possible to the type of fracture. This means that the surgeon should have a deep knowledge of the elbow anatomy and of the fracture patterns (a preoperative CT scan study with reconstruction is often recommended).

We can conclude that the correct choice of the approach is the first basic step to obtain good functional results and minimize complications.

The strategic choice of the approach should be mainly based on:

1. Obtaining *adequate exposure,* allowing the best management of all the potential surgical difficulties.
   A posterior cutaneous incision, named the "universal approach" for its maximal versatility, permits to treat every type of distal humerus fracture. For this reason in trauma reconstruction, the approach is posterior in the great majority of cases. More rarely, a lateral or medial skin incision, or sometimes both of them, is performed.
   Olecranon osteotomy can be considered the gold standard in elbow trauma for the treatment of complex intra-articular fractures of the distal humerus. However, in elderly and low-demand patients with severe comminution, if the decision can be to replace the fractured distal humerus with a linked total elbow

prosthesis, the recommended approach is the triceps on. In fact, excision of the fractured condyles creates a distal working space that permits to preserve the entire extensor mechanism decreasing time in surgery and triceps-related complications and enhancing rapid restoration of elbow strength and motion.

For the exposure, it is also important to remember to try to take advantage from possible associated lesions whenever possible. If there are an open fracture and a triceps defect, a triceps-splitting approach should be considered; if there is an olecranon fracture, it can be used instead of an osteotomy; if in a coronal shear fracture there is a lesion of the lateral collateral ligament or a fracture of the lateral column, these injuries can be exploited to facilitate dislocation through an extensile posterolateral exposure.

2. *Versatility* with possibility of extensile option and possible conversion from ORIF to replacement if necessary. It is useful to remember that the TRAP or Bryan-Morrey approach is especially attractive when the decision to proceed with internal fixation or arthroplasty (DHH or TEA) needs to be taken intraoperatively.

We think that the algorithm proposed (Figs. 24.1 and 24.2) can help the surgeon in deciding among many different approaches, guiding the choice to the more appropriate exposure for the specific pattern of fracture.

In conclusion, we want to highlight the importance of reconstructive surgery. We need to remember that the initial and the final steps of exposure and reconstruction should be considered as important as the fixation in obtaining good results and minimizing the complications in elbow trauma surgery.

References

1. Muller ME (1991) The comprehensive classification of fractures of long bones. In: Muller ME, Allgower M, Schneider R et al (eds) Manual of internla fixation, 3rd edn. Springer, Berlin, pp 118–150
2. Morrey BF (2002) Masters techniques in orthopaedic surgery: limited and extensile triceps reflecting and exposures of the elbow. Lippincott, Williams & Wilkins, Wolters Kluwer, Philadelphia, pp 3–25
3. Morrey BF (2009) Surgical exposures of the elbow. In: Morrey BF (ed) The elbow and its disorders, 4th edn. W.B. Saunders Co, Philadelphia, pp 115–142
4. Dubberley JH, Faber KJ, Macdermid JC, Patterson SD, King GJ (2006) Outcome after open reduction and internal fixation of capitellar and trochlear fractures. J Bone Joint Surg Am 88(1):46–54
5. Ring D, Jupiter JB, Gulotta L (2003) Articular fractures of the distal part of the humerus. J Bone Joint Surg Am 85-A(2):232–238
6. Mansat P, Morrey BF (1998) The column procedure: a limited lateral approach for extrinsic contracture of the elbow. J Bone Joint Surg Am 80–11:1603–1615
7. O'Driscoll SW (2000) The triceps-reflecting anconeus pedicle (TRAP) approach for distal humeral fractures and nonunions. Orthop Clin North Am 31:91–101
8. Athwal GS, Rispoli DM, Steinmann SP (2006) The anconeus flap transolecranon approach to the distal humerus. J Orthop Trauma 20:282–285
9. Campbell WC (1932) Incision for exposure of the elbow joint. Am J Surg 15:65–67
10. O'Driscoll SW, Jupiter JB, Cohen MS, Ring D, McKee MD (2003) Difficult elbow fractures: pearls and pitfalls. Instr Course Lect 52:113–134
11. Gschwend N (1981) Our operative approach to the elbow joint. Arch Orthop Trauma Surg 98:143–146
12. Bryan RS, Morrey BF (1982) Extensive posterior exposure of the elbow: a triceps-sparing approach. Clin Orthop Relat Res 166:188–192
13. Wolfe SW, Ranawat CS (1990) The osteo-anconeus flap. An approach for total elbow arthroplasty. J Bone Joint Surg Am 72(5):684–688
14. Alonso-Llames M (1972) Bilaterotricipital approach to the elbow. Its application in the osteosynthesis of supracondylar fractures of the humerus in children. Acta Orthop Scand 43:479–490
15. Cobb TK, Morrey BF (1997) Total elbow arthroplasty as primary treatment for distal humeral fractures in elderly patients. J Bone Joint Surg Am 79:826–832
16. Wilkinson JM, Stanley D (2001) Posterior surgical approaches to the elbow: a comparative anatomic study. J Shoulder Elbow Surg 10(4):380–382
17. Dakouré PWH, Ndiaye A, Ndoye JM, Sané AD, Niane MN, Sèye SIL, Dia A (2007) Posterior surgical approaches to the elbow: a simple method of comparison of the articular exposure. Surg Radiol Anat 29(8):671–674

Suggested Readings

Celli A, Celli L (2008) Elbow surgical approaches. In: Celli A, Celli L, Morrey BF (eds) Treatment of elbow lesions. Springer-Verlag Italia, Milano, pp 39–59

Laakso RB, Forcada-Calvet P, Ballesteros-Betancourt JR, Liusa-Pérez M, Antuna S (2012). In: Stanley D, Trail I (eds) Surgical Approacnes to the Elbow. Edinburgh, Churchill Livingstone Elsevier, pp 91–105

25 Principles of Fixation for Distal Humerus Fractures

Davide Blonna and Enrico Bellato

Fractures of the distal humerus are common and are increasing in frequency as the average age of our population increases.

Nonoperative management is rarely indicated and reserved for undisplaced fractures, for patients for whom anesthesia is deemed to pose too high of a risk, and for patients not mentally fit for surgery. Nonoperative treatment commonly results in poor outcomes due to nonunion, malunion, and joint stiffness [1–4].

The alternative to conservative treatment is surgery with reduction and fixation using plates or wires. Early reports on open reduction and internal fixation (ORIF), however, were unsatisfactory because the plates were bulky, difficult to contour, and rarely able to provide good distal fixation [5, 6]. On the other hand, other techniques, such as Kirschner wire fixation, did not provide adequate stability to treat bicolumnar distal humeral fractures [7, 8].

Modern operative fixation techniques and systems have progressively led to good results. Robinson [3] compared 273 surgically treated patients with 47 nonoperatively treated patients and stated that the latter were almost six times more likely to experience a nonunion. In the study performed by Srinivasan [9] of 29 fractures that occurred in patients over the age of 75, good to excellent results were seen in 57 % of the patients treated with ORIF and in 25 % of the patients treated nonoperatively. Conversely, poor results were seen in 10 % of the patients treated operatively and in 37.5 % of the patients treated conservatively. Zagorski [10] compared 29 patients treated with ORIF. Thirteen of these 29 were treated conservatively, and authors observed excellent or good results in 76 % of the patients of the first group versus observing satisfactory results only in 8 % of the second group of patients. A pooled analysis of these last two studies showed that patients treated conservatively experience three times the risk of having unacceptable result [11].

> **Key Point**
> Surgical treatment is indicated in the majority of cases since it provides better outcomes compared to conservative treatment.

D. Blonna (✉)
Department of Orthopaedics and Traumatology, University of Turin Medical School, Mauriziano-Umberto I Hospital, Largo Turati 62, Turin 10128, Italy
e-mail: davide.blonna@virgilio.it

E. Bellato
Department of Orthopaedics and Traumatology, University of Turin Medical School, CTO-Maria Adelaide Hospital, Via Zuretti 29, Turin 10126, Italy
e-mail: bellatoenrico@gmail.com

The online version of this chapter (doi:10.1007/978-88-470-5307-6_25) contains supplementary material, which is available to authorized users.

F. Castoldi et al. (eds.), *Simple and Complex Fractures of the Humerus*,
DOI 10.1007/978-88-470-5307-6_25, © Springer-Verlag Italia 2015

25.1 Which Type of Fixation?

Fixation of distal humeral fractures has evolved from the use of Kirschner wires and lag screws to modern double-plate fixation resulting in a dramatic improvement in outcomes.

Ulusal [12] compared the results of three different surgical techniques: double plates (seven patients), multiple Kirschner wires (eight patients), and multiple screws (seven patients); the mean Mayo Elbow Performance Scores (MEPS) were 88, 55, and 72, respectively, and the authors concluded that ORIF with double plates was superior. Papaioannou [13] reported the results achieved by two groups of patients, one treated with minimal osseous reconstruction (screw and pins) and the other with double plates; the risk of poor outcomes was three times higher after the first treatment ($p<0.01$). Screw reconstruction and fracture fixation by pins resulted in a high percentage of implant failures in Södergard's study [14].

These and other studies have led to the conclusion that plate fixation is the procedure of choice in the adult population, while Kirschner wire fixation remains the treatment of choice for pediatric supracondylar fractures [15–17].

Key Point
Plate fixation is the procedure of choice in the adult population, while Kirschner wire fixation is the treatment of choice in pediatric supracondylar fractures.

25.2 Which Type of Plates?

Distal humeral fracture fixation can be achieved basically with three types of plates: (1) 3.5 mm straight standard plates that are intraoperatively contoured, (2) perpendicular precontoured plates (Fig. 25.1), and (3) parallel precontoured plates (Fig. 25.2). The plates moreover can be placed with or without the locking screw principle.

The use of one-third tubular plates is not recommended because they are too weak and prone to breakage, particularly in cases of metaphyseal comminution [18–20].

Different authors advocate the use of locking compression plates (LCPs) because they are more reliable in humeri with decreased bone quality or in the presence of a metaphyseal comminution and because they are based on the principle of an internal fixator [21]. However, even though they have been proven to achieve better fixation and outcomes when used for other types of fractures, the use of locking plates for distal humeral fractures is debated. There is a lack of evidence to recommend for or against the use of LCP. Schuster [22] used cadaver specimens of different bone mineral densities to compare the stiffness of conventional reconstruction plates, surgeon-contoured 3.5 mm LCPs, and precontoured distal humerus LCPs. Results were not significantly different between the three groups even though the failure rate was lower in the precontoured distal humerus plate group. In particular, there was no statistical difference between LCPs and conventional reconstruction plates, but the author concluded that, in case of low bone density, LCPs should be chosen over other hardware. Korner [23] showed no difference in stiffness between LCPs and non-locking conventional reconstruction plates placed in a perpendicular configuration. Reising [24] and Greiner [25] reported good results, but the evidence level of their studies is type IV. Other authors prefer not using LCP to prevent the problem of incorrect screw positioning due to the fixed angles of the hardware [26, 27].

Quite recently, implant manufacturers have started producing specially precontoured distal humeral plates. Despite being more costly, these plates are preferable since they may reduce the duration of surgery and since their fracture-specific screw patterns allow high-density screw placement into the distal humeral articular segment [22, 24, 28]. Low distal humerus fractures with articular comminution seem to be best treated with precontoured plates [29]. Athwal [28] reported the results of 32 patients affected by AO C-type fractures treated with precontoured non-locking plates. He stated that a high rate of union with good outcomes can be expected but was also concerned about the high rate of complications (a total of 24 complications occurred in 17 patients, including nerve injuries, wound problems, and intra-articular screw penetration). Celli [30] reported excellent

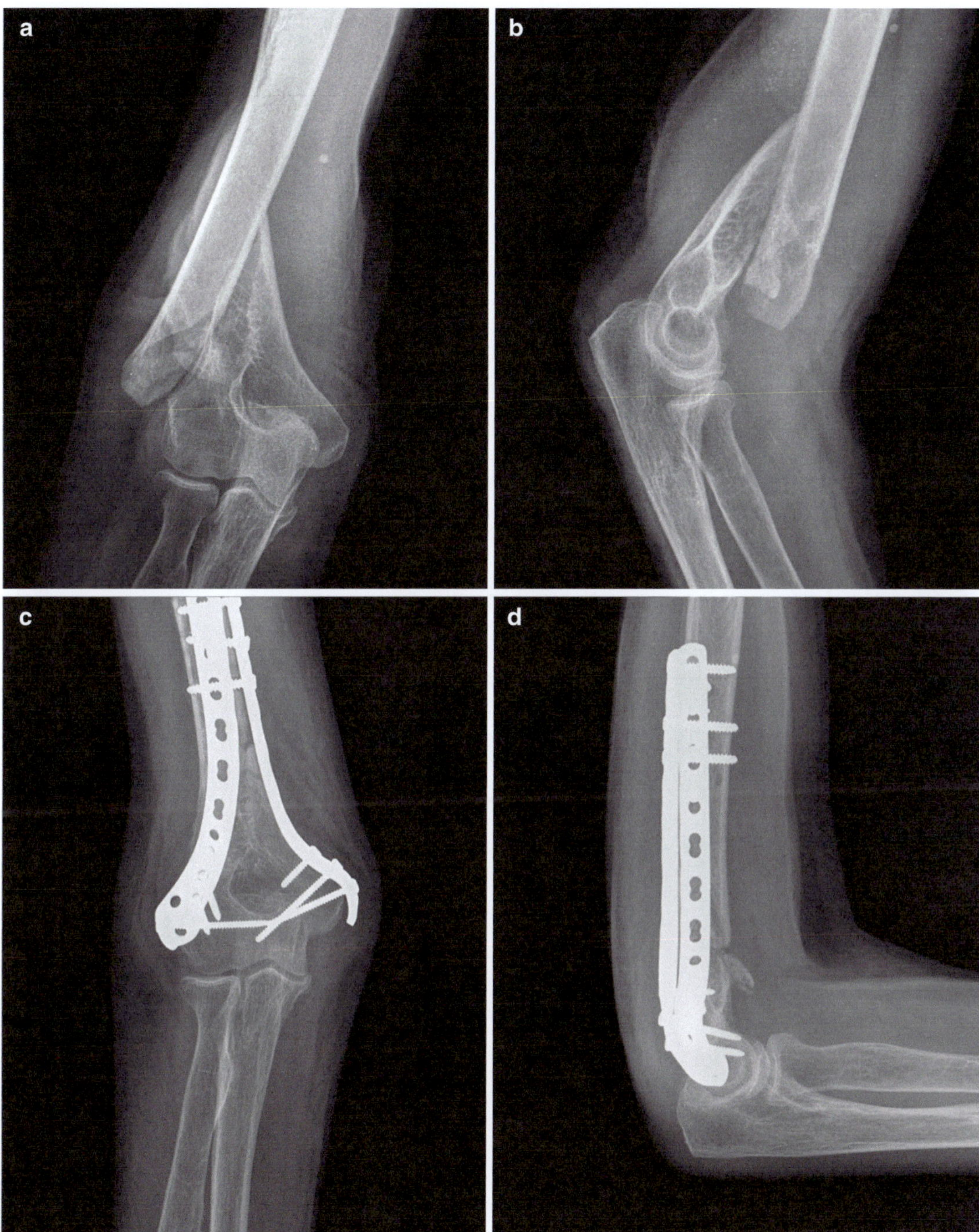

Fig. 25.1 Two precontoured anatomic perpendicular plates are used to fix a distal humeral fracture. In this case, the use of perpendicular plates can be indicated since the fracture does not affect the articular surface. (**a**, **b**) Preoperative x-rays, showing displaced distal humeral fracture; (**c**, **d**) Postoperative x-rays showing anatomical reduction and plate fixation

and good results achieved in 16 patients and unsatisfactory results in 2, but the study was a retrospective, multi-surgeon series with a relatively short follow-up period. Theivendran [31] reported good functional results and a high union rate but pointed out that screw extraction can be difficult when the implant is removed. Contrary to this, Koonce [32] stated that perpendicular

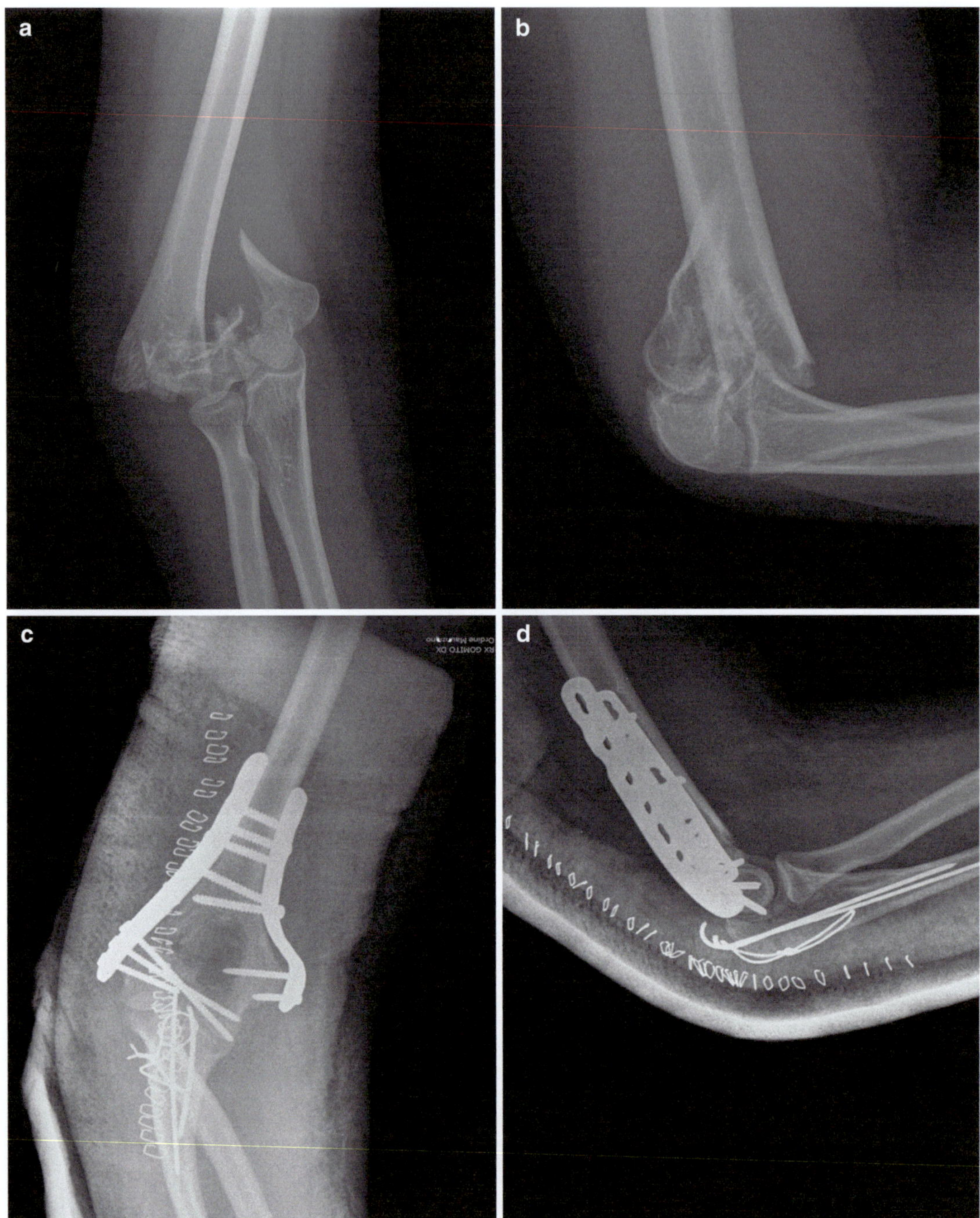

Fig. 25.2 Two precontoured anatomic parallel plates are used to fix this distal humeral fracture affecting the articular surface of the humerus. Using these plates, fractures with comminution of the articular surface can be successfully treated. (**a**, **b**) Preoperative x-rays, showing displaced distal humeral fracture with comminution of the articular surface; (**c**, **d**) Postoperative x-rays showing anatomical reduction and plate fixation

conventional reconstruction plate constructs provided similar stiffness and load to failure properties to precontoured locking plate systems regardless of plate configuration.

Finally, plate length is also important: plates should end at different levels proximally to avoid the formation of a stress riser in the humeral diaphysis [26].

Key Point
Precontoured anatomic plates seem to provide better outcomes through superior biomechanical properties.

25.3 How Many Plates?

It is now widely accepted that good fixation requires two plates, either parallel or perpendicular [11, 18, 33, 34]. In distal humeral fractures, one plate is usually not enough to guarantee good stability, while in other fractures (e.g., proximal tibia and distal femur) the introduction of LCPs has obviated the need for bicolumnar fixation. The use of a single lateral plate should be avoided or limited to well-selected cases where the fracture does not affect both the lateral and medial columns of the distal humerus.

Some clinical studies reported adequate fixation of extra-articular distal humerus fractures using a single-plate technique [4, 35, 36], but some degree of cortical contact was present, and this probably influenced the outcome. Tejwani [37] performed a biomechanical study to compare the stiffness and the strength provided either by standard double-plate fixation or by single-locking plate fixation in cases of comminuted extra-articular distal humeral fractures. The first construct was significantly stiffer than the second in anterior bending, posterior bending, and lateral bending, while there were no significant differences in axial compression and torsion.

However, different results have been recently reported by Meloy [38]. The authors compared the traditional dual-column plating with a single-column posterolateral small-fragment precontoured locking plate used as a neutralization device with at least five screws in the short distal segment in fracture extra-articular cases (AO A2 and A3 types). The two groups had similar union rates and alignment, but the second was characterized by a better range of motion with less complications.

A third posterolateral plate may be used to increase the fixation rigidity [39, 40]. Some authors believe that it is mainly indicated for low transcondylar fractures and those with a coronal shear component, which are best stabilized using posterior to anterior screws [34].

Key Point
Two plates either parallel or perpendicular are preferred to a single-plate configuration.

25.4 Which Plate Configuration?

Three options of plate localization have been described:

- Perpendicular plating (Fig. 25.1): This technique evolved after a publication by Jupiter in 1985 [41]; the posterior plate is the lateral one. It needs to be placed as close as possible to the capitulum articular surface without causing impingement, so that it can gain the best possible purchase of its screws in the distal fragment.
- Parallel plating (Fig. 25.2): This concept was conceived because some surgeons felt that the orthogonal plating technique provided inadequate fixation of the distal fragments and not enough stability between the intra-articular distal fragments and the humeral shaft [14, 19, 42–44]. Based on these observations, the Mayo Clinic group proposed the idea of parallel plating [33, 45]. The lateral plate is applied along the supracondylar ridge in the sagittal plane and is characterized by a "J" shape to accommodate the anterior angulation of the lateral epicondyle; it needs to be placed as distal as possible to the edge of the capitulum. The surgeon must evaluate the elbow in full extension and pay attention that the plate does not impinge on the radial head. The medial plate is placed along the supracondylar ridge that curves around the medial epicondyle; it is better if distal tip of the plate lies superior to the most prominent portion of the medial epicondyle. Actually, the two plates are not perfectly parallel, rather they are offset dorsally such that the angle between them is usually between 150° and 160°. This allows the placement of at least four long screws passing through the distal fragments from medial to lateral and vice versa [46].
- Triple plating: It is a combination of the two techniques. It is used in cases with severe comminution where additional fixation is required. Typically, the third plate is applied along the

lateral aspect of the lateral column [47, 48]. However, it does not seem to confer greater stiffness and is technically difficult [34].

To date, the first two plate configurations have typically been used. Historically, the treatment with conventional reconstruction plates in a perpendicular configuration has been recommended by the AO group [49, 50]. However, this approach has been widely criticized—mainly because obtaining adequate screw purchase and length in a posteroanterior direction through a posterolateral plate can be difficult (especially with osteopenic bone) [51]. Several studies support either the parallel plating technique [28, 30, 31, 52, 53] or the orthogonal plating technique [24, 25, 54–56].

25.4.1 Studies Supporting the Parallel Configuration

Schemitsch [18] created a metaphyseal supracondylar osteotomy to reproduce a distal humeral fracture in eight upper extremities from cadavers. He then created a gap and tested the plate reconstruction with and without cortical contact. In the former configuration, the plates provided equivalent rigidity, while in the later configuration, the parallel plates showed higher stiffness in axial compression, without any difference in ultimate load to failure.

Zalavras [57] stressed the fact that the fracture model used in his study was characterized by an extensive metaphyseal defect for which he used, in contrast to previous studies, plates from a single elbow fixation system in order to avoid bias. Screw loosening occurred in all posterior plates of orthogonal constructs but in none of the parallel plate constructs.

Arnander [58] osteotomized two groups of artificial humeri. The specimens were subject to static loading only in the sagittal plane in an anteroposterior direction, and the parallel system had superior strength and stiffness as compared to the orthogonal system.

Stoffel [59] tested on cadavers two elbow plating systems with locking screws (the perpendicular 3.5 mm LCP distal humerus plating system and the parallel Mayo Clinic Congruent elbow plate system). They were tested for their stiffness (in compression and internal/external rotation), plastic deformation, and failure in torsion and showed that the parallel construct had significantly higher stiffness in axial compression and external rotation than the orthogonal construct. However, the different plating systems might be a confounding factor.

In Penzkofer's biomechanical study [60], three different implant configurations on artificial humeri were compared to each other: parallel plating and orthogonal plating either with a posteromedial plate or with a posterolateral plate. All three plate configurations provided enough mechanical stability to start early postoperative rehabilitation; the parallel configuration achieved the highest bending stiffness in extension, while in flexion the highest bending stiffness was provided by the construct with a posterolateral plate. However, the author concluded that a parallel plate configuration provides the highest stability since extension is the most demanding load situation for the elbow.

25.4.2 Studies Supporting the Perpendicular Configuration

One of the first studies evaluating the perpendicular configuration was carried out by Helfet [61], who stated that it was biomechanically optimal. However, he compared this construct with cross screws or the single "Y" plate.

Jacobson [34] evaluated the rigidity of five internal fixation constructs. There was no significant difference in torsional stiffness of the five constructs. The configuration with a medial pelvic reconstruction plate combined with a posterolateral dual compression plate had significantly greater relative bending stiffness in the sagittal plane than the other constructs. However, this difference could be a consequence of the stronger plate used in the orthogonal group and as opposed to the plate orientation.

Got [62] evaluated bone density of ten pairs of cadaver elbows and randomly assigned them to either the parallel or the perpendicular configuration group. These two constructs were tested in cases of comminuted intra-articular fractures. He demonstrated that the two constructs had similar biomechanical properties, while the perpendicular configuration had greater torsional resistance.

25.4.3 Studies Showing No Difference Between the Two Options

Kollias [63] compared in a cadaveric study precontoured non-locking parallel plates versus a 90° non-locking construct. He found a trend toward more stiffness of the parallel construct in anteroposterior, mediolateral, and torsional testing, but statistical significance was not achieved. He concluded by suggesting both configurations but stressing that his results were in line with the biomechanical literature supporting the use of a parallel configuration.

Schwartz [64] created a bicolumnar fracture in ten artificial humeri: five were randomly fixed with parallel plates and the other five were fixed with orthogonal plates. Both configurations seemed to provide similar stabilization under physiological loads: there were no differences between constructs both under longitudinal strain (for torsion, varus/valgus or flexion-extension) and under transverse strain. However, this study does have some limitations, e.g., the low number of specimens and the different plate systems used.

Key Point

A parallel plate configuration seems to provide better biomechanical properties compared to a perpendicular plate configuration.

As we can see, all the references cited above are biomechanical studies. Only two clinical studies have been recently carried out.

Shin [51] described the results of 17 patients treated by perpendicular plating and 18 by parallel plating techniques. All patients were affected by closed intra-articular distal humerus fractures (AO C type) and were randomly assigned to one of the two groups. Different types of plates were used, but the material was the same (titanium). A single surgeon carried out all surgeries within 5 days of injury (except for one patient), and all patients followed the same postoperative rehabilitation protocol. In the perpendicular plating group, the arc of flexion averaged 106° ± 23° postoperatively (mean elbow flexion of 119° ± 16° and mean extension of 13° ± 9°), while in the parallel plating group the arc of flexion averaged 112° ± 19° (mean elbow flexion of 121° ± 15° and mean extension of 10° ± 8°). The Mayo Elbow Performance Scores (MEPS) were 91.5 and 94.3, respectively. Bony union occurred at 6.3 months and at 5.4 months after surgery, respectively, and nonunion was observed only in two patients of the first group. The author reported five complications in the first group and seven in the second one. Even though no significant differences were recorded between the two groups, the author concluded that the two nonunions in the perpendicular group may suggest a more rigid fixation provided by two parallel plates.

Lee [65] performed a prospective, randomized, comparative study including 67 patients affected by AO C-type intra-articular distal humerus fractures randomly divided into two groups: 32 in the perpendicular group (using a locking compression distal humerus plate) and 35 in parallel group (using a precontoured anatomic plate). All surgeries were performed by the same surgeon, and all patients followed the same postoperative and rehabilitation protocol. The operating time, the time to fracture union, the presence of a step or gap at the articular margin, the varus/valgus angulation, the functional recovery, and the complications were recorded. No articular defects >1 mm were detected. Bony union was achieved at a mean of 6.1 months in the first group and 5.8 months in the second group, and no patients were affected by nonunion. The mean arc of motion at last follow-up was 98° ± 20° versus 100° ± 23°, respectively. The VAS, DASH, and MEP scores were 2 ± 1.3 versus 2 ± 1.7, 25.2 ± 9.8 versus 22.9 ± 8.7, and 85.1 ± 28.2 versus 89.7 ± 30.1, respectively. Three patients in the perpendicular group and two patients in the parallel group experienced heterotopic ossification: one of the latter two needed resection with arthrolysis and implant removal after 11 months. Two patients with screw loosening in the parallel group had a secondary procedure; however, fracture stability was not affected. Eight patients in the perpendicular group and 13 in the parallel group required surgery to remove hardware, the main reason for which being the prominence of the olecranon plate or lateral plate in the parallel group. The author concluded that no significant differences were found between the two methods with respect to clinical outcomes and complications. Nevertheless, the perpendicular configuration may provide additional stability in cases of coronal shear fractures, while the parallel configuration may provide more stability at the most distal portion of the humerus thanks to a higher number of screws.

25.5 Authors' Preferred Approach

A good outcome after surgical treatment for a fracture of the distal humerus is the result of the integration of several factors:

- Detailed preoperative evaluation
- Careful management of the soft tissues
- Adequate visualization of the fracture
- Proper fixation technique
- Early postoperative mobilization

Detailed Preoperative Evaluation. All patients undergoing surgery for fractures of the distal humerus should be evaluated with CT scans with 2D and 3D reconstructions (Fig. 25.3).

Careful Management of the Soft Tissues. Careful management of soft tissues means: (1) using full-thickness flaps from the skin to the fascial plane (Fig. 25.4); (2) preserving the triceps when possible, preferring the triceps-on technique (Video 25.1); and (3) maintaining the upper limb extended and hanging over the head for 12 h after surgery to facilitate the resolution of edema (Fig. 25.5).

Adequate Visualization of the Fracture. Fixation devices with superior biomechanical properties are not useful if we are not able to properly see the fracture and obtain an anatomic reduction. This is especially important in

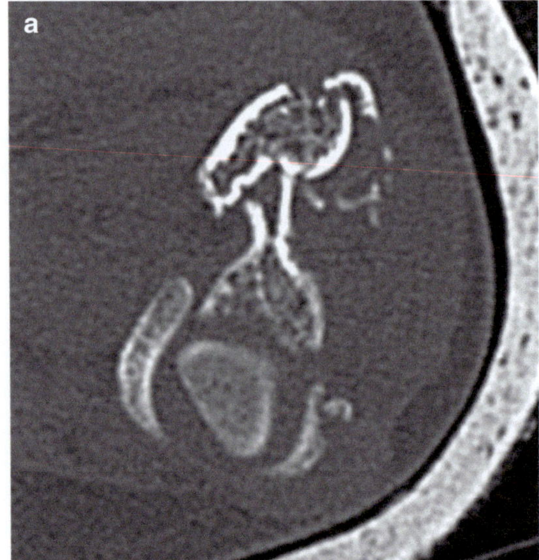

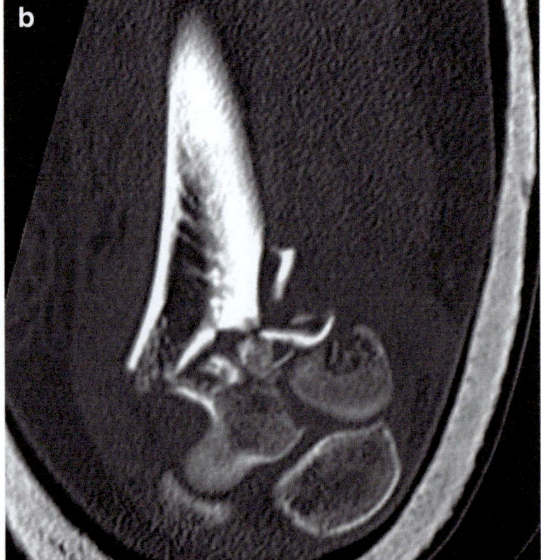

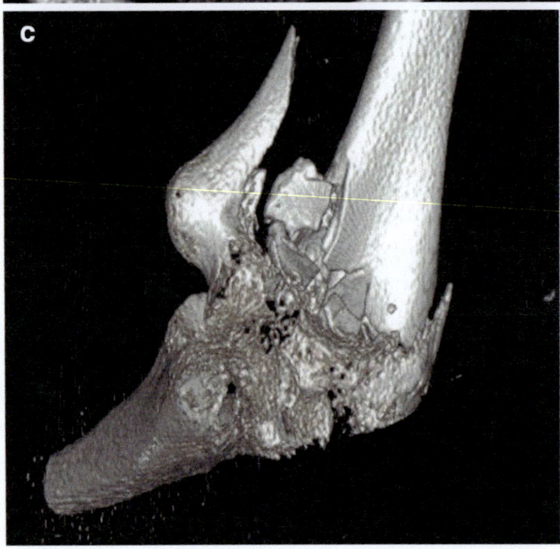

Fig. 25.3 Accurate preoperative planning is mandatory to successfully treat comminuted fractures of the distal humerus: 2D and 3D reconstructions should be obtained in all the cases. (**a**, **b**) preoperative x-rays, showing displaced distal humeral fracture with comminution of the articular surface. (**c**) postoperative xrays showing anatomical reduction and plate fixation

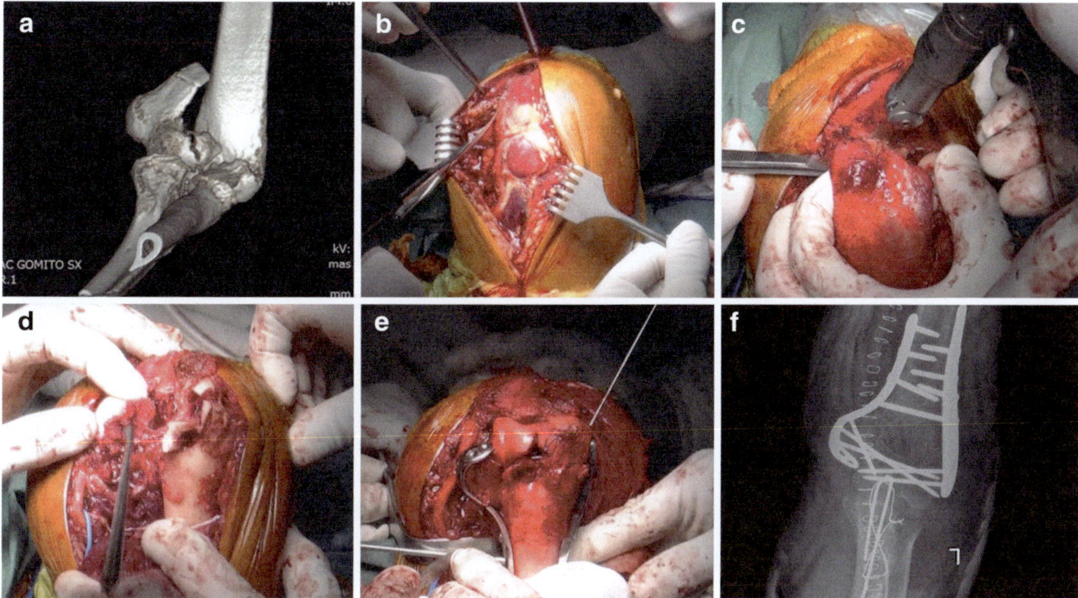

Fig. 25.4 A transolecranon osteotomy used to fix a fracture with comminution of the articular surface. (**a**) 3D CT scan showing the comminution of the trochlea. (**b**) Posterior approach to the elbow with two deep flaps that reach the fascia. (**c**) Olecranon osteotomy performed using a saw. (**d**) Through the osteotomy, the comminution of the articular surface is assessed. (**e**) Two parallel anatomic plates are used to fix the fracture. (**f**) Postoperative X-ray

fractures with comminution of the articular surface. When in doubt, always favor a transolecranon approach to the distal humerus, which provides excellent exposure of the articular surface of the trochlea.

The blind pursuit of a minimally invasive approach can lead to an insufficient reduction of the articular surface.

Proper Fixation Technique. In our experience, the treatment with perpendicular plate configurations has been replaced by the parallel plate configurations that have significantly reduced our rate of nonunions and malunions (Fig. 25.6).

Our results have significantly improved since we have embraced the principles stated by O'Driscoll [33]. He stated that the key principles to successful ORIF are:

- Maximizing fixation in the distal fragments
- Ensuring that all fixation in the distal segment contributes to stability at the supracondylar level

This can be done by achieving eight technical objectives:

1. Each screw should pass through a plate.
2. Each screw should engage a fragment on the opposite side that is also fixed to a plate.
3. As many screws as possible should be placed in the distal fragments.
4. Each screw should be as long as possible.
5. Each screw should engage as many articular fragments as possible.
6. The screws should lock together by interdigitation, thereby creating a fixed-angle structure and linking the columns together.
7. The plates should be applied such that compression is achieved at the supracondylar level for both columns.
8. The plates used must be strong enough and stiff enough to resist breaking or bending before union occurs at the supracondylar level.

In our personal experience, when these objectives are not achieved, an increase in the rate of complications is commonly observed (Fig. 25.7).

Early Postoperative Mobilization. Except for very rare cases, all patients begin passive and active motion 24 h after surgery without the use of braces but remain in an elastic bandage that limits extreme movements. The elastic bandage is removed at the removal of the stitches, three weeks after the surgery. The patient is informed that he/she cannot lift weights until bone healing occurs.

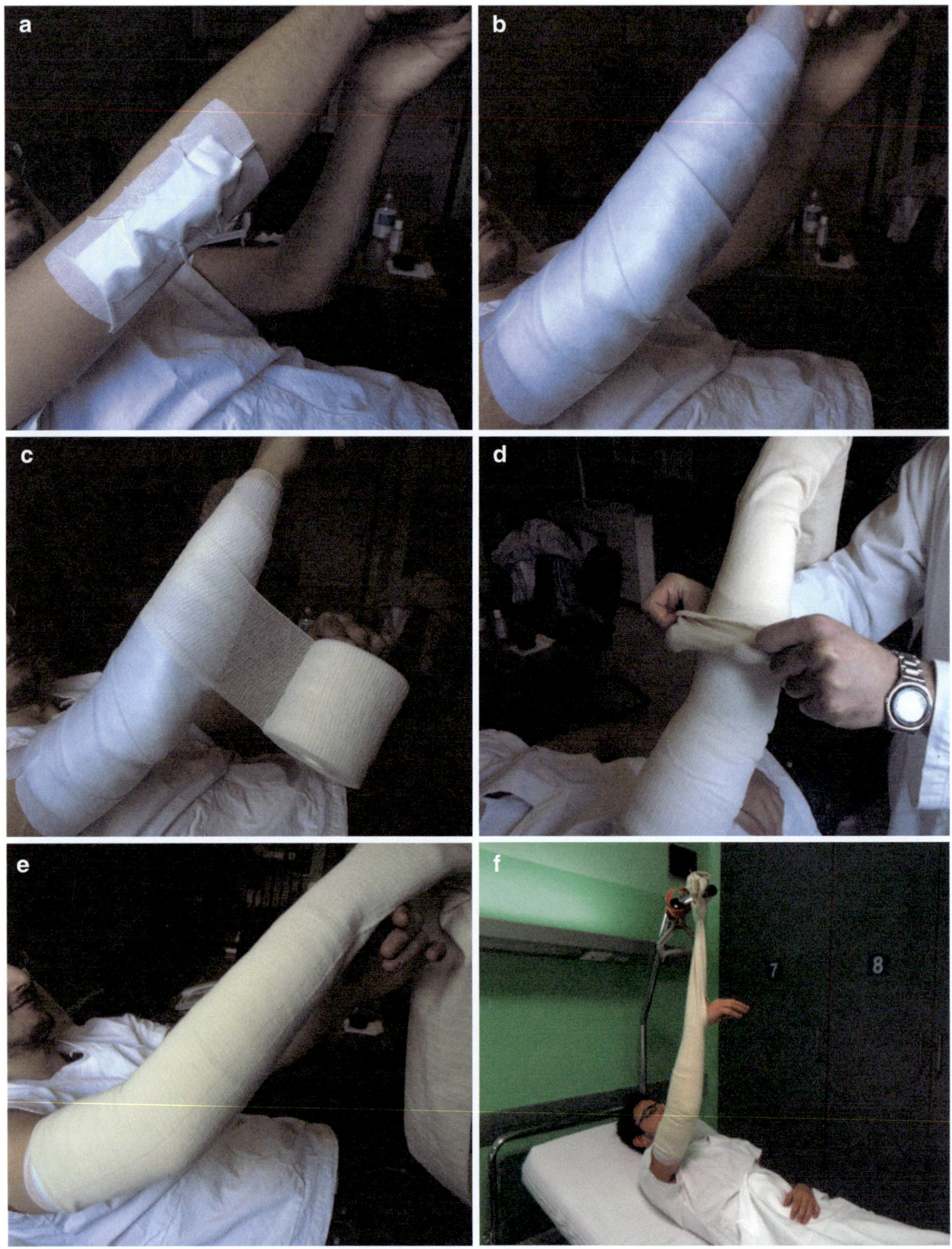

Fig. 25.5 Postoperative management to reduce edema and swelling. (**a**) a steril plaster is plased over the skin incision; (**b**) a soft cotton cast padding is position with the elbow in extension and than; (**c**) coverd by a single layer of peha-half adhesive bandage; (**d-e**) a tubular bandage is wraped over the arm and the arm is hang over the head of the patient for 12 hours (**f**)

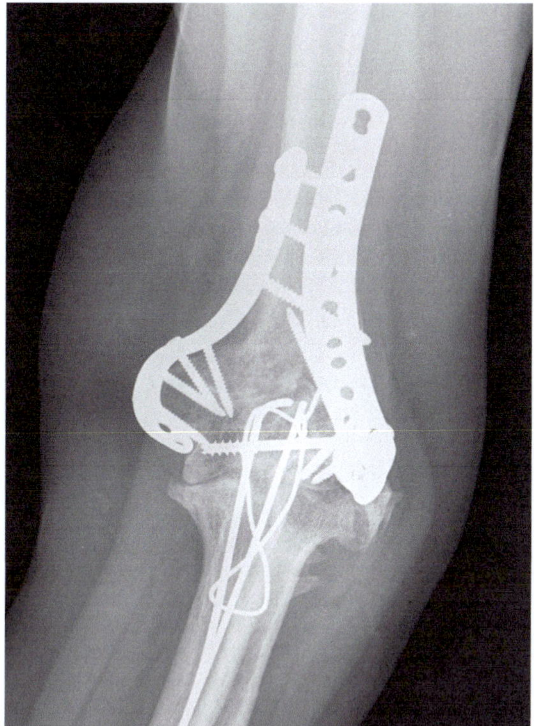

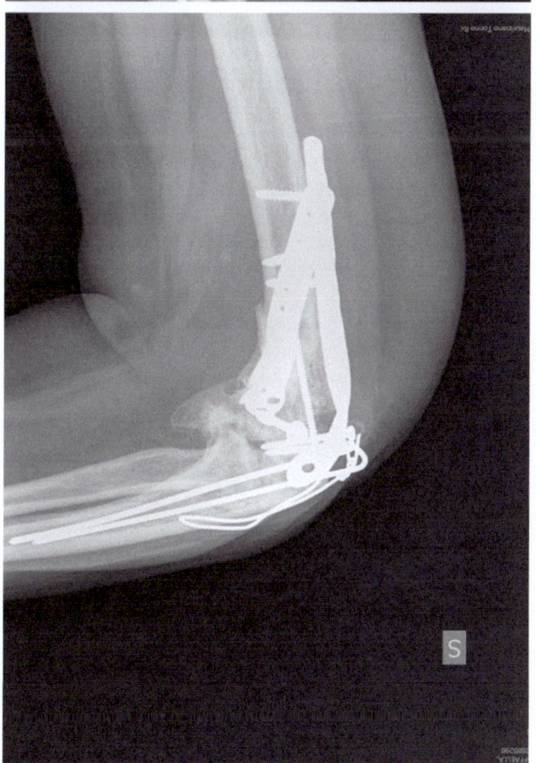

Fig. 25.6 Perpendicular plate configuration with a failure of the fixation

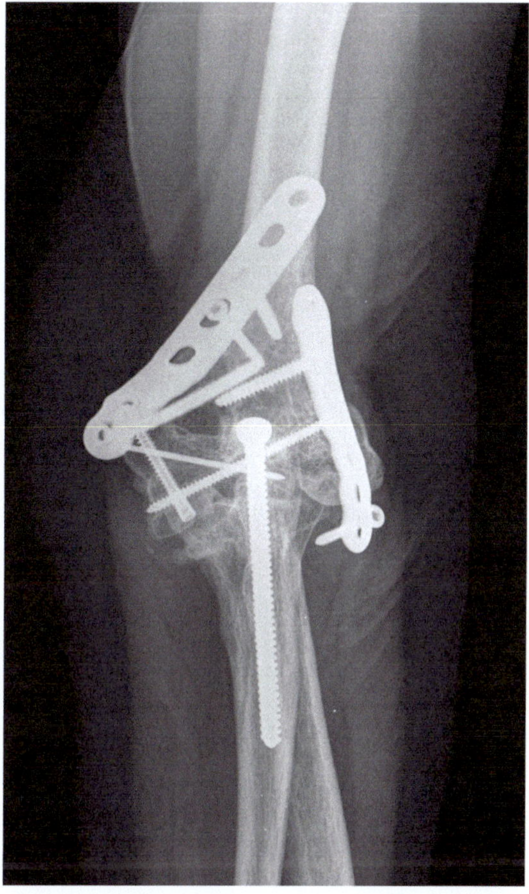

Fig. 25.7 Parallel plate configuration with a failure of the fixation. The fixation of this distal humeral fracture has been performed without achieving the technical objectives. Only few screws have been used, and not all the screws passed through the plates. With these screws, interdigitation was not achievable

> **Key Point**
> By following simple principles, the complication rate can be reduced drastically. The use of parallel anatomic plates has definitely brought radical positive changes in our practice.

References

1. Brown RF, Morgan RG (1971) Intercondylar T-shaped fractures of the humerus. Results in ten cases treated by early mobilisation. J Bone Joint Surg Br 53:425–428

2. Garcia JA, Mykula R, Stanley D (2002) Complex fractures of the distal humerus in the elderly. The role of total elbow replacement as primary treatment. J Bone Joint Surg Br 84:812–816
3. Robinson CM, Hill RM, Jacobs N, Dall G, Court-Brown CM (2003) Adult distal humeral metaphyseal fractures: epidemiology and results of treatment. J Orthop Trauma 17:38–47
4. Waddell JP, Hatch J, Richards R (1988) Supracondylar fractures of the humerus – results of surgical treatment. J Trauma 28:1615–1621
5. Riseborough EJ, Radin EL (1969) Intercondylar T fractures of the humerus in the adult. A comparison of operative and non-operative treatment in twenty-nine cases. J Bone Joint Surg Am 51:130–141
6. Miller WE (1964) Comminuted fractures of the distal end of the humerus in the adult. J Bone Joint Surg Am 46:644–657
7. McKee MD, Jupiter JB (1994) A contemporary approach to the management of complex fractures of the distal humerus and their sequelae. Hand Clin 10:479–494
8. McKee M, Jupiter J, Toh CL, Wilson L, Colton C, Karras KK (1994) Reconstruction after malunion and nonunion of intra-articular fractures of the distal humerus. Methods and results in 13 adults. J Bone Joint Surg Br 76:614–621
9. Srinivasan K, Agarwal M, Matthews SJ, Giannoudis PV (2005) Fractures of the distal humerus in the elderly: is internal fixation the treatment of choice? Clin Orthop Relat Res 434:222–230
10. Zagorski JB, Jennings JJ, Burkhalter WE, Uribe JW (1986) Comminuted intraarticular fractures of the distal humeral condyles. Surgical vs. nonsurgical treatment. Clin Orthop Relat Res 202:197–204
11. Nauth A, McKee MD, Ristevski B, Hall J, Schemitsch EH (2011) Distal humeral fractures in adults. J Bone Joint Surg Am 93:686–700
12. Ulusal AE, Boz U, Sertöz Z, Ustaoğlu RG (2006) Approaches to distal humeral fractures in adults and comparison of treatment results. Acta Orthop Traumatol Turc 40:22–28
13. Papaioannou N, Babis GC, Kalavritinos J, Pantazopoulos T (1995) Operative treatment of type C intra-articular fractures of the distal humerus: the role of stability achieved at surgery on final outcome. Injury 26:169–173
14. Södergård J, Sandelin J, Böstman O (1992) Postoperative complications of distal humeral fractures. 27/96 adults followed up for 6 (2–10) years. Acta Orthop Scand 63:85–89
15. Brauer CA, Lee BM, Bae DS, Waters PM, Kocher MS (2007) A systematic review of medial and lateral entry pinning versus lateral entry pinning for supracondylar fractures of the humerus. J Pediatr Orthop 27:181–186
16. Zamzam MM, Bakarman KA (2009) Treatment of displaced supracondylar humeral fractures among children: crossed versus lateral pinning. Injury 40:625–630
17. Gordon JE, Patton CM, Luhmann SJ, Bassett GS, Schoenecker PL (2001) Fracture stability after pinning of displaced supracondylar distal humerus fractures in children. J Pediatr Orthop 21:313–318
18. Schemitsch EH, Tencer AF, Henley MB (1994) Biomechanical evaluation of methods of internal fixation of the distal humerus. J Orthop Trauma 8:468–475
19. Henley MB, Bone LB, Parker B (1987) Operative management of intra-articular fractures of the distal humerus. J Orthop Trauma 1:24–35
20. Henley MB (1987) Intra-articular distal humeral fractures in adults. Orthop Clin North Am 18:11–23
21. Korner J, Lill H, Müller LP, Rommens PM, Schneider E, Linke B (2003) The LCP-concept in the operative treatment of distal humerus fractures–biological, biomechanical and surgical aspects. Injury 34(Suppl 2):B20–B30
22. Schuster I, Korner J, Arzdorf M, Schwieger K, Diederichs G, Linke B (2008) Mechanical comparison in cadaver specimens of three different 90-degree double-plate osteosyntheses for simulated C2-type distal humerus fractures with varying bone densities. J Orthop Trauma 22:113–120
23. Korner J, Diederichs G, Arzdorf M et al (2004) A biomechanical evaluation of methods of distal humerus fracture fixation using locking compression plates versus conventional reconstruction plates. J Orthop Trauma 18:286–293
24. Reising K, Hauschild O, Strohm PC, Suedkamp NP (2009) Stabilisation of articular fractures of the distal humerus: early experience with a novel perpendicular plate system. Injury 40:611–617
25. Greiner S, Haas NP, Bail HJ (2008) Outcome after open reduction and angular stable internal fixation for supra-intercondylar fractures of the distal humerus: preliminary results with the LCP distal humerus system. Arch Orthop Trauma Surg 128:723–729
26. Sanchez-Sotelo J, Torchia ME, O'Driscoll SW (2008) Complex distal humeral fractures: internal fixation with a principle-based parallel-plate technique. Surgical technique. J Bone Joint Surg Am 90(Suppl 2 Pt 1):31–46
27. Maratt JD, Peaks YS, Doro LC, Karunakar MA, Hughes RE (2008) An integer programming model for distal humerus fracture fixation planning. Comput Aided Surg 13:139–147
28. Athwal GS, Hoxie SC, Rispoli DM, Steinmann SP (2009) Precontoured parallel plate fixation of AO/OTA type C distal humerus fractures. J Orthop Trauma 23:575–580
29. Wong AS, Baratz ME (2009) Elbow fractures: distal humerus. J Hand Surg Am 34:176–190
30. Celli A, Donini MT, Minervini C (2008) The use of pre-contoured plates in the treatment of C2-C3 fractures of the distal humerus: clinical experience. Chir Organi Mov 91:57–64

31. Theivendran K, Duggan PJ, Deshmukh SC (2010) Surgical treatment of complex distal humeral fractures: functional outcome after internal fixation using precontoured anatomic plates. J Shoulder Elbow Surg 19:524–532
32. Koonce RC, Baldini TH, Morgan SJ (2012) Are conventional reconstruction plates equivalent to precontoured locking plates for distal humerus fracture fixation? A biomechanics cadaver study. Clin Biomech (Bristol, Avon) 27:697–701
33. O'Driscoll SW (2005) Optimizing stability in distal humeral fracture fixation. J Shoulder Elbow Surg 14:186S–194S
34. Jacobson SR, Glisson RR, Urbaniak JR (1997) Comparison of distal humerus fracture fixation: a biomechanical study. J South Orthop Assoc 6: 241–249
35. Levy JC, Kalandiak SP, Hutson JJ, Zych G (2005) An alternative method of osteosynthesis for distal humeral shaft fractures. J Orthop Trauma 19:43–47
36. Moran MC (1997) Modified lateral approach to the distal humerus for internal fixation. Clin Orthop Relat Res 340:190–197
37. Tejwani NC, Murthy A, Park J, McLaurin TM, Egol KA, Kummer FJ (2009) Fixation of extra-articular distal humerus fractures using one locking plate versus two reconstruction plates: a laboratory study. J Trauma 66:795–799
38. Meloy GM, Mormino MA, Siska PA, Tarkin IS (2013) A paradigm shift in the surgical reconstruction of extra-articular distal humeral fractures: single-column plating. Injury 44:1620–1624
39. Jupiter JB (1995) Complex fractures of the distal part of the humerus and associated complications. Instr Course Lect 44:187–198
40. Ring D, Jupiter JB (1999) Complex fractures of the distal humerus and their complications. J Shoulder Elbow Surg 8:85–97
41. Jupiter JB, Neff U, Holzach P, Allgöwer M (1985) Intercondylar fractures of the humerus. An operative approach. J Bone Joint Surg Am 67:226–239
42. Letsch R, Schmit-Neuerburg KP, Stürmer KM, Walz M (1989) Intraarticular fractures of the distal humerus. Surgical treatment and results. Clin Orthop Relat Res 241:238–244
43. Holdsworth BJ, Mossad MM (1990) Fractures of the adult distal humerus. Elbow function after internal fixation. J Bone Joint Surg Br 72:362–365
44. Wildburger R, Mähring M, Hofer HP (1991) Supraintercondylar fractures of the distal humerus: results of internal fixation. J Orthop Trauma 5:301–307
45. Sanchez-Sotelo J, Torchia ME, O'Driscoll SW (2007) Complex distal humeral fractures: internal fixation with a principle-based parallel-plate technique. J Bone Joint Surg Am 89:961–969
46. Goel DP, Pike JM, Athwal GS (2010) Open reduction and internal fixation of distal humerus fractures. Oper Tech Orthop 20:24–33
47. Gofton WT, Macdermid JC, Patterson SD, Faber KJ, King GJ (2003) Functional outcome of AO type C distal humeral fractures. J Hand Surg Am 28: 294–308
48. Jupiter JB, Mehne DK (1992) Fractures of the distal humerus. Orthopedics 15:825–833
49. Rüedi T, Buckley R, Moran C (2007) AO principles of fracture management, 2nd edn. Thieme Verlag, New York
50. Helfet DL, Schmeling GJ (1993) Bicondylar intraarticular fractures of the distal humerus in adults. Clin Orthop Relat Res 292:26–36
51. Shin SJ, Sohn HS, Do NH (2010) A clinical comparison of two different double plating methods for intraarticular distal humerus fractures. J Shoulder Elbow Surg 19:2–9
52. Atalar AC, Demirhan M, Salduz A, Kiliçoğlu O, Seyahi A (2009) Functional results of the parallel-plate technique for complex distal humerus fractures. Acta Orthop Traumatol Turc 43:21–27
53. Rebuzzi E, Vascellari A, Schiavetti S (2010) The use of parallel pre-contoured plates in the treatment of A and C fractures of the distal humerus. Musculoskelet Surg 94:9–16
54. Aslam N, Willett K (2004) Functional outcome following internal fixation of intraarticular fractures of the distal humerus (AO type C). Acta Orthop Belg 70:118–122
55. Chi-Fat C, Grace Y, Frankie KL (2009) Fixation of distal humeral fracture in elderly patient by locking compression plate. Zhongguo Xiu Fu Chong Jian Wai Ke Za Zhi 23:1285–1289
56. Liu JJ, Ruan HJ, Wang JG, Fan CY, Zeng BF (2009) Double-column fixation for type C fractures of the distal humerus in the elderly. J Shoulder Elbow Surg 18:646–651
57. Zalavras CG, Vercillo MT, Jun BJ, Otarodifard K, Itamura JM, Lee TQ (2011) Biomechanical evaluation of parallel versus orthogonal plate fixation of intra-articular distal humerus fractures. J Shoulder Elbow Surg 20:12–20
58. Arnander MW, Reeves A, MacLeod IA, Pinto TM, Khaleel A (2008) A biomechanical comparison of plate configuration in distal humerus fractures. J Orthop Trauma 22:332–336
59. Stoffel K, Cunneen S, Morgan R, Nicholls R, Stachowiak G (2008) Comparative stability of perpendicular versus parallel double-locking plating systems in osteoporotic comminuted distal humerus fractures. J Orthop Res 26:778–784
60. Penzkofer R, Hungerer S, Wipf F, von Oldenburg G, Augat P (2010) Anatomical plate configuration affects mechanical performance in distal humerus fractures. Clin Biomech (Bristol, Avon) 25: 972–978
61. Helfet DL, Hotchkiss RN (1990) Internal fixation of the distal humerus: a biomechanical comparison of methods. J Orthop Trauma 4:260–264

62. Got C, Shuck J, Biercevicz A et al (2012) Biomechanical comparison of parallel versus 90-90 plating of bicolumn distal humerus fractures with intra-articular comminution. J Hand Surg Am 37:2512–2518
63. Kollias CM, Darcy SP, Reed JG, Rosvold JM, Shrive NG, Hildebrand KA (2010) Distal humerus internal fixation: a biomechanical comparison of 90° and parallel constructs. Am J Orthop 39: 440–444
64. Schwartz A, Oka R, Odell T, Mahar A (2006) Biomechanical comparison of two different periarticular plating systems for stabilization of complex distal humerus fractures. Clin Biomech (Bristol, Avon) 21:950–955
65. Lee SK, Kim KJ, Park KH, Choy WS (2013) A comparison between orthogonal and parallel plating methods for distal humerus fractures: a prospective randomized trial. Eur J Orthop Surg Traumatol. 2013 Aug 7.

26 Elbow Prosthesis in Distal Humeral Fractures

Roberto Rotini, Michele Cavaciocchi, Graziano Bettelli, and Lorenzo Zaccarelli

26.1 Introduction

Fractures of the distal humerus are not common: they represent 0.5 % of all fractures [1]. Recent studies showed that these fractures affect with high frequency an osteoporotic old population, with a mean age of 63 years and a male-to-female ratio of 29:71; Palvanen et al. [2] observed an increase in the distal humeral fractures in the Finnish female population older than 60 years from 11/100,000 in 1970 to 30/100,000 in 1995, with a rise of 9 % in patients older than 80 years: thus, distal humeral fractures can be considered as fragility fractures of the elderly [1].

The main cause is a fall from standing height in 70 % of the cases, while high-energy traumas or sport traumas represent just 30 %.

These fractures are often very unstable and usually need surgery. The surgical treatment of elbow fractures has considerably evolved over the last 30 years: the new techniques of fixation and prosthetic implants confined conservative treatment to a marginal role.

Despite these evolutions, the literature indicates an incidence of 20–25 % of unsatisfactory results after osteosynthesis of a distal humeral fracture in an elderly population [3], due to the often severe and disabling sequelae like loss of reduction, nonunion, stiffness, and posttraumatic arthrosis.

Although ORIF is nowadays the first treatment option, also in osteoporotic patients, an unstable fixation has more disadvantages than a prosthesis that warrants an early mobilization, a faster recovery of autonomy in daily life activities, and reproducible results in terms of range of movement and pain control [4, 5].

Indications for a primary prosthesis are also strengthened by the increased technical difficulties when performing secondary prosthesis (in malunited fractures and nonunions) and by the worse functional results if compared with those of a primary implant in elbow fracture [6].

The elbow prostheses currently used in distal humeral fractures are the linked *total elbow arthroplasty (TEA)* and the *distal humeral hemiarthroplasty* (DHH).

The linked TEA has an absolute indication in cases with joint instability and in the ones with loss of the condyles (where the collateral ligaments have their origin) [7].

The indications for DHH are the comminuted intra-articular fractures where an ORIF is not technically feasible or cannot achieve absolute stability and the patient is not fit for a TEA because of the active age and the high/moderate functional needs [8].

The advantages of a DHH if compared with a TEA are the avoidance of the ulnar implant, that is, the prosthesis component more susceptible to aseptic loosening, and the absence of the

R. Rotini (✉) • M. Cavaciocchi • G. Bettelli
L. Zaccarelli
Shoulder and Elbow Surgery Unit,
Rizzoli Orthopaedic Institute,
Via G.C. Pupilli, nr 1, Bologna 40136, Italy
e-mail: roberto.rotini@ior.it;
michele.cavaciocchi@ior.it; graziano.bettelli@ior.it;
lorenzo.zaccarelli@gmail.com

F. Castoldi et al. (eds.), *Simple and Complex Fractures of the Humerus*,
DOI 10.1007/978-88-470-5307-6_26, © Springer-Verlag Italia 2015

components connection, eliminating the polyethylene wear problems.

The market, nowadays, offers to the surgeon convertible prosthesis systems, allowing the passage from DHH to TEA intraoperatively or, if necessary, during a revision surgery, leaving the humeral stem in place [9–11].

26.2 Indications

26.2.1 TEA

The articular comminuted fractures of the distal humerus in elderly and low-demand patients (usually with an age higher than 70 years) in which an ORIF cannot achieve stability represent the main indication for TEA, most of all in case of comorbidities like osteoporosis, low humeral bone stock, rheumatoid arthritis, or long-term steroid treatment. In these patients, TEA allows an early autonomy recovery, with good short- and midterm results for range of motion and pain.

Before choosing a prosthesis, the surgeon must carefully evaluate the skin conditions, to exclude abrasions or open fracture and to assess the presence of neurological defects.

The fracture pattern should be assessed by a CT scan with bidimensional and three-dimensional reconstructions (plain X-rays usually underrate the comminution of the articular part of the humerus).

Based on AO classification of fractures, C2 and C3 fractures in patients older than 70 years are the elective indications for TEA. In the same patient group, the authors consider as relative indication for TEA also fracture types A3.3, B3.3, and A2.3 [12], especially in cases with pre-existing degenerative arthropathy (Fig. 26.1).

26.2.2 DHH

This prosthesis is indicated in unreconstructible fractures of the distal humerus when the following two conditions are met:

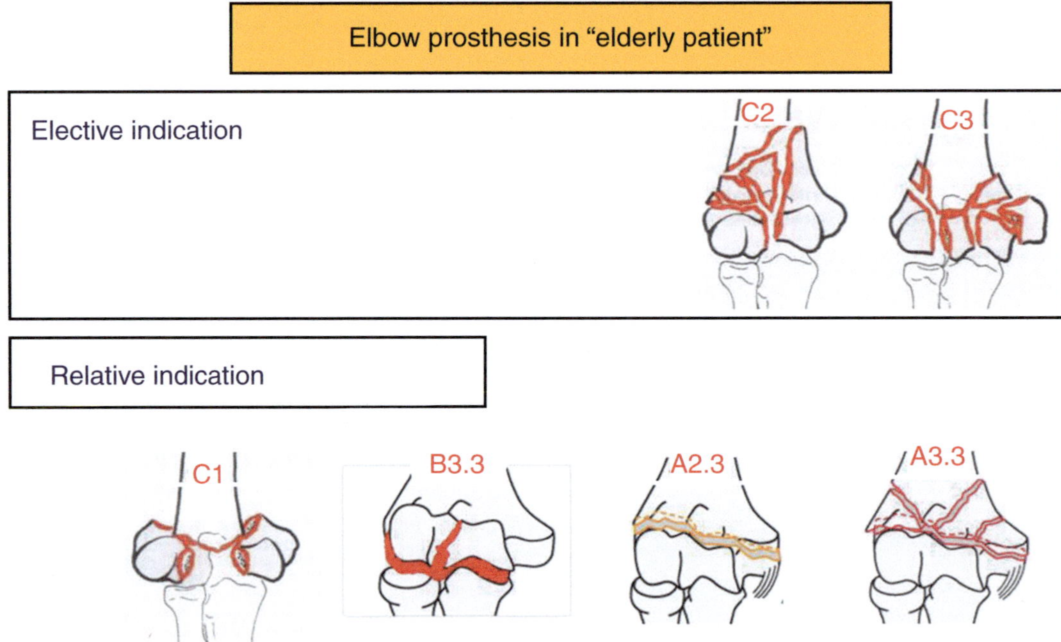

Fig. 26.1 Fractures of the distal humerus, basing on AO classification [12], in which, in low-demand patients, the prosthesis is indicated

- Integrity or stable fixation of the medial and lateral *humeral columns* with presence/validity of the medial collateral ligament (MCL) and of the lateral ulnar collateral ligament (LUCL)
- Integrity of the coronoid and of the radial head

26.3 Contraindications

The main contraindications for a prosthetic implant in the elbow are critical wounds, open fracture, history of previous joint infection, neurological or vascular diseases, and muscle deficiency of the elbow flexors and/or extensors.

Other contraindications are a noncompliant patient (who would be unable to follow a rehabilitation program and to respect the limitations in the use of the elbow, most of all in TEA implants) and immunosuppression or immunodeficiency.

26.4 Surgical Technique

In the authors' preferred technique, the patient is placed in supine position, with the arm above the chest (the lateral position is preferred sometimes if an ORIF of both columns is planned).

During the anesthesia procedure, intravenous antibiotic is administered (2 g of cefazolin or 600 mg of clindamycin in case of allergy to cephalosporins).

A sterile tourniquet is placed at the arm. Under regional or general anesthesia, a posterior median skin incision is performed.

The ulnar nerve is protected and widely isolated for the possible anterior transposition. The key point of this technique is the triceps management that the authors carry out according to the following diagram.

26.4.1 TEA

- More followed method: *triceps-sparing approach* (Fig. 26.2)
  The removal of bone fragments creates enough space for all the steps of the prosthetic implant, in both the humeral and the ulnar side (this is the most uncomfortable passage of the implant). By this method, the triceps remains intact, and the first phase of the rehabilitation is quicker and more effective.
- Alternative methods: *triceps splitting, triceps reflecting*
  The use of these techniques depends on the surgeon confidence, but splitting and reflecting are mainly indicated in case of prosthesis implant in degenerative diseases.

26.4.2 DHH

- Conservation of the medial and lateral collateral ligaments is mandatory.
- More followed method: *triceps-sparing approach*
  This technique combines the advantages of leaving the extensor mechanism intact with an adequate exposure of both humeral columns for the plating needs.

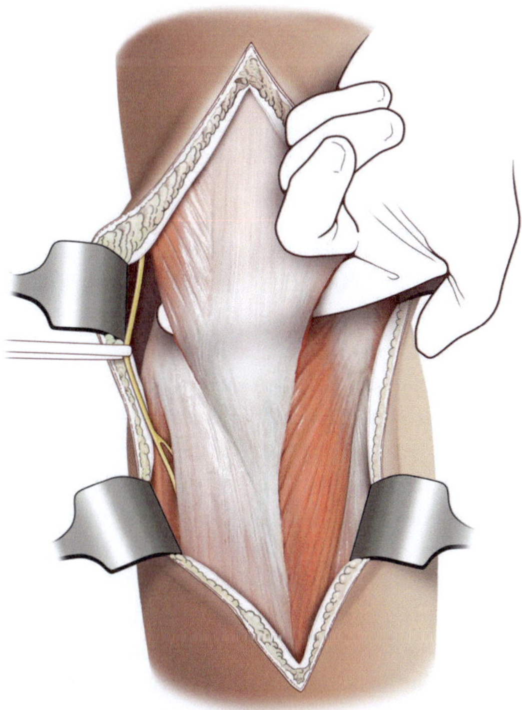

Fig. 26.2 Triceps-sparing approach (Designed by School of Anatomical Drawing of Rizzoli Orthopaedic Institute)

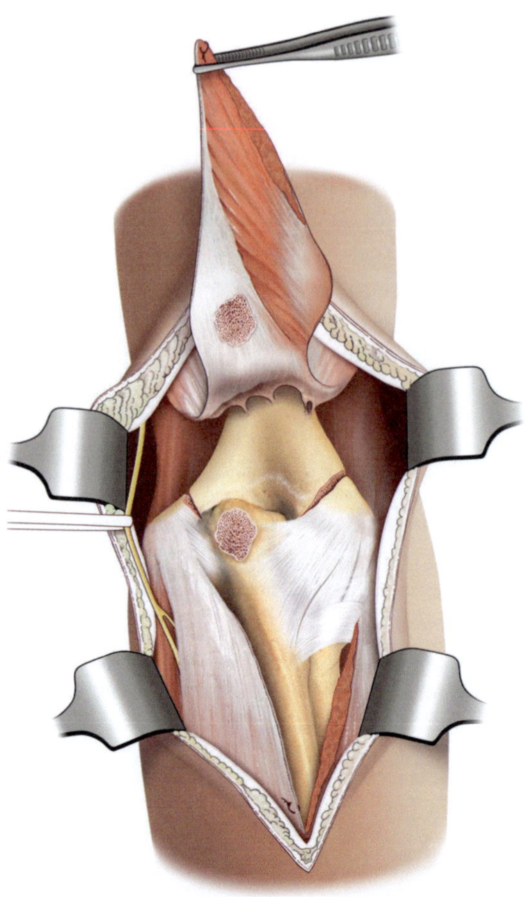

Fig. 26.3 TRAP approach (Designed by School of Anatomical Drawing of Rizzoli Orthopaedic Institute)

- Hughes et al. [8, 13] described a lower incidence of complications with olecranon osteotomy.
- *TRAP approach* (Fig. 26.3)
  The authors prefer this technique to olecranon osteotomy, if a wide exposure of the columns is needed for their fixation.

Once the bone surface is exposed, the fracture pattern is evaluated, and the bone fragments are recovered and used to determine the size and the depth of the prosthesis; the depth of the humeral component is evaluated by the flange of the implant staying on the roof of the coronoid fossa.

A radial head prosthesis is implanted only in case of degenerative arthritis, but usually the proximal radius is conserved. The ulna is prepared with dedicated rasps and reamers, after the resection of the olecranon tip, to improve direct access to the medullary canal.

The trial components are very useful to check the implant alignment and the articulation in TEAs and to verify the feasibility of column fixation and of collateral ligament repair in DHHs.

The *cementation technique* is another key point of this surgery. After a careful canal lavage, the authors prefer the use of bony cement restrictors in the ulna and a plastic cement restrictor in the humerus to obtain a correct pressurization. Antibiotic-loaded cement is inserted under pressure by a cement gun with a thin nozzle (which can be cut in the suitable length). Cementation should be performed with the elbow in extension. When the prosthesis is correctly in place, a thin bone graft is inserted between the flange and the anterior humeral cortex.

In linked TEAs, if possible, tensioning of the collateral ligaments should be carried out, to improve the soft tissue balance and to reduce the load stress on the system.

In DHHs, the *reconstruction of MCL and LUCL is mandatory*. A correct reconstruction of the columns is necessary and is performed exploiting the hole (if available, like in Tornier Latitude implant) of the articular component. If a *TRAP approach* has been done, the anconeus is strongly sutured, and the triceps-olecranon contact is recreated by transosseous stitches with high-resistance sutures (Figs. 26.4, 26.5, 26.6 and 26.7*: case and surgical technique*).

The ulnar nerve, if conflicting with the prosthesis, is anteriorly translocated, and the skin is closed in layers over two drains.

26.5 Postoperative Care

At the end of the surgical procedure, an elbow splint is placed preferably in extension. In case of wound problems, few days of rest from kinesis are indicated.

If a *triceps-sparing approach* has been performed, active extension and flexion can be immediately allowed.

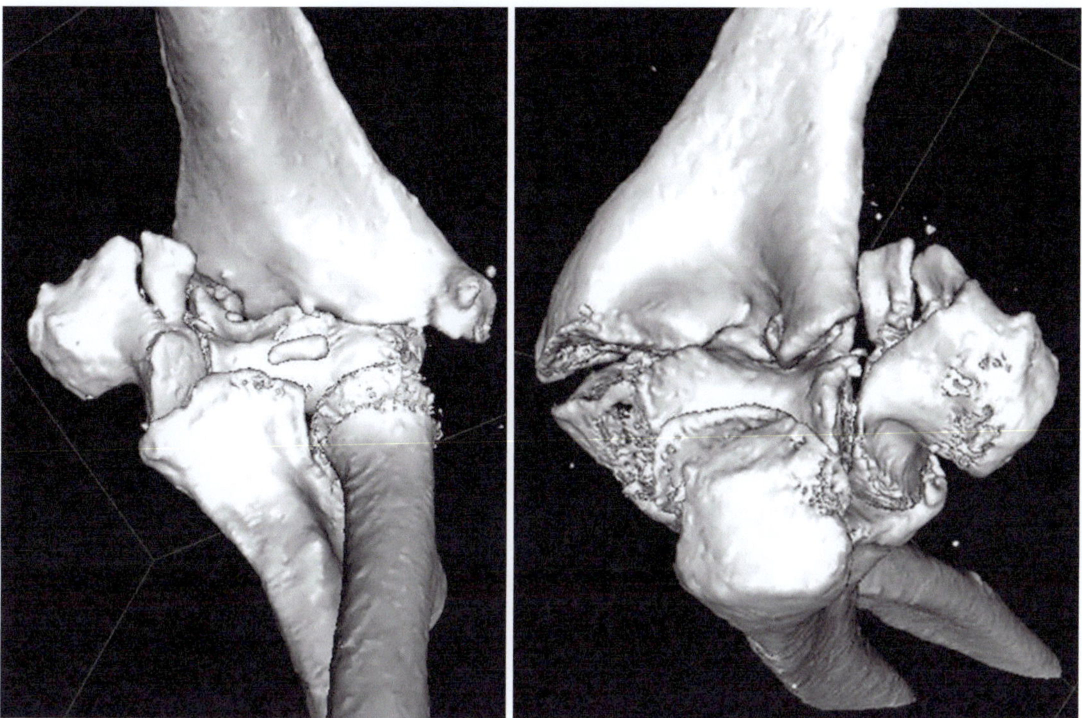

Fig. 26.4 Distal humeral fracture 3D CT scan images (anterior and posterior visions)

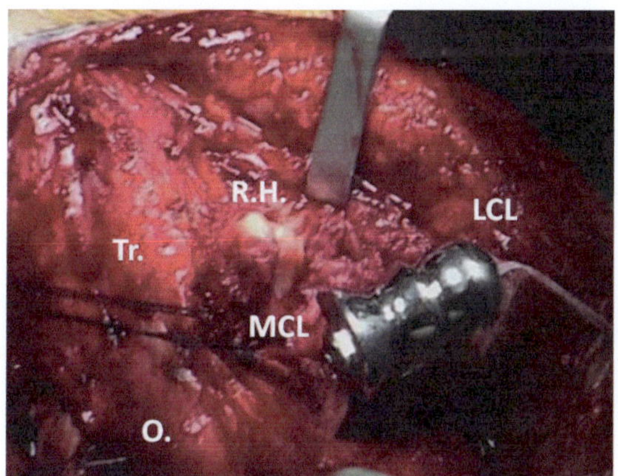

Fig. 26.5 DHH in situ with triceps-sparing approach. *Tr.* triceps dislocated, *O.* olecranon, *MCL* medial collateral ligament, *RH* radial head, *LCL* lateral collateral ligament

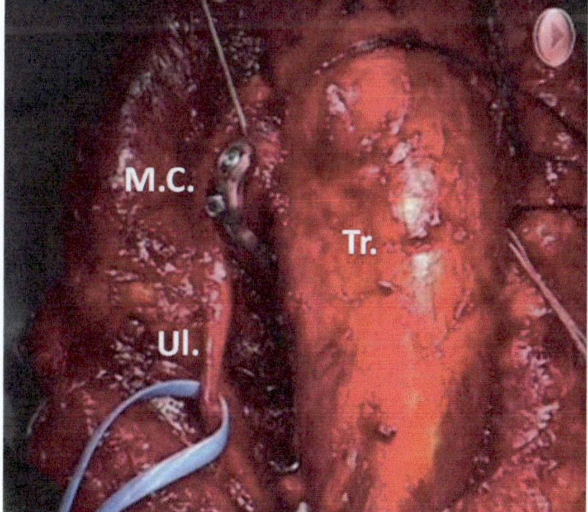

Fig. 26.6 ORIF of medial column, triceps in anatomic position. *MC* medial column, *Ul* ulnar nerve, *Tr* triceps

If the triceps has been detached (*TRAP approach*), it should be protected by a splint in flexion for 4 weeks performing exercises in active flexion and passive or gravity-assisted extension, avoiding a flexion over 100°.

Usually, in linked TEA, the passive movement in flexion and extension begins the day after the operation and is progressively increased. This movement can be performed by a therapist or by a CPM machine. The patient is also taught how

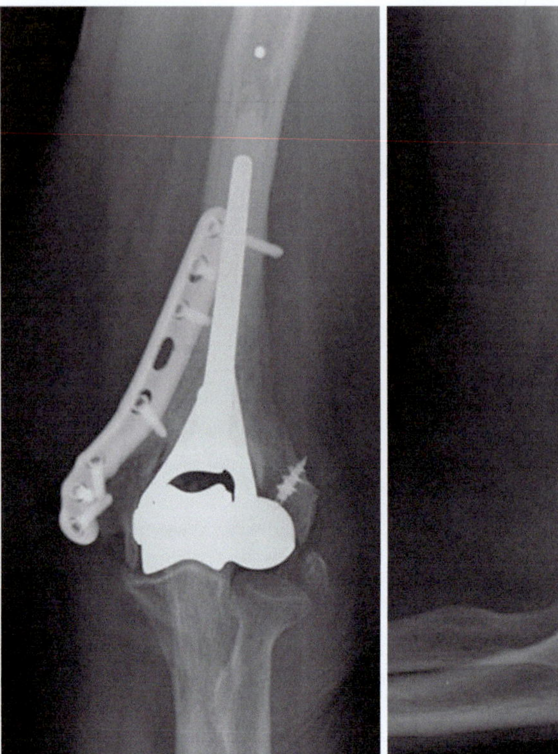

Fig. 26.7 Elbow X-rays after 1 year: DHH, plate for medial column reconstruction and suture anchor for LCL reconstruction

to perform *self-assisted exercises* in flexion, extension, pronation, and supination, using the contralateral arm.

In DHH, the rehabilitation must be more careful, avoiding varus and valgus stress on the reconstructed collateral ligaments, so the preferred protocol includes only self-assisted mobilization in flexion, extension, pronation, and supination after a detailed explanation of the exercises to do and of the movements to avoid. After 3 weeks of full-time splinting (with the only exceptions of self-assisted mobilization, wound care, suture removal, and personal hygiene), the rehabilitation program begins with passive and then active movement.

The recovery of the normal activities of daily living should be complete in 3 months. Weight lifting must be limited to 2–3 kg, with a further restriction to 1 kg if the effort has to be repeated.

26.6 Complications

After an elbow prosthesis, there can be major or minor complications.

Minor complications include:

- *Ulnar nerve apraxia*. The entity of nerve damage ranges from transient numbness to deep neuropathy. It can be caused by excessive traction on the nerve or by ischemia due to aggressive nerve isolation. Thermal damage during cementation is possible; however, it is very rare if the appropriate cautions are observed.
- *Wound problems*. Their occurrence is more frequent in patients affected with rheumatoid arthritis or under corticosteroid therapy. Extensive dissection of the superficial tissues and excessive wound traction are additional causes.
- *Instability*. This complication can be present only in DHH when a correct reconstruction of the collateral ligaments has not been obtained.
- *Triceps insufficiency*. It can take place when the muscle is detached and not correctly reconstructed or in case of *triceps-splitting* procedure with possible boutonniere-type lesion [14].

Major complications can be:

- *Periprosthetic fractures*. These can be intraoperative or postoperative. The former can be favored by bad bone quality or by too vigorous maneuvers, and the latter usually are due to trauma or sometimes to rehabilitation stresses in case of bad bone quality. A special condition to be considered when implanting an elbow prosthesis is the presence of a shoulder prosthesis in the same limb, as this can cause a significant risk of interprosthetic fractures with low-energy trauma, quite difficult to treat [15–17].

- *Aseptic loosening.* Mechanical failure of the prosthesis components is strictly consequent to the cementation technique. Progresses in the development of prostheses with stem coating and a careful respect of pressurized cementation techniques should restrict chances for this complication in the future.
- *Infection.* In the past, this complication had unacceptably high incidences (up to 12 % [18, 19]). The current occurrence is about 2–3.3 % [20], still higher if compared to prosthetic implants of other major joints.

Conclusions

In view of the anatomic complexity of the elbow joint, displaced and comminuted distal humeral fractures still represent a challenge for the orthopedic surgeon.

Even though double-plate internal fixation is the treatment to be preferred, in the elderly patient this method is often difficult to perform and bears high risks of failure due to the low mechanical bone quality. The elbow functional limitation consequent to a possible failure of fixation can restrict the normal activities of daily living to such an extent in the elderly to impair his or her independence.

Therefore, with the aim to conserve a good level of autonomy in elderly patients, Cobb and Morrey [3] in 1997 suggested the elbow prosthesis as a solution. The results reported by several authors [4, 5, 21–26] who followed this indication allow nowadays to include the elbow prosthesis among the surgical techniques to be considered in elderly patients. This surgical procedure however is not free from possible complications, well evidenced in the literature [27].

The higher incidence of *complications* is related to the *ulnar component* (aseptic loosening, periprosthetic fractures, polyethylene wear), and this has prompted the development of distal humeral hemiarthroplasty.

It is of paramount importance for the surgeon to carefully evaluate the features of the patients in which to consider an elbow prosthesis. A *patient* should be *compliant* not only in following a careful rehabilitation protocol but also in avoiding weight lifting with the operated limb.

A recent paper from the Mayo Clinic [28] has shed light on the fact that, although instructed about the permanent activity restrictions to observe, 94 % of the patients have performed moderate-level activities (carrying groceries, gardening, leaf raking) and 40 % high-level activities (dirt shoveling, snow shoveling, putting luggages overhead).

The *management of the triceps* represents a key point for the success of this complex surgical act. There is consensus about the use of the *triceps-sparing approach* in TEA in fracture cases, while there is still open debate about the approach to prefer DHH. The *triceps-sparing approach* is the authors' preferred method considering the respect of the anatomy of the extensor mechanism and the consequently shorter functional recovery. This approach moreover does not impair the conversion of a DHH, in case of instability, into a TEA.

Some authors [8] indicate olecranon osteotomy as the ideal approach for DHH as it allows a better view and would warrant in time a superior ligamentous stability if compared to the *triceps-sparing approach.* The authors of the present chapter prefer the *TRAP approach* over the *olecranon osteotomy* as it allows an equally wide visualization of the two columns and does not bear the risk of olecranon nonunion.

There is consensus in *DHH* technique about the point that *fixation of the columns* and *collateral ligament repair* are the key steps for success. About timing of the surgical steps, it is the authors' opinion that it is useful to put the prosthetic implant in place first, as this will provide a stable base over which, in the following steps, internal fixation of the columns and reconstruction of the collateral ligaments will be performed.

In patients aged over 65 years, TEA is superior to ORIF for both elbow range of motion and pain, especially in short-term (<2 years) follow-up [4, 5].

References

1. Court-Brown CM, Aitken SA, Forward D, O'Toole RV (2010) The epidemiology of fractures. In: Bucholz RW, Court-Brown CM, Heckman JD, Tornetta P (eds) Rockwood and Green's fractures in adults, 7th edn. Lippincott Williams and Wilkins, Philadelphia
2. Palvanen M, Niemi S, Parkkari J, Kannus P (2003) Osteoporotic fractures of the distal humerus in elderly women [letter]. Ann Intern Med 139:W-61
3. Cobb TK, Morrey BF (1997) Total elbow arthroplasty as primary treatment for distal humeral fractures in elderly patients. J Bone Joint Surg Am 79(6):826–832
4. McKee MD, Veillette CJH, Hall JA, Schemitsch EH, Wild LM, McCormack R, Perey B, Goetz T, Zomar M, Moon K, Mandel S, Petit S, Guy P, Leung I (2009) A multicenter, prospective, randomized, controlled trial of open reduction and internal fixation versus total elbow arthroplasty for displaced intra-articular distal humeral fractures in elderly patients. J Shoulder Elbow Surg 18:3–12
5. Kamineni S, Morrey BF (2004) Distal humeral fractures treated with noncustom total elbow replacement. J Bone Joint Surg Am 86-A(5):940–947
6. Kaminemi S (2009) Chapter 56. Distal humeral fractures – acute total elbow arthroplasty. In: The elbow and its disorders, 4th edn. Saunders Elsevier, Philadelphia, pp 800–813
7. Rotini R, Antonioli D, Marinelli A, Guerra E (2007) Disegno e selezione dell'impianto nella protesi totale di gomito. GIOT 33(suppl1):S139–S143
8. Hughes JS, Parsons M (2007) Chapter 30. Distal humeral hemiarthroplasty. In: Yamaguchi K, King GJ, McKee MD, O'Driscoll SW (eds) Advanced reconstruction elbow. American Academy of Orthopaedic Surgeons, Rosemont, pp 219–228
9. Gramstad GD, King GJ, O'Driscoll SW, Yamaguchi K (2005) Elbow arthroplasty using a convertible implant. Tech Hand Up Extrem Surg 9(3):153–163
10. King GJ, Yamaguchi K, O'Driscoll SW (2007) Chapter 36. Convertible total elbow arthroplasty: the latitude prosthesis. In: Yamaguchi K, King GJ, McKee MD, O'Driscoll SW (eds) Advanced reconstruction elbow. American Academy of Orthopaedic Surgeons, Rosemont, pp 277–285
11. King GJ (2009) Chapter 52. Convertible total elbow arthroplasty. In: Morrey BF, Sanchez-Sotelo J (eds) The elbow and its disorders, 4th edn. Saunders Elsevier, Philadelphia, pp 754–764
12. Hessmann MH, Ring DC (2007) Distal humerus. In: Ruedi TP, Buckley RE, Moran CG (eds) AO principles of fractures management, Thieme; Stuttgart, New York pp 609–625. ISBN 978-3-13-117442-0
13. Smith GC, Hughes JS (2013) Unreconstructable acute distal humeral fractures and their sequelae treated with distal humeral hemiarthroplasty: a two-year to eleven-year follow-up. J Shoulder Elbow Surg 22(12):1710–1723. doi:10.1016/j.jse.2013.06.012. Epub 2013 Sep 20
14. Celli A, Arash A, Adams RA, Morrey BF (2005) Triceps insufficiency following total elbow arthroplasty. J Bone Joint Surg Am 87(9):1957–1964
15. Gill DRJ, Cofield RH, Morrey BF (1999) Ipsilateral total shoulder and elbow arthroplasties in patients who have rheumatoid arthritis. J Bone Joint Surg 81-A:1128–1137
16. Mavrogenis AF, Angelini A, Guerra E, Rotini R (2011) Humeral fracture between a total elbow and total shoulder arthroplasty. Orthopedics 34(4):315–318. 10.3928/01477447-20110228-21
17. Plausinis D, Greaves C, Regan WD, Oxland TR (2005) Ipsilateral shoulder and elbow replacements: on the risk of periprosthetic fracture. Clin Biomech 20:1055–1063
18. Gutow AP, Wolfe SW (1994) Infection following total elbow arthroplasty. Hand Clin 10:521–529
19. Morrey BF, Bryan RS (1983) Infection after total elbow arthroplasty. J Bone Joint Surg 65-A: 330–338
20. Cheung EV, Adams RA, Morrey BF (2008) Reimplantation of a total elbow prosthesis following resection arthroplasty for infection. J Bone Joint Surg Am 90(3):589–594. doi:10.2106/JBJS.F.00829
21. Gambirasio R, Riand N, Stern R, Hoffmeyer P (2001) Total elbow replacement for complex fractures of the distal humerus. An option for the elderly patient. J Bone Joint Surg Br 83(7):974–988
22. Garcia JA, Mykula R, Stanley D (2002) Complex fractures of the distal humerus in the elderly. The role of total elbow replacement as primary treatment. J Bone Joint Surg Br 84(6):812–816
23. Frankle MA, Herscovici D Jr, DiPasquale TG, Vasey MB, Sanders RW (2003) A comparison of open reduction and internal fixation and primary total elbow arthroplasty in the treatment of intraarticular distal humerus fractures in women older than age 65. J Orthop Trauma 17(7):473–480
24. Charissoux JL, Mabit C, Fourastier J, Beccari R, Emily S, Cappelli M, Malingue E, Mansat P, Hubert L, Proust J, Bratu D, Veillard D, Grandmaison FL, Apard T, Martinel V, Bonnevialle N (2008) Comminuted intra-articular fractures of the distal humerus in elderly patients. Rev Chir Orthop Reparatrice Appar Mot 94(4 Suppl):S36–S62. doi:10.1016/j.rco.2008.03.005. Epub 2008 May 19. [Article in French]
25. Prasad N, Dent C (2008) Outcome of total elbow replacement for distal humeral fractures in the elderly: a comparison of primary surgery and surgery after failed internal fixation or conservative treatment. J Bone Joint Surg Br 90(3):343–348. doi:10.1302/0301-620X.90B3.18971
26. Mehlhoff TL, Bennett JB (2011) Distal humeral fractures: fixation versus arthroplasty. J Shoulder

Elbow Surg 20(2 Suppl):S97–S106. doi:10.1016/j.jse.2010.11.012
27. Cil A, Veillette CJ, Sanchez-Sotelo J, Morrey BF (2008) Linked elbow replacement: a salvage procedure for distal humeral nonunion. J Bone Joint Surg Am 90(9):1939–1950. doi:10.2106/JBJS.G.00690
28. Barlow JD, Morrey BF, O'Driscoll SW, Steinmann SP, Sanchez-Sotelo J (2013) Activities after total elbow arthroplasty. J Shoulder Elbow Surg 22(6):787–791. doi:10.1016/j.jse.2013.01.023. Epub 2013 Mar 13

27 External Fixation: When and How

Antonio M. Foruria and Jesus Cobos

27.1 Introduction

Although a rigid external fixator applied on the distal humerus can be used in the general situations for which these devices have been designed (i.e., open fractures with extensive soft tissue damage or infections), there are specific indications and considerations to be taken when these devices are used in the context of elbow pathology.

The pathological elbow joint has a tendency to develop stiffness; specific hinged elbow external fixators have been designed with the aim of maintaining motion at the same time the joint is stabilized and the soft tissues protected. There are several hinged elbow fixators on the market [1]:

- The Dynamic Joint Distractor (DJD) II: a simple device with an integrated hinge and a low profile. The stability can be increased by bilateral application, but this configuration is seldom needed. Concentric joint reduction is required before fixation to the ulna.
- The Orthofix Elbow Fixator: similar to the DJD, it is integrated by linked components with central connecting units. It can be used only by unilateral configuration and bigger in size.
- The OptiROM Elbow Fixator: it has a comfortable unilateral design; multiple adjustable linkages feature it; therefore, it has less frame stability.
- Compass Universal Hinge: a multiplanar device based on the Ilizarov concept, composed by radiolucent arcs with bilateral hinges. It is the fixator with more frame stability but less patient comfort. It is also and the most difficult to apply.

The concept of an articulating fixator about the elbow is based on the normal ulno-humeral kinematics, which approximate a simple hinged joint. Recreating the anatomic axis of rotation with a hinged fixator allows concentric ulno-humeral motion while protecting the joint surfaces and periarticular soft tissues from loads [2].

A hinged fixator stabilizes the elbow joint in varus and valgus stress, neutralizes rotational forces around the forearm preventing elbow rotatory instability, and, at the same time, allows a congruent elbow flexion and extension [3]. If required, it is also possible to protect the articular cartilage adding joint distraction. Given the above-mentioned advantages, hinged external fixators are indicated in a wide spectrum of elbow problems, including both traumatic and reconstructive pathologies. In our opinion, it is imperative that surgeons treating elbow diseases are familiar with their indications, surgical technique, potential complications, and postoperative care.

Elbow hinged external fixators are used commonly along with other reconstructive procedures performed simultaneously, so the reported results

A.M. Foruria, MD, PhD (✉) • J. Cobos
Department of Orthopedic Surgery Fundación,
Shoulder and Elbow Reconstructive Surgery Unit.
Jiménez Díaz, Avda. Reyes Católicos, 2,
Madrid 28040, Spain
e-mail: antonio.foruria@gmail.com;
jesuscobosmorales@gmail.com

F. Castoldi et al. (eds.), *Simple and Complex Fractures of the Humerus*,
DOI 10.1007/978-88-470-5307-6_27, © Springer-Verlag Italia 2015

cannot be attributed exclusively to the frame; there are no comparative studies randomizing patients to receive either external fixation or braces or splinting, and the procedures in which a hinged external fixator is used are also uncommon. On this context, our aim is to provide the necessary information to the reader to be able to use these devices with confidence in the selected group of patients that can benefit from this technique.

27.2 Indications

Hinged elbow external fixators are used in a wide variety of elbow pathology including acute and chronic instability and severe elbow arthropathy and as an adjuvant to control elbow motion.

27.2.1 Acute Elbow Instability [1]

1. Fracture-dislocations, including terrible triads (the combination of elbow dislocation, radial head fracture, and coronoid fracture) and posteromedial rotatory instability (combined ligamentous injury and anteromedial facet coronoid fracture)
2. Radial head and medial collateral ligament disruption with subsequent valgus instability
3. Comminute olecranon or distal humerus fractures
4. Extensive post-contracture release of a stiff joint (see below)

Persistent instability that is present either acutely or in the early postoperative period is an indication for a hinged external fixator to maintain concentric reduction, protect the bony and ligament repair, and allow early postoperative motion [4]. In this setting, the fixator should be used to protect a suboptimal reconstructive procedure allowing immediate postoperative rehabilitation and in cases of persistent subluxation despite ligamentous and fracture repair. Several authors have reported their experience with hinged external fixators in acute elbow fracture-dislocations with reasonable good results [5, 6].

Missing the opportunity to further stabilize and protect the elbow can lead to the prescription of a prolonged period of immobilization with the subsequent high risk of joint stiffness. On the other hand, in some instances we could be too optimistic about our repairs, and persistent subluxation can be easily missed intraoperatively; realizing a suboptimal joint congruency in the postoperative X-rays is present can lead us to proceed to a second procedure for ligament and/or fracture re-repair along with external fixation. When this is necessary, good results can still be obtained if the reoperation is performed within the first 6 weeks after the injury [7]. Without ignoring the potential complications related to the use of this device, we believe a more liberal use of hinged external fixators in the more severe complex elbow instability cases, along with a thorough intraoperative exam including the use of fluoroscopy, will prevent complications and improve the final outcome.

Hinged external fixation is also indicated in the setting of acute gross instability that cannot be splinted in concentric reduction in a patient who is unable to tolerate a prolonged surgical procedure.

27.2.2 Chronic Elbow Instability [7, 8]

There are two major types of chronic elbow instability, subluxation and dislocation, and both can be treated with a hinged fixator.

Chronic subluxation is a difficult problem that requires reconstruction of the bony and soft tissue elbow stabilizators when possible and the application of an external fixation. As mentioned before, this is particularly effective when performed before 6 weeks after the injury [7]. The presence of extensive posttraumatic joint degeneration would require other reconstructive procedures as distraction interposition arthroplasty or total elbow arthroplasty.

Chronic complete elbow dislocation requires excision of all fibrous tissue and release of contracted soft tissues, including the capsule, the medial and lateral collateral ligaments, and possibly the triceps, before joint reduction. The induced instability will be neutralized with a hinged fixator to allow immediate motion and to protect the repaired collateral ligaments. The application of distraction can be useful to start immediate concentric motion [8].

27.2.3 Severe Elbow Arthropathy

Distraction interposition arthroplasty has been developed from two procedures, distraction and biologic resurfacing of the joint, both used to treat incapacitating elbow pain and loss of motion. This procedure has been used for posttraumatic, postinfectious, and hemophilic arthropathies and rheumatoid arthritis; in general, this procedure is indicated for patients with severe intra-articular pathology who are too young to undergo total elbow prosthesis [9].

In this procedure, the articular surface of the humerus or the ulna is debrided and covered by a biologic material such as fascia lata or Achilles tendon allograft or autologous deep dermal skin. Subsequently, the addition of joint distraction by the means of an external fixator allows early motion and minimizes shear forces across the interposed tissue, protecting the collateral ligaments of the elbow [1, 9].

27.2.4 Control of Motion

Elbow contracture releases often require extensive excision of soft tissues, including sometimes heterotopic bone, hypertrophic capsule, and osteophytes and sometimes even the collateral ligaments [10]. On this context, the joint may be rendered unstable, requiring the application of a hinged fixator to allow controlled motion.

An uncommon use of hinged fixation is protecting elbow motion and/or repair in the obese patient, because the use of bracing and splinting may be difficult [3, 11].

27.2.5 Contraindications

The contraindications for the hinged external fixation of the elbow are the general of this kind of devices:

- Absolute contraindications: local infection in the pin site, cellulitis, and osteomyelitis; large disturbance of the anatomy for a high-energy trauma or inflammation; or a noncompliant patient
- Relative contraindications: internal fixation or the presence of other kinds of devices which may make the correct positioning of the pins or the correct position of the external fixator difficult

27.3 Relevant Anatomy

Being familiar with elbow anatomy is paramount when using external fixation. Of special interest is recognizing the location of important neurovascular structures, as the radial nerve, and being familiar with ligamentous attachments and their bony landmarks, as these are the reference we will use to reproduce the axis of rotation.

Since the recognition of both varus and valgus stabilities is restored with a half-pin lateral fixation configuration in the absence of collateral ligaments [3], medial frames or transfixing pins or wires have been mostly abandoned. As a consequence, the majority of mayor vessels and nerves are safe during the procedure with the exception of the radial nerve. The radial nerve is the main noble structure at risk during surgery, and its injury generally occurs with the placement of the humeral half pins. In this regard, knowing its location with respect to identifiable bone landmarks is probably the main concept that needs to be clarified. Studies performed by Kamineni et al. [12] identified the distance between the lateral epicondyle and the point where the radial nerve crosses the humerus in the mid-lateral plane to be 1.4–1.7 times the inter-epicondylar distance for a given patient. Based on this finding, an "absolute safe zone" has been described for humeral pin placement and is defined as equivalent in length to the patient's own transepicondylar distance, when projected proximally from the lateral epicondyle (Fig. 27.1). The ulnar nerve is usually safe, but a too proud ulnar half pin or a careless placement of the axis pin guide could put this structure at risk.

The elbow axis of rotation is located with the aim of bony landmarks. On the lateral aspect of the capitellum, the axis crosses a tubercle present at the site of origin of the lateral collateral ligament, which represents the geometric center of curvature of the capitellum. On the medial aspect

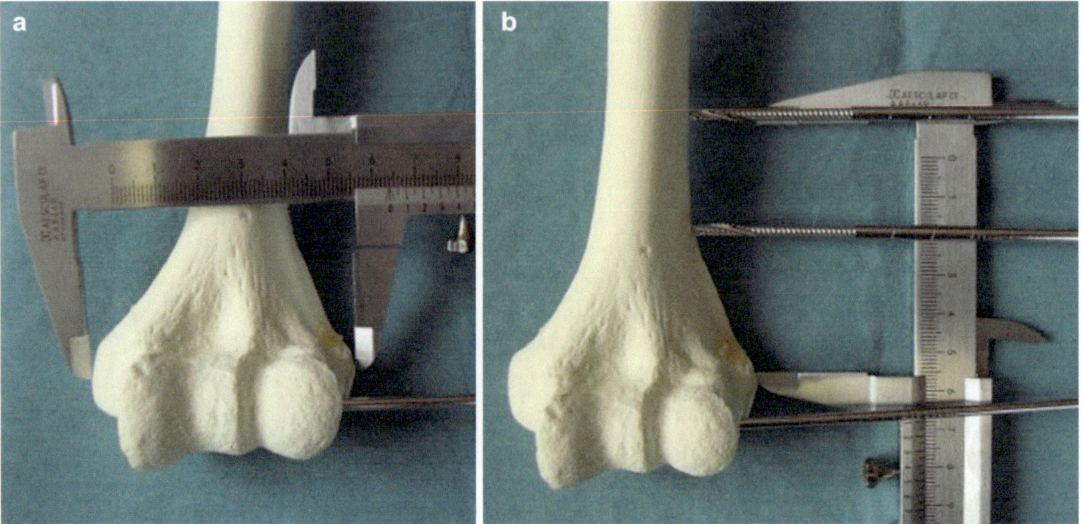

Fig. 27.1 "Absolute safe zone" defined as equivalent in length to the patient's own transepicondylar distance (**a**), when projected proximally from the lateral epicondyle (**b**)

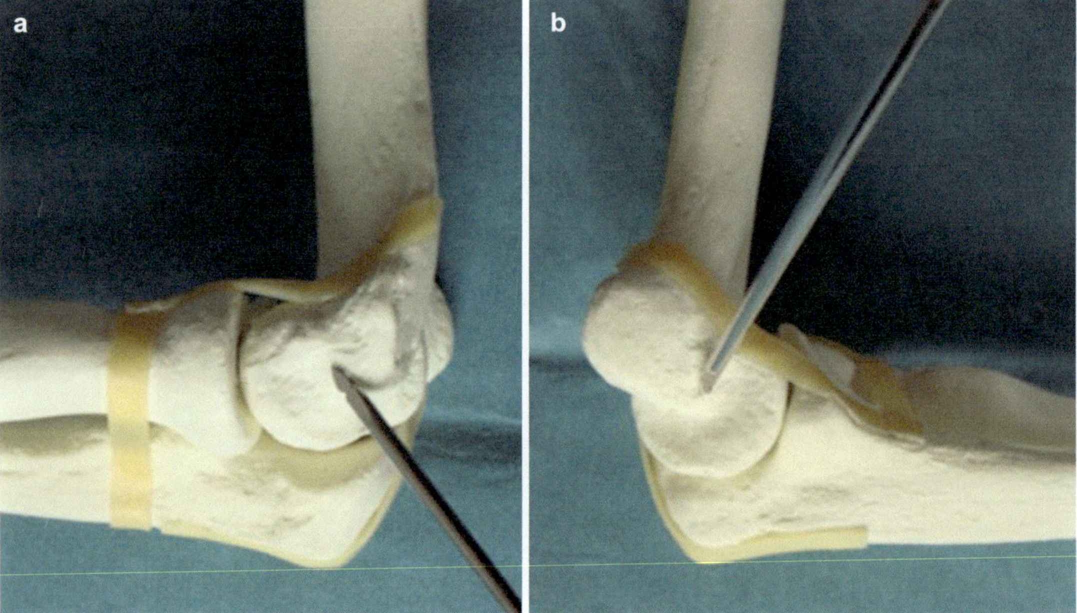

Fig. 27.2 Landmarks for flexion axis pin insertion. (**a**) Site of origin of the lateral collateral ligament representing the geometric center of curvature of the capitellum. (**b**) Site of the humeral origin of the medial ulnar collateral ligament representing the center of curvature of the medial contour of the trochlea. See text for more details

of the distal humerus, the axis of rotation lies just anterior and inferior to the medial epicondyle. This corresponds to the center of curvature of the medial contour of the trochlea and is the locus of the humeral origin of the medial ulnar collateral ligament (Fig. 27.2).

27.4 Surgical Technique

We commonly use the DJD II (Stryker, Kalamazoo, MI) because of its simple surgical technique and reduced size; several configurations can be used, including a lateral frame with lateral half pins, a medial frame with half pins, and transfixing pins with bilateral frames. As mentioned before, mechanical stability is restored with a half-pin lateral fixation configuration [3], so we do not use medial frames. We describe in this section the surgical technique for the lateral unilateral hinged external fixator (Fig. 27.3).

27.4.1 Setup and Patient Positioning

We usually place the patient supine in the operating table with the forearm across the chest, although the use of a radiolucent arm board or hand table can be also useful. Fluoroscopy enters parallel to the table from the feet. A small tourniquet is used as proximal as possible, making sure it will not interfere with the fixator frame; this is especially important in small persons. The field is prepared and draped, and the indicated repair-reconstruction procedure performed; the external fixation is generally the last steps of the whole surgery. In choosing the skin approach, it should be taken into account the lateral placement of the fixator and the necessity of identifying correctly the bony landmarks used for axis pin insertion (Fig. 27.2).

27.4.2 Axis Identification and Frame Orientation

The tubercle present at the site of origin of the lateral collateral ligament, which represents the geometric center of curvature of the capitellum, is identified. Medially, the axis of rotation lies just anterior and inferior to the medial epicondyle; this corresponds to the center of curvature of the medial contour of the trochlea and is the locus of the humeral origin of the medial ulnar collateral ligament. If a medial exposure/cutaneous flap has been performed, the medial landmark is easily identified. When only a lateral approach is being used, the medial landmark can be palpated through the skin using the medial epicondyle as a reference that can be confirmed with the aid of a fluoroscope; a slight nonanatomic axis does not alter the elbow kinematics [11], so we usually do not perform a medial approach specifically for this purpose (Fig. 27.2) and have not had any complications on this regard.

Once the axis is located, the pointed tip of the axis target guide is placed on the medial side, with the cannulated stylus guide on the lateral side; the axis pin is then inserted through the guide in the distal humerus with a mallet or power tool.

The fixator frame is then placed on the axis pin with the distraction mechanism oriented distally; the proximal bar is aligned with the anterior humeral cortex.

27.4.3 Humeral Pin Insertion

The "absolute safe zone" (the inter-epicondylar distance proximal to the axis guide) demarcates the area of the humerus where the pins will be inserted. Before pin insertion, the skin should be positioned back anatomically where it will be sutured, and then a stab incision is performed for pin insertion. A 4 mm (3 mm in small bones) self-drilling self-taping pin is inserted proximally engaging both humeral cortices through the specific pin guide. A pin-rod coupling is placed and tightened with a wrench. A second pin is inserted distally using the same procedure including the pin guide, avoiding the olecranon fossa. Once both pins are rigidly coupled to the proximal rod, the axis pin can be removed.

27.4.3.1 Technical Points

- Before proximal pin insertion, it is useful to plan where both pins are going to be positioned. This is of special interest in small persons, as a too distally placed proximal pin can make impossible to correctly place and orientate the pin guide for the distal humeral pin.
- As opposed to other external fixation techniques, humeral and ulnar pins spatial position is determined by the spatial position of the

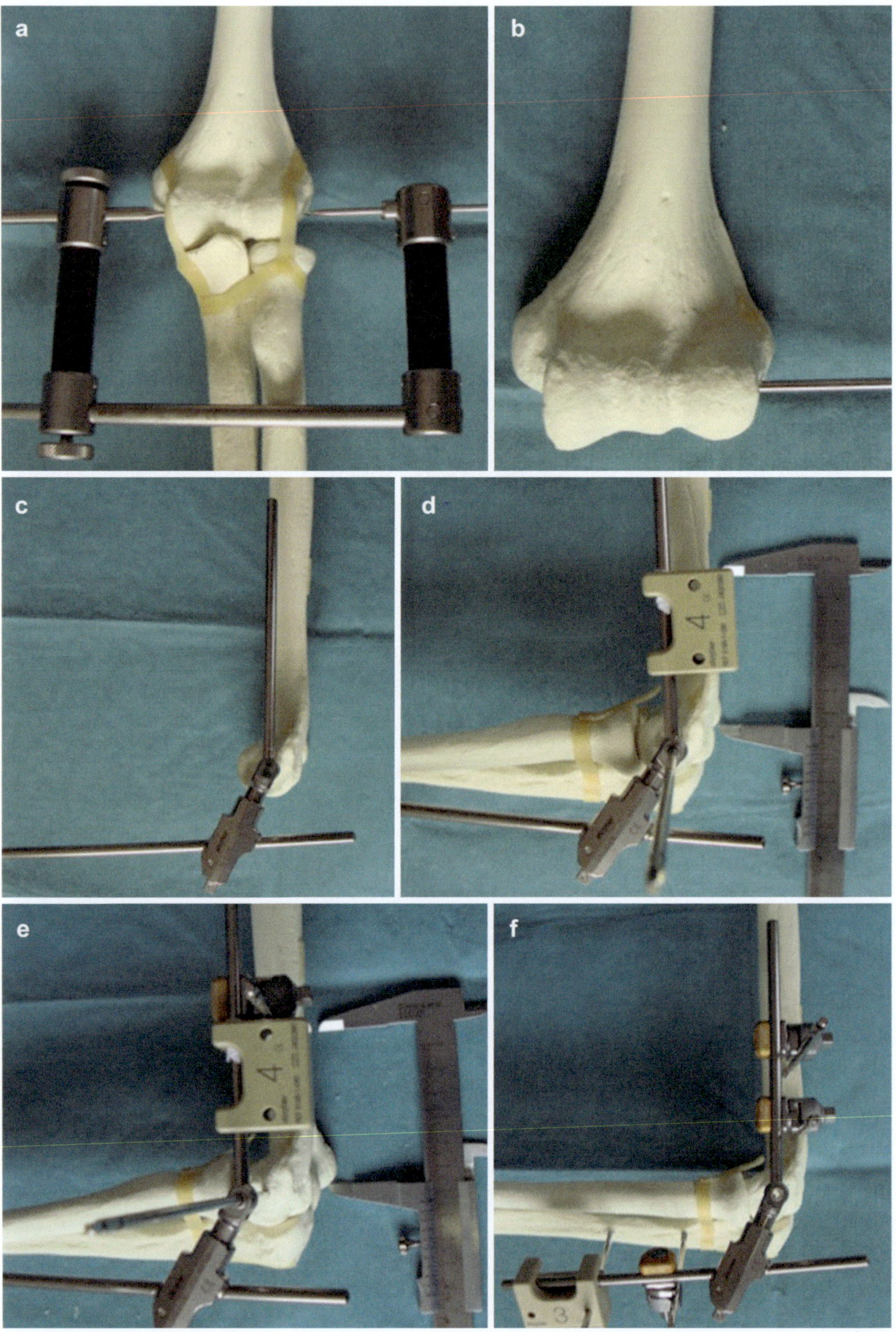

Fig. 27.3 Surgical technique for elbow hinged external fixation. (**a**) Axis pin guide placement. (**b**) Axis pin inserted in the distal humerus. (**c**) External fixation frame inserted on the axis pin and with its humeral rod aligned with the anterior humeral cortex. (**d**) Humeral pin guide placed within the margins of the "absolute safe zone." (**e**) Distal humeral pin insertion through the pin guide. (**f**) Ulnar pin insertion

frame; as a consequence, not using the pin guides or sliding the frame along the axis pin once the humeral pin has been inserted will change the pin-frame distance, changing the orientation of the frame as a consequence when the coupling system is tightened.

- The pins do not need to be parallel. The pin guide can be rotated over the humeral rod to gain access to a better bone purchase. By providing proper pin to rod distance, an independent pin placement is possible.
- The pin guide is positioned so the pin is located posterior to the rod, increasing its distance from the radial nerve.

27.4.4 Ulnar Pin Insertion

Three millimeter self-taping self-drilling pins are used for the ulna. The technique is similar to that described for the humeral pins. We insert the proximal pin first and then the distal one, always with the aid of the pin guide. It can be difficult to "feel" the ulnar second cortex penetration, so we recommend checking with fluoroscope the correct position of the pins at the end of the procedure.

27.4.5 Distraction

The amount of separation between articular surfaces is determined by the calibrations on the distraction unit. Two to three mm is usually enough to protect the articular surfaces and the bony repairs.

The skin is closed and a bandage applied.

27.5 Postoperative Care

The patient should be informed of the pin and wound daily care. The postoperative care must be tailored for each individual. In patients treated for elbow stability problems, our main indication, we do all possible efforts to maintain the external fixator a minimum of 4 weeks and try not to remove it before 6 weeks after surgery. We teach our patients range of motion exercises in both flexion and extension and prono-supination, to be performed with the elbow at the side of the body. They start this program the day after the surgery performing the exercises during a few minutes five to six times a day. As time goes by, we encourage them to increase the frequency and intensity of exercises. We advise not to take any weight or manipulate any object with the operated elbow. Serial X-rays are taken at 10 days, 3 weeks, and 6 weeks after surgery.

After the sixth to eighth weeks, we proceed to fixator removal under regional blockade or general anesthesia. This is a good moment for gentle manipulation to help the patient gaining some degrees of motion. The manipulation should be done before fixator removal to preventing any additional damage. Stability and congruity are evaluated under fluoroscopy. After this, the patient can initiate formal progressive physical therapy.

Postoperative care after distraction interposition arthroplasty is similar to the one described above. Physical therapy starts the day after the surgery; the external fixator is also removed at 6 weeks with gentle manipulation as needed; therapy with the use of static splinting if necessary is also implemented.

27.6 Complications

27.6.1 Minor Complications

1. Pin tract infection. This complication can occur in up to 5 % of pin sites. Usually, local erythema and non-purulent drainage are present, but the pin is not loose. In addition, cellulitis around the pin can be also frequent. They can be treated with oral antibiotics, as an oral first- or second-generation cephalosporin, for 2 weeks or even for the entire duration of the fixation, and care of the pin tract with daily local cures [13].
2. Some patients need skin release around the humeral pin site to improve their motion. This can be made easily with local anesthesia.

27.6.2 Major Complications

1. Pin loosening is a major complication. It may require debridement of pin sites and placement of new pins in healthy tissue and oral antibiotics. Some patients may require early removal of the fixator.
2. Purulent drainage with associated deep sepsis and/or osteomyelitis is a rare complication. It requires open irrigation, debridement, and 6-week course of antibiogram-guided antibiotics to eradicate the infection.
3. Loss of reduction can occur from improper placement of the fixator axis or from hardware failure. Periodic radiographic evaluation is important. In these cases, fixator replacement may be necessary.
4. The occurrence of a fracture is a very infrequent complication. It involves usually the ulna and is related to a vigorous therapy. Using smaller-diameter pins (3 mm) for the ulna can help to reduce the stress riser effect. When the fracture occurs, internal fixation with plating may be necessary.

27.6.3 Nerve Injuries

Ulnar nerve can be at risk during the surgical procedure because of an injudicious placement of the axis pin guide or medial humeral half pins, over-penetration of lateral humeral or ulnar half pins, and increased elbow flexion after a contracture release. Ulnar nerve injury can be avoided with precise pin insertion and protection and/or transposition of the nerve [1].

As mentioned before, for laterally based unilateral frames, care must be taken to protect the radial nerve during the application of the most proximal pin. The radial nerve crosses the humerus in the mid-lateral plane at a distance of 1.4–1.7 times the inter-epicondylar distance projected proximally over the lateral epicondyle, and this location makes it vulnerable to injury with placement of the humeral pins superior to the elbow [13, 14]. Injury to the posterior interosseous has been reported as an infrequent complication [15].

Conclusions

Hinged elbow external fixation is a surgical resource indicated in complex elbow fracture-dislocations, elbow instability, and chronic degenerative disorders along with other reparative or reconstructive techniques. Recognizing its value is paramount to avoid suboptimal treatment of these conditions and to open the spectrum of treatment in elbow degenerative diseases. Recognizing the importance of working in safe areas when implanting this device and following the recommendations given about the surgical technique are mandatory to obtain a rewarding result in the difficult situations in which it is indicated.

References

1. Tan V, Daluiski A, Capo J, Hotchkiss R (2005) Hinged elbow external fixators: indications and uses. J Am Acad Orthop Surg 13(8):503–514. Epub 2005/12/07
2. Deland JT, Garg A, Walker PS (1987) Biomechanical basis for elbow hinge-distractor design. Clin Orthop Relat Res 215:303–312. Epub 1987/02/01
3. Kamineni S, Hirahara H, Neale P, O'Driscoll SW, An KN, Morrey BF (2007) Effectiveness of the lateral unilateral dynamic external fixator after elbow ligament injury. J Bone Joint Surg Am 89(8):1802–1809. Epub 2007/08/03
4. Kolb W, Guhlmann H, Windisch C, Marx F, Markgraf E, Koller H et al (2008) Complex osteoligamentary injuries of the elbow. Treatment with a hinged external fixator. Unfallchirurg 111(8):584–586, 8–91. Epub 2008/06/28. Komplexe osteoligamentare Verletzungen des Ellenbogens. Therapie mit dem Bewegungsfixateur externe
5. Frank J, Howorka A, Marzi I (2011) Treatment of complex elbow injuries with the hinged fixation device DJD II. Technique and results. Orthopade 40(4): 316–322. Epub 2011/02/26. Behandlung komplexer Ellenbogenverletzungen mit dem Bewegungsfixateur DJD II. Technik und Ergebnisse
6. Schep NW, De Haan J, Iordens GI, Tuinebreijer WE, Bronkhorst MW, De Vries MR et al (2011) A hinged external fixator for complex elbow dislocations: a multicenter prospective cohort study. BMC Musculoskelet Disord 12:130. Epub 2011/06/11
7. Sorensen AK, Sojbjerg JO (2011) Treatment of persistent instability after posterior fracture-dislocation of the elbow: restoring stability and mobility by internal fixation and hinged external fixation. J Shoulder Elbow Surg 20(8):1300–1309. Epub 2011/10/11
8. Jupiter JB, Ring D (2002) Treatment of unreduced elbow dislocations with hinged external fixation. J Bone Joint Surg Am 84-A(9):1630–1635. Epub 2002/09/05

9. Larson AN, Morrey BF (2008) Interposition arthroplasty with an Achilles tendon allograft as a salvage procedure for the elbow. J Bone Joint Surg Am 90(12):2714–2723. Epub 2008/12/03
10. Foruria AM, Augustin S, Morrey BF, Sanchez-Sotelo J (2013) Heterotopic ossification after surgery for fractures and fracture-dislocations involving the proximal aspect of the radius or ulna. J Bone Joint Surg Am 95(10):e66. Epub 2013/05/17
11. Morrey BF (2012) Ligament injury and the use of hinged external fixators at the elbow. Instr Course Lect 61:215–225. Epub 2012/02/04
12. Kamineni S, Ankem H, Patten DK (2009) Anatomic relationship of the radial nerve to the elbow joint: clinical implications of safe pin placement. Clin Anat 22(6):684–688. Epub 2009/07/29
13. Cheung EV, O'Driscoll SW, Morrey BF (2008) Complications of hinged external fixators of the elbow. J Shoulder Elbow Surg 17(3):447–453. Epub 2008/03/04
14. Baumann G, Nagy L, Jost B (2011) Radial nerve disruption following application of a hinged elbow external fixator: a report of three cases. J Bone Joint Surg Am 93(10):e51. Epub 2011/05/20
15. Tomaino MM, Sotereanos DG, Westkaemper J, Plakseychuk A (1999) Posterior interosseous nerve palsy following placement of the compass elbow hinge for acute instability: a case report. J Hand Surg Am 24(3):554–560. Epub 1999/06/05

28 The Malunion and Nonunion of Distal Humerus Fractures

Andrea Celli

The incidence of complex articular fractures of the distal humeral in adults has increased and will be growing in the future due to the greater incidence of high-energy trauma and to the higher percentage of elderly population [1]. The distal humerus and the entire elbow joint have complex anatomy (three articulations in a small space) with a high degree of mechanical force crossing the articular surface from the forearm to the shoulder. This leads to an increased risk of complications after intra- and extra-articular fractures of the distal humerus. The two major complications that influence daily living activities are stiffness and instability with pain. These clinical aspects are often related to the malunion or nonunion of the distal humerus. The risk of malunion or nonunion following fractures is influenced by a variety of factors: biology, in particular the blood supply of the metaphysis; the nonanatomic reduction of the fracture; and the methods of osteosynthesis and mechanical failure.

28.1 Distal Humerus Malunion

Malunions of distal humerus fractures occur fairly often following closed-treated fractures and occasionally after open reduction and internal fixation. Frequently, different planes can be involved (transversal, coronal, and sagittal planes). The intra-articular or extra-articular areas can also be involved. The most common deformities in the supracondylar area associated with distal humeral fractures are varus malunion and extension malunion. Both of these are related to elbow deformity (clinical assessment) with or without loss of range of motion. The malunion of intra-articular fractures is associated with loss of range of motion in flexion-extension. The stiffness depends on the extent and nature of the articular surface deformity. The common intra-articular deformities are related to a reduction of the trochlea shape and to the malposition of the capitellum. Both the latter lead to maltracking of the olecranon and radial head onto the articular surface of the humerus.

28.1.1 Extra-articular Malunion

28.1.1.1 Varus Malunion

The malunion of the cubitus varus is the most common cause of deformity following fractures of the extra-articular area in the distal humerus in children. Clinically, these patients present with deformity in the varus of the elbow with or without loss of range of motion (Fig. 28.1). The cosmetic deformity often influences daily living activities and can increase the risk of secondary instability.

It is well described that varus deformity causes the medialization of the olecranon and triceps

A. Celli
Department of Orthopaedic Surgery,
Shoulder and Elbow Unit, Hesperia Hospital,
Via Emilia Est 380/1, Modena 41124, Italy
e-mail: celli.lg@libero.it

F. Castoldi et al. (eds.), *Simple and Complex Fractures of the Humerus*,
DOI 10.1007/978-88-470-5307-6_28, © Springer-Verlag Italia 2015

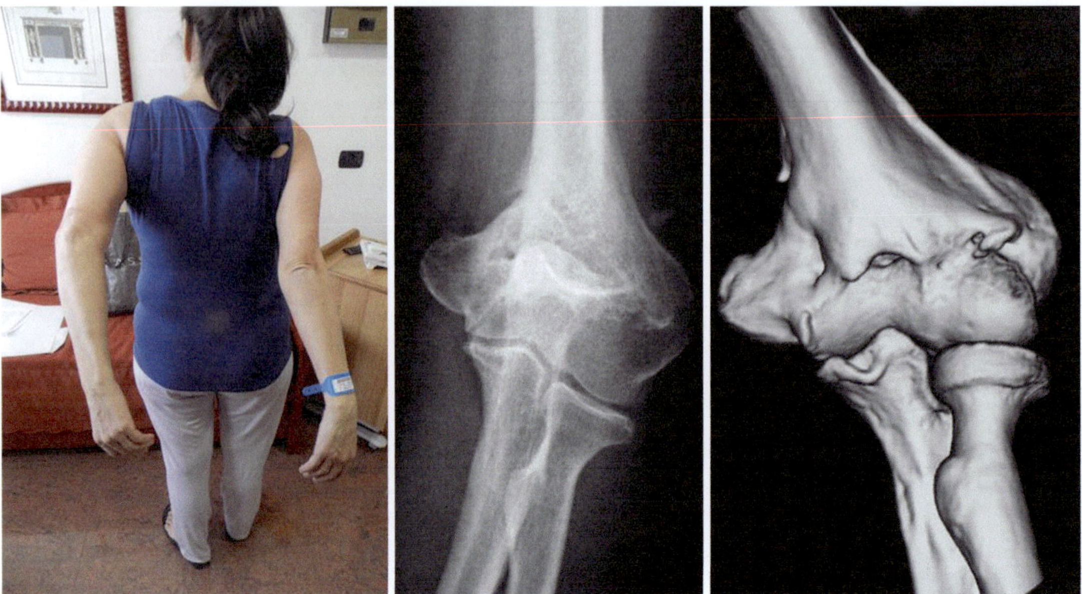

Fig. 28.1 Deformity in the varus of the elbow with loss of range of motion following supracondylar fracture. The angulation and the level of the osteotomy are determined in the preoperative X-ray and CT scan evaluations

insertion. This results in the triceps muscles being forced to become medial with respect to the mechanical axis of the elbow. This situation increases stress on the lateral collateral ligament complex which may lead in time to posterolateral rotatory instability. The clinical signs of this situation will be increased pain and clicking during the flexion and extension movements. The surgical indication is related not only to the deformity with snapping of the medial triceps with or without ulnar nerve symptoms but also to the posterolateral instability when the forearm is in full supination. The more common surgical treatment is osteotomy with internal fixation and ligament reconstruction or retention in cases of lateral ligament deficiency.

This surgical procedure can be performed in supine or lateral position (we prefer the lateral decubitus). A posterior skin incision is performed, and the ulnar nerve is identified and decompressed to the medial epicondyle through the two heads of the flexor carpi ulnaris. The medial intermuscular septum is excised, and the ulnar nerve is moved to a position anterior to the epicondyle in order for it to be in a safe position during the procedure. The triceps tendon is lifted from the posterior surface of the humerus, and the anterior muscles are also detached from the humerus to expose the osteotomy site all around the humeral bone. The lateral side of the triceps is reflected together with the anconeus muscle, and the lateral ligament complex is exposed. The osteotomy can be performed with or without triceps splitting. The angulation and the level of the osteotomy (three-cut osteotomy) are determined in the preoperative X-ray evaluations. A goniometer is useful to determine the correct angulation and level of the lateral closing wedge osteotomy. Distal cutting is performed as distally as possible above the olecranon fossa. The depth of the osteotomy is marked with electrocautery, and an oscillating saw is used to perform the three levels of bone cuts, while the anterior tissue and muscles are moved out of the way. A cut is made, and the triangular bone block shape is removed leaving a lateral edge to the cortex, to improve the stability of the reduction. The distal and proximal cutting levels are reduced to recover the anatomic axis in the frontal and sagittal planes. The proximal aspect of the lateral humeral cortex is modeled to adjust it to the lateral spike of the distal fragment. The fixation can

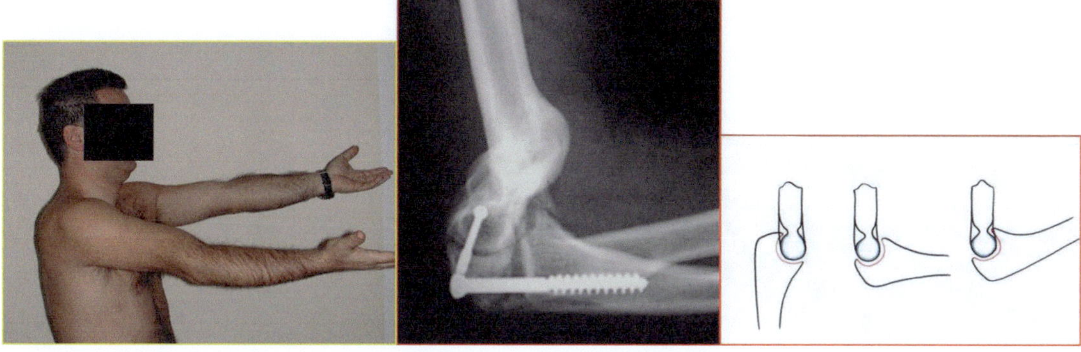

Fig. 28.2 The loss of humerus antiversion, also known as "gunshot deformity," is clinically defined, and it is related to hyperextension and loss of flexion

be performed with 3.5-mm screws placed from lateral to medial, or a precontoured plate can be used on the medial side or on both sides; this will improve stability in particular in adults. A cortical bone graft can be also carried out in conjunction, to improve healing in adults. Usually, at this point the tension of the lateral ligament complex can be found to be inadequate, and reconstruction or augmentation is then advised, depending on tissue quality. A postoperative program has to then be carried out to optimize bone healing and ligament reconstruction. The arm is held in a hinge elbow brace with the forearm pronated for 6–8 weeks (depending on the kind of ligament reconstruction) with limited range of motion. Finally, the brace is removed, and the full range of motion is allowed. The full range of activities with strengthening will be allowed after 4–6 months depending on the healing progress.

28.1.1.2 Extension Malunion

The extension malunion is the posterior angulation of the distal humerus on the sagittal plane. The loss of humerus antiversion, also known as "gunshot deformity," is clinically defined and is related to hyperextension and loss of flexion (Fig. 28.2). Two major groups of surgical procedures can be performed in adults: osteotomy to correct the posterior angulation and recontouring arthroplasty. Osteotomy can be considered in cases of high-degree retroversion of the distal humerus with clinical deformity, as previously described.

A radical debridement of the posterior and anterior compartments can be achieved by an open Outerbridge-Kashiwagi operation as a "house-keeping procedure" [2] which includes olecranon tip resection, transhumeral fenestration, and coronoid tip resection.

Recontouring arthroplasty can be performed with either open or arthroscopic techniques. Preoperative evaluations should include a physical examination to assess the range of motion loss and an examination of the extra-articular deformity and the intra-articular status of the distal humerus by means of imaging studies. Imaging studies (X-rays and CT scan) allow an evaluation of the nature and degree of malunion and to identify any associated loose bodies or heterotopic ossifications. The aim of open and arthroscopic procedures is to increase the range of motion and not to alter the retroversion of the distal humerus with no change in the clinical aspect. The remodeling procedure has to be performed on both sides of the ulno-humeral articulation, following the anterior capsulectomy and the remodeling of the coronoid and radial head fossa, and also on the ulnar side to reduce the coronoid apex. Following these surgical steps, an increase in range of motion can be obtained. Posterior capsulectomy with incision of the posterior band of the medial collateral ligament associated with ulnar nerve neurolysis is an advanced technique to improve range of motion in terms of flexion and to reduce the risk of secondary neuropathy.

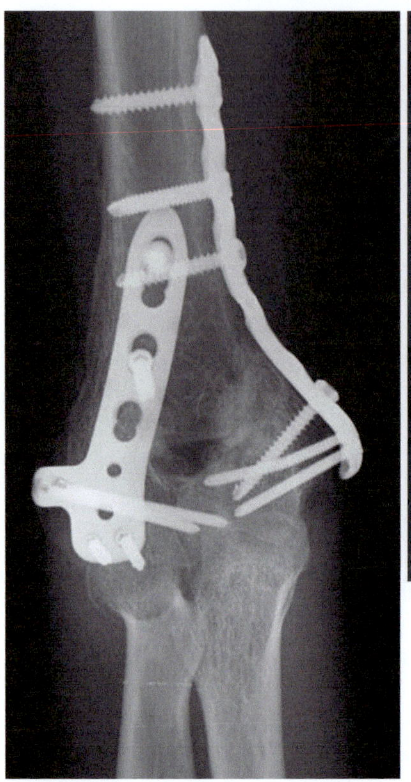
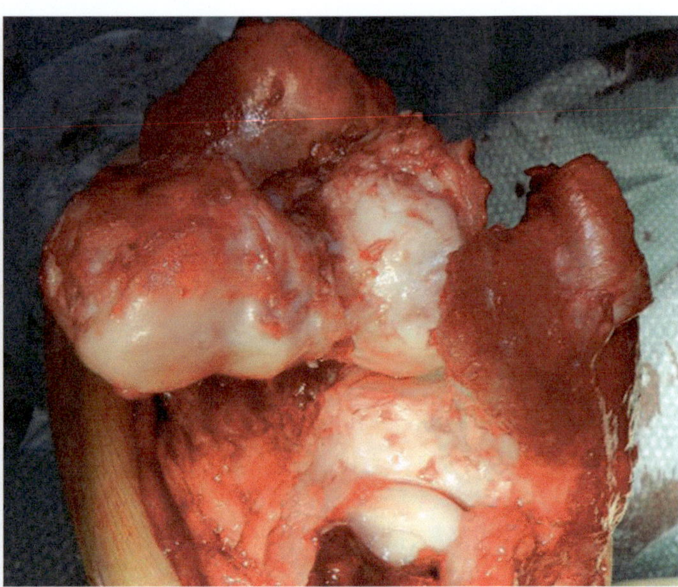

Fig. 28.3 Preserved joint congruency with limited articular damage (less than 50 %). The articular deformity is not further compromised by severe joint destruction, avascular necrosis, or secondary degenerative changes

28.1.2 Intra-articular Malunion

Intra-articular malunions involve the articular surface (shape, orientation, dimension, and axis of rotation) of the trochlea and capitellum humeri. The most common intra-articular deformity is secondary to the loss of orientation and dimension of the trochlea shape with or without change in angulation of the rotational axis. Clinically, patients lose flexion-extension range of motion due to the incongruency between the olecranon and the trochlea. If the intra-articular malunion is associated with an extra-articular deformity, the elbow becomes stiff due to the malunion of the three axes within the elbow (diaphyseal, intercondylar, and rotational axes). Imaging studies are useful to assess the status of the articular surface and its deformity. Computer tomography with three-dimensional reconstructions reproduces the elbow joint and allows the investigator to understand the nature of the articular deformity and the alignment between the olecranon and trochlea and the radial head and the capitellum humeri. Different surgical options (ulno-humeral arthroplasty, interposition arthroplasty, or elbow prosthesis) are available for this group of patients with distal humerus deformities depending on the nature and extent of the articular changes and on patient age.

28.1.2.1 Surgical Techniques for Preserved Joint Congruency with Limited Articular Damage (Less Than 50 %) (Fig. 28.3)

Ulno-humeral arthroplasty can be performed following open or arthroscopic techniques. This surgical procedure is indicated if the articular deformity is not further compromised by severe joint destruction, avascular necrosis, or secondary degenerative changes.

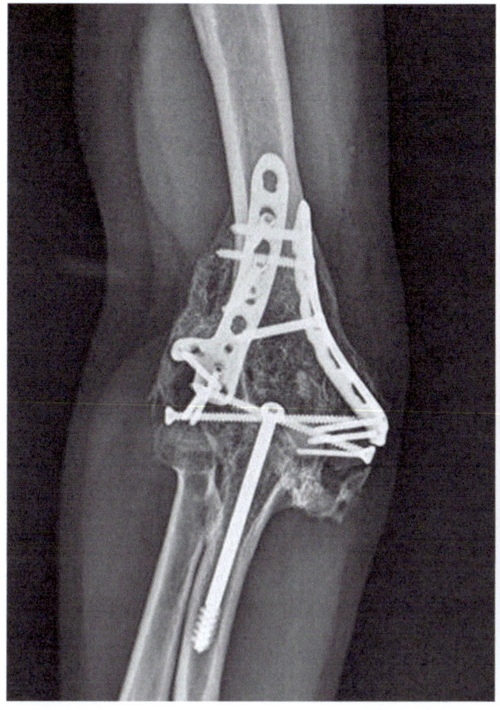

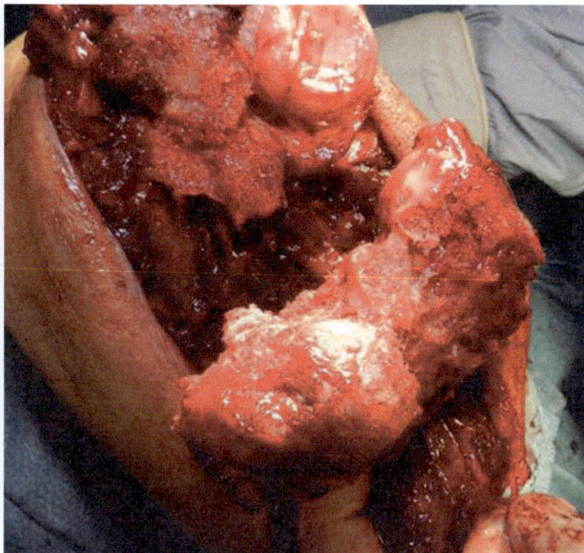

Fig. 28.4 Lost joint congruency with extensive articular damage (more than 50 %). Severe joint destruction of the articular surface that involves more than half of the joint surface and with significant incongruity between the trochlea and olecranon

The open technique can be performed using a posterior midline skin incision; the ulnar nerve is isolated, and triceps splitting is performed. The posterior compartment is exposed, and the articular bone surface of the distal humerus and olecranon is reshaped. The anterior compartment can be exposed using medial and lateral column procedures, and the anterior bone remodeling is then adjusted. The arthroscopic procedure follows the same open surgical steps. The standard setups and portals are made. We usually isolate the ulnar nerve through a medial skin incision just above the ulnar nerve groove. Posterior debridement is performed with standard approaches, the capsula is lifted from the bone to create a space, and bone remodeling is performed with a 5-mm round burr, on both sides of the joint to reduce impingement and maltracking of the ulno-humeral joint.

Remodeling of the anterior is routinely performed using blunt retractors to help with visualization and to protect the nearby neurovascular structures.

Once the bony debridement and remodeling are completed, the anterior and posterior capsulae are excised. The medial capsula can be excised through a medial skin incision performed to isolate the ulnar nerve.

The aim of both surgical techniques is to improve the range of motion without altering the articular surface.

28.1.2.2 Surgical Techniques for Lost Joint Congruency with Extensive Articular Damage (More Than 50 %) (Fig. 28.4)

Interposition arthroplasty is indicated for severe joint destruction or avascular necrosis of the articular surface that involves more than half of the joint surface or with significant incongruity between the trochlea and olecranon or between the radial head and the capitellum humeri.

Usually, the trochlea is altered in conformity and size due to the reduction with high-compression screws. In these cases, the trochlea needs to be treated with a broad remodeling technique to recover an adequate size and congruency with the olecranon. Following this broad remodeling, the use of interposition tissue can be useful to interpose within the articular joint. Tissues commonly used are the Achilles tendon (for allografts) or the fascia (for autografts or allografts). The medial and lateral collateral ligaments can be reconstructed using a portion of the tissue grafts. External joint distraction is also performed in conjunction to protect the reconstruction for 5–6 weeks and to allow early mobility.

In cases of severe joint destruction that cannot be recovered with conservative procedures, elbow replacement can be considered.

Elbow replacement (total or hemi) may be the principal indication for older patients with lower mobility requirements. In selected cases, this course of action offers reliable improvements in pain relief and mobility even if it does introduce the potential for complications related to the mechanical failure of the implant or of the soft tissues.

Recently, hemi-humeral arthroplasty has been introduced with anatomic designs that reproduce the trochlea surface. From our experience, this is correctly indicated in cases of preserved olecranon articular surface and ligaments, but little information is available from the literature, on medium- and long-term follow-up.

The surgical technique to implant the hemi- or total elbow prosthesis (arthroplasty) can be performed using a posterior midline approach. The ulnar nerve should be isolated, and the extensor mechanism is prepared using a splitting or preserving approach to expose the articular bone surface.

28.1.3 Outcomes of Malunion

There is limited information about the outcomes of surgical correction of distal humerus malunions, but most of these procedures have been performed in the young or adult populations with high degrees of varus and retroversion deformity. Elbow stiffness and instability are the most common clinical, surgical sequelae following a malunion of the distal humerus [3]. The treatment, which is technically demanding, since it requires great surgical experience, includes correct osteotomy or debridement with recontouring arthroplasty. The primary goal is to restore the original anatomic morphology and stability of the elbow, to allow motion without pain. In the preoperative planning stages, a CT scan should be performed to assess the joint congruency and intra-articular bone deformity. Moreover, the choice of surgical treatment must take into account patient age and extent of disabilities.

McKee et al. [4] reported 13 patients treated with osteotomy and bone graft associated with capsular release. The mean age of patients was 40 years, and the mean follow-up time was 25 months (ranging from 12 to 60 months). According to the Mayo Elbow Performance Score (MEPS), 2 were excellent, 3 good, and 8 fair. All the osteotomies healed with an average range of mobility between 25° and 122°. Other experiences have been reported in the literature with good results in osteotomy healing and useful outcomes in elbow motion and pain relief [5–8].

A variety of procedures have been described for operative humerus osteotomy; Lim et al. [9] analyzed the results of three-dimensional corrective osteotomy in the middle-aged population. Twenty consecutive patients underwent corrective osteotomy at an average age of 47.9 years (range, 41–55 years). The osteotomy was fixed with single plating in eight patients and with double plating in 12. The average follow-up was 23 months (range, 18–109 months). Osseous union was radiographically demonstrated in all patients at an average of 17.5 weeks. Delayed union of further than 12 weeks was observed in 15 patients (75 %). The average time to union in the single-plating group was 21.0 weeks compared with 15.1 weeks in the double-plating group. Failure of fixation occurred in two patients who had single plating. The average final MEPS was 90.3 points (range, 70–100 points).

Hahn et al. [10] reported their experience using a corrective dome osteotomy performed in 19 adult patients. The mean age was 31.1 years, and the mean follow-up was 41 months. None of the patients had recurrence of deformity. An excellent result was achieved in 13 patients and good in 6. They therefore concluded that corrective dome osteotomy with stable fixation is a valid option in cases of distal humerus deformity also among adults.

Gong et al. [11] reported their experience with 12 consecutive patients treated with lateral oblique closing wedge osteotomy with a larger contact area and stable fixation. The mean age at the time of the surgery was 39 years (range, 31–48 years). The minimum follow-up was 15 months. All patients achieved healing of the osteotomy and regained preoperative arcs of elbow motion at a mean of 7 weeks. The final MEPS and Disabilities of the Arm, Shoulder and Hand questionnaire (DASH) averaged 95.4 points and 5.5 points, respectively. The conclusion of their report was that humerus osteotomy and fixation with lateral plating is a sound technique for humerus deformities in adults, with early recovery of elbow motion and satisfactory deformity correction.

The outcomes of recontouring arthroplasty were reported in patients with a lesser amount of extra-articular or intra-articular deformities.

Husband and Hastings [12] used this technique on seven patients with a mean age of 32 years at 38-month follow-up. They were able to recover functional arc of motion in six patients with a mean range of 117°.

Mansat and Morrey [13] reported 37 patients treated with the column procedure. At 43 months of mean follow-up, they reported a satisfactory result in 82 % of cases, while 89 % improved the range of motion with a mean arc of 94°. More recently, Stans et al. [14] reported 37 patients treated with capsular release and bony debridement at 15 months of mean follow-up. They described an improvement in elbow motion in 75 % of cases with an average arc of 94°.

Capsular release and bone recontouring can be also performed using either open or arthroscopic procedures. Most of these cases are analyzed as part of a posttraumatic series, and it is difficult to agree whether the stiffness in the elbow is the consequence of distal humerus malunion from the simple contracture with heterotopic ossifications.

In 2000, Cohn et al. [15] reported their experience with the treatment of osteoarthritis (primary and posttraumatic) in the elbow, comparing open and arthroscopic debridement. The outcomes of 18 patients treated by the Outerbridge-Kashiwagi (O-K) open procedure and 26 patients treated by arthroscopic debridement and fenestration of the olecranon fossa were compared at mean follow-up of 35 months. At the end of their study, they found that both procedures were effective, with no major complications. Patients treated by arthroscopic debridement and fenestration achieved better relief of pain, whereas those patients undergoing the O-K open procedure achieved significantly greater improvement in range of motion. In the same years, Kim and Shin [16] reported their series of 63 patients focused on arthroscopy for limited elbow range of motion. The mean range of motion was 79° before surgery. Patients with posttraumatic stiffness had a more marked reduction in extent and total range of motion (73°) compared to those with degenerative stiffness (86°) before surgery. However, no significant differences were found in the postoperative range of motion (posttraumatic stiffness, 123°, and degenerative stiffness, 121°). In 2011, Cefo and Eygendaal [17] reported their experience with 27 patients with posttraumatic stiff elbow treated by arthroscopic release. The mean preoperative range of motion was 99°, and after surgery, improved significantly to 125°, they reported one postoperative superficial infection of the lateral portal but no vascular or neurological complications. The conclusion of the study was that arthroscopic capsular release of the elbow is a safe and reliable option for patients with posttraumatic elbow stiffness without intrinsic broad deformity.

Recently, Charalambous and Morrey [18] published a systematic review on the treatment options for posttraumatic stiff elbow. They described how arthroscopic treatment for posttraumatic conditions is a challenging procedure. Good results with improvement in range of motion and daily living activities have been reported in the literature, but the fact that it carries with it a steep learning curve in order to avoid complications, in particular in the posttraumatic conditions, has to be borne in mind.

In cases of severe intra-articular malunion, interposition arthroplasty can be performed; Cheng and Morrey [19] reported the outcomes of this technique in 13 patients at 63 months of mean follow-up. They found 62 % of satisfactory results based on to the Mayo Elbow Performance Index. Four cases were subsequently revised as requiring total elbow arthroplasty.

In cases of severe damage of the articular surface, total elbow arthroplasty is the primary indication, mostly for older patients.

In the young portion of the population with severe deformity of the articular surface as a consequence of posttraumatic lesions, total elbow arthroplasty may be considered as a salvage procedure. In a recent Mayo experience [20], this indication was correlated with a higher risk of complications and implant failure than the degenerative conditions. The most important factors to be considered are the possibility of using alternative, non-replacement techniques and patient choice.

28.2 Distal Humerus Nonunion

The incidence of nonunion in distal humeral fractures has been reported as approximately ranging between 10 and 25 % [21–25]. Poor surgical technique with inadequate fixation was found to be the principal risk factor for fracture nonunion. Other factors are related to severe soft tissue injuries that reduce bone blood supplies or to poor bone condition of the distal humerus. The nonunion can be located at the supracondylar level (extra-articular zone) or in the intra-articular zone involving the trochlea and the capitellum. The nonunion at the supracondylar level is affected by inadequate stable fixation and also by the limited blood supply at this level [26]. In the normal elbow, mechanical forces from the articular surface are transferred to the diaphysis crossing the supracondylar region. In cases of unstable fixation of the supracondylar fracture, the flexion-extension motion can develop the hardware failure with a secondary windshield-wiper effect on the fracture (Fig. 28.5). Additional joint stiffness can worsen the failure of the fracture

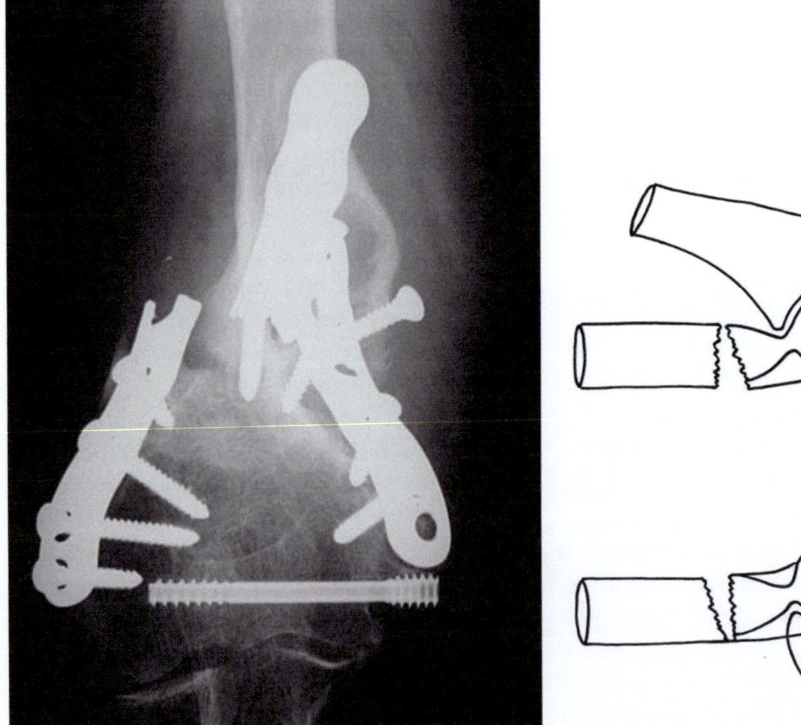

Fig. 28.5 The unstable fixation of the supracondylar fracture associated to the flexion-extension early motion can develop the hardware failure with a secondary windshield-wiper effect on the fracture as shows by two *arrows*

reduction. The movement occurs through the nonunion site rather than through the joint [27] with excessive loads being transmitted through the supracondylar region.

Risk factors for bone nonunion also include smoking and the use of medication that may impact on bone formation. An investigation for symptoms and signs of infection can be performed in all cases of nonunion to exclude their concomitant presence. Imaging evaluations should start with an analysis of the previous X-rays in order to assess the quality of the initial fixation and to determine the amount of bone loss. Recent radiographs will help to determine the status of the internal fixation and the bone quality and loss to help with planning treatment. Computer tomography with 3D reconstruction is a useful tool when a further internal fixation is planned, because it provides a better understanding of the remaining bone condition and the degree of the associated malunion.

Major surgical options available for treatment of distal humerus nonunions are internal fixation with bone graft and elbow replacement, and in some rare and particular cases elbow arthrodesis can be performed. The choice will depend on the level of nonunion (intra-articular or extra-articular region) and on the concomitant presence of an intra-articular malunion or degenerative joint disease. Finally, it will depend on patient age and activity levels.

28.2.1 Internal Fixation

This is the treatment of choice for the majority of patients with intra-articular or extra-articular distal humerus nonunion. The principal goal of internal fixation is to achieve an anatomic reduction and stable internal fixation and to stimulate bone healing using a bone graft. To avoid stress on the nonunion area, it is useful to release the associated joint contracture. In intra-articular nonunions, the anatomic reconstruction of the articular surface and the recovery of the dimension and orientation of the trochlea and capitellum are the most important aspects to consider. In cases of large bone loss, inadequate to recover a correct dimension of the trochlea, a cortical iliac bone graft can be used, associated with interposition arthroplasty.

The aim of a reconstruction in the intra-articular region is to recover the congruencies between the humeral surface and the olecranon and the radial head. In the supracondylar region, the treatment of the nonunion has to recover the correct orientation of the distal humerus in both the frontal and sagittal planes. A bone graft at the supracondylar level can be useful to improve the healing process, and occasionally, a metaphysis shortening can be applied in cases of bone reabsorption. In these cases, the correct orientation of the distal fragment relative to the diaphysis can be difficult to obtain, especially with more extensive bone loss. The problems with the reduction at the supracondylar level are related to the attempt to avoid nonanatomic reduction with excessive flexion or extension, valgus/varus, or malrotation defects between the diaphysis and articular surfaces.

An adequate surgical exposure can help the visualization of the degree of the nonunion. For intra-articular nonunions, when nonunited previous olecranon osteotomy is present, this should be used to expose the articular surface. If other surgical exposure techniques have been used, such as triceps reflecting or splitting, and if incomplete healing of the extensor mechanism to the olecranon is detected, the same approach should be used. For extra-articular nonunions with an intact extensor mechanism as a consequence of an attempt to preserve the triceps, the same approach can be used on both sides of the triceps without violating the extensor mechanism. Olecranon osteotomy provides an excellent exposure for intra-articular distal humerus nonunions and allows extensive exposure of the trochlea surface including the anterior compartment. The anterior and posterior capsular release of the contracture is important for reducing stress being transmitted to the nonunion site, which may contribute to fixation failure.

The two plates provide a stable fixation of the distal humerus reconstruction after nonunion when applied laterally and medially with multiple distal long screws that, in most cases, will be

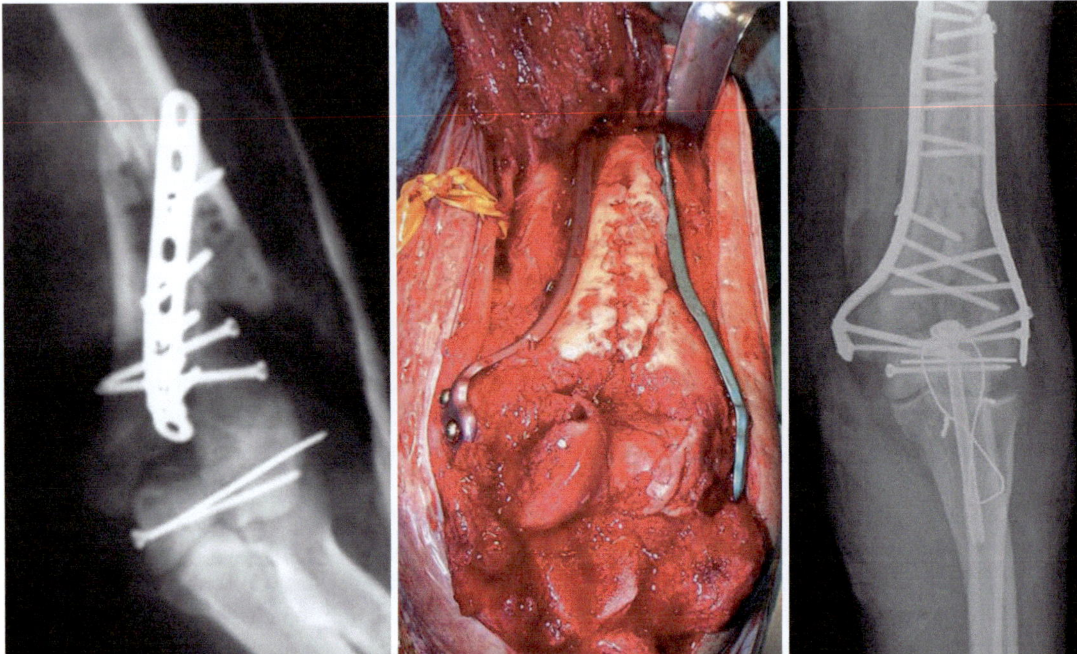

Fig. 28.6 The principal goal of the intra-articular or extra-articular distal humerus nonunion is to achieve an anatomic reduction and stable internal fixation (two plates) and to stimulate bone healing using bone graft

interdigitated together to increase mechanical stability. Compression forces should be applied at the supracondylar level to avoid reducing the articular surface of the trochlea. A bone graft can be applied after the reduction at the supracondylar level using a cortical cancellous stabilized with screws or heavy sutures (Fig. 28.6).

28.2.2 Joint Replacement

Elbow arthroplasty use has increased in the last few decades as it is seen as an effective treatment option for selected patients with distal humerus nonunion. The primary indications for elbow replacement (total and hemi) are irreversible damage of the articular surface of the distal humerus and extensive bone loss (Fig. 28.7). Most of these patients are unable to use their upper limb in their daily living activities. Gross instability with pain can be related to a nonunion after unstable osteosynthesis or to severe joint stiffness after failed reduction of the intra-articular fractures, which is known as an intrinsic malunion.

Patient selection, in the preoperative decision-making stages, is an important factor to consider to reduce the risk of complications. Total elbow arthroplasty is reserved for the older population or for sedentary patients with low levels of activity and only in selected cases among the young, active category of patients as a salvage procedure. Also, it is important in the preoperative planning stages to exclude an infection to avoid the risk of secondary septic loosening of the components.

During the surgical technique, it is important to preserve the extensor mechanism to improve the postoperative recovery time and reduce pain and risk of triceps insufficiencies. In humeral hemiarthroplasty, the reconstruction of both ligaments and columns is an important surgical step to recover an adequate elbow congruency while avoiding the risk of secondary instability.

Elbow replacement should be considered as a useful surgical option for the treatment of distal humerus nonunions, but it should be considered as a salvage procedure with limitations in daily living activities and with a high risk of complications if the patient selection is not correct.

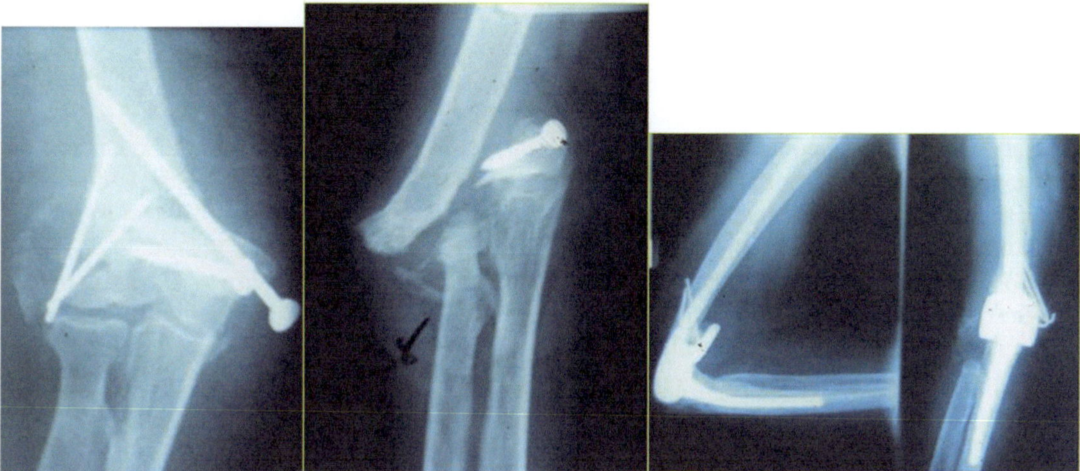

Fig. 28.7 Elbow replacement should be considered as a useful surgical option for the treatment of distal humerus nonunions in selected cases with irreversible damage of the articular surface and with extensive bone loss

28.2.3 Outcomes of Nonunion

There are several studies on the outcomes of distal humerus treatment using a new internal fixation and bone graft protocol published in the last few decades. In the 1980s, Mitsunaga et al. [28] reported 25 patients treated with internal fixation for nonunion of distal humerus fractures. At mean follow-up of 8 months, they recovered satisfactory results in seven patients.

Union was obtained in 22 patients, and the reoperation rate was 24 % at a mean follow-up time of 7.7 months for revision of the fixation or bone graft. Ackerman and Jupiter [29] reported their experience with 20 patients (11 were considered to have a reactive nonunion and nine, a nonreactive nonunion) with a mean age of 43 years. At 42 months of mean follow-up, they reported satisfactory results based on the MEPS in seven patients. They recovered a high percentage of union of around 94 %.

In conclusion, they observed how the results in the extra-articular nonunion category were much better than those in the intra-articular nonunion category. They also observed that those patients reported to have a long-term disability also achieved successful union.

The outcomes of nonunion treatment have improved with the introduction of better fixation systems associated to capsular release aimed at reducing stress on the side the nonunion is on.

Helfet et al. [30] reported their experience with 52 patients with delayed union or nonunion of the distal humerus. Thirteen nonunions were at the intercondylar level, 27 were at the supracondylar one, and 6 cases were in the transcondylar area. The last six patients presented with nonunion at the lateral and medial condylar level. The average time to clinical assessment was 18 months. Union was achieved in 94 % of patients (the average time to union was 6 months), but 30 % of patients required additional surgery to improve their range of motion, address the ulnar nerve, or remove areas of wearing. They concluded that open reduction through extensive exposure and rigid internal fixation consistently results in healing of the nonunion of the distal part of the humerus.

McKee et al. [4] described their experience in 13 patients with mean age of 40 years at mean follow-up of 25 months. Based on the MEPS, they recovered two excellent, eight good, and three fair results.

Ring et al. [31] described outcomes in 15 patients with unstable nonunion in which the hand and forearm could not be supported against gravity. The average time from the original fracture to the initial treatment of the nonunion was 7 months. At mean follow-up of 51 months, they achieved union in 12 patients; of these, six patients required additional surgery to improve motion. Three nonunions failed to heal and were treated with total elbow arthroplasty. Based on the MEPS, satisfactory results were observed in 11 patients. They concluded that unstable nonunions of the distal part of the humerus can be treated successfully with the use of rigid internal fixation, joint contracture release, and bone grafting. Ali et al. [32] reported their experience with 16 patients with mean age of 42 years and at mean follow-up of 39 months. The MEPS was excellent in 11, good in two, fair in two, and poor in one. They reported one failure with an infected nonunion that required a subsequent bone graft to obtain union. They observed that the most important factor to obtain union of a distal humeral fracture is the adequacy of fixation.

Regarding total elbow replacement used for the treatment of nonunion of the distal humerus, different experiences have been reported, the majority of which comes from the Mayo Clinic. In 1995, Morrey and Adams [33] published their experience using linked semi-constrained prosthesis design for the treatment of distal humerus nonunions on 36 consecutive patients with a mean age of 68 years. At average follow-up of 50.4 months (24–127 months), 31 patients (86 %) had satisfactory results, three (8 %) had fair, and two (6 %) had poor results, and in terms of pain, 91 % had no or only mild discomfort after the procedure. Motion had improved compared to the preoperative state, recovering a mean arc ranging between 16° and 127° after surgery. There were seven complications (deep infection, synovitis, ulnar neuropathy, and worm polyethylene bushes).

In 2008 and 2009, Cil et al. and Sanchez-Sotelo and Morrey [34, 35] reported a new series of total elbow arthroplasties performed in nonunion cases at the Mayo Clinic. Ninety-one consecutive patients (92 elbows) underwent elbow replacement; the results were analyzed at a mean follow-up of 6.5 years. Joint stability had been restored in all patients. Sixty-seven (74 %) patients had no or mild pain, and 20 (22 %) had a fair or poor MEPS. A total of 44 complications occurred in 40 elbows, and there were 32 reoperations. Factors that increased the risk of implant failure were patient age of less than 65 years, two or more prior surgical procedures, and a history of infection. The rate of prosthetic survival without removal or revision for any reason was 96 % at 2 years, 82 % at 2 years, and 65 % at both 10 and 15.

LaPorte et al. [36] reported their experience using the linked semi-constrained prosthesis for nonunion of the distal humerus following failure of internal fixation on 12 patients at mean follow-up of 63 months; 11 patients had good pain relief and a good or excellent functional result: mean arc of motion was 134–18°.

In 2011, Espiga et al. [37] reported their experience on using elbow replacement in patients older than 70 years and with nonunion of the distal humerus. Six patients underwent this procedure for symptomatic nonunion of the distal humerus. At a mean follow-up of 40 months, the mean range of motion in terms of flexion-extension was between 15° and 125°. Only one patient had moderate pain, and all six were satisfied with the procedure.

28.3 Prevention of Malunion and Nonunion

- Reduction of the articular distal humeral fragment to recover anatomic congruency and mechanical axis in the sagittal and frontal planes
- Stable fixation of distal humerus using two parallel or orthogonal plates and screws
- Avoiding aggressive mobilization or stress of the metaphyseal area (Fig. 28.8)

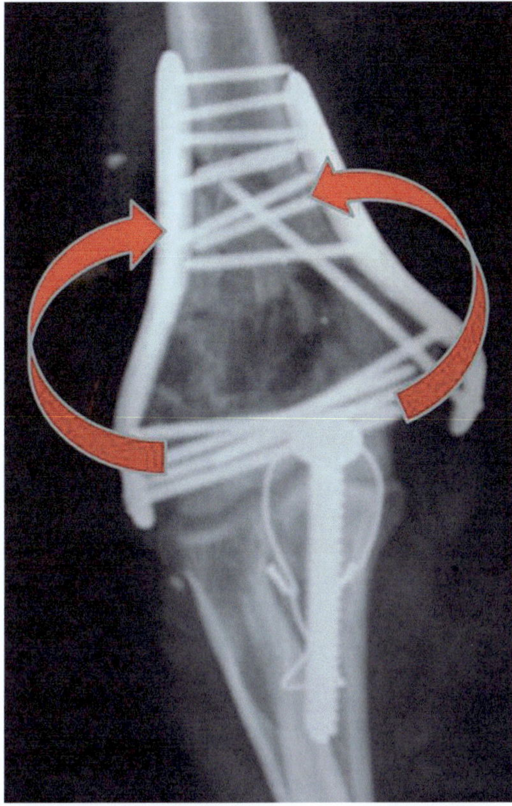

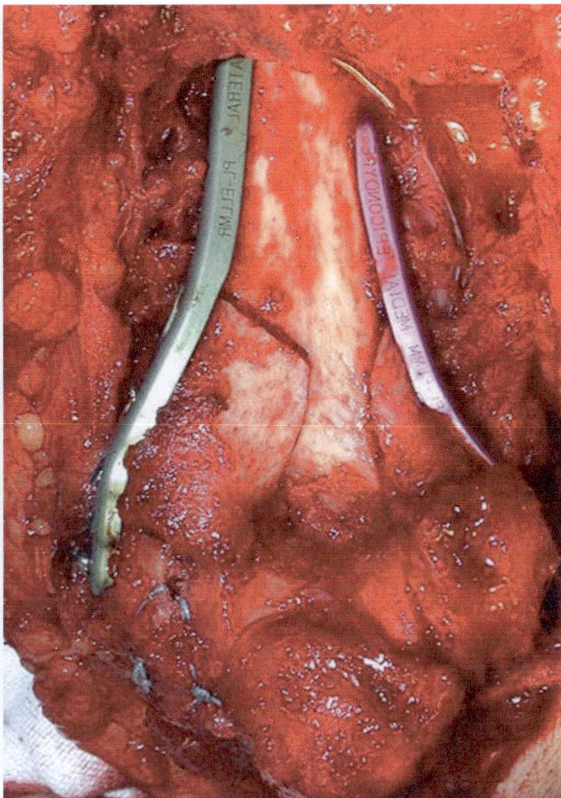

Fig. 28.8 Reduction of the articular distal humeral fragment and stable fixation of distal humerus using two plates allow to reduce the mechanical stress on the metaphysis (the two *arrows* show the transfer of the forces from the articular surface to the diaphysis)

28.4 Treatment of Malunion and Nonunion

- Check for a correlation between the malunion and instability with pain and between the intra-articular malunion and severe stiffness.
- Precise preoperative imaging studies to assess the articular deformity and the congruity with the olecranon and radial head.
- Exclude a subacute infection of the malunion or nonunion areas.
- The main treatment is to restore the articular congruencies and joint stability.
- In selected cases, total or hemi-elbow arthroplasty should be considered as a salvage procedure.

References

1. Court-Brown CM, Caesar B (2006) Epidemiology of adult fractures: a review. Injury 37(8):691–697
2. Kashiwagi D (1975) Outerbridge Kashiwagi arthroplasty for osteoarthritis of the elbow, the elbow joint. Kashiwagi D (ed) Elsevier Science publishers (Biomedical Division), Amsterdam, pp 177–188
3. Muller LP, Hansen M, Morrey BF, Prommersberger KJ, Rommens PM (2008) The surgery of neglected distal humerus fractures in children and adult. In Celli A, Celli L, Morrey BF (eds), treatment of elbow lesion. Springer, New York, pp 221–230
4. McKee M, Jupiter J, Toh CL, Wilson L, Colton C, Karras KK (1994) Reconstruction after malunion and nonunion of intra-articular fractures of the distal humerus. Methods and results in 13 adults. J Bone Joint Surg Br 76(4):614–621

5. Cobb TK, Linscheid RL (1994) Late correction of malunited intercondylar humeral fractures. Intra-articular osteotomy and tricortical bone grafting. J Bone Joint Surg Br 76(4):622–626
6. Davids JR, Maguire MF, Mubarak SJ, Wenger DR (1994) Lateral condylar fracture of the humerus following posttraumatic cubitus varus. J Pediatr Orthop 14(4):466–470
7. Tricot M, Duy KT, Docquier PL (2012) 3D-corrective osteotomy using surgical guides for posttraumatic distal humeral deformity. Acta Orthop Belg 78(4):538–542
8. Skaggs DL, Glassman D, Weiss JM, Kay RM (2011) A new surgical technique for the treatment of supracondylar humerus fracture malunions in children. J Child Orthop 5(4):305–312
9. Lim TK, Koh KH, Lee do K, Park MJ (2011) Corrective osteotomy for cubitus varus in middle-aged patients. J Shoulder Elbow Surg 20(6):866–872
10. Hahn SB, Choi YR, Kang HJ (2009) Corrective dome osteotomy for cubitus varus and valgus in adults. J Shoulder Elbow Surg 18(1):38–43
11. Gong HS, Chung MS, Oh JH, Cho HE, Baek GH (2008) Oblique closing wedge osteotomy and lateral plating for cubitus varus in adults. Clin Orthop Relat Res 466(4):899–906
12. Husband JB, Hastings H (1990) The lateral approach for operative release of post-traumatic contracture of the elbow. J Bone Joint Surg Am 72(9):1353–1358
13. Mansat P, Morrey BF (1998) The column procedure: a limited lateral approach for extrinsic contracture of the elbow. J Bone Joint Surg Am 80(11):1603–1615
14. Stans AA, Maritz NG, O'Driscoll SW, Morrey BF (2002) Operative treatment of elbow contracture in patients twenty-one years of age or younger. J Bone Joint Surg Am 84-A(3):382–387
15. Cohen AP, Redden JF, Stanley D (2000) Treatment of osteoarthritis of the elbow: a comparison of open and arthroscopic debridement. Arthroscopy 16(7):701–706
16. Kim SJ, Shin SJ (2000) Arthroscopic treatment for limitation of motion of the elbow. Clin Orthop Relat Res 375:140–148
17. Cefo I, Eygendaal D (2011) Arthroscopic arthrolysis for posttraumatic elbow stiffness. J Shoulder Elbow Surg 20(3):434–439
18. Charalambous CP, Morrey BF (2012) Posttraumatic elbow stiffness. J Bone Joint Surg Am 94(15):1428–1437
19. Cheng SL, Morrey BF (2000) Treatment of the mobile, painful arthritic elbow by distraction interposition arthroplasty. J Bone Joint Surg Br 82(2):233–238
20. Celli A, Morrey BF (2009) Total elbow arthroplasty in patients forty years of age or less. J Bone Joint Surg Am 91(6):1414–1418
21. McKee MD, Wilson TL, Winston L, Schemitsch EH, Richards RR (2000) Functional outcome following surgical treatment of intra-articular distal humeral fractures through a posterior approach. J Bone Joint Surg Am 82-A(12):1701–1707
22. Pajarinen J, Björkenheim JM (2002) Operative treatment of type C: intercondylar fractures of the distal humerus: results after a mean follow-up of 2 years in a series of 18 patients. J Shoulder Elbow Surg 11(1): 48–52
23. Sanders RA, Raney EM, Pipkin S (1992) Operative treatment of bicondylar intraarticular fractures of the distal humerus. Orthopedics 15(2):159–163
24. Soon JL, Chan BK, Low CO (2004) Surgical fixation of intra-articular fractures of the distal humerus in adults. Injury 35(1):44–54
25. Korner J, Lill H, Müller LP, Hessmann M, Kopf K, Goldhahn J, Gonschorek O, Josten C, Rommens PM (2005) Distal humerus fractures in elderly patients: results after open reduction and internal fixation. Osteoporos Int 16(Suppl 2):S73–S79
26. Yamaguchi K, Sweet FA, Bindra R, Morrey BF, Gelberman RH (1997) The extraosseous and intraosseous arterial anatomy of the adult elbow. J Bone Joint Surg Am 79:1654
27. Jupiter JB, Goodman LJ (1992) The management of complex distal humerus nonunion in the elderly by elbow capsulectomy, triple plating, and ulnar nerve neurolysis. J Shoulder Elbow Surg 1(1):37–46
28. Mitsunaga MM, Bryan RS, Linscheid RL (1982) Condylar nonunions of the elbow. J Trauma 22(9): 787–791
29. Ackerman G, Jupiter JB (1988) Non-union of fractures of the distal end of the humerus. J Bone Joint Surg Am 70(1):75–83
30. Helfet DL, Kloen P, Anand N, Rosen HS (2003) Open reduction and internal fixation of delayed unions and nonunions of fractures of the distal part of the humerus. J Bone Joint Surg Am 85-A(1): 33–40
31. Ring D, Gulotta L, Jupiter JB (2003) Unstable nonunions of the distal part of the humerus. J Bone Joint Surg Am 85-A(6):1040–1046
32. Ali A, Douglas H, Stanley D (2005) Revision surgery for nonunion after early failure of fixation of fractures of the distal humerus. J Bone Joint Surg Br 87(8): 1107–1110
33. Morrey BF, Adams RA (1995) Semiconstrained elbow replacement for distal humeral nonunion. J Bone Joint Surg Br 77(1):67–72
34. Cil A, Veillette CJ, Sanchez-Sotelo J, Morrey BF (2008) Linked elbow replacement: a salvage procedure for distal humeral nonunion. J Bone Joint Surg Am 90(9):1939–1950
35. Sanchez-Sotelo J, Morrey BF (2009) Linked elbow replacement: a salvage procedure for distal humeral nonunion. Surgical technique. J Bone Joint Surg Am 91(Suppl 2):200–212
36. LaPorte DM, Murphy MS, Moore JR (2008) Distal humerus nonunion after failed internal fixation: reconstruction with total elbow arthroplasty. Am J Orthop 37(10):531–534
37. Espiga X, Antuña SA, Ferreres A (2011) Linked total elbow arthroplasty as treatment of distal humerus nonunions in patients older than 70 years. Acta Orthop Belg 77(3):304–310

29 Terrible Triad

Davide Blonna

29.1 Definition

The terrible triad injury pattern is a variant of traumatic posterolateral elbow instability, characterized by three elements: (1) posterior dislocation of the elbow, (2) fracture of the radial head, and (3) fracture of the coronoid (Fig. 29.1). The definition of "terrible" was coined to emphasize its clinical prognosis which is frequently associated with very poor functional results after either conservative treatment or surgery.

29.2 Pathogenesis

The terrible triad is the result of an indirect trauma to the elbow, characterized by an injury on the hand, with a combination of compression on the elbow, valgus stress, and forearm supination with respect to the humerus (Video 29.1). This dynamic of the trauma is usually the result of a fall to the ground onto an outstretched hand which is resting on the ground and with the elbow extended in an attempt to slow the fall.

Depending on several factors, the first of which being the degree of flexion and pronation of the elbow during the trauma, the elbow may suffer a spectrum of pathologies ranging from a "simple dislocation" (not associated with fractures) to a terrible triad. The basic principle of the interaction between the degree of flexion and pronation of the elbow and severity of the instability is relatively simple.

> **Tip**
> The elbow is more stable in flexion and pronation and less stable in extension and supination.

In extension and supination, the major stabilizers of the elbow resisting posterolateral dislocation are the soft tissues (lateral collateral ligament and anterior capsule). In flexion and pronation, the stability of the elbow is further reinforced by the bony stabilizers (coronoid and radial head). As a consequence, the elbow is more stable in flexion and pronation, while it is less stable in extension and supination.

A trauma in extension and supination is thus able to dislocate the elbow with lower kinetic energies without affecting the bony stabilizers of the elbow. If the elbow instead undergoes a trauma in this position of greater stability, in flexion and pronation, the dislocation occurs only after a fracture of the primary (coronoid) and secondary

D. Blonna
Department of Orthopaedics and Traumatology, University of Turin Medical School, Mauriziano-Umberto I Hospital, Largo Turati 62, Turin 10128, Italy
e-mail: davide.blonna@virgilio.it

The online version of this chapter (doi:10.1007/978-88-470-5307-6_29) contains supplementary material, which is available to authorized users.

F. Castoldi et al. (eds.), *Simple and Complex Fractures of the Humerus*,
DOI 10.1007/978-88-470-5307-6_29, © Springer-Verlag Italia 2015

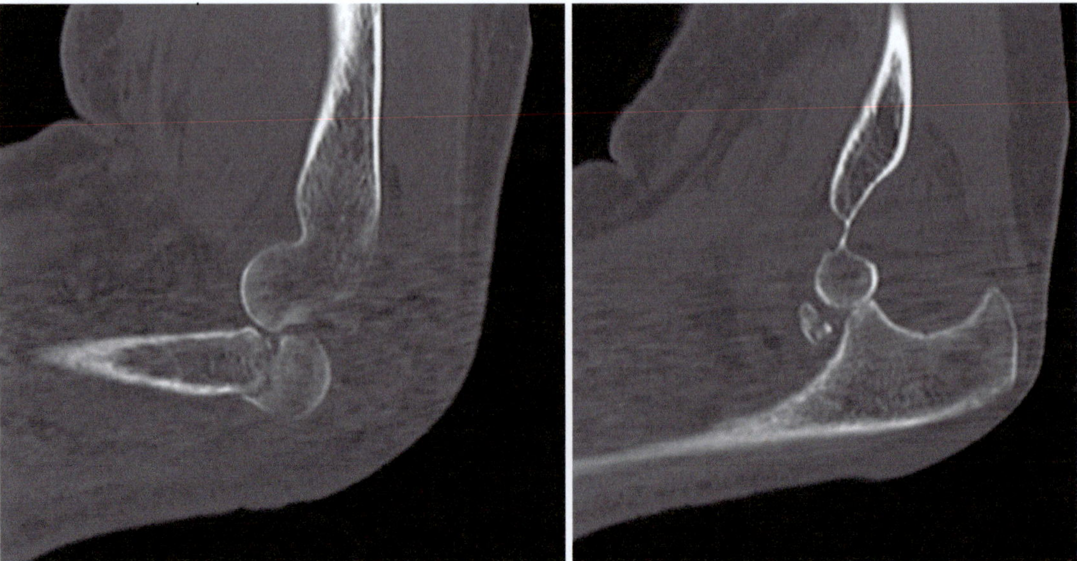

Fig. 29.1 CT scan showing a typical terrible triad pattern of fracture, characterized by a fracture of the coronoid, a fracture of the radial head, and a posterior dislocation of the elbow

stabilizer of the elbow (radial head). This explains why the terrible triad occurs most frequently with high-energy trauma or with lower-energy trauma in patients affected by osteoporosis.

In addition to the degree of flexion and supination of the elbow, the degree of valgus stress and compression of the elbow also influences the type and severity of elbow instability. The greater the trauma component of valgus stress as compared to the compression, the greater the damage to the medial collateral ligament and radial head, versus the damage to the coronoid.

29.3 Principles of Biomechanics Applied to the Terrible Triad

> **Tip**
> The residual instability is a critical concept in understanding the treatment of a terrible triad.

The terrible triad is characterized by an impairment of primary and secondary stabilizers of the elbow, frequently resulting in a *residual instability* of the elbow. The residual instability is defined as the degree of instability after reduction of the terrible triad. The primary stabilizers of the elbow, pertaining to the terrible triad, are the joint capsule, the lateral collateral ligament, and the coronoid. The radial head, which under normal conditions is a secondary stabilizer, becomes a primary stabilizer in circumstances where the coronoid is deficient.

The degree of involvement of these structures, however, varies from case to case, significantly affecting the degree of residual instability and therefore the treatment and prognosis of the terrible triad. The concept of residual instability is vital and determines the outcome of our conservative or surgical treatment.

The degree of residual instability depends on the interaction of several elements:

- Extent of the coronoid fracture
- Extent of the radial head fracture
- Potential for spontaneous healing of the primary and secondary stabilizers

29.4 Fracture of the Coronoid

The extent of the coronoid fracture is the most important factor in predicting the degree of residual instability of the elbow. The classification of

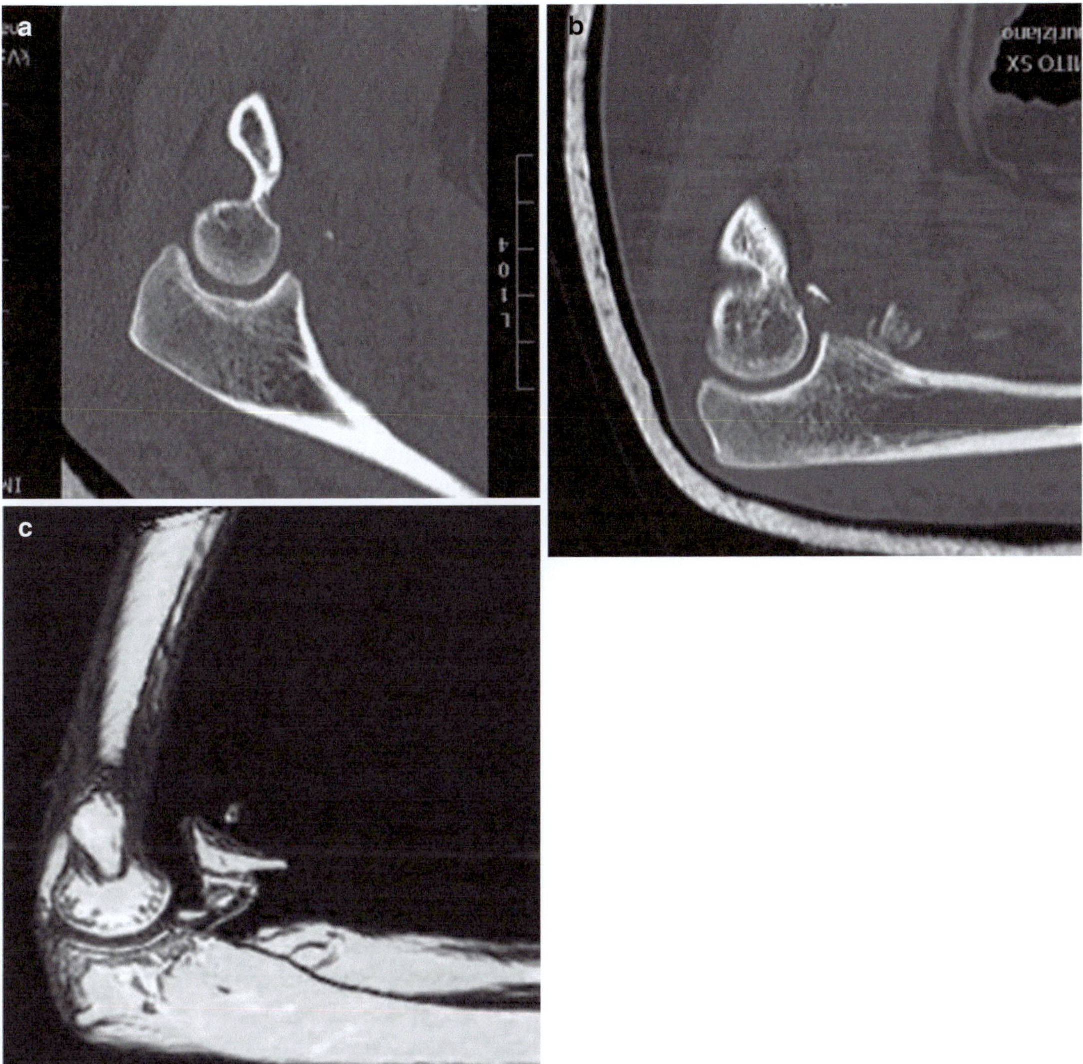

Fig. 29.2 CT scan showing a type I (**a**), type II (**b**), and type III (**c**) fracture of the coronoid according to the Regan-Morrey classification

Ragan-Morrey [1] is probably the most used and divides the fractures into three groups depending on the extent of the fracture of the coronoid (Fig. 29.2).

29.4.1 Type I

Fracture of the apex (Fig. 29.2a). The elbow after reduction usually shows no signs of residual posterolateral instability, even with severe impairment of the radial head. If there is a complete lesion of the medial collateral ligament associated with a fracture of the radial head, a residual valgus instability can occur and must be diagnosed early. In case of type I coronoid fracture, the coronoid remains an efficient primary stabilizer of the elbow and the radial head a secondary stabilizer. That means that the function of the radial head is not mandatory for posterolateral stability. The elbow remains stable even under unfavorable conditions such as extension and supination. The stability of this condition allows the elbow to be mobilized early and to allow physiological healing of the lateral collateral ligament.

29.4.2 Type II

> **Tip**
> Terrible triad with a type II fracture of the coronoid is at high risk of inadequate treatment and subsequent complications.

Fracture affecting 50 % of the coronoid (Fig. 29.2b). The elbow has significant residual posterolateral instability in extension and supination, if the function of the radial head is compromised. Conservative treatment in this case must be weighed carefully and is closely linked to the function of the radial head, which in this context is a primary stabilizer. If the radial head is only partially affected by the fracture or has a fracture that is likely to heal well, conservative treatment may be indicated, but the patient must be followed closely with clinical and radiographic follow-up for early detection of residual posterolateral instability. A concomitant lesion of the medial collateral ligament increases the degree of residual instability by adding residual valgus instability.

In our experience, patients affected by a terrible triad with a type II fracture of the coronoid comprise the cases where there is the greatest risk of inadequate treatment and subsequent complications.

29.4.3 Type III

Fracture affecting more than 50 % of the coronoid (Fig. 29.2c) (base of the coronoid). In these cases, the elbow is unstable posterolaterally also at more than 45° of flexion and in pronation. The radial head is usually not able to provide sufficient stability to the elbow even after a proper reconstruction or prosthetic replacement. In these cases, coronoid reconstruction, suture of the external collateral ligament, and reconstruction or replacement of the radial head are recommended. In some cases, even proper surgical treatment cannot guarantee the absence of residual instability, and it is necessary to use an external fixator which is kept in place for 4–6 weeks.

29.5 Extent of the Fracture of the Radial Head

The extent of radial head involvement is of great importance since it can become the primary stabilizer in terrible triad cases. The radial head becomes a primary stabilizer against valgus instability in concomitant lesions of the medial collateral ligament and a stabilizer against posterior instability in the event of type II and III coronoid fractures.

In these cases, it is essential to restore the function of the radial head through reconstruction or prosthetic replacement. The function of the radial head is of such importance in the terrible triad such that our inclination is to prefer a prosthetic implant that provides excellent primary stability rather than a suboptimal reconstruction. For the same reason, we prefer an anatomic prosthesis which ensures better initial stability rather than bipolar prosthesis.

> **Tip**
> The radial head becomes a primary stabilizer against valgus instability in case of concomitant lesion of the medial collateral ligament and a crucial stabilizer against posterior instability in the event of type II and III coronoid fractures.

The study of the type of fracture of the radial head is vital to predict the degree of residual instability of the elbow affected by a terrible triad. The involvement of the anterosuperior aspect of the radial head, the comminution of the fragments, and a fracture with displacement of the neck are negative prognostic factors in which we recommend a prosthetic replacement. One or two fragments without involvement of the neck are potentially reducible and fixable with screws or a precontoured plate (Fig. 29.3). The final goal is to obtain good primary stability of the elbow, thus allowing early mobilization.

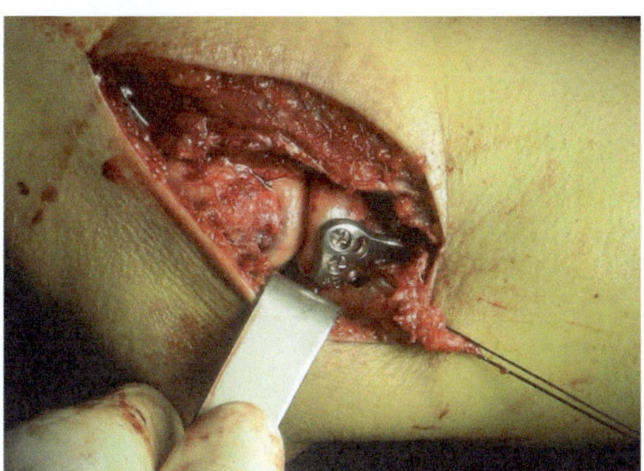

Fig. 29.3 Intraoperative picture of a radial head fixation using a precontoured plate

29.6 Potential for Spontaneous Healing of Primary and Secondary Stabilizers of the Elbow

The primary and secondary stabilizers of the elbow may heal spontaneously. This applies mostly to the lateral and medial collateral ligament. Between the two collateral ligaments, the medial collateral ligament is the one that has the most potential for spontaneous healing. The reasons for this difference are not known with certainty, but it is likely due to the continuous varus stress in which the elbow is subjected during activities of daily living. During the activities of everyday life such us grabbing objects to bring them to the mouth, the elbow undergoes a varus stress that leads to a constant force on the lateral collateral ligament, causing a failure of the healing. This stress is greater in cases of the residual elbow instability.

> **Tip**
> The medial collateral ligament has good potential for spontaneous healing.

Valgus stress is much less common during the activities of daily living. So, the medial collateral ligament has a greater potential for spontaneous healing. The potential for spontaneous healing has important consequences in the decision-making process. In cases of conservative treatment, the immobilization period should be approximately 3 weeks to ensure initial healing of the lateral and medial collateral ligaments. After 3 weeks of immobilization, a brace is usually prescribed to protect the elbow against varus stress for up to 2 months after the trauma.

29.7 Assessment of Residual Instability

The degree of residual instability after reduction of a terrible triad is dependent on the combination of different elements (coronoid fracture, radial head fracture, soft tissue insufficiency). While the contribution of each element to the degree of residual instability may be relatively easy to predict, predicting the result of the contributions of the various elements in combination is rarely possible.

> **Tip**
> There are two main types of residual instability:
> - A residual posterolateral instability
> - A residual valgus instability

It is for this reason that it is important to assess the degree of residual instability before deciding on the type of treatment. *The assessment of residual instability is the focus of our therapeutic choice* and, therefore, must be done correctly and repeated several times intraoperatively.

The assessment of residual instability is based on the concept that there are two main types of residual instability once a terrible triad is reduced: residual *posterolateral instability* and residual *valgus instability*:

1. Residual posterolateral instability
   This is the most common type of instability due to an insufficient coronoid, radial head, anterior capsule, and lateral collateral ligament. It is assessed with the patient supine using the *lateral pivot shift test* [2]. After reducing the dislocation of the elbow, under anesthesia, with the patient supine, the elbow is moved from its position of greater stability (in flexion and pronation) to its position of greater instability

(in extension and supination) (Video 29.2). During this progression, the examiner will assess angles of extension and supination of the elbow, at which the elbow appears to subluxate or dislocate. In this manner, the examiner is able to measure the degree of residual posterolateral instability. If the elbow does not dislocate or subluxate, the examiner can add a valgus stress to increase the instability of the elbow.

2. Residual valgus instability

   This is a less common instability, after a terrible triad, due to a complete lesion of the medial collateral ligament and a failure of the radial head. After reducing the terrible triad, the examiner measures the degree of valgus instability with the elbow flexed to approximately 20°, with the forearm in pronation. We recommend to administer this test under a fluoroscope since this helps to reduce false positives. The test is performed in pronation, also to avoid false-positive results, due to a concomitant posterolateral instability (Video 29.3).

29.8 Treatment

The treatment of a terrible triad is highly variable and includes conservative treatment, fixation or replacement of the radial head, fixation of the coronoid, reinsertion of the lateral collateral ligament, and the application of an external fixator. Deciding which treatment to choose from can be challenging.

As mentioned earlier, our treatment of a terrible triad is based on the evaluation of the residual instability while adhering to these concepts:

(a) Avoid undertreatment.
(b) Closed follow-up.
(c) Prefer a stiff elbow than an unstable elbow.
(d) Immediate postoperative passive and active motion.

Our protocol is shown in Fig. 29.4.

29.8.1 Closed Reduction

> **Tip**
> The reduction should be done under anesthesia to allow immediate assessment of residual instability.

Although reduction under anesthesia is not essential, since terrible triad dislocations are usually reduced without difficulty, the use anesthesia allows immediately assessment of the degree of residual instability. The degree of residual instability can also be evaluated if the patient is awake or can be postponed until immediately before surgery, but nonetheless, whenever possible, we prefer to do so as soon as the patient is anesthetized and under fluoroscopic control. The reduction of the dislocation of the elbow, in terrible triad cases, is usually easy since the radial head and the coronoid are fractured and the elbow is unstable. In these cases, traction in a semi-extended (20°) position is usually sufficient to reduce the elbow. In cases with type I coronoid fractures or a marginal fracture of the radial head, the reduction may be more difficult. In these cases, we recommend disengaging the radial head from the capitulum humeri, by applying prono-supinating movements of the forearm and by applying a force in varus during the traction of the elbow.

29.8.2 Conservative Treatment

Conservative treatment is rarely indicated for a terrible triad. Excluding patients in poor general

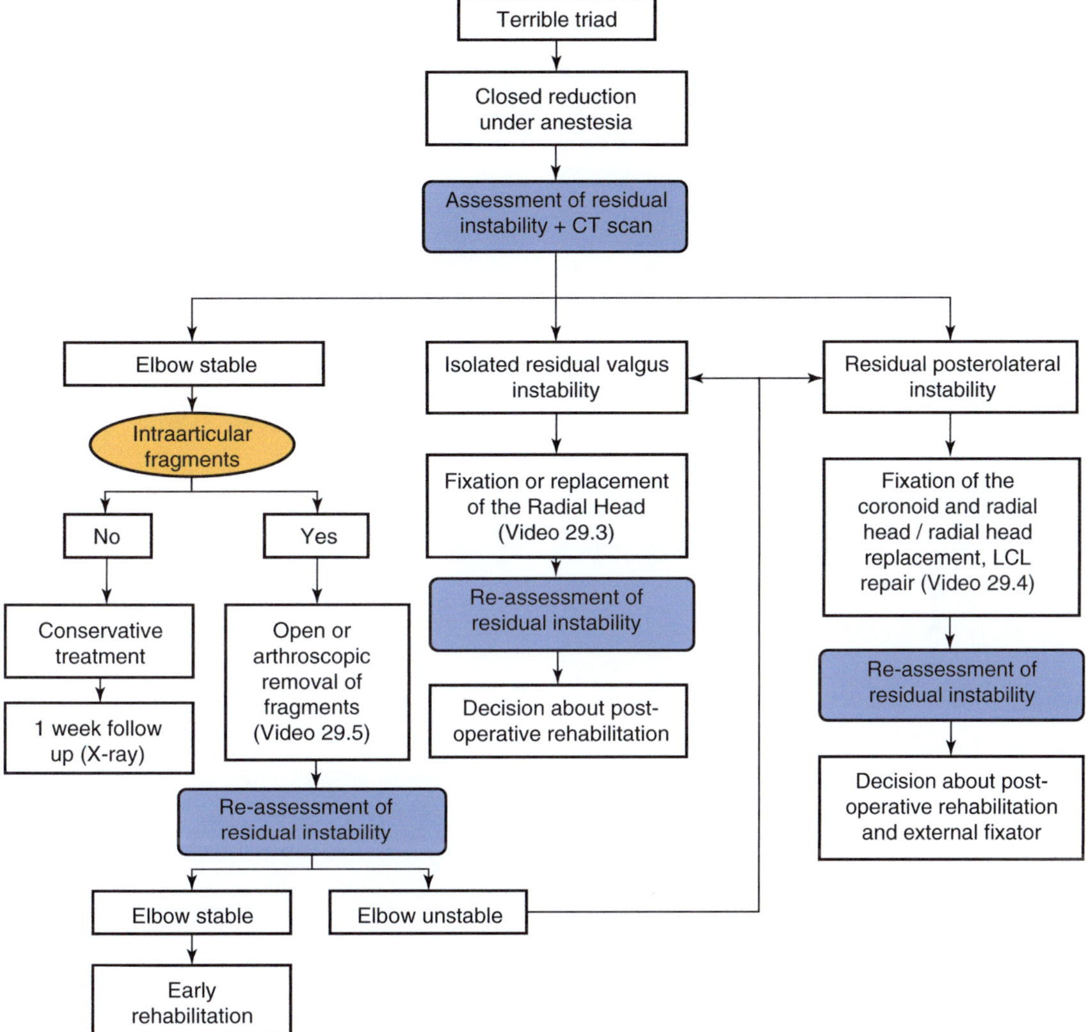

Fig. 29.4 Flow chart used in decision-making for terrible triad injuries. See also Videos 29.4 and 29.5

medical health for whom surgery is absolutely contraindicated, conservative treatment may be indicated in patients with a type I fracture of the coronoid with an undisplaced fracture of the radial head. For these, the elbow is immobilized at about 90–110° of flexion in pronation (Fig. 29.5).

29.8.3 Surgical Approach

Tip
The Kaplan approach to the lateral elbow is indicated in most of the cases.

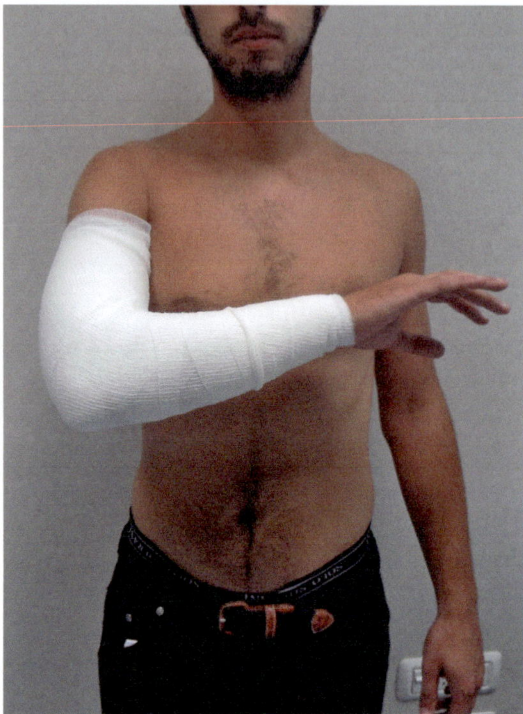

Fig. 29.5 The patient is immobilized at 90–110° of flexion with the forearm in pronation

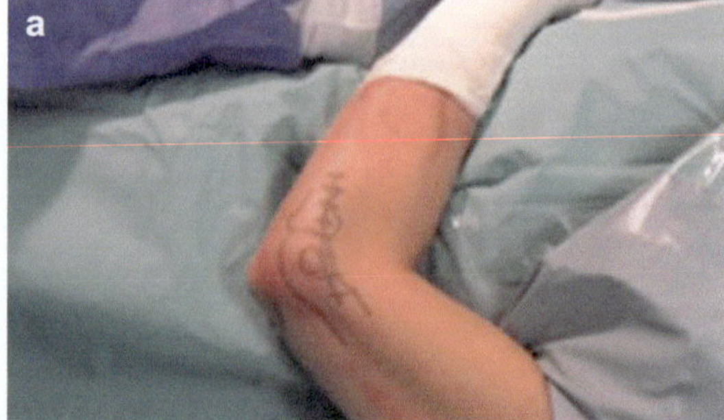

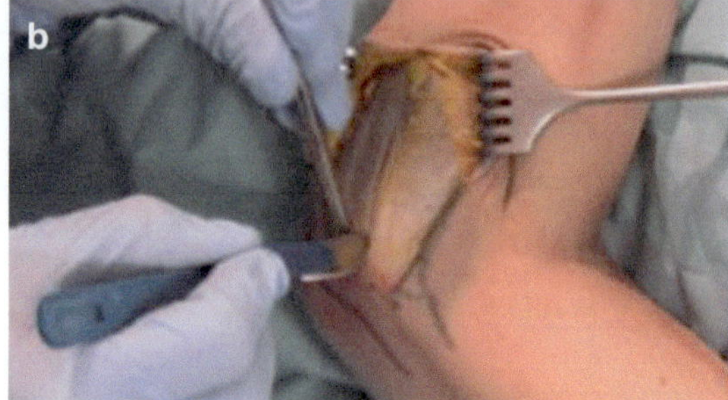

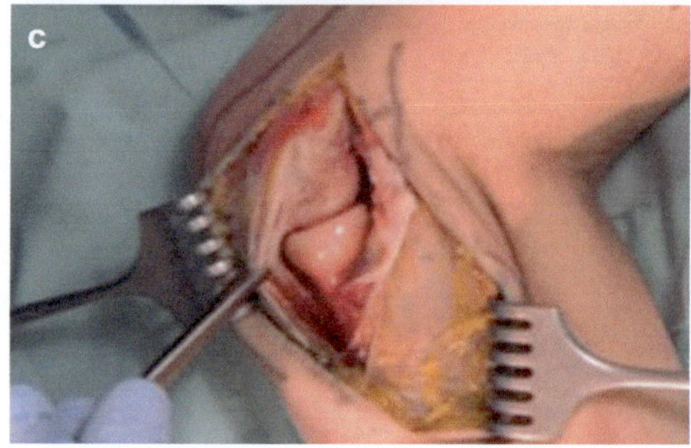

Fig. 29.6 The Kaplan approach to the lateral elbow (**a**). The incision is made in line with the interval between the extensor carpi radialis brevis (ECRB) muscle and the extensor digitorum muscle (**b**). The Kaplan approach allows the preservation of the most posterior component of the muscles and tendons that act as a hammock, significantly limiting the posterolateral instability of the radial head (**c**)

In cases in which surgical treatment is indicated, the type of surgical approach depends on the type of fracture associated with the terrible triad. In our experience, in about 90 % of our cases, lateral access to the elbow is enough to properly address the terrible triad. Among the lateral approaches to the elbow, we prefer the Kaplan approach [3] which has the great advantage of not further damaging the lateral collateral ligament and the extensor-supinator group (Fig. 29.6, Video 29.4). For this approach, the incision is made in line with the interval between the extensor carpi radialis brevis (ECRB) muscle and the extensor digitorum muscle. In contrast to the Kocher approach (between the anconeus and extensor carpi ulnaris), the Kaplan approach crosses the tendon and muscles in a longitudinal manner (split) allowing the preservation of the most posterior component of the muscles that acts as a hammock, significantly limiting the posterolateral instability of the radial head. Through this approach, it is possible to address type I to type III coronoid fractures without significant comminution and medial extension of the fracture. Although the visualization of the coronoid is suboptimal through this approach, the concomitant fracture of radial head improves the visualization.

In cases involving a concomitant olecranon fracture, we recommend a posterior approach to the elbow. This permits reconstruction of the ulna and management of both the medial and lateral sides of the elbow.

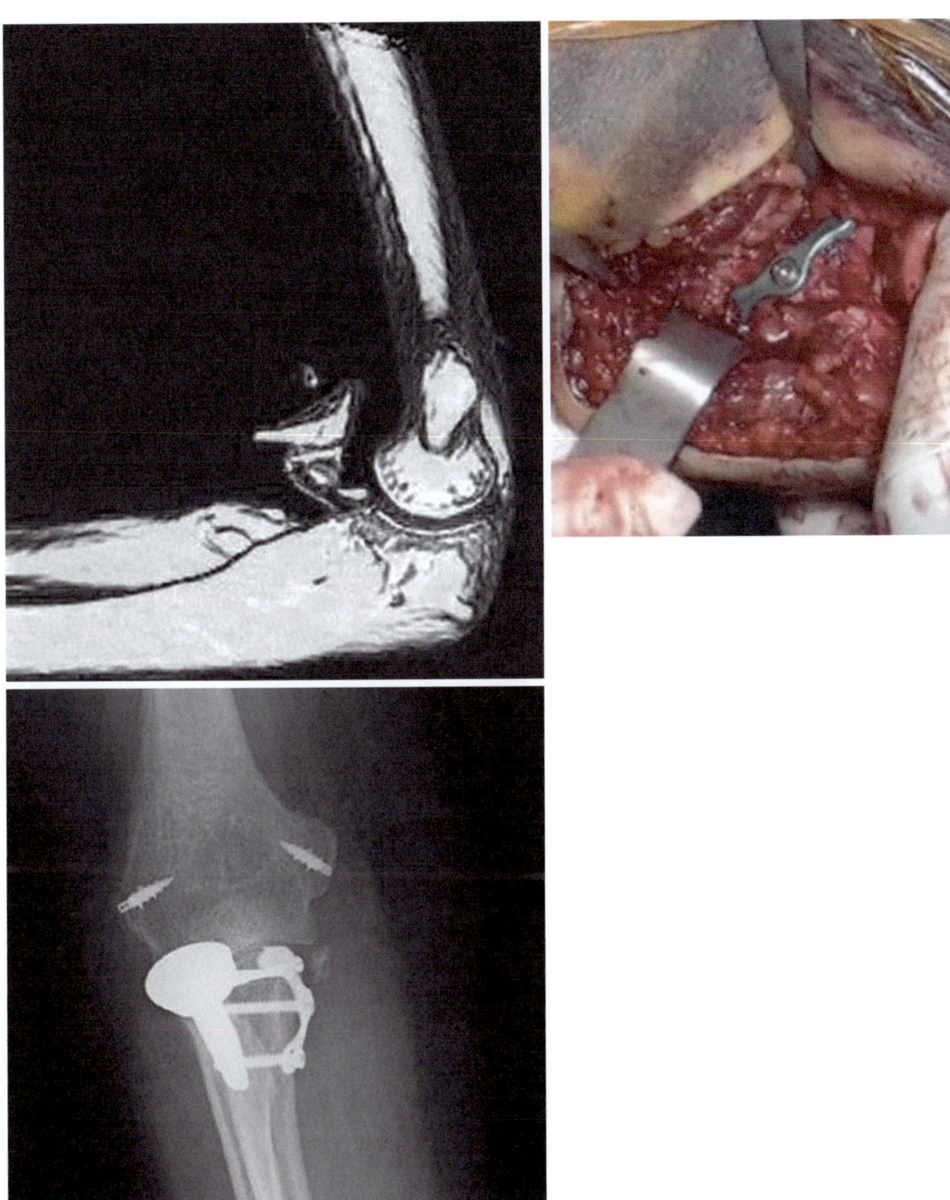

Fig. 29.7 Type III coronoid fracture and comminution of the radial head. The patient was treated with a radial head replacement, precontoured coronoid plate, and sutures of the medial and lateral collateral ligaments

A medial approach to the elbow is reserved for cases in which the coronoid is too challenging to reconstruct using the Kaplan approach. This usually happens in cases with comminution and medial extension of the coronoid fracture (Fig. 29.7).

29.8.3.1 Fixation of the Coronoid

The reconstruction of the coronoid, in most cases, is feasible from a lateral approach. The visualization of the coronoid from the lateral side is greater in cases with large fractures of the radial head. In cases with a type I fracture of the coronoid, we recommend the simple removal of the tip without retensioning the anterior capsule. In cases with a fracture of types II and III, the reconstruction can be performed using anterograde or retrograde cannulated screws. In cases of fixation using a retrograde screw placed from the back of the ulna, a cruciate ligament reconstruction guide can be used in order to simplify the procedure. In isolated cases, the fracture can be synthesized by using a medial approach and a precontoured plate (Fig. 29.7).

29.8.3.2 Fixation and Replacement of the Radial Head

It is likely that the stability of the radial head is the most important factor that determines a successful outcome after surgical treatment for a terrible triad. This is due to the fact that between the coronoid and the radial head, the treatment of the radial head is definitely more reliable. While the coronoid fragment can be difficult to repair and can heal in a suboptimal way, the radial head allows easier surgical management, better exposure, and more surgical options (screw fixation, precontoured plate, and prosthetic replacement).

The choice between reconstruction and prosthetic replacement depends on several factors. The elements that we consider most important are:

- Involvement of the radial neck (subcapital fracture)
- Comminution of the fragments
- Degree of residual instability
- Age of the patient

An elderly patient, severe residual instability, comminution of the fracture fragments, and a subcapital fracture are elements that guide us toward a prosthetic replacement.

Particular care should be taken in the implantation of a radial head prosthesis in order to avoid overstuffing. In terrible triad cases, the elbow can show severe intraoperative instability. Under such conditions, the surgeon may be tempted to seek greater stability by increasing the prosthetic offset. This error causes an overstuffing or overlengthening of the radial head resulting in chronic pain. In order to avoid this error, we suggest measuring the correct prosthetic offset by positioning the elbow in a neutral position (to avoid the varus position typical of the limb resting on the abdomen with the patient is in a supine position) and to stabilize the ulna on the trochlea of the humerus with one hand. If there are doubts, we recommend an intraoperative image intensifier control. In cases with gross medial instability (usually in cases with medial coronoid fractures), we recommend treating the medial instability before deciding on the height of the radial head replacement.

> **Tip**
> Do not rely on radial head implant offset to increase stability of the elbow.

29.8.3.3 External Collateral Ligament Repair

A posterolateral dislocation of the elbow is always associated with a lateral collateral ligament injury. Frequently, the ligament is avulsed from its insertion on the lateral epicondyle. After completing the reconstruction of the coronoid and/or treatment of the radial head, the collateral ligament is reinserted into the epicondyle using transosseous sutures or 5 mm anchors loaded with high-resistance nonabsorbable sutures. Using the Kaplan approach, the lateral collateral ligament is not identified directly, but nevertheless is reinserted together with the extensor-supinator group to the epicondyle with Mason-Allen stitches.

29.8.3.4 Postoperative Care

After surgery, the residual instability of the elbow has to be evaluated. If the elbow is also stable in extension, we recommend the placement of an elastic bandage to allow immediate active and passive mobilization. The patients are instructed to avoid maximal extension for 30 days after surgery. To reduce the risk of heterotopic ossification, prophylactic indomethacin is prescribed for 21 days. In cases of persistent elbow instability despite surgical intervention, the placement of an external fixator may be indicated.

29.8.4 Complications

The conservative and surgical treatment of the terrible triad, even if the choice of treatment and the surgical technique have been optimal, can be associated to a high number of complications. The most frequent complications are residual instability, heterotopic ossification, stiffness, and arthritis. In our experience, correct surgical treatment is able to reduce the complication rate to below 20 %.

References

1. Regan W, Morrey B (1989) Fractures of the coronoid process of the ulna. J Bone Joint Surg Am 71: 1348–1354
2. O'Driscoll SW (1999) Elbow instability. Acta Orthop Belg 65(4):404–415
3. Kaplan EB (1941) Surgical approaches to the proximal end of the radius and its use in fractures of the head and neck of the radius. J Bone Joint Surg 23:86

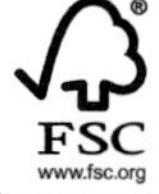

MIX
Papier aus verantwortungsvollen Quellen
Paper from responsible sources
FSC® C105338

If you have any concerns about our products,
you can contact us on
ProductSafety@springernature.com

In case Publisher is established outside the EU,
the EU authorized representative is:
Springer Nature Customer Service Center GmbH
Europaplatz 3, 69115 Heidelberg, Germany

Printed by Libri Plureos GmbH
in Hamburg, Germany